P9-CEK-373

Focus on PHARMACOLOGY
Essentials for Health Professionals

Jahangir Moini, MD, MPH

Professor, Florida Metropolitan University
Epidemiologist, Brevard County Health Department

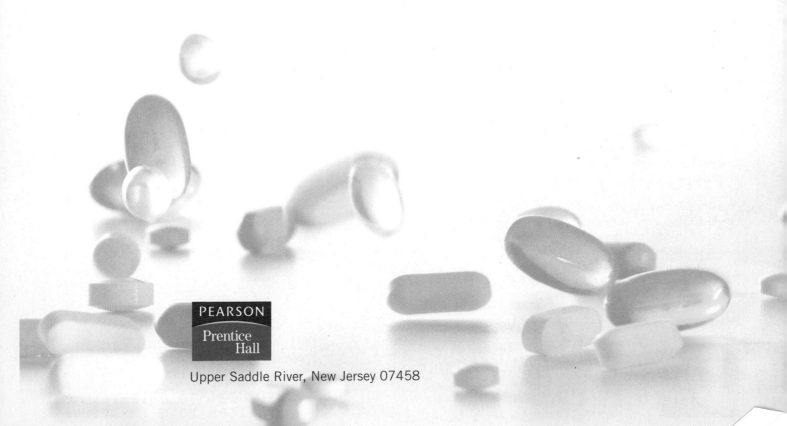

PEARSON

Prentice Hall

Upper Saddle River, New Jersey 07458

Library of Congress Cataloging-in-Publication Data

Moini, Jahangir, (date)
  Focus on pharmacology: essentials for health professionals/
Jahangir Moini.—1ˢᵗ ed.
    p. cm.
  Includes index.
  ISBN 0-13-171642-5
  1. Pharmacology.   2. Allied health personnel   I. Title.
[DNLM: 1. Pharmacology—methods.   2. Allied Health Per-
sonnel.   3. Pharmacokinetics.   4. Pharmacologic Actions.
QV 4 M712f 2008]
  RM300.M63 2008
  615'.1—dc22
                                              2007006152

Publisher: Julie Levin Alexander
Assistant to Publisher: Regina Bruno
Executive Editor: Mark Cohen
Managing Editor: Melissa Kerian
Editorial Assistant: Nicole Ragonese
Media Product Manager: John J. Jordan
Development Editor: Jennifer Maybin
Managing Production Editor: Patrick Walsh
Production Liaison: Christina Zingone
Production Editor: Francesca Monaco/Preparè
Manufacturing Manager: Ilene Sanford
Manufacturing Buyer: Pat Brown
Design Coordinator: Mary Siener

Interior Designer: Amanda Kavanagh
Cover Design: Robert Aleman
Director of Marketing: Karen Allman
Marketing Manager: Harper Coles
Media Project Manager: Stephen Hartner
Media Production: Horus Development
Composition: Preparè
Printing/Binding: Quebecor World/Versailles
Cover Printer: Phoenix Color Corp.
Cover Image: Jupiter Images Royalty Free

Notice: Care has been taken to confirm the accuracy of the information presented in this book. The authors, editors, and the publisher, however, cannot accept any responsibility for errors or omissions or for the consequences of the application of the information in this book and make no warranty, express or implied, with respect to its contents.

The authors and the publisher have exerted every effort to ensure that drug selections and dosages set forth in this text are in accord with current recommendations and practice at time of publication. However, in view of ongoing research, changes in government regulations, and the constant flow of information relating to drug therapy and drug reactions, the reader is urged to check the package insert of all drugs for any change in indications of dosage and for added warnings and precautions. This is particularly important when the recommended agent is a new and/or infrequently employed drug.

The authors and publisher disclaim all responsibility for any liability, loss, injury, or damage incurred as a consequence, directly or indirectly, of the use and application of any of the contents of this volume.

Pearson Prentice Hall™ is a trademark of Pearson Education, Inc.
Pearson® is a registered trademark of Pearson plc
Prentice Hall® is a registered trademark of Pearson Education, Inc.

Pearson Education Ltd., *London*
Pearson Education Australia PTY, Limited, *Sydney*
Pearson Education Singapore, Pte. Ltd
Pearson Education North Asia Ltd., *Hong Kong*
Pearson Education, Canada, Ltd., *Toronto*
Pearson Educación de Mexico, S.A. de C.V.
Pearson Education–Japan, *Tokyo*
Pearson Education Malaysia, Pte. Ltd
Pearson Education Upper Saddle River, *New Jersey*

10 9 8 7 6 5 4 3
ISBN-13:978-0-13-171642-1
ISBN-10:0-13-171642-5

Dedication

This book is dedicated to my precious daughters, Mahkameh and Morvarid.

Preface

Pharmacology is often a challenging subject for allied health students. To the rescue comes this text uniquely designed to use a *focused* approach to learning pharmacology. Introductory chapters lay the groundwork for learning this subject by explaining the history of pharmacology, discussing the legal and ethical principles involved, illustrating drug administration techniques, reviewing math, and explaining drug calculations. The chapters that follow focus on drugs specific to body systems, pharmacotherapy of certain age groups (pediatrics and geriatrics), or broad drug categories such as antibiotics.

Structured Presentation of Pharmacologic Principles

Each drug chapter focuses on drugs used to treat a certain body system and its associated disorders. The chapters open with a concise review of anatomy and physiology, providing a foundation for understanding the actions, effects, and uses of each drug. These pharmacologic principles are succinctly explained by using clearly identifiable headings in question format that help focus students' attention on the most important points about a drug class or an individual drug:

✻ **How do they work?**

✻ **How are they used?**

✻ **What are the adverse effects?**

✻ **What are the contraindications and interactions?**

✻ **What are the most important points patients should know?**

Sometimes these question headings focus on a class of drugs, for example, beta-adrenergic blockers. Other times, the question headings focus on a *prototype* (representative) drug—that is, the drug that was either the first developed in the class or is the most widely used drug in its class. Whichever approach is taken in the chapter, the five-question headings are used so students can easily focus on the key "need-to-know" drug information.

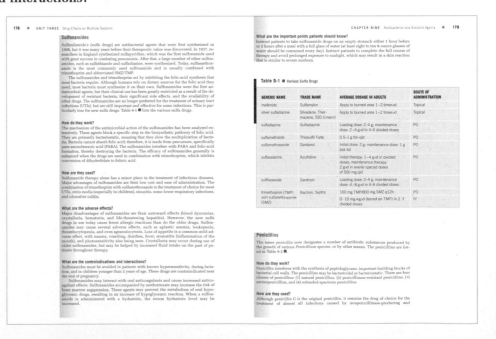

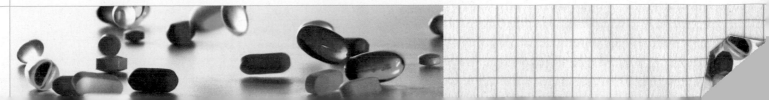

Teach-and-Test Approach

Learning small amounts of information and testing themselves on what they've just learned is a proven way for students to retain new information. This text includes a large number of exercises, implemented in three ways: (1) chapter-opening *Practical Scenarios* with critical thinking questions; (2) within-chapter *Apply Your Knowledge* questions; and (3) end-of-unit *Checkpoint Reviews.* This approach makes learning about pharmacology an engaging, interactive process. The Teach-and-Test approach truly differentiates the text from others and has been positively received by educators.

PRACTICAL SCENARIO

Each chapter opens with a short scenario involving a fictional patient with a real-life problem concerning medications. A list of two or three questions follows. Students are invited to ponder the answers to the questions as they read the chapter. After completing the chapter, individual students can write short answers to the questions, or the class as a whole can discuss the answers.

PRACTICAL SCENARIO

Pharmacy technicians must always be careful when using mathematical equations for compounding. Phil, a pharmacy technician who only recently began working in a pharmacy, is asked by the pharmacist to use a powdered drug and mix it with a solution so that the amount of drug is 3%. Phil converts 3% to a decimal (0.03) so that he can more easily mix the proper amount. He then mixes 0.03 g of the powdered drug into 100 mL of solution. When the pharmacist checks the mixture, he finds that Phil's solution is much too weak.

Critical Thinking Question
1. What miscalculation did Phil make when mixing the solution?
2. When Phil prepares the medication, which rights of administration should he follow?

✳ Apply Your Knowledge 3.1

The following questions focus on what you have just learned about pharmaceutical terminology. *See Appendix E for the correct answers.*

FILL IN THE BLANK
Select terms from your reading to fill in the blanks.

1. A root is the main part of a word that gives the word its _____ _____.
2. The most common combining vowel is _____.
3. A prefix is a structure at the _____ of a word that modifies the meaning of the _____.
4. The combining vowel in the term *hyperlipoproteinemia* is the letter _____.
5. A suffix is a word ending that modifies the meaning of the _____.

MATCHING
Match the lettered meaning to the numbered word part.

WORD PART	MEANING
1. _____ -pathy	a. Study of
2. _____ -itis	b. Half
3. _____ -semi	c. Disease
4. _____ -logy	d. Inflammation
5. _____ anti-	e. Life
6. _____ bio-	f. Against

APPLY YOUR KNOWLEDGE

The second implementation of the "teach-and-test" approach includes exercises that are strategically placed *within* the chapters (rather than at the end). These exercise sections, called *Apply Your Knowledge,* appear after each component of the chapter content, including anatomy and physiology, and the individual pathophysiology/pharmacology sections.

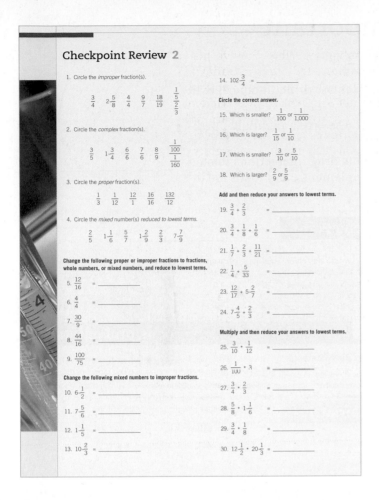

The exercise sections include a variety of exercises in which students need to recall and apply the content they just learned. Exercise types include fill-in-the blank, labeling, matching, and multiple choice, as well as more pharmacology-specific exercises such as dosage calculations and drug name exercises (sound-alike and look-alike and generic-to-brand). The goal in these sections is to provide the student with an immediate review of all vital content. All drugs and drug classes mentioned in the content are "tested" in these exercise sections.

CHECKPOINT REVIEWS

The third component of our teach-and-test approach is unit "tests" called *Checkpoint Reviews*. These review questions reflect the format on most certifying and licensing exams, and include multiple choice and essay questions. Answers to the Apply Your Knowledge and Checkpoint Reviews are found at the end of the book in Appendix E.

Drug Dosing Information

Each drug chapter includes tables of all drugs discussed in the chapter, arranged by drug classes and formatted to include generic and trade names, adult dosing, and route of administration.

Table 18-1 ■ Organonitrates and Other Anginal Medications

GENERIC NAME	TRADE NAME	USUAL DOSE FOR ADULT	ROUTES OF ADMINISTRATION
Nitrates			
nitroglycerin	Nitrolingual	0.4–0.8 mg PRN	Translingual spray
	Nitrostat	0.15–0.6 mg PRN	Sublingual
	Nitro-Bid	2.5–6.5 mg tid or qid	PO
isosorbide dinitrate	Isordil, Sorbitrate, Dilatrate-SR	2.5–40 mg tid	Sublingual
isosorbide mononitrate	Imdur, ISMO	20 mg bid	PO
erythrityl tetranitrate	Cardilate	10–30 mg tid	PO
pentaerythritol tetranitrate	Peritrate, Duotrate	10–20 mg tid or qid	30-80 mg/d
Beta-Adrenergic Blockers			
atenolol	Tenormin	25–50 mg/d, may increase to 100 mg/d	PO
propranolol	Inderal	10–90 mg bid or qid	PO
	Vascor	200–400 mg/d	PO
Calcium Channel Blockers (See Table 17-3 Class IV for other calcium channel blockers used as antidysrhythmics.)			
verapamil	Calan, Calan SR, Covera-HS, Isoptin, Isoptin SR, Verelan, Verelan PM	80 mg q6–8h, may increase up to 320–480 mg/d in divided doses (Covera-HS must be given once daily at bedtime.)	PO

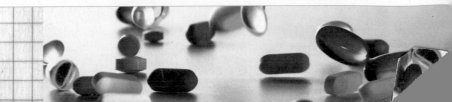

Special Populations and Important Drug-Related Points

✻ **Focus Points:** These marginal features highlight significant or difficult concepts in pharmacology.

✻ **Focus on Pediatrics** and **Focus on Geriatrics:** Each of these boxes highlights pediatric or geriatric information specific to pharmacology.

✻ **Focus on Natural Products:** This boxed feature highlights drug interactions related to complementary and alternative medicines. Herbs, supplements, and foods are included in these boxes.

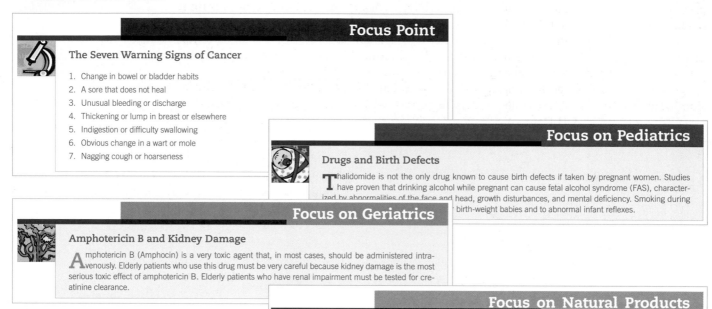

Focus Point

The Seven Warning Signs of Cancer

1. Change in bowel or bladder habits
2. A sore that does not heal
3. Unusual bleeding or discharge
4. Thickening or lump in breast or elsewhere
5. Indigestion or difficulty swallowing
6. Obvious change in a wart or mole
7. Nagging cough or hoarseness

Focus on Pediatrics

Drugs and Birth Defects

Thalidomide is not the only drug known to cause birth defects if taken by pregnant women. Studies have proven that drinking alcohol while pregnant can cause fetal alcohol syndrome (FAS), characterized by abnormalities of the face and head, growth disturbances, and mental deficiency. Smoking during birth-weight babies and to abnormal infant reflexes.

Focus on Geriatrics

Amphotericin B and Kidney Damage

Amphotericin B (Amphocin) is a very toxic agent that, in most cases, should be administered intravenously. Elderly patients who use this drug must be very careful because kidney damage is the most serious toxic effect of amphotericin B. Elderly patients who have renal impairment must be tested for creatinine clearance.

Focus on Natural Products

Interactions Between Gossypol and Amphotericin B

The herb gossypol, which is derived from cottonseed oil, may be used to treat endometriosis in women. It may also be used by both men and women to prevent pregnancy. Gossypol used with amphotericin B (Amphocin) may increase risk of renal toxicity.

Other Elements

Each chapter includes:

✻ Chapter Objectives
✻ Key Terms with pronunciations
✻ Chapter Capsule: A review of each chapter objective with bulleted summaries of the key information for each objective

The focused teach-and-test approach of this textbook provides allied health students with the perfect blend of concise content and an enjoyable—even fun—learning process. Pharmacology and fun have never been joined in the same sentence—until now!

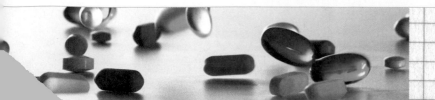

Acknowledgments

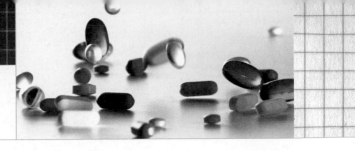

This textbook is the culmination of the efforts of many people, including my students of many years who inspired me to write it. Thank you to Julie Levin Alexander (Publisher), and to Mark Cohen (Executive Editor), who believed in this project from the start, and included dedicated professionals on the editorial team to help produce it. Elena Mauceri (Publishing Consultant) worked tirelessly for several years to develop the initial vision for this project. Jennifer Maybin (Developmental Editor) supplied the guidance and leadership to keep everyone on task and to be certain it reached its fruition on time. The design staff at Prentice Hall, especially Amanda Kavanagh (Designer), created a magnificent text design. Overseeing the production process with finesse was Christina Zingone (Production Liaison). The staff at Preparé provided expert guidance in all aspects of the art and production process.

My special thanks go to Greg Vadimsky, who has been beside me from the initiation of the proposal and the project until the end. He also assisted me in completing the Instructor's Manual, CD-Rom, and PowerPoint presentation. Melissa Kerian has been invaluable in helping me with the media as the Managing Editor.

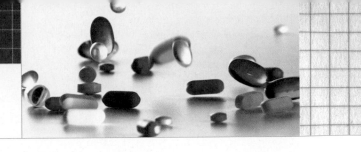

About the Author

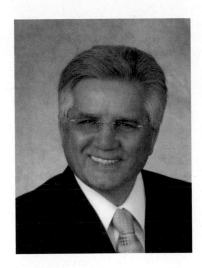

Jahangir Moini, MD, MPH, was assistant professor at Tehran University School of Medicine for 9 years, teaching medical and allied health students. The author is a professor and former director (for 15 years) of allied health programs at Florida Metropolitan University (FMU). Dr. Moini reestablished the medical assisting program in 1990 and the associate degree program for pharmacy technicians in 2000 at FMU's Melbourne campus. He also established several other new allied health programs for FMU.

Dr. Moini is actively involved in teaching and helping students prepare for service in various health professions, including the roles of pharmacy technicians, medical assistants, and nurses. He has worked with the Brevard County Health Department as an epidemiologist and health educator consultant since 1990, offering continuing education courses and keeping nurses up to date on the latest developments related to pharmacology, medication errors, immunizations, and other important topics. He has been a published author of various allied health books since 1999.

Contributors/Reviewers

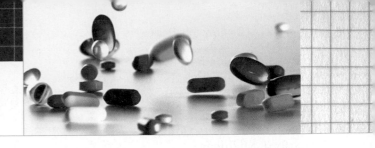

CONTRIBUTORS

Karen Bills, PharmD, CPH
Walgreens
Melbourne, Florida

Maggie Carpenter, PharmD
Sea Pines Hospital
Melbourne, Florida

Jeffrey R. Mabry, DMD
West Palm Beach, Florida

Stephanie K. Mullen, RN, MSN, CPNP
Medical College of Wisconsin
Milwaukee, Wisconsin

Susan Neil, MBA, RNP, LMIF
Melbourne, Florida

Mahkameh Moini, DMD
West Palm Beach, Florida

Norman Tomaka, CRPh, LHCRM
Walgreens
Melbourne, Florida

Greg Vadimsky, Pharmacy Technician
Melbourne, Florida

THANK YOU TO OUR REVIEWERS

Patricia J. Allee, RN
Blinn College
Brenham, Texas

Kristen Anderson, RN, BSN
Southwest Wisconsin Technical College
Fennimore, Wisconsin

Deborah Bedford, CMA
North Seattle Community College
Seattle, Washington

Susan Boggs, RN, CNOR
Piedmont Technical College
Greenwood, South Carolina

Vince Druash, CMA, BS
Medical Careers Institute
Virginia Beach, Virginia

Judy Ehninger, MA
Lehigh Carbon Community College
Schnecksville PA 18078

Rosemary Fischer, RN, BSN, MS
Retired from Alfred State College
Alfred, New York

Steve Forshier, RT(R), MEd
Pima Medical Institute
Mesa, Arizona

Nancy D. Glass, RN, PhD
Austin Community College
Austin, Texas

Robyn Gohsman, RMA, CMAS, AAS
Medical Careers Institute
Newport News, Virginia

Henry Gomez, MD
ASA Institute
Brooklyn, New York

Jeanette Goodwin, CMA, BSN
Southeast Community College
Lincoln, Nebraska

Corrine C. Harmon, RN, MS, EdD, AOCN
Clemson University
Clemson, South Carolina

Elizabeth Hoffman, MAEd, CMA, CPT, (ASPT)
Baker College of Clinton Township
Clinton Township, Michigan

Robin Kern, RN, BSN
Moultrie Technical College
Moultrie, Georgia

Len Lichtblau, PhD
University of Minnesota School of Nursing
Edina, Minnesota

Douglas Lytle, PhD, MBA
Widener University
Pottstown, Pennsylvania

David Martinez, RHE, BA
International Business College
El Paso, Texas

Nancy Matyunas, PharmD
Jefferson Community & Technical College
Louisville, Kentucky

Gayle Mazzocco, RN, CMA, BSN
Oakland Community College
Waterford, Michigan

Carol McMahon, RN, BSN, MEd
Capital Community College
Simsbury, Connecticut

Michele G. Miller, MEd, CMA, COMT
Lakeland Community College
Kirtland, Ohio

Lisa Nagle, BSed, CMA
Augusta Technical College
Augusta, Georgia

Eva Ruth Oltman, CMA, CPC, EMT, LMR, MA
Kentucky Community & Technical College System
Prospect, Kentucky

Christopher Owens, PharmD, BCPS
Idaho State University
Pocatello, Idaho

Steve Peterson, CPhT, MEd
Apollo College
Scottsdale, Arizona

Diane Premeau, RHIA, CHP, MBA
Chabot College
Fremont, California

Myra Resnick, RN
Southwestern College
Florence, KY

Jackie Smith, RN, CPhT
National College of Business and Technology
Pounding Mill, Virginia

Karen Snipe, CPhT, MAEd
Trident Technical College
Charleston, South Carolina

Pat Stroupe, RN, MSN
Waukesha County Technical College
Pewaukee, Wisconsin

Joe Tinervia, CPhT, MBA
Community Care College
Tulsa, Oklahoma

Robert Tralongo, RRT-NPS, MBA
Molloy College
Rockville Centre, New York

Jana Tucker, CMA, LPRT
Salt Lake Community College
Salt Lake City, Utah

Gail Tuohig, RN, PhD
St. Mark's Hospital
Salt Lake City, Utah

Lori Warren, RN, CPC, CCP, CLNC, MA
Spencerian College
Jefferson, Indiana

Tonia Webster, RN, CMA
Southwest Wisconsin Technical College
Platteville, Wisconsin

Mary Ann Woods, RN, CMA, MS, PhD
Fresno City College
Fresno, California

Judith Wulff, RN, BSN
D.G. Erwin Technical Center
Tampa, Florida

MEDIA REVIEWERS

Joyce B. Benedetti, RN, MS, JD, CMA-AC
Allan Hancock College
Santa Maria, California

Peggy Bush, PhD, RPh
Durham Technical Community College
Durham, North Carolina

Carol Buttz
Dakota County Technical College
Rosemount, Minnesota

Jennifer Chang, BS, MS
College of Marin
Kentfield, California

June A. Griffith, PharmD, CGP
Florida Community College
Jacksonville, Florida

Lynda Harkins, PhD
Texas State University-San Marcos
San Marcos, Texas

Anne P. LaVance, BS, CPhT
Delgado Community College
New Orleans, Louisiana

Vivian C. Lilly, PhD, MBA, RN
North Harris College
Houston Texas

Patricia McLane, RHIA, MA
Schoolcraft Collage
Garden City, Michigan

Michele G. Miller, MEd, CMA, COMT
Lakeland Community College
Kirtland, Ohio

Lisa Nagle, BSed, CMA
Augusta Technical College
Augusta, Georgia

Geraldine Twomey, MEd, RRT, RN
North Shore Community College
Danvers, Massachusetts

Contents

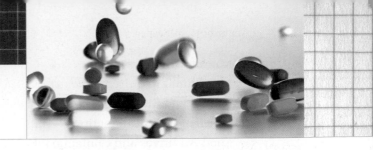

Unit 4   Effects of Drugs on Specific Systems 293

Focus on PHARMACOLOGY

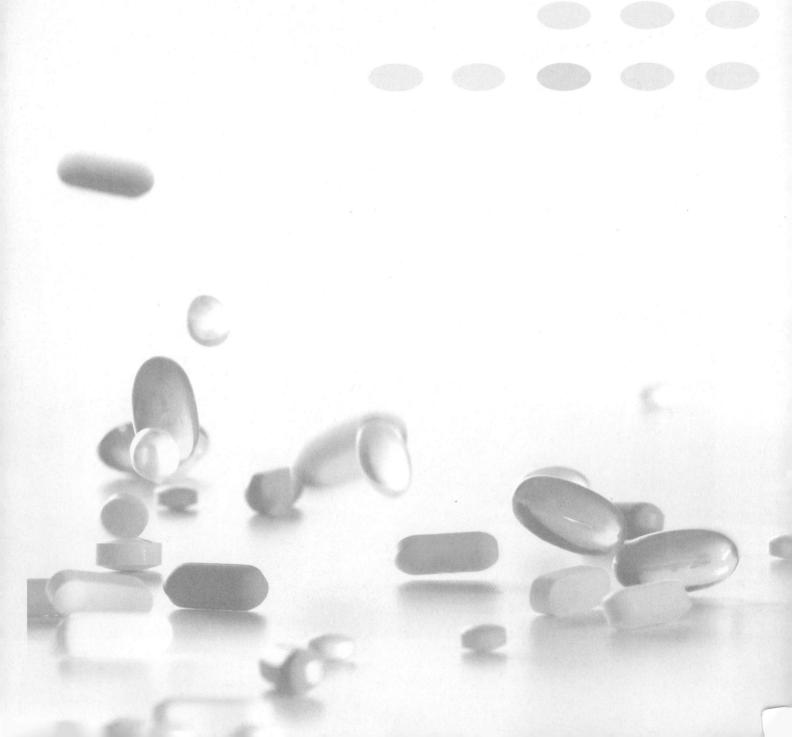

Unit 1

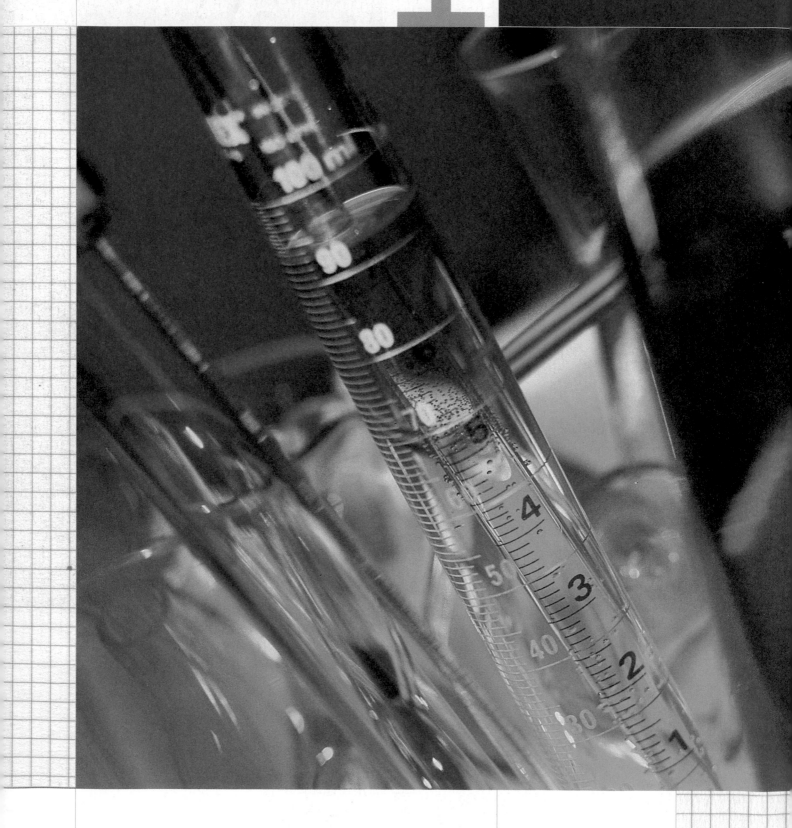

GENERAL PRINCIPLES

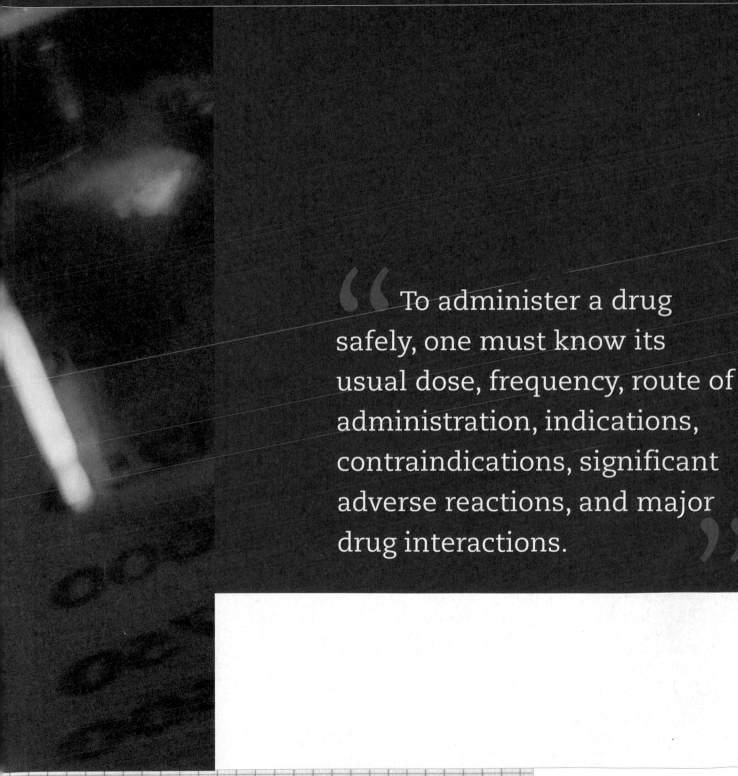

" To administer a drug safely, one must know its usual dose, frequency, route of administration, indications, contraindications, significant adverse reactions, and major drug interactions. "

Chapter 1

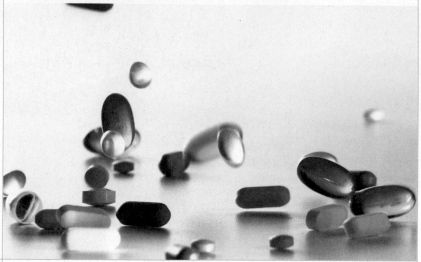

Introduction and Principles of Pharmacology

Key Terms

PRACTICAL SCENARIO

A 73-year-old man with a 25-year history of alcoholism was prescribed the sedative phenobarbital by his family physician after he reported anxiety and trouble sleeping. The patient was also taking the anticoagulant warfarin (Coumadin) that had been prescribed by his cardiologist. Warfarin is a drug that is metabolized more rapidly when given with phenobarbital. This patient was later brought into the emergency department (ED) with a possible hemorrhagic stroke.

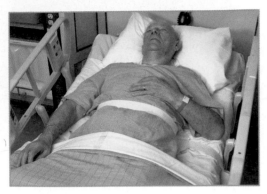

Critical Thinking Questions

1. Explain how alcohol, warfarin, and phenobarbital may be related to the patient's possible stroke.
2. How might the patient's age be related to the drug toxicity?
3. How could the family physician have helped prevent this emergency?

Introduction

Pharmacology is the study of drugs, including their action and effects in living body systems. Drugs do not create effects in the body, but they do modify physical processes by mimicking or blocking effects of substances found within the body. The term *drug* is defined as "any substance or product that is used or intended to be used to modify or improve a physiologic or pathologic condition." The terms *medication* and *medicine* refer to drugs mixed in a formulation with other ingredients to improve the stability, taste, or physical form to allow appropriate administration of the active drug.

Pharmacology deals with all of the drugs used in society today—those that are legal, illegal, prescription, and over-the-counter (OTC) medications. Health-care professionals should be well informed about each medication before administering or dispensing it to a patient and should consider what drugs the patient is taking (whether prescribed or self-administered for medical or recreational reasons). To administer a drug safely, one must know its usual dose, frequency, route of administration, indications, contraindications, significant adverse reactions, and major drug interactions. Knowledge of the patient's medication allergies, weight, and liver and kidney function are also essential.

Pharmacodynamics refers to the biochemical and physiologic effects of drugs and mechanisms of drug action (the effects of a drug on the body or organism). **Pharmacokinetics** is the study of the absorption, distribution, biotransformation **(metabolism**—the sum of chemical and physical changes in the tissues, consisting of anabolism and catabolism), and excretion of drugs (Figure 1-1 ■). Each of these factors is related to the concentration of the drug, its metabolites, and mechanism of action.

Pharmacognosy is the study of drugs derived from herbal and other natural sources. By studying the compositions of natural substances and how the body reacts to them, one gains better knowledge for developing purified versions. **Pharmacotherapeutics** is the study of how drugs may best be used in the treatment of illnesses and which drug is most or least appropriate to use for a specific disease. **Toxicology** is the study of poisons and poisonings; almost all drugs are capable of being toxic. Toxicology deals with the toxic effects of substances on the living organism. Pharmacodynamics, pharmacokinetics, and toxicology are the principal subjects of pharmacology that will be discussed in depth.

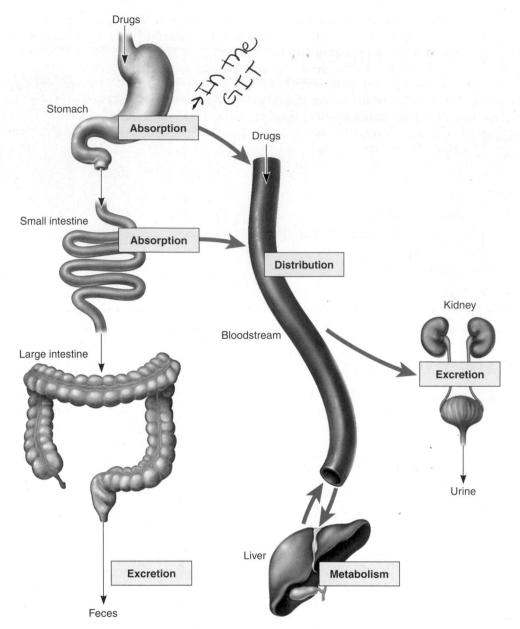

Figure 1-1 ■ The four processes of pharmacokinetics (that is, movement) are absorption, metabolism, distribution, and excretion.

Pharmacodynamics

The pharmacodynamics process describes all matters concerned with the pharmacologic actions of a drug, whether they are determinants of **therapeutic** effects (those effects meant to treat a disease or disorder) or **adverse effects** (harmful effects). A basic understanding of the factors that control drug concentration at the site of action is important for the optimal use of drugs. Blood is the most commonly sampled fluid used to characterize the pharmacologic actions of drugs. The drugs must dissolve before being absorbed. Then they are able to pass through the small intestine and enter the blood circulation. Some of these drugs are absorbed and metabolized before reaching the site of action. The factors that may influence onset, duration, and intensity of drug effects include absorption, metabolism, reabsorption, excretion, site of action, and observed response. Usually there are correlations between pharmacokinetics and pharmacodynamics that demonstrate the relationship between drug dose and blood, or other biological fluid concentrations. Pharmacokinetics and pharmacodynamics can determine the **dose-effect relationship** (also called *dose-response relationship*), which is the relationship between the dose of a drug (or other agent) that produces therapeutic effects and the potency of the effects on the person (Figure 1-2 ■). A graph is used to illustrate the relationship: The response is plotted along the *y*-axis and the dose along the *x*-axis. The resulting plotted relationship is a characteristic curve, as the figure shows. The body's response to a drug (or toxic agent) increases as its overall exposure to the substance increases (for example, in the case of toxic agents, a small dose of carbon monoxide may cause drowsiness; a large dose can be fatal).

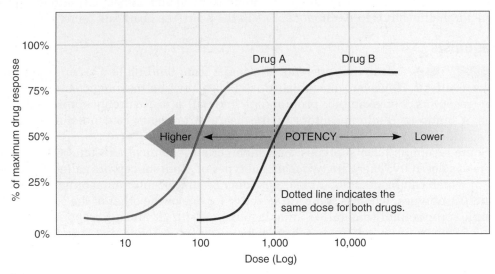

A

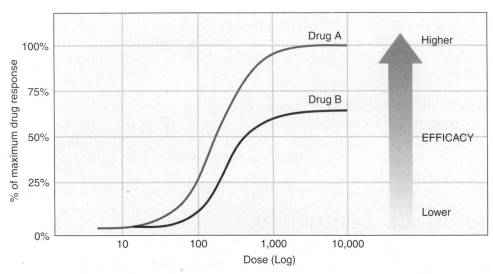

B

Figure 1-2 ■ The dose-effect relationship. Along the *x*-axis is the drug dose, which increases from left to right. Along the *y*-axis is the maximum response for each drug (%). (A) These curves show drug potency. Drug A's curve is to the left of drug B's curve, which indicates that drug A has a higher potency. This means that a smaller dose of drug A will produce the same effect as a larger dose of drug B. (B) These curves show drug efficacy (or effectiveness). Drug A reaches a maximum response of 100% at the same dose as drug B, which reaches a maximum response of about 60%. Therefore, drug A's efficacy (or effectiveness) is greater than that of drug B.

MECHANISM OF DRUG ACTIONS AND RECEPTORS

Drugs produce their effects by altering the function of the cells and tissues of the body or of organisms such as bacteria. Each drug has a specific affinity (attractive force) for a target receptor. The cell recipient is known as a **receptor**, usually a specific protein, situated either in cell membranes on cell surfaces, or within the cellular cytoplasm. However, some drugs act on intracellular receptors; these include corticosteroids, which act on cytoplasmic steroid receptors. As drugs bind to their specific receptors, one of two actions are produced—an agonist or antagonist action.

Agonists

An **agonist** is a drug that binds to a receptor and produces a stimulatory response that is similar to what an endogenous substance (such as a hormone) would have done if it were bound to the receptor. For example, adrenaline is an agonist at beta (β)-adrenoceptors. When adrenaline binds to β-adrenoceptors in the heart, the heart rate increases.

Antagonists

An **antagonist** is a drug that prevents an agonist from binding to a receptor and thus blocks its effects. However, antagonists do not have any pharmacologic actions mediated by receptors. For example, propranolol (Inderal) is a β-adrenoceptor antagonist. When it binds to β-adrenoceptors in the heart, it prevents catecholamine-induced tachycardia (for example, in response to exercise).

Some receptors have subtypes for which certain chemical substances have some degree of selectivity. There are two main subtypes of β-adrenoceptors called β_1 and β_2, both of which can respond to adrenaline. Some β-adrenoceptor antagonists act at both β_1 and β_2 subtypes, whereas some are selective for one or the other of the subtypes. For example, propranolol (Inderal) is an antagonist at both β_1 and β_2 receptors, whereas atenolol (Tenormin) is relatively selective for β_1 receptors. Note that selectivity of this kind is only relative. Although a drug such as atenolol acts primarily on β_1 receptors, at high enough concentrations, it can have effects on β_2 receptors as well.

VARIOUS FACTORS THAT AFFECT DRUG ACTIONS

Drug actions depend on various factors that are important in determining the correct drugs for a patient. These factors include age, sex, body weight, diurnal body rhythms, diseases, allergies, psychological factors, drug half-life, tolerance, drug toxicity, and drug interactions.

Drug Half-Life

A drug's **half-life** ($t^{1}\!/_{2}$) is defined as the time taken for the blood or plasma concentration of the drug to decrease from full to one-half (50%). The half-life is the major determinant of the duration of drug action. The longer the half-life of the drug, the longer the drug remains in the body.

The half-life of each drug may be different; for example, a drug with a short half-life of 2 or 3 hours must be administered more often than one with a longer half-life of 12 hours. Another method of explaining drug action is shown in Figure 1-3 ■, a graphic depiction of the plasma concentration of the drug versus time.

Age

Drug effects may vary in patients according to their different metabolic rates. Age often affects metabolic rates. Drug dosages may need to be adjusted in children or eldery patients. The rule of thumb with pediatric and geriatric individuals is "start low and go slow!"

Gender

Male and female patients respond to drugs differently. Drugs administered intramuscularly are absorbed faster by men than by women. Such drugs remain in women's tissues longer than in men's tissues because women have higher body fat content.

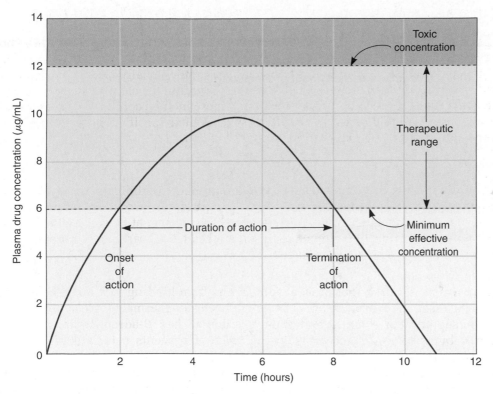

Figure 1-3 ■ Plasma concentration of a drug versus time. The onset of action occurs at 2 hours; the duration of action is 6 hours; peak plasma concentration is 10 mcg/mL; and the time to reach peak drug effect is 5 hours.

Body Weight

Body weight is an important factor for drug action. The same dosage of medication can have varied effects in patients whose weights differ. Some medication doses must be adjusted based on body weight and body surface area, especially in children. Calculation of correct dosage of drugs based on body weight is discussed in Chapter 7.

Diurnal Body Rhythms

Diurnal, or circadian, rhythms can affect the intensity of a person's response to a drug. For example, at night the circadian clock sets the stage for sleep. By administering sleep-inducing medications at night, the drug actions may be more pronounced. In contrast, administering corticosteroids during the day is meant to mimic the circadian variations in endogenous cortisol.

Diseases

Because the liver is the major site of detoxification and the kidneys are the major sites of elimination of chemical substances, a person with liver or kidney disease may respond differently to medications than does a healthy individual.

Focus on Geriatrics

Drug Elimination in Elderly Patients

Acute or chronic diseases that affect liver architecture or function also markedly affect hepatic metabolism of some drugs. Elderly patients with chronic active hepatitis, cirrhosis of the liver, or drug-induced hepatitis can have markedly affected drug elimination. Consequently, some drugs such as diazepam may cause coma in severely liver-damaged patients when given in ordinary doses.

✳ Apply Your Knowledge 1.1

The following questions focus on what you have just learned about pharmacodynamics. *See Appendix E for the correct answers.*

MULTIPLE CHOICE

Choose the correct answer from choices a–d.

1. Pharmacodynamics means:

   a. Study of the biotransformation of drugs

   b. Study of drugs, including their actions and side effects

   c. Study of the biochemical and physiologic effects of drugs

   d. Study of drugs derived from herbal and other natural sources

2. The specific cell recipient is known as a(an):

   a. Receptor

   b. Affinity

   c. Agonist

   d. Bioavailability

3. Which of the following factors may influence intensity of drug effects?

   a. Drug price

   b. Metabolism

   c. Drug allergy

   d. Tolerance

4. Which of the following drugs are affected by diurnal body rhythms?

   a. Antiemetics

   b. Sedatives

   c. Analgesics

   d. Antacids

5. Propranolol is an antagonist at which of the following receptors?

   a. α and β receptors

   b. α_1 and α_2 receptors

   c. β_1 and β_2 receptors

   d. β_1 and α_1 receptors

FILL IN THE BLANK

Select terms from your reading to fill in the blanks.

1. The factors that may influence onset, duration, and intensity of drug effects include _____, _____, _____, _____, and _____.

2. A special drug that has a specific affinity for a particular cell is known as a _____.

3. The longer the half-life of the drug, the longer the plasma _____ will remain within the therapeutic range.

4. Drugs administered intramuscularly are absorbed faster by _____. They remain in women's tissues _____ than in men's tissues because women have higher _____ content.

5. The liver and kidneys are the major sites of _____ and _____ chemical substances.

Pharmacokinetics

Pharmacokinetics, as noted earlier in this chapter, is the study of the action of drug absorption, drug distribution, drug metabolism, and drug excretion.

DRUG ABSORPTION AND SYSTEMIC AVAILABILITY

The process of drug movement into the systemic circulation is **absorption**. Absorption depends on the drug's ability to cross cell membranes and resist extensive breakdown by the stomach, liver, and intestines. Presystemic metabolism occurs when enzymes in the GI tract begin to break down the drug before it is absorbed. Presystemic metabolism affects the amount of drug that reaches the systemic circulation intact and the speed at which this happens—a concept termed **bioavailability**.

Bioavailability depends on pharmaceutical factors (such as the rate at which a tablet or capsule dissolves or the use of binding products in formulating the medication) and variable factors that affect GI absorption (such as food in the stomach, other drugs taken concurrently, intestinal motility, or certain disease states). The extent of bioavailability depends mostly on absorption and somewhat on presystemic metabolism. Lipid-soluble drugs (for example, diazepam and phenytoin) and weak acids (such as acetylsalicylic acid and penicillin V) may be absorbed directly from the stomach. Weak bases (for example, morphine and atropine) are not normally absorbed from the site. The small intestine is the primary site of absorption because of the very large surface area across which drugs may diffuse. Acids (such as ibuprofen and warfarin) are normally absorbed more extensively from the intestines than from the stomach, even though the intestines have a higher pH.

Factors That Affect the Rate of Drug Absorption

In the GI tract, many factors influence the rate of drug absorption, including:

1. **Acidity of the Stomach**—Aspirin and other drugs that have an acidic pH are easily absorbed in the stomach's acidic environment. The small intestine, which has an alkaline environment, more readily absorbs alkaline medications. The pH of the stomach tends to be changed by milk products and antacids. Some drugs are not absorbed properly as a result. For this reason, infants who are consuming milk or formula may need to be given certain medications on an empty stomach.

2. **Physiochemical Properties**—The rate of a drug's absorption may be greatly affected by the rate at which the drug is made available to the biologic fluid at the administration site. Some of the factors that affect a drug's rate of **dissolution** (the process of dissolving) from a solid form include intrinsic physiochemical properties, such as solubility and thermodynamics (having to do with energy).

3. **Presence of Food in the Stomach or Intestine**—The rate and extent of drug absorption may be greatly influenced by the presence of food. An empty stomach increases the rate of absorption of some medications, whereas food in the stomach decreases the absorption rate. However, if a medication causes irritation to the stomach, the patient should eat food with the medication; the food serves as a buffer to decrease irritation.

4. **Routes of Administration**—Routes that protect drugs from chemical decomposition that may occur in the stomach or liver include sublingual (under the tongue), buccal (in the folds of the cheeks), and rectal (within the rectum). Orally administered drugs are usually absorbed in the upper GI tract. They are immediately exposed to metabolism by liver enzymes before they reach the systemic circulation. This exposure is called the **first-pass effect**. Once the drug is in the liver, it is partly metabolized before being sent to the body where systemic effects occur. As a result, medications that are metabolized too quickly in the liver should not be given orally. Alprenolol (Alfeprol), dopamine (Intropin), and lidocaine (Xylocaine) are some examples of drugs that exhibit first-pass metabolism. To determine the suitability of a drug for each patient, it is crucial that the route of administration be

correctly chosen. Depending on the degree of first-pass elimination and the formulation of some drugs, oral administration is feasible for some drugs and not for others. Drugs that are directly injected into the bloodstream via the veins or arteries bypass the process of absorption and are distributed throughout the body. The time before the drug becomes effective for these injections is typically short compared with other types of injections. Also, drugs may be injected deeply into skeletal muscle. The vascularity of the muscle site and lipid solubility of the drug determine the rate of absorption. Because the subcutaneous region is less vascular than the muscle tissues, subcutaneous injections (given beneath the skin) are absorbed less rapidly. Transdermal injections (such as those used for tuberculin skin testing), transdermal patches, and otic or ophthalmic administration are other routes. Topical drugs may be absorbed through several layers of skin for a local effect. Transdermal nitroglycerin (Nitrostat, Nitro-Bid) is absorbed rapidly and provides sustained blood levels after application to the skin, in the form of either an ointment or a transdermal patch. Some drugs such as morphine patches (Duramorph) also provide certain systemic effects like pain relief. Drugs administered in low concentrations tend to be less rapidly absorbed than those administered in high concentrations.

DRUG DISTRIBUTION

Many drugs are bound to circulating proteins, usually albumin (acid drugs), but also globulins (hormones), lipoproteins (basic drugs), and acid glycoproteins (basic drugs). Only the fraction of drugs that are not bound to protein can bind to cellular receptors, pass across tissue membranes, and gain access to cellular enzymes, thus being distributed to body tissue, metabolized, and excreted (for example, by the kidneys). Changes in protein binding can therefore sometimes cause changes in drug **distribution** (the passage of an agent through blood or lymph to various body sites). The initial rate of distribution of a drug is heavily dependent on the blood flow to various organs. Lipid-soluble drugs enter the central nervous system (CNS) rapidly. Because of the blood-brain barrier, certain drugs are poorly distributed to the CNS because they pass through the barrier.

DRUG METABOLISM

Most drug metabolism occurs in the liver (although it may also occur in the kidneys, nerve cells, and plasma) through the same biochemical pathways and reactions that affect nutrients, vitamins, and minerals. The first-pass effect is an important mechanism that influences drug action and metabolism. Metabolism accomplishes the conversion of small and large molecules, as well as biodegration of foreign substances. Substances absorbed across the intestinal wall enter blood vessels. This is known as *hepatic portal circulation*, a process that carries blood directly to the liver (Figure 1-4 ■).

Enzymes act on most drugs in the body and convert drugs to metabolites during metabolism. **Biotransformation** is the process of conversion of drugs. Biotransformation may be divided into four main stages:

1. **Oxidation**—combination with oxygen
2. **Reduction**—a reaction with a substance that involves the gaining of electrons
3. **Hydrolysis**—the cleaving of a compound into simpler compounds with the uptake of the hydrogen and hydroxide parts of a water molecule
4. **Conjugation**—the combination of substances with glucuronic or sulfuric acid, terminating biologic activity and making them ready for excretion

All of these activities occur primarily in the liver via metabolizing enzymes called *microsomal enzymes.* One of these enzymes is cytochrome P-450, which has an essential role in drug metabolism. The end products of metabolism are called *metabolites,* which may be active or inactive. *Active* metabolites may contribute to a drug's pharmacologic action or its adverse effects. Toxic drug action can be influenced by drug metabolism, which includes duration of drug effects, drug interactions, drug activation,

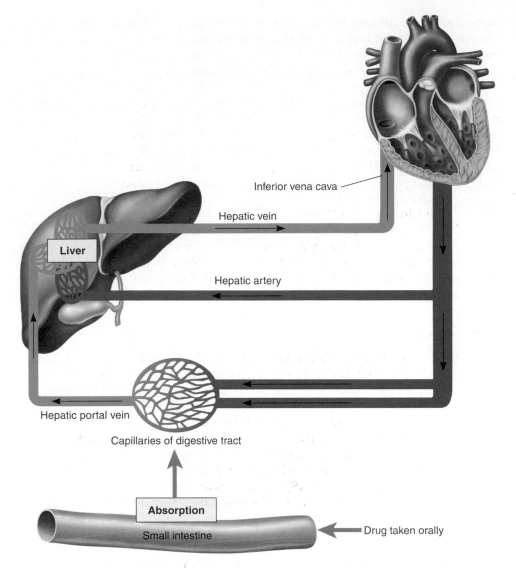

Figure 1-4 ■ First-pass effect. Oral drugs are absorbed through the intestinal wall and enter the hepatic portal circulation. They are taken directly to the liver for metabolism before reaching the heart and circulating throughout the body.

drug toxicity, and adverse effects (often referred to as **side effects**). Side effects are defined as results of drug (or other) therapy that are beyond the desired therapeutic effects. Side effects are usually (but not always) undesirable.

DRUG EXCRETION

The main route of drug **excretion**, the last stage of pharmacokinetics that removes drugs from the system, is via the kidneys. The kidneys remove waste and harmful agents in the blood circulation. Because most drugs are excreted by the kidneys, diseases of the kidneys can significantly prolong the duration of drug action. Drugs that affect the kidneys and the processes the kidneys use to remove substances from the body are discussed in Chapter 21.

Other routes of excretion include:

✻ Lungs—important for the excretion of alcohol

✻ Breast milk—important for the excretion of aspirin, barbiturates, and other drugs

✻ Sweat, tears, urine, and feces—excretions that may be alarming if the patient is not expecting the orange-red discoloration caused by phenazopyridine or rifampicin

✳ Bile—leading to the recirculation of compounds such as chloramphenicol (its inactive metabolites are reactivated by hydrolysis in the gut), morphine, rifampicin, tetracycline, and digitoxin

✳ Saliva—sometimes used in monitoring drug concentrations in body fluids

To aid in the proper excretion of drugs, the patient should follow these guidelines:

✳ Take medications as ordered.

✳ Cough and breathe deeply after general anesthesia to help eliminate anesthetics more quickly.

✳ Chew gum or suck on hard candy to decrease the unpleasant effects of drugs that are eliminated through saliva.

✳ Increase intake of fluids because this will increase filtration of the urine and increase blood volume, thereby assisting in proper excretion.

✳ Maintain proper diet and amount of physical activity because both of these speed drug excretion.

✳ Keep skin clean to help avoid irritation from drugs that are eliminated through the sweat glands.

✳ Discuss use of all medications, including OTC drugs, with your physician to avoid possible risks to the fetus if you are pregnant.

✳ Apply Your Knowledge 1.2

The following questions focus on what you have just learned about pharmacokinetics. *See Appendix E for the correct answers.*

MULTIPLE CHOICE
Select the correct answer from choices a–d.

1. Lipid-soluble drugs may be absorbed directly from which of the following parts of the digestive system?

   a. Mouth
   b. Stomach
   c. Ilium of small intestine
   d. Sigmoid colon

2. The initial rate of distribution of a drug is most dependent on the:

   a. Concentration of urine
   b. Insufficiency of vitamin C in the blood
   c. Blood glucose level
   d. Blood flow to various organs

3. The term *biotransformation* means the process of:

   a. Conversion of drugs
   b. Distribution of urea in the serum
   c. Oxidation of aldehyde
   d. Conversion of protein to amino acid

4. Which of the following drugs may be excreted in breast milk?

   a. Paraldehyde

   b. Aspirin

   c. Digitoxin

   d. Morphine

5. Which of the following organ systems of the body is involved in the last stage of pharmacokinetics?

   a. Stomach

   b. Liver

   c. Kidneys

   d. Brain

FILL IN THE BLANK

Select terms from your reading to fill in the blanks. Answers to some questions may be the same.

1. The four key pharmacokinetic parameters that aid in the design of a rational dosing regimen are _____, _____, _____, and _____.

2. Drug absorption is affected by stomach acidity, the presence of _____ in the stomach or intestines, _____ properties, and _____ of administration.

3. The last stage of pharmacokinetics is _____, which is accomplished mainly by the _____.

4. The four main groups of biotransformations include _____, _____, _____, and _____.

Other Pharmacologic Principles

Many of the concepts applicable in the study of pharmacology apply equally to unforeseen or inadvertent reactions, including adverse drug reactions, adverse effects, drug allergies, drug interactions, and idiosyncratic reactions.

TOXICITY AND OVERDOSE

Toxicity is the state of being noxious and refers to a drug's ability to poison the body. There may be an antidote for the poison—a drug that has the opposite effect and can reverse the toxic symptoms. Sometimes, through medication errors or poor judgment, or as a result of attempted suicide, a patient may receive a drug **overdose**, a toxic dose of the drug that causes harm. This can be dangerous because any drug can act like a poison if taken in too large a dose.

ADVERSE DRUG REACTIONS AND ADVERSE EFFECTS

An *adverse drug reaction (ADR)* has been defined as any response to a drug that is noxious, unintended, and occurs at doses normally used in man for the prophylaxis, diagnosis, or therapy of disease (World Health Organization, 1984). Clinical responses to an ADR include discontinuing the drug, modifying the dose, hospitalizing the patient, or providing supportive measures. An example of an ADR is severe nausea, vomiting, or diarrhea.

ADRs occur in people of all ages. They are a major cause of morbidity and mortality, especially among elderly patients. Little attention has been given to the incidence of ADRs in neonates, infants, children, and adolescents. Before release of a new drug, few (if any) studies are undertaken in children because of issues including ethics, responsibility, cost, and regulations. This often leads prescribers to estimate dosage and hence increases the risk of ADRs in this young population. Today, ADRs are a significant issue in elderly and pediatric patients.

The term *side effect* is frequently used by health-care professionals and often appears in drug advertisements and consumer information. It refers to effects not necessarily intended. But side effects can be beneficial. Therefore, if one is referring to harmful, unexpected effects, the more accurate term to use is *adverse effect*.

DRUG INTERACTIONS

A *drug interaction* occurs when the effects of one drug are altered by the effects of another drug. The interaction can result in either an increased or a decreased effect of the object drug. For example, amiodarone (Cordarone) inhibits cytochrome P-450 isoenzyme, leading to reduced metabolism of warfarin (Coumadin) and increased anticoagulant effects. The drug carbamazepine (Tegretol) reduces the anticoagulant effect of warfarin by increasing its liver metabolism.

Occasionally in an interaction, the effects of both drugs are altered, as occurs in the complex interaction of phenytoin (Dilantin) with phenobarbital (Luminal). Although drug interactions usually result in an ADR, in some cases an interaction is beneficial. One example of this beneficial effect is the pharmacodynamic synergy between diuretics and angiotensin-converting enzyme (ACE) inhibitors in the treatment of hypertension.

IDIOSYNCRATIC REACTIONS

When a patient experiences a unique, strange, or unpredicted reaction to a drug, it is termed an *idiosyncratic reaction*. Idiosyncratic reactions may be caused by underlying enzyme deficiencies resulting from genetic or hormonal variation. For example, carisoprodol (Soma) may cause idiosyncratic reactions such as transient quadriplegia, dizziness, or temporary loss of vision.

ANAPHYLACTIC SHOCK

An idiosyncratic, sudden, and severe allergic reaction that may be life threatening is termed **anaphylactic shock**. It can cause a sharp loss of blood pressure, urticaria (lesions known as *hives* or *wheals*), paralysis of the diaphragm, and swelling of the oropharynx; the end result may be cardiac collapse. Anaphylactic shock, a true medical emergency, occurs so swiftly and with such severity that controlled clinical studies of treatment have never been possible. Prevention is, of course, most important. A history of previous allergic reactions to drugs, vaccines, serum, or blood transfusions must be obtained from anyone about to undergo treatment to prevent or at least be prepared for the slightest hazard of this kind. Patients who are predisposed to allergic reactions should wear an alerting bracelet or necklace (for example, Medic-Alert®). Epinephrine (adrenaline) is frequently injected to combat anaphylactic shock, but must be administered soon after shock begins.

ALLERGIC REACTIONS

Drug allergy is an abnormal response characterized by:

✳ Occurrence in a small number of individuals
✳ Previous exposure to either the same or a chemically related drug
✳ Rapid development of an allergic reaction after reexposure
✳ Production of clinical manifestations of an allergic reaction

The term *hypersensitivity* is often used synonymously with allergy.

The diagnosis of a drug allergy is often difficult to establish because there are no reliable laboratory tests that can identify the relevant drug, and in some cases, the symptoms can imitate infectious disease symptoms. A health-care practitioner must clarify whether the patient is experiencing a true allergic reaction or drug intolerance. For example, administration of penicillin by injection may cause a severe allergic reaction, which may be life threatening. Conversely, when a patient takes penicillin orally, allergy to the substance may cause nausea and vomiting to an intolerable degree. Allergic reactions to drugs generally follow the type I–IV classification as listed in Table 1-1 ■.

Table 1-1 ■ **Allergic Drug Reactions**

TYPE	EXAMPLES OF DRUGS OR CLASSES OF DRUGS
I. Immediate hypersensitivity	Penicillins, streptomycin, local anesthetics, neuromuscular-blocking drugs, radiologic contrast medicine
II. Antibody-dependent, cytotoxic	Quinine, quinidine, rifampicin, metronidazole
III. Complex-mediated	Anticonvulsants, antibiotics, hydralazine, diuretics
IV. Cell-mediated or delayed-hypersensitivity	Local anesthetic creams, antihistamine creams

TOLERANCE

Drug **tolerance** is the development of resistance to the effects of a drug such that the drug's doses must be continually raised to elicit the desired response. Tolerance is often experienced in relation to drugs of abuse. Drugs that commonly produce tolerance are opiates, nitrates, barbiturates, alcohol, and tobacco. Cross-tolerance occurs when a person develops a resistance to chemically similar drugs. *Dependence*, a frequently confused term, refers to a drug's ability to stimulate pleasure centers in the brain, causing the patient to desire more or continued use of the drug.

CUMULATIVE EFFECT

When the body is not able to metabolize and excrete one dose of a drug completely before the next dose is given, a *cumulative effect* occurs. With repeated doses, the drug starts to collect in the blood and body tissues, resulting in cumulative toxicity. Cumulative toxicity may occur rapidly, such as with ethyl alcohol, or slowly over time, such as with lead poisoning.

SYNERGISM

The combined action of two or more agents that produce an effect greater than that which would have been expected from the two agents acting separately is called *synergism*. Some drug interactions exhibit synergism, which, depending on the circumstances, may be beneficial or harmful. For example, the combination of the antibacterial drug trimethoprim with sulfamethoxazole (Bactrim, Septa) is more effective for treating infections than either drug acting alone. However, the combination of aspirin and the anticoagulant warfarin (Coumadin) can act synergistically to reduce blood clotting to the extent of spontaneous hemorrhage if doses are not carefully monitored.

POTENTIATION

An interaction between two drugs that causes an effect greater than that which would have been expected from the additive properties of the drugs involved is called *potentiation*. For example, alcohol potentiates the sedating effects of the tranquilizer diazepam (Valium) when the two drugs are ingested at the same time.

Focus Point

Allergy History

Ask all patients if they have a history of allergies, such as hay fever, rashes, or asthma, or have had unusual reactions to any drugs taken orally or by injection in the past.

✳ Apply Your Knowledge 1.3

The following questions focus on what you have just learned about toxicology. *See Appendix E for the correct answers.*

MATCHING

Match the lettered term to the numbered description. Some descriptions may have more than one lettered term.

DESCRIPTION	TERM
1. _____ Types of allergic drug reactions	a. . Immediate hypersensitivity
2. _____ Any response to a drug that is noxious, unintended, and occurs at normal doses	b. Laboratory tests
	c. Medical emergency
3. _____ Not reliable for diagnosing a drug allergy	d. Antibody-dependent cytotoxic
4. _____ A unique, strange, or unpredicted reaction to a drug	e. Idiosyncratic reaction
	f. Complex-mediated
5. _____ Anaphylactic shock is a true case	g. Cell-mediated or delayed hypersensitivity
	h. Adverse drug reaction

FILL IN THE BLANK

Select terms from your reading to fill in the blanks.

1. A type II allergic drug reaction is also known as a cytotoxic or _____ reaction.

2. Penicillin and streptomycin most often cause a(an) _____ allergic drug reaction.

3. Diuretics have been known to cause type III, or _____ allergic drug reactions.

4. Cell-mediated or _____ reactions can result from the use of local anesthetic or antihistamine creams.

5. Administration of penicillin by injection can possibly cause a(an) _____ allergic drug reaction.

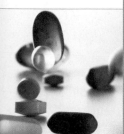

Chapter Capsule

This section repeats the objectives from the beginning of the chapter and then provides a summary of the most important concepts for that objective. Use this section as a quick review and to check your knowledge.

Objective 1: Define and differentiate the terms *pharmacodynamics* and *pharmacokinetics*.

- The study of the biochemical and physiologic effects of drugs and the mechanism of drug action

Objective 2: Explain the mechanism of drug action.

- Alters the normal function of the cells and tissues of the body by mimicking or blocking the effects of normal endogenous substances
- Specific cells (known as receptors) are chosen because the drug has a specific affinity for a particular cell
- Each receptor type attracts a specific group of drugs capable of binding to the receptor, thereby producing a pharmacologic effect

Objective 3: List various factors that affect drug action.

- Age
- Gender
- Body weight
- Diurnal body rhythms
- Diseases
- Drug half-life, absorption, administration route, distribution, metabolism, and excretion

Objective 4: Discuss the main site variables that affect drug absorption.

- Acidity of the stomach—acidic drugs such as aspirin are easily absorbed here; the pH of the stomach tends to be changed by milk products and antacids, thus some drugs are not absorbed properly; certain medications should be given on an empty stomach to ensure proper absorption
- Physiochemical properties—factors that affect the rate of drug dissolution from a solid form, including intrinsic physiochemical properties, such as solubility and rate of dissolution
- Presence of food in the stomach or intestine—an empty stomach increases the rate of absorption of some medications; food in the stomach decreases the absorption rate
- Routes of administration—sublingual (under the tongue), buccal (inner lining of the cheeks), and rectal (within the rectum); orally administered drugs are usually absorbed in the upper GI tract and are immediately exposed to metabolism via liver enzymes before reaching systemic circulation (the first-pass effect)

Objective 5: Define the systemic bioavailability of a drug.

- The amount of administered drug that reaches the systemic circulation intact and the speed at which this happens

Objective 6: Describe the metabolism of drugs.

- Mostly occurs in the liver, but some occurs in the plasma, kidneys, and cells; at synapses; or within nerves
- First-pass effect—influences drug action and metabolism (the amount of drug that is able to reach the systemic circulation)
- Substances absorbed across the intestinal wall enter blood vessels (known as the hepatic portal circulation) and are carried with the blood directly to the liver
- Most drugs are acted on by enzymes (such as cytochrome P-450) and converted to metabolic derivatives (biotransformation)
- Biotransformation—divided into oxidation, reduction, hydrolysis, and conjugation

Objective 7: Explain the excretion of drugs through the kidneys.

- The main route of excretion
- Remove waste and harmful agents in the blood circulation, including the majority of drugs
- Diseases of the kidneys—significantly prolong the duration of drug action

Objective 8: Define the term *idiosyncratic reaction*.

- A unique, strange, or unpredicted reaction to a drug
- May be caused by enzyme deficiencies resulting from genetic or hormonal variation, allergy, or sensitivities

Objective 9: Explain adverse drug reactions and adverse effects.

- Adverse drug reactions (ADRs)—any responses to a drug that are noxious and unintended and occur at doses normally used in humans for the prophylaxis, diagnosis, or therapy of disease
- ADRs—occur in people of all ages; a significant issue concerning children and elderly patients
- Adverse effects—ADRs that are sometimes called side effects; the term *side effect* implies that the adverse reaction is insignificant, medically trivial, or acceptable
- Use of the term *side effect* should be avoided if possible; *adverse effect* is the preferred term

Objective 10: Define the term *drug allergy*.

- A hypersensitivity reaction
- Characterized by:
  - ❏ Occurrence in only a few individuals
  - ❏ Previous exposure to either the same or a chemically related drug
  - ❏ Rapid development of an allergic reaction after reexposure
  - ❏ Production of clinical manifestations of an allergic reaction

Internet Sites of Interest

- An encyclopedia of medical and pharmacology terms, health news, and information on disorders can be found at Science Daily's Web site: **www.sciencedaily.com/**
- The FDA's Web site **www.fda.gov/cder/drug/** includes new drug approvals, prescription and over-the-counter drug information, drug safety and side-effect information, and more.
- INCHEM posts a study on the effects of human exposure to various chemicals and toxicity tests. The report was prepared in conjunction with the World Health Organization. See: **www.inchem.org**
- Medscape Pharmacists contains a wealth of information about drugs, natural therapies, FDA drug warnings, and even continuing education programs for health professionals at: **www.medscape.com/pharmacists**
- The topic of drug allergies can be found on the National Institutes of Health's MedLink site: **www.nlm.nih.gov/medlineplus**. Search the site for "drug allergies."
- An excellent article on adverse drug reactions and treatment options is offered by Riedl and Casillas in *American Family Physician*. 2003; 68:1781–90. It is available at: **www.aafp.org**. Search for this article from the journal's home page.

Chapter Objectives

After completing this chapter, you should be able to:

1. Discuss legal and ethical requirements regarding the use, dispensing, and administration of medications.

2. Explain how the need for drug control evolved.

3. Discuss the poisoning disaster that led to legislation requiring testing for the purity, strength, effectiveness, safety, and packaging quality of drugs.

4. Explain the major points of the thalidomide disaster of 1962.

5. List the provisions of the Controlled Substances Act.

6. Differentiate between each of the five schedules for controlled substances.

7. Define *orphan drug* and list some examples.

8. Discuss the federal regulatory agencies that deal with food, drugs, and disease control.

9. Explain which level of government primarily controls pharmacy licensure.

10. Define *ethics* as it relates to pharmacology.

Chapter 2

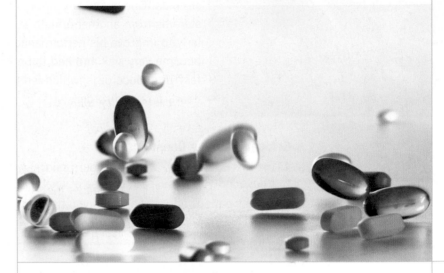

Law and Ethics of Medication Administration

Key Terms

Abuse potential (page 25)

Anabolic steroids (an-uh-BOL-lik-STAYR-oidz) (page 27)

Controlled substances (page 22)

Designer drugs (page 24)

Ethics (page 33)

Interstate commerce (page 23)

Legend drugs (page 23)

Nuclear pharmacy (page 30)

Orphan drugs (page 27)

Reimportation (ree-im-por-TAY-shun) (page 27)

PRACTICAL SCENARIO

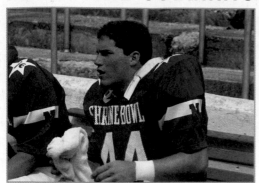

Anabolic steroids are very popular among today's athletes who want to gain the competitive edge over others by building muscle. The evening news often contains stories of professional athletes testing positive for anabolic steroids. One such 20-year-old male athlete illegally obtained anabolic steroids from another athlete at his school and began injecting them regularly to improve his performance in college football. During the season, he became very sick and had to be hospitalized. His physician diagnosed infective endocarditis, which led to inflammation of the inner lining of his heart, a fatal disorder.

Critical Thinking Questions

1. If this young man had been your patient, what changes in the patient over time may have led you to suspect his use of anabolic steroids?
2. What patient education would you have given this patient?
3. How can you explain the link between steroid use and infective endocarditis?

Introduction

All health-care workers who deal with dispensing, preparing, and administering medications must be familiar with the legal and ethical requirements that relate to these procedures. In the United States, the early 1900s marked the beginnings of drug legislation. Today, federal regulations are in place to help protect the consumer from the harmful effects of improperly using drugs; however, drug-related adverse effects still occur even with "approved" over-the-counter (OTC) and prescription drugs. The use of frankly dangerous or illicit drugs is prohibited by state and federal governments. The sale and distribution of drugs in the United States is controlled primarily by two major legislative acts, the Federal Food, Drug, and Cosmetic Act (FDCA) and the Federal Controlled Substances Act (CSA). These acts give the Food and Drug Administration (FDA) and other federal and state agencies the power to enforce legislative decisions. The FDCA is predominantly concerned with fixing the rules and regulations by which drugs are imported, manufactured, distributed, and sold in the United States. The CSA is part of the Comprehensive Drug Abuse Prevention and Control Act of 1970, which, as the title suggests, is concerned with the prevention and control of the abuse of certain drugs called **controlled substances**—or those drugs whose possession and use are controlled by the Act.

The CSA is administered and enforced by the Department of Justice under the attorney general and is a unit of the Federal Bureau of Investigation, known as the Drug Enforcement Administration (DEA). Although the two agencies have separate missions, they do cooperate in the administration of the federal drug abuse treatment program. The DEA is required to obtain the expert scientific advice of the FDA when seeking to add a substance to the list of controlled substances.

These two acts are supplemented on the federal level by a series of legislative acts designed to address specific problems, including the Poison Prevention Packaging Act of 1970 and the Federal Hazardous Substances Act.

The Need for Drug Control

During the nineteenth century, there was virtually no regulation of the sale of drugs in the United States. Opium was readily and legally available OTC in pharmacies, grocery and general stores, and from mail order houses. The medications containing opium were advertised extensively in newspapers. Labels often did not reveal the contents. No law required that the contents of a drug be stated.

Case after case of addiction to opiates and fatal delay in seeking medical treatment—caused by reliance on the claims of charlatans or drug-clouded perceptions—occurred (Figure 2-1 ■). To combat this situation, Congress passed the first Pure Food and Drug Act in 1906.

Federal Law

Congress found the authority to pass drug legislation within its constitutional right to control **interstate commerce**—that is, the commerce, traffic, transportation, and exchange between states of the United States. The purpose of the Federal Food, Drug, and Cosmetic Act of 1938 was the same then as it still is today: to limit interstate commerce of drugs to those that are safe and effective.

The act (which is described more completely later in this chapter) requires that drugs comply with the standards of safety and efficacy, whereas the earlier Pure Food and Drug Act of 1906 focused on standards of strength and purity, as well as proper labeling that indicated the kind and amount of ingredients present. In 1912, Congress passed the Sherley Amendment, prohibiting the use of fraudulent therapeutic claims.

To fulfill the obligation undertaken in 1912, Congress adopted the Federal Narcotic Drug Act in 1914. This law became popularly known as the Harrison Narcotic Act.

SULFANILAMIDE DISASTER OF 1937

A manufacturer decided to market the antimicrobial *sulfanilamide* in a liquid form for sore throats and mixed the sulfanilamide with diethylene glycol, which is the same ingredient used today as antifreeze in car radiators. Because sulfanilamide was poorly soluble in known solvents, drug marketers rushed to be the first to find a suitable solvent and develop a liquid version of the drug, particularly for use in young children. Diethylene glycol was chosen because of its pleasant color and taste. However, it was a deadly poison, and because no clinical safety or efficacy studies were required prior to marketing, this fact went overlooked until patients started dying. There were 107 reported deaths from this product. The 1938 Food, Drug, and Cosmetic Act, which followed this disaster, prevented the marketing of new drugs before they had been properly tested for purity, strength, effectiveness, safety, and packaging quality. This act gave the FDA the authority to approve or deny new drug applications. As a result of this law and further legislation, the FDA now approves the investigational use of drugs on humans and ensures that all approved drugs are safe and effective.

THE DURHAM–HUMPHREY AMENDMENT OF 1951

The Durham–Humphrey Amendment of 1951 exempted certain drugs from the requirement that their labeling must contain adequate directions for use. These drugs, which could be taken safely only under medical supervision, were exempted provided they were sold pursuant to the order of a licensed physician or administered under a prescriber's supervision. The Durham–Humphrey Amendment of 1951 prohibits the dispensing of legend drugs without a prescription. Federal law requires **legend drugs** (prescription drugs) to bear the following statement, "Caution: Federal law prohibits dispensing without prescription." Nonlegend, OTC, drugs were not restricted for sale and use under a physician's supervision. They were deemed safe for use by the public for self-limited use in minor conditions. Their sale is not restricted and their use is thought, in most cases, to require neither prescription nor medical supervision.

THALIDOMIDE DISASTER OF 1962

In 1962, thalidomide, used both as a sleeping pill and antinausea agent during pregnancy, was being widely used abroad. Before it could be approved for use in the United States, its adverse effects on developing fetuses were discovered. Meanwhile, women in other countries who took thalidomide during their first trimester of pregnancy delivered babies with severe deformities including malformed or missing limbs.

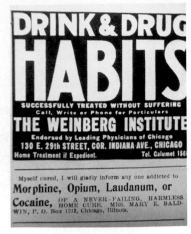

Figure 2-1 ■ During the nineteenth century in the United States, OTC opium could be purchased at pharmacies and grocery stores. As a result, addiction became a problem, leading to programs such as the one advertised in this poster. However, in 1906, the Pure Food and Drug Act put an end to the sale of unsafe or untested drugs such as opium.

These events led to the passage of the Kefauver–Harris Amendment in 1962. Currently, thalidomide has limited availability in the United States for the treatment of leprosy, bone marrow transplantation, acquired immunodeficiency syndrome (AIDS), and several other conditions.

Focus on Pediatrics

Drugs and Birth Defects

Thalidomide is not the only drug known to cause birth defects if taken by pregnant women. Studies have proven that drinking alcohol while pregnant can cause fetal alcohol syndrome (FAS), characterized by abnormalities of the face and head, growth disturbances, and mental deficiency. Smoking during pregnancy has been linked to smaller birth-weight babies and to abnormal infant reflexes.

Apply Your Knowledge 2.1

The following questions focus on what you have just learned about drug control, federal law, and early legislation that related to drug control. *See Appendix E for the correct answers.*

FILL IN THE BLANK
Select terms from your reading to fill in the blanks.

1. To combat the lack of drug product regulation in the United States, Congress passed the _____ of 1906.

2. The purpose of the Federal Food, Drug, and Cosmetic Act was to limit _____ of drugs to those that are _____ and _____.

3. In 1937, the deadly poison mixed with sulfanilamide was _____, used as _____ today.

4. The dispensing of legend drugs without a _____ was prohibited by the Durham–Humphrey Amendmen of 1951.

5. Thalidomide caused severe _____ in children whose mothers took the drug during the _____ trimester of pregnancy.

DRUG ABUSE CONTROL AMENDMENT OF 1965

This amendment, the effective precursor of the Drug Abuse Control Act, permitted only certain authorized registrants to manufacture stimulant drugs. This drug abuse control legislation provided the first guidelines for determining the classifications of drugs subject to abuse. By and large, they were incorporated into the 1970 act, which follows.

COMPREHENSIVE DRUG ABUSE PREVENTION AND CONTROL ACT OF 1970

One of the primary functions of this act was to encompass all federal laws dealing with narcotic drugs, stimulants, depressants, and abused **designer drugs** that did not fit the historical classifications. (*Designer drugs* are defined as drugs produced by a minor modification in the chemical structure of an existing drug, resulting in a new substance with similar pharmacologic effects. Scientists also call these drugs *analogues.*) This act also served to consolidate the government's enforcement activities that had previously been handled by various competing agencies. For example, the Bureau of Narcotics and the Bureau of Drug Abuse Control became the Bureau of Narcotics and Dangerous Drugs (BNDD). Finally, in 1973, all agencies involved in drug abuse control and the enforcement of drug abuse laws were combined into one agency, the Drug Enforcement

Administration (DEA). The DEA, housed within the Department of Justice, became the nation's sole legal drug enforcement agency.

The Comprehensive Drug Abuse Prevention and Control Act of 1970, also called the Controlled Substances Act (CSA), became effective on May 1, 1971. This law was designed to:

✳ Provide increased research into and prevention of drug abuse and drug dependence

✳ Provide for the treatment and rehabilitation of drug abusers and drug-dependent persons

✳ Improve the administration and regulation of the manufacture, distribution, and dispensing of controlled substances by legitimate handlers of these drugs to help reduce their widespread dispersion into illicit markets

Drugs covered by this act have a potential for causing drug dependence, abuse, or both, and are classified according to their use and **abuse potential** (possibility of causing abuse or dependence in a user).

Drugs with the potential for abuse are classified into five schedules: I, II, III, IV, and V. Drugs in Schedule I have the highest potential for abuse and addiction, and those in Schedule V have the least potential.

Schedule I: These drugs have a high potential for abuse, and they are not accepted for medical use in the United States. Properly registered individuals may use Schedule I substances for research, analysis, or instruction purposes.

Schedule II: These drugs also have a high potential for abuse, but they are currently accepted for medical use in the United States. The abuse of these drugs may result in severe psychological or physical dependence. The quantity of the substance in a drug product often determines the schedule that will control it. For example, amphetamines (Figure 2-2 ■) and codeine usually are classified in Schedule II; however, specific products containing smaller quantities of Schedule II substances, most often manufactured in combination with a noncontrolled substance, are controlled by Schedules III and IV. An example would be Tylenol mixed with codeine, which is considered a Schedule III drug.

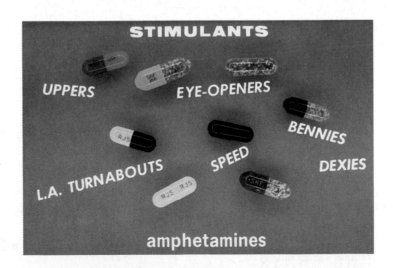

Figure 2-2 ■ Amphetamines, Schedule II drugs, have a high abuse potential and are sold illegally under many street names.

Focus Point

Keeping Medications Safe in the Hospital

All restricted substances must be stored in locked storage facilities to prevent access by unauthorized persons. The nurse in charge of the shift or the pharmacy technician working directly under the supervision of the in-charge pharmacist carries the keys to the locked storage.

Schedule III: These drugs have less abuse potential than those in Schedules I and II and cause only low to moderate physical dependence if abused. They have accepted medical uses in the United States. Schedule III drugs contain limited quantities of certain narcotic and nonnarcotic agents.

Schedule IV: These drugs have only slight abuse potential and accepted medical uses in the United States. They are still more potent than Schedule V drugs and require a prescription.

Schedule V: These drugs have the lowest abuse potential of all the controlled substances and consist of preparations containing limited quantities of certain narcotic drugs that are generally used for antitussive and antidiarrheal purposes. Schedule V drugs are OTC preparations that may be sold without a prescription to individuals 18 years or older. Diphenoxylate hydrochloride with atropine sulfate (Lomotil), which is listed as a Schedule V drug, is an exception: It requires a prescription. Paregoric (a drug that causes emesis, or vomiting) is now restricted to prescription sales only and is included in Schedule III (Table 2-1 ■).

Table 2-1 ■ Drug Schedules

SCHEDULE	ABUSE POTENTIAL	PRESCRIPTION REQUIREMENTS	EXAMPLES
I	High abuse potential; no accepted medical use	No prescription permitted	Heroin, lysergic acid (LSD), marijuana, mescaline, and peyote
II	High abuse potential; accepted medical use	Prescription required; no refills permitted without a new written prescription	Cocaine, codeine, methamphetamine (Desoxyn), methadone hydrochloride (Methadose), morphine (Astramorph), opium (deodorized), methylphenidate (Ritalin), and secobarbital (Seconal)
III	Low to moderate abuse potential; accepted medical use	Prescription required; 5 refills permitted in 6 months	Certain drugs compounded with small quantities of narcotics; also other drugs with high potential for abuse (Tylenol with codeine tablets), and certain barbiturates
IV	Low abuse potential; accepted medical use	Prescription required; 5 refills permitted in 6 months	Barbital, chloral hydrate (Noctec), diazepam (Valium), chlordiazepoxide (Librium), and pentazocine hydrochloride (Talwin)
V	Low abuse potential; accepted medical use	No prescription required for patients 18 years or older	Cough syrups with codeine, diphenoxylate hydrochloride with atropine sulfate (Lomotil)*, and kaolin/pectin/opium (Parepectolin)*

* These Schedule V drugs *do* require a prescription.

Focus Point

Ensuring Specificity of Orders

An order or prescription must clearly state the specific circumstances and conditions under which the drug may be given. Health-care providers must not accept conditions that are nonspecific (for example, "if needed," "if indicated," or "as warranted").

ORPHAN DRUG ACT OF 1983

Substantial evidence of both safety and effectiveness is required before a new drug can be marketed in the United States; this requirement causes the drug development process to be extremely expensive, lengthy, and difficult. Therefore, because drug companies are businesses trying to make money, they are more likely to invest the millions of dollars and years of research necessary to secure approval for drugs that would be used to treat millions of people with common diseases and disorders. This means that effective new drugs for rare diseases would likely go undeveloped. Recognizing this as a problem in drug research and development, the government passed the Orphan Drug Act of 1983, which offers federal financial incentives to nonprofit and commercial organizations to develop and market drugs to treat rare diseases that affect fewer than 200,000 people in the United States—that is, **orphan drugs**.

This act offers a 7-year patent exclusivity on drug sales and tax breaks to induce drug companies to undertake development and manufacturing of such drugs. Since going into effect, more than 100 orphan drugs have been approved, including those used to treat AIDS, cystic fibrosis, blepharospasm (uncontrolled, rapid blinking), and snake bites.

THE PRESCRIPTION DRUG MARKETING ACT OF 1987

This act prohibits the **reimportation** (importation of a drug into the United States that was originally manufactured here) of a drug by anyone but the manufacturer. It also deals with safety and competition issues raised by secondary drug markets and prohibits the trading or sale of drug samples, the distribution of samples except by mail or common carrier, and the distribution of samples to persons other than those licensed to prescribe them.

SAFE MEDICAL DEVICES ACT OF 1990

This act requires that medical device users report to manufacturers and the FDA occurrences in which a medical device has contributed to or caused the death or illness of, or serious injury to, a patient. The illness or injury must be life-threatening, or result in permanent impairment of body function or permanent damage to body structures. Medical devices may include dialyzers, electronic equipment, implants, monitors, restraints, syringes, catheters, in vitro diagnostic test kits and reagents, disposables, components, parts, accessories, related software, thermometers, ventilators, and other types of devices.

ANABOLIC STEROIDS CONTROL ACT OF 1990

Anabolic steroids are hormonal substances related to estrogen, progestins, testosterone, and corticosteroids, which promote muscle growth. Athletes sometimes use these agents to increase their physical performance. This act, which became effective in February 1991, placed anabolic steroids under the CSA's regulatory provisions. It is important because it reflects an essential change of direction for drug abuse control.

Focus Point

Ensuring Clarity of Orders

Health-care providers must ensure that orders and prescriptions clearly include in writing the drug's name, dosage, route, and frequency of administration. The order must be signed with clear notation of the prescribing physician's name.

OMNIBUS BUDGET RECONCILIATION ACT (OBRA) OF 1990

This act requires that pharmacists offer to counsel Medicaid and Medicare patients about drug information and potential adverse effects for all new and refilled prescriptions. OBRA '90 reduced state entitlements to reimbursement from the federal government and also requires states that seek such reimbursement to adopt programs directly affecting the pharmacy profession. Only costs for drugs approved as "safe and effective" are reimbursed with just a few exceptions. States must require pharmacists who provide services under this program to give consulting services. These pharmacists may discuss with their patients dosage form, dosage, route of administration, duration of drug therapy, name and description of medication, interactions with other drugs or food, therapeutic contraindications, common adverse effects, proper storage, self-monitoring of medication therapy, special directions for and precautions to be taken, and action in the event of a missed dose.

Focus on Geriatrics

Checklists for Elderly Patient Care

The Omnibus Budget Reconciliation Act was implemented by many nursing home–care facilities to establish a checklist for patients, including:

- Yearly reevaluation of health, memory, hobbies, habits, and the ability to walk, talk, comprehend, communicate, dress, and bathe
- Assistance in finding a doctor, if needed, plus the right to be informed about treatment programs, which can be refused if desired

✳ Apply Your Knowledge 2.2

The following questions focus on what you have just learned about orphan drugs and recent drug legislation. *See Appendix E for the correct answers.*

MULTIPLE CHOICE
Choose the correct answer from choices a–d.

1. Examples of orphan drugs include those used to treat:
   a. Cancer
   b. Shark bite
   c. Bronchospasms
   d. AIDS

2. Medical devices include:
   a. Ventilators
   b. Implants
   c. Both a and b
   d. None of the above

3. Anabolic steroids are:
   a. Hormonal substances

b. Vitamins

c. Minerals

d. Electrolytes

4. Under OBRA, pharmacists may discuss which of the following with Medicare or Medicaid patients?

a. Drug interactions

b. Hobbies

c. Bathing

d. Memory

5. Which act prohibits the reimportation of a drug into the United States?

a. Orphan Drug Act of 1983

b. Safe Medical Devices Act of 1990

c. Prescription Drug Marketing Act of 1987

d. Omnibus Budget Reconciliation Act of 1990

FILL IN THE BLANK

Select terms from your reading to fill in the blanks. Some terms may be used more than once.

1. Drug abuse control legislation enacted by the _____ provided the first guidelines for determining the classifications of drugs subject to abuse.

2. _____ are defined as drugs produced by a minor modification in the chemical structure of an existing drug, resulting in a new substance with similar pharmacologic effects.

3. _____ is another name scientists use for designer drugs.

4. The act that was designed to provide increased research into and prevention of drug abuse and drug dependence, provide for the treatment and rehabilitation of drug abusers and drug-dependent persons, and improve the administration and regulation of the manufacture, distribution, and dispensing of controlled substances by legitimate handlers of these drugs is the _____

5. Drugs in Schedule _____ have the highest potential for abuse and addiction, and those in Schedule _____ have the least potential.

6. Schedule _____ drugs also have a high potential for abuse, but they are currently accepted for medical use in the United States.

7. Schedule _____ drugs have the potential to cause only low to moderate physical dependence if abused.

8. Paregoric is now restricted to prescription sales only and is included in Schedule _____.

9. The Orphan Drug Act offers a 7-year _____ on drug sales and tax breaks to induce drug companies to undertake development and manufacturing of such drugs.

10. The distribution of samples except by mail or common carrier is prohibited by the _____.

Focus Point

Maintaining Reasonable Standards of Care

The law requires all health-care professionals to maintain reasonable standards regarding medication management duties, always mindful of the patient's care.

OCCUPATIONAL SAFETY AND HEALTH ACT OF 1970 (REVISED IN 1992)

This act, originally signed in 1970 by President Richard M. Nixon, is administered by the Occupational Safety and Health Administration (OSHA), which is part of the Department of Labor. In the late 1980s, the medical industry became involved with OSHA-related publicity, surrounding the threat of human immunodeficiency virus (HIV) infection as it extended to health-care workers. OSHA's mission is to ensure workplace safety and a healthy workplace environment. The HIV-AIDS crisis provoked improvements in protection of health-care workers who cared for patients with the disease. Prior to HIV-AIDS, OSHA had been focusing more directly on viral hepatitis and other pathogens as they affected medical staff members. In July of 1992, OSHA's Final Ruling on Bloodborne Pathogens became fully effective. Medical facilities must now comply with the Bloodborne Pathogens Standard and be able to prove their compliance to OSHA inspectors (Figure 2-3 ■). Common OSHA violations include missing or improper labeling of hazardous chemicals, lack of eyewash facilities; inadequate documentation of annual and initial employee training, lack of proof of destruction of hazardous waste, deficient records of the required Written Exposure Control Plan and Emergency Action Plan, missing records of hepatitis B vaccinations on declaration forms, inadequate annual hazard assessment, and neglected posting of OSHA Form 300A during the required time period.

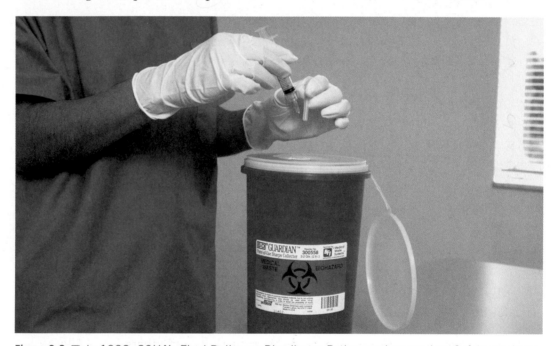

Figure 2-3 ■ In 1992, OSHA's Final Ruling on Bloodborne Pathogens became law. Safety measures such as sharps containers for the disposal of needles and syringes were implemented to stem the spread of HIV-AIDS and other bloodborne diseases.

The first specialty area in the pharmacy profession, for which a special regulation at the state level has been established, is the area of **nuclear pharmacy** (a specialty area of pharmacy dealing with radioactive materials for nuclear studies). In nuclear medicine, exposure to chemotherapy requires safety procedures and special precautions. Most regulations make it unlawful for any persons to provide nuclear pharmaceutical services unless they are under a qualified nuclear pharmacist's supervision.

THE HEALTH INSURANCE PORTABILITY AND ACCOUNTABILITY ACT (HIPAA) OF 1996

This act, known as HIPAA, was signed into law in August of 1996 by President Bill Clinton, amending the Internal Revenue Service Code of 1986 (also known as the Kassebaum–Kennedy Act). Each of its four administrative simplification parts has generated various standards and rules, with different compliance deadlines from 2000 to 2005. The four parts are as follows:

1. Electronic Health Transaction Standards—Standard code sets must be adopted by health organizations and used in all health transactions. All parties to any transaction must use and accept the same coding systems, which describe diseases, injuries, and other health problems (as well as their symptoms, causes, and actions taken). The goal is to reduce mistakes, duplication, and costs.

2. Unique Identifiers—HIPAA aims to reduce multiple identification numbers when organizations deal with each other, to reduce confusion, errors, and costs.

3. Security and Electronic Signature Standards—Physical storage and maintenance, transmission, and individual health information access standards were improved by this section, governing all individual health information that is maintained or transmitted (Figure 2-4 ■). The loophole is that this section applies only to transactions adopted under HIPAA.

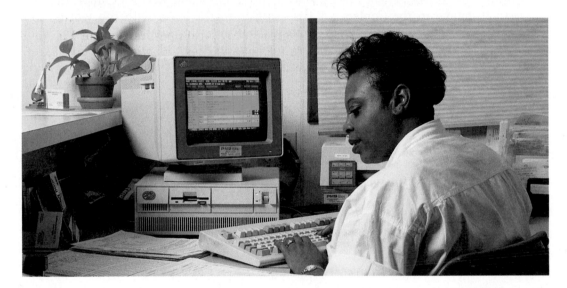

Figure 2-4 ■ Electronic transmission and storage of medical records is protected by HIPAA.

4. Privacy and Confidentiality Standards—This section limits nonconsensual use and release of private health information (now called *protected health information*). It gives patients new rights to access their medical records and to be informed of others who have accessed them. It also restricts most disclosure of health information to the minimum required for the intended purpose. This section also developed new civil and criminal sanctions for the improper use or disclosure of health information and new requirements for access to records by researchers and others.

Federal Regulatory Agencies

The FDA is responsible for cosmetics, medicines, medical devices, radiation-emitting products, food and drugs used for farm animals, domestic and imported food, bottled water, and wine beverages that contain less than 7% alcohol. The DEA oversees controlled substances, including the investigation and prosecution of those who grow or manufacture these substances for illegal distribution. The Centers for Disease Control and Prevention (CDC) oversees foods and foodborne diseases.

FOOD AND DRUG ADMINISTRATION

The FDA is a branch of the U.S. Department of Health and Human Services and controls all drugs for legal use. All drug administration laws are initiated, implemented, and enforced by the FDA.

DRUG ENFORCEMENT ADMINISTRATION

The DEA enforces controlled substance laws and regulations and prosecutes individuals (and organizations) who grow, manufacture, or distribute illegal substances. It also targets people who use violence in the coercion of others to help them in their illegal activities and distributes information about illegal substances to educate the public. The DEA also works with other governments to assist global drug trafficking enforcement.

CENTERS FOR DISEASE CONTROL AND PREVENTION

The CDC provides statistics and information to health professionals about the treatment of common and rare diseases worldwide. Its services include investigating, identifying, preventing, and controlling disease. The CDC's primary function is to issue infection control regulations. Established in 1946 as the Communicable Disease Center, the CDC changed its name to the Centers for Disease Control in 1970, with the words "and Prevention" added in 1992. Congress requested, however, that the initials "CDC" remain the same. This agency has been actively involved in the war against AIDS and HIV.

✱ Apply Your Knowledge 2.3

The following questions focus on what you have just learned about OSHA, HIPAA, and federal regulatory agencies. *See Appendix E for correct answers.*

FILL IN THE BLANK
Select terms from your reading to fill in the blanks. Some terms may be used more than once.

1. The division of the Department of Labor that ensures workplace safety and a healthy workplace environment is the

   _____.

2. Lack of labeling or improper labeling of hazardous chemicals, lack of eyewash facilities, and missing documentation of initial or annual employee training are examples of _____ violations.

3. Mistakes, effort duplication, costs, confusion, or errors are areas that _____ focuses on reducing.

4. Private health information is now called _____.

5. Aside from enforcing controlled substance laws and regulations, the _____ also targets people who use _____ in the _____ of others to help aid their illegal activities.

NAME THAT ACRONYM
Write out names of agencies whose acronyms are listed here.

1. OSHA _____
2. HIPAA _____
3. FDCA _____
4. FDA _____
5. CSA _____

6. DEA _____
7. OTC _____
8. AIDS _____
9. BNDD _____
10. OBRA _____

State Law

State governments, not the federal government, are the main regulators of laws that regulate pharmacy practice. Each state is concerned with protecting the health, safety, and welfare of its citizens. Pharmacy laws, while differing from state to state, are based on the same goals, objectives, and principles of pharmaceutical practice.

State law requires minimal qualifications for individuals involved with pharmacy practice—no one may practice pharmacy without a license except those exempted by the state legislation that creates the licensing requirement. Licensed individuals must successfully complete state board of pharmacy requirements. These boards are part of the licensing division of state health departments.

Pharmacy licensure is difficult to gain and not easily revoked. After due process, and for just cause as set out in the appropriate legislation, the state can suspend, revoke, or terminate a pharmacist's license. The practice of licensed pharmacists is safeguarded by federal and state constitutions as a property right. Certificates of registration are granted for one or two years in most states.

Health-care providers must use prescription pads only for writing prescriptions for medications. The prescription pad must be secured at all times. Some states allow medication administration by allied health professionals; other states do not. Therefore, health-care workers must know the laws of the state in which they work. It is also important to understand the rulings that apply to phoning in prescriptions to pharmacists.

Certificates of registration, or pharmacy licenses, can be canceled or revoked only under special circumstances. Depending on the type of state law violation, a pharmacist's license may be suspended or revoked permanently. An example is the dispensing of a scheduled drug without a prescription or proper documentation. The National Association of Boards of Pharmacy (NABP) developed a Model State Pharmacy Practice Act (MSPPA), which offers flexibility to the states that adopt it, but provides a greater degree of uniformity between states.

Ethics in Clinical and Pharmacy Practice

Ethics are standards of behavior and include concepts of right and wrong beyond what legal considerations are in any given situation. Health-care professionals are expected to act in ways that reflect society's ideas of right and wrong, even if such behavior is not enforced by law. Allied health professionals must use confidentiality in all areas concerning medications and their administration.

Although drug companies, by law, may provide free supplies of medications to physicians for promoting sales (Figure 2-5 ■), these samples may not be sold. A sample drug is marked "sample," bears a federal legend (Rx), and requires a prescription. Some manufacturers may also provide drug coupons that discount the price of a specific prescribed drug, but these coupons cannot be sold or traded. Samples should be stored immediately where they are not accessible to patients and organized by indication and expiration date. Health-care professionals may not legally supply medicine samples to family, friends, or themselves. Other ethical considerations cover pharmacists' or other health-care providers' professional relationships with their patients and dispensing of medications that may be against their personal beliefs.

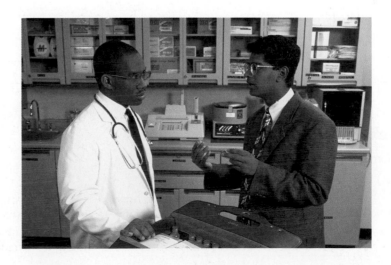

Figure 2-5 ■ Pharmaceutical company representatives provide drug samples to physician offices. These samples may not be sold.

✺ Apply Your Knowledge 2.4 ▬▬▬▬▬

The following questions focus on what you have just learned about state law and ethics in clinical and pharmacy practice. *See Appendix E for the correct answers.*

MATCHING

Match the lettered term to the numbered description.

DESCRIPTION

1. _____ Govern pharmacy practice
2. _____ Controlled by DEA
3. _____ Standards of behavior beyond a situation's legal considerations
4. _____ Must be used by allied health professionals in all areas that concern medications and their administration
5. _____ Drug samples bearing the federal "Rx" legend and requiring this
6. _____ Requiring prescription pads

TERM

a. Ethics
b. Confidentiality
c. Prescription
d. Medications
e. Substance laws and regulations
f. State

MULTIPLE CHOICE

Choose the correct answer from among choices a–d.

1. The medical industry became involved in the late 1980s with OSHA-related publicity surrounding the threat of:
   a. Latex gloves
   b. HIV infection
   c. Polio
   d. Hepatitis C

2. In July of 1992, OSHA's final ruling on this problem became fully effective:
   a. Bloodborne pathogens
   b. HIV
   c. Influenza
   d. Latex gloves

3. The first specialty area in the pharmacy profession, for which a special regulation at the state level has been established, is:
   a. HIV testing and drug prescribing
   b. Marketing and dispensing of samples
   c. Nuclear pharmacy
   d. Pharmacy technician training

4. Physical storage and maintenance, transmission, and individual health information access standards were improved by HIPAA's:
   a. Unique identifiers provision
   b. Electronic Health Transaction Standards
   c. Privacy and Confidentiality Standards
   d. Security and Electronic Signature Standards

5. All foods and foodborne diseases are overseen by the:
   a. CDC
   b. FDA
   c. DEA
   d. OSHA

Chapter Capsule

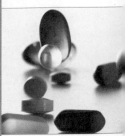

This section repeats the objectives from the beginning of the chapter and then provides a summary of the most important concepts for that objective. Use this section as a quick review and to check your knowledge.

Objective 1: Discuss legal and ethical requirements regarding the use, dispensing, and administration of medications.

- Federal regulations: protect consumers from potential for harm from both legal and illicit drugs
- FDA: controls all drug administration laws

Objective 2: Explain how the need for drug control evolved.

- Absence of laws requiring drug testing or drug labeling in the early nineteenth century
- Pure Food and Drug Act of 1906: developed to require safety and efficacy of drugs

Objective 3: Discuss the poisoning disaster that led to legislation requiring testing for the purity, strength, effectiveness, safety, and packaging quality of drugs.

- Sulfanilamide mixed with diethylene glycol, sold to the public in liquid form for upper respiratory infections: resulted in 107 reported deaths
- Food, Drug, and Cosmetic Act, created in 1938: gave the FDA authority to approve or deny new drug applications
- FDA: approves investigational use of drugs on humans; ensures safety and efficacy of all approved drugs

Objective 4: Explain the major points of the thalidomide disaster of 1962.

- Thalidomide (used in other countries), tested for marketing in the United States as a sleeping pill or antinausea medication for pregnant women
- Discovery of birth defects (severe deformities) in the children of many women of other countries who took thalidomide during their first trimester of pregnancy
- Kefauver–Harris Amendment passed in 1962: limited thalidomide use to treatment of leprosy, bone marrow transplantation, AIDS, and some other conditions

Objective 5: List the provisions of the Controlled Substances Act.

- Provides increased research into and prevention of drug abuse and drug dependence
- Provides treatment and rehabilitation of drug abusers and drug-dependent persons
- Regulates manufacture, distribution, and dispensing of controlled substances
- Applies schedules to drugs with potential for causing drug dependence, abuse, or both

Objective 6: Differentiate between each of the five schedules for controlled substances.

- Schedule I—High abuse potential; not accepted for medical use in the United States
- Schedule II—High abuse potential; accepted for medical use in the United States
- Schedule III—Low to moderate abuse potential; accepted for medical use in the United States
- Schedule IV—Slight abuse potential; accepted for medical use in the United States
- Schedule V—Lowest abuse potential of all; includes OTC preparations

Objective 7: Define *orphan drug* and list some examples.

- Used to treat diseases that affect fewer than 200,000 people in the United States
- Provides a 7-year monopoly on the sale and breaks on taxes given to manufacturers
- 100 orphan drugs approved, including those used to treat AIDS, cystic fibrosis, uncontrolled rapid blinking, and snake bites

Objective 8: Discuss the federal regulatory agencies that deal with food, drugs, and disease control.

- Food and Drug Administration (FDA): controls drugs for legal use
- Drug Enforcement Administration (DEA): enforces controlled substance laws, regulations, and more
- Centers for Disease Control and Prevention (CDC):

  ❑ Provides statistics and information about treatment of common and rare diseases worldwide

  ❑ Provides facilities and services for investigating, identifying, preventing, and controlling disease

  ❑ Issues infection control regulations

Objective 9: Explain which level of government primarily controls pharmacy licensure.

- States: main regulators of laws governing pharmacy practice
- Licensing required of practicing pharmacies except if exempted by state legislation that creates licensing requirements

Objective 10: Define *ethics* as it relates to pharmacology.

- Expectation of health-care professionals to act in ways that reflect society's ideas of right and wrong, even if such behavior is not enforced by law
- Guarantee of confidentiality in all areas that concern medications and their administration
- Security and proper use of prescription pads

Internet Sites of Interest

- The National Institutes of Health (NIH) Web site, **www.nlm.nih.gov/**, provides information on ethical considerations in research studies. Search for "ethics."
- The abuse of pain medications has led some health-care providers to limit the appropriate use of pain medications in patients who need them. See a discussion among government agents about this issue at: **www.usdoj.gov/dea/pubs/pressrel/pr102301.html**
- Read about laws enforced by the FDA at: **www.fda.gov/opacom/laws**
- Find information about the Orphan Drug Act at: **www.fda.gov/orphan/oda.htm**
- Access an overview of the FDA at: **www.emedicinehealth.com/fda_overview/article_em.htm**

Chapter Objectives

After completing this chapter, you should be able to:

1. Explain abbreviations used in pharmacology.
2. Describe how drugs are named.
3. Describe five sources of drug derivation.
4. Explain preparations of oral drugs.
5. Define solid drug forms.
6. Describe topical drugs.
7. Explain gaseous drugs.
8. List seven component parts of a prescription.
9. Define standing orders.

Chapter 3

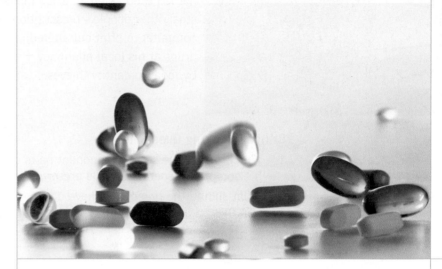

Terminology, Abbreviations, and Dispensing Prescriptions

Key Terms

Alkaloids (AL-kuh-loyds) (page 44)

Approved name (page 43)

Chemical name (page 43)

Generic name (page 43)

Glycoside (GLY-ko-side) (page 44)

Parenteral (puh-REN-teh-rul) (page 46)

Proprietary name (page 43)

Sustained release (page 46)

Trade name (page 43)

PRACTICAL SCENARIO

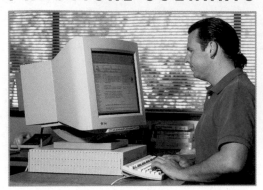

Pharmacy technicians, as well as pharmacists, must always be on guard when dispensing prescriptions for people seeking to defraud their pharmacy and illegally obtain medications. One such individual, a 25-year-old named Brad, used a device that scanned for wireless Internet signals to steal other people's prescription painkiller information. Then he used his computer to print out altered prescriptions and illegally obtain prescription drugs at his local pharmacy. Prescription drug information is highly prized by today's identity thieves.

Critical Thinking Questions

1. Which one of the seven component parts of a prescription could Brad not provide in his computer-generated bogus prescription?
2. What should the pharmacist have done if she had any suspicions about the prescription itself or suspected that the physician's signature was a forgery?

Introduction

Learning the language of medicine is essential for all fields of the health-care industry. Medical terminology originated primarily from Greek and Latin prefixes, roots, and suffixes, which are known as *word parts.* There are also new terms that are derived from the universal language of English. A majority of terms related to surgery and diagnosis have Greek origins, and most anatomic terms come from Latin origins. To learn medical terminology, it is very helpful to memorize word parts and rules for creating words. By understanding how word parts are combined, it is possible to determine the meaning of medical words.

Health-care professionals who are involved with pharmacology must be familiar with word building, common medical terms, and abbreviations. They must understand general pharmacology terms and concepts.

In this chapter, terminology and abbreviations, drug names, sources of drugs, drug forms, and drug dispensing will be reviewed in detail.

Pharmaceutical Terminology

Allied health-care professionals who must deal with pharmaceutical agents need to be familiar with medical and pharmaceutical terminology. They must understand roots, prefixes, suffixes, and combining vowels.

A *root* is the main part of a word that gives the word its central meaning. It is the basic foundation of a word that can be made more complex through the addition of other word parts. A *prefix* is a structure at the beginning of a word that modifies the meaning of the root; Table 3-1 ■ shows some common general prefixes. A *suffix* is a word ending that modifies the meaning of the root; Table 3-2 ■ gives some common general suffixes.

Medical terms are formed from many different word parts. These parts are often joined by vowels known as *combining vowels.* The most common combining vowel is the letter *o* and occasionally, the letter *i.* For example, *o* serves as a combining vowel in the term *hyperlipoproteinemia* (hyper / lip /*o*/ protein / emia).

Table 3-1 ■ **Some Common General Prefixes**

PREFIX	MEANING	EXAMPLE
alb-	white	albinism
ante-	before	antepartum
anti-	against	antibiotic
bi-	two, both	bilateral
bio-	life	biology
ecto-	outside	ectoplasm
endo-	into, within	endoscopic
epi-	upon, above	epidermic
multi-	many	multinuclear
myo-	muscle	myocarditis
poly-	many	polyarthritis
semi-	half	semiconscious
ultra-	beyond, excessive	ultrasound

Table 3-2 ■ **Some Common General Suffixes**

SUFFIX	MEANING	EXAMPLE
-ectomy	excision, removal	hysterectomy
-emesis	vomit	hyperemesis
-gram	record	electrocardiogram
-ism	condition	cryptorchidism
-itis	inflammation	appendicitis
-logy	study of	microbiology
-oma	tumor	carcinoma
-pathy	disease	hemopathy
-phobia	abnormal fear	photophobia
-scope	instrument used to view	oscilloscope
-stomy	surgical creation of a new opening	colostomy
-tomy	incision, cutting	phlebotomy

✳ Apply Your Knowledge 3.1

The following questions focus on what you have just learned about pharmaceutical terminology. *See Appendix E for the correct answers.*

FILL IN THE BLANK
Select terms from your reading to fill in the blanks.

1. A root is the main part of a word that gives the word its _____ _____.

2. The most common combining vowel is _____.

3. A prefix is a structure at the _____ of a word that modifies the meaning of the _____.

4. The combining vowel in the term *hyperlipoproteinemia* is the letter _____.

5. A suffix is a word ending that modifies the meaning of the _____.

MATCHING
Match the lettered meaning to the numbered word part.

WORD PART	MEANING
1. _____ -pathy	a. Study of
2. _____ -itis	b. Half
3. _____ -semi	c. Disease
4. _____ -logy	d. Inflammation
5. _____ anti-	e. Life
6. _____ bio-	f. Against

Abbreviations Used in Pharmacology

Abbreviations are shortened forms of words representing commonly used medical terms. Many such abbreviations are used in all areas of health-care practice. It is essential for health-care professionals to be familiar with the most common abbreviations used for writing prescriptions (Table 3-3 ■), and the abbreviations associated with various measurements (Table 3-4 ■), as well as general medical abbreviations (Table 3-5 ■).

Table 3-3 ■ Abbreviations Commonly Used in Prescriptions

ABBREVIATION	MEANING	ABBREVIATION	MEANING
ā ā, aa	of each	bin	twice a night
ac	before meals	c̄ (with straight line)	with
ad	to, up to	cap, caps	capsule
ad lib	as desired	comp	compound
a.m., AM	morning	d	day
amt	amount	dil	dilute
aq	water	disp	dispense
bid, BID	twice a day	elix	elixir

Table 3-3 ■ Abbreviations Commonly Used in Prescriptions

ABBREVIATION	MEANING	ABBREVIATION	MEANING
hr	hour	qid, QID	four times a day
IM	intramuscular	q2h	every 2 hours
inj, INJ	inject	QN	every night
IV	intravenous	qs, qv	as much as you wish (sufficient quantity)
liq	liquid	s̄ (with straight line)	without (sine)
mixt	mixture	SIG	write on label
noct	at night	sol	solution
non rep	do not repeat, no refills	sp	spirits
NPO	nothing by mouth (*nulla per os*)	sos	if necessary
oint	ointment	stat	immediately
pc	after meals	supp	suppository
per	through or by	syr	syrup
p.m., PM	afternoon	top	topically
po, PO	by mouth	tab	tablet
PR	through the rectum	tid	three times a day
prn, PRN	as needed	tr., tinct	tincture
PULV	powder	vo	verbal order
q	every	×	times
qh	every hour		

Note: See Internet Sites of Interest at the end of this chapter for the Institute for Safe Medical Practices (ISMP) Web site, which provides a list of medical abbreviations that are frequently misinterpreted and involved in harmful errors and thus should not be used.

Table 3-4 ■ Abbreviations Commonly Used for Measurements

ABBREVIATION	MEANING	ABBREVIATION	MEANING
°C	celsius	mEq	milliequivalent
cm	centimeter (2.5 cm = 1 in)	mg	milligram
°F	Fahrenheit	mL	milliliter
fl	fluid	No.	number
g, gm	gram	oz	ounce
gtt	drops	T	temperature
lb	pound	Tbs, Tbsp	tablespoon
kg	kilogram (1 kg = 2.2 lb)	tsp	teaspoon
L	liter	w/v	weight in volume
mcg	microgram		

Table 3-5 ■ General Medical Abbreviations

ABBREVIATION	MEANING	ABBREVIATION	MEANING	ABBREVIATION	MEANING
AP	anterior–posterior	EENT	eyes, ears, nose, throat	N	nitrogen
BE	barium enema	ECG	electrocardiogram	Na	sodium
BP	blood pressure	FBS	fasting blood sugar	OB	obstetrics
Bx	biopsy	Fe	iron	P	pulse
C	carbon	FUO	fever of unknown origin	PERRLA	pupils equal, round, reactive to light and accommodation
Ca	calcium, cancer	GI	gastrointestinal		
CAD	coronary artery disease	GU	genitourinary	PO	orally
		Gyn	gynecology	Pt	patient
C&S	culture and sensitivity	H	hydrogen	R	respirations, right
cath.	catheter	H&P	history and physical	r	take
CBC	complete blood count	Hgb	hemoglobin	RBC	red blood cell
CC	chief complaint	HBV	hepatitis B virus	R/O	rule out
CHF	congestive heart failure	HCT	hematocrit	ROM	range of motion
c/o	complains of	Hg	mercury	SOB	shortness of breath
CO	carbon dioxide	Hib	*Haemophilus influenzae* type B	T	temperature
COPD	chronic obstructive pulmonary disease	Hx, hx	history	TIA	transient ischemic attack
CVA	cerebral vascular accident	I	iodine	Tx	treatment
CXR	chest x-ray	IM	intramuscular	UA	urinalysis
D&C	dilatation & curettage	IUD	intrauterine device	UTI	urinary tract infection
		IV	intravenous	VS, vs	vital signs
DOB	date of birth	K	potassium	WBC	white blood cell
DPT	diphtheria-pertussis-tetanus	LMP	last menstrual period	WNL	within normal limits
		MI	myocardial infarction	wt	weight
Dx	diagnosis	MMR	measles-mumps-rubella	y/o, yo	years old
EEG	electroencephalogram				

✳ Apply Your Knowledge 3.2

The following questions focus on what you have just learned about abbreviations used in pharmacology. *See Appendix E for the correct answers.*

MULTIPLE CHOICE

Choose the correct answer from choices a–d.

1. The abbreviation for *water* is:
   a. dil
   b. mist
   c. aq
   d. ac

2. The abbreviation *qh* means:

   a. Every hour

   b. Every other day

   c. Every night

   d. As needed

3. The abbreviation *sos* means:

   a. Immediately

   b. Suppository

   c. If needed

   d. As much as you wish

4. The abbreviation *ad lib* means:

   a. Through or by

   b. As desired

   c. As much as you wish

   d. As needed

5. The abbreviation *pc* means

   a. Before meals

   b. After meals

   c. By mouth

   d. Powder

FILL IN THE BLANK

Select terms from your reading to fill in the blanks.

1. The abbreviation for *nothing by mouth* is _____ and for *treatment is* _____.

2. Write the meanings of *SIG;* ×; stat, qid: _____, _____, _____, and _____.

3. The abbreviation of *powder* is _____.

4. The abbreviation *bid* means _____.

5. The abbreviation *mcg* means _____.

Drug Names

Each drug may have three different types of names: the **chemical name** (describing the chemical makeup of a drug), the generic name (also called **approved name** or *nonproprietary name*), and the **proprietary name** (also called *brand* or **trade name**). For example, the chemical name of amoxicillin, a commonly prescribed antibacterial antibiotic, is hydroxybenzyl-penicillin. Its **generic name** (also known as a drug's *official* or *approved name*) is amoxicillin, a name much simpler than its chemical name. All drugs have a generic name, which is not protected by copyright. Amoxicillin is marketed under dozens of proprietary names, including Alphamox, Amohexal, and Amoxil. This proprietary name is assigned by the manufacturer and is protected by copyright. Because there is only one generic name per drug, the use of a drug's generic name is encouraged over trade names to avoid confusion. Drugs are also classified by their therapeutic use. For example, Tylenol is the brand name of the generic drug acetaminophen, which is classified as an analgesic and an antipyretic agent.

Sources of Drug Derivation

There are basically five sources of drugs: (1) plants, (2) animals (including humans), (3) minerals or mineral products, (4) synthetics (chemical substances), and (5) engineered (investigational) sources. Today, chemicals and even human tissues such as those used in stem-cell therapy can be manipulated to create new drug sources.

PLANTS

Plant sources are grouped by their physical and chemical properties. **Alkaloids** are organic nitrogen-containing compounds that are alkaline and usually bitter tasting. They are combined with acids to make a salt. Atropine sulfate, nicotine, and morphine sulfate are examples of these chemical compounds. An important cardiac **glycoside** (an organic compound that yields sugar and nonsugar substances when hydrolyzed) is digoxin. Digoxin is made from digitalis, a derivative of the foxglove plant.

HUMANS AND OTHER ANIMALS

Animal sources, such as the body fluids and glands of animals, can act as drugs. The drugs obtained from animal sources include hormones such as adrenaline, insulin, and thyroid hormones. Enzymes such as pancreatin and pepsin are also from animal sources.

MINERALS

Minerals from the Earth and soil are used to provide inorganic materials unavailable from plants and animals. They are used as they occur in nature. Examples include sodium, iodine, potassium, iron, and gold, which are used to prepare medications. Sodium chloride (table salt) is one of the best known examples in this group. Gold is prescribed to prevent severe rheumatoid arthritis, and coal tar is used to treat seborrheic dermatitis and psoriasis.

SYNTHETIC SOURCES

Certain drugs may come from living organisms (organic substances) or nonliving materials (inorganic substances). These drugs are known as synthetic or manufactured drugs. They have evolved from the application of chemistry, biology, and computer technology. Because they do not exist in nature, these medications come from artificial substances. Examples of synthetic drugs include oral contraceptives, meperidine (Demerol), and sulfonamides. Certain organic drugs such as penicillin are semisynthetic and are made by altering their natural compounds or elements. Some drugs are both organic and inorganic, such as propylthiouracil, which is an antithyroid hormone.

ENGINEERED SOURCES

The newest area of drug origin is gene splicing, or *genetic engineering*. The newer forms of insulin for use in humans have been produced with this technique. Tissue plasminogen activator for heart attack victims is also being developed via this method. Growth hormones (bovine or porcine somatotropin) are being produced from bacteria that has received the appropriate gene (human, cow, or pig). Another new and experimental treatment is gene therapy, which involves replacing a gene that is missing or not functioning correctly with a correct gene. The first successful gene therapy was used in 1990 to treat an immune system defect in children. Genetically engineered products, featuring modified DNA, are being produced to treat malignant brain tumors, cystic fibrosis, and HIV. The public seems to be greatly interested in this new way of developing a wide range of new drugs.

✳ Apply Your Knowledge 3.3

The following questions focus on what you have just learned about drug names and sources of drug derivation. *See Appendix E for the correct answers.*

FILL IN THE BLANK

Select terms from your reading to fill in the blanks.

1. Name five sources of drugs: _____, _____, _____, _____, and _____.

2. The proprietary name of a drug is also called the _____ or _____ name.

3. The drugs obtained from human or animal sources include _____ and _____.

4. The official name of a drug is also called the _____ name.

5. Alkaloids are organic nitrogen-containing compounds that are alkaline and usually have a _____ taste.

MULTIPLE CHOICE

Choose the correct answer from choices a–d.

1. Which of the following drugs is an important cardiac glycoside?
   a. Morphine sulfate
   b. Nicotine
   c. Digoxin
   d. Atropine sulfate

2. Coal tar is an example of a mineral drug that is used for:
   a. Rheumatoid arthritis
   b. Rheumatic fever
   c. Peptic ulcer
   d. Psoriasis

3. Which of the following is an example of synthetic sources of drugs?
   a. Progesterone
   b. Insulin
   c. Oral contraceptives
   d. Gold preparations

4. The first successful gene therapy was used in 1990 to treat which of the following systems of the body (in children)?
   a. Reproductive
   b. Immune
   c. Digestive
   d. Respiratory

5. A proprietary name is also known as a(n):
   a. Trade name
   b. Generic name
   c. Approved name
   d. Chemical name

Drug Forms

Pharmaceutics is the science of formulating drugs into different types of preparations such as tablets, ointments, injectable solutions, or eye drops. It also includes studying the ways in which various drug forms influence pharmacokinetic and pharmacodynamic activities of the active drug.

Many drugs are available in different formulations. This variety assists the prescriber in choosing a formulation that is best suited for the individual patient and route of administration. Formulations, such as oral pills and tablets, injectable medications, or rectally or vaginally administered drugs, also determine whether a drug acts locally or is absorbed into the systemic circulation. Failure to administer the drug in the correct form results in a medication error. Using an incorrect form can also cause damage to body cells. Therefore, allied health-care professionals need to learn about the various drug preparations and their uses. Drug dosage forms are classified according to their physical state (for example, liquid or solid) and chemical composition. Various forms of drug preparations allow for oral, topical, mucous membrane, or **parenteral** use (introduction of a drug outside of the gastrointestinal [GI] tract; generally in injectable form), and for miscellaneous drug delivery systems.

Some substances can undergo a change of state or phase, from solid to liquid (melting) or from liquid to gas (vaporization). Certain drugs are soluble in water, some are soluble in alcohol, and others are soluble in a mixture of liquids.

PREPARATIONS FOR ORAL USE

An oral drug may appear in solid form (for example, tablets, capsules, or powders) or liquid forms (solutions, elixirs, or suspensions). Disintegration of the solid dose form must occur before *dissolution,* a process by which a drug goes into solution and becomes available for absorption. The form of drug dose is important because the more rapid the rate of dissolution, the more readily the compound crosses the cell membrane and is absorbed into the systemic circulation to be circulated to the site where it acts. Oral drugs in liquid form are therefore more rapidly available for GI absorption than those in solid form.

Solid Drugs

The route for administering a medication depends on its form, its properties, and the effect desired. Solid forms of drugs are widely used in drug treatment. The solid forms are also a convenient way to take unpleasant-tasting or irritating drugs. Solid drugs include pills, tablets, capsules, **sustained-release** tablets and capsules (that are specially coated so that they dissolve at specific times), enteric-coated tablets and capsules, caplets, gelcaps, powders, granules, and troches or lozenges (Figure 3-1 ■). Some plasters are also considered to be solid drugs, although they generally are semisolids.

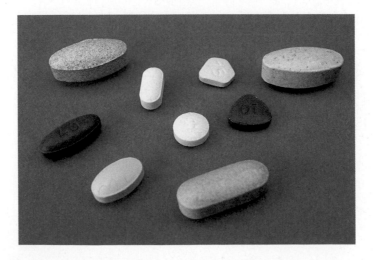

Figure 3-1 ■ Solid drug forms.

PILLS

A single-dose unit of medicine made by mixing the powdered drug with a liquid such as syrup and rolling it into a round or oval shape is called a *pill*.

TABLETS

A *tablet* is a pharmaceutical preparation made by compressing the powdered form of a drug and bulk-filling material under high pressure (Figure 3-2 ■). Tablets may appear as simple white disks or may be multilayered or coated with a film to mask an unpleasant taste. Special forms of tablets include sublingual tablets and enteric-coated tablets. Most tablets are intended to be swallowed whole for dissolution and absorption from the GI tract. Some are intended to be dissolved in the mouth, dissolved in water, or inserted as suppositories. Many times tablets are mistakenly called pills. Tablets come in various sizes, shapes, colors, and compositions. The various forms of tablets include chewable, sublingual, buccal, enteric-coated, and buffered tablets. Chewable tablets contain a flavored or sugar base and must be chewed. They are commonly used for antacids and antiflatulents and for children who cannot swallow medication. Sublingual tablets must be dissolved under the tongue for rapid absorption; an example is nitroglycerin for angina pectoris. Buccal tablets are placed between the cheek and the gum until they are dissolved and absorbed.

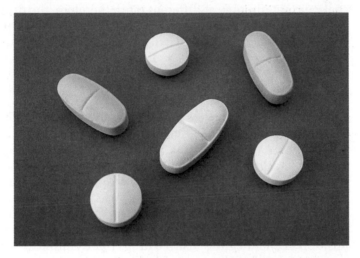

Figure 3-2 ■ Examples of tablets.

CAPSULES

A *capsule* is a medication dosage form in which the drug is contained in an external shell (Figure 3-3 ■). Capsule shells are usually made of hard cylindrical gelatin and enclose or encapsulate powder, granules, liquids, or some combinations of these. Liquids may be placed in soft gelatin capsules; examples are vitamin E capsules and cod liver oil capsules. They are used when medications have an unpleasant odor or taste.

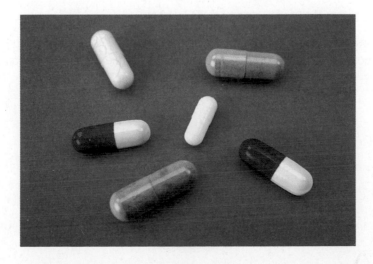

Figure 3-3 ■ Examples of capsules.

Focus on Geriatrics

Coated Aspirin Tablets

Some patients, particularly elderly people who have stomach ulcers, cannot take certain medications, such as aspirin. Therefore, these patients should be given enteric-coated aspirin tablets.

Capsules can be pulled apart, and the entire contents can be added as powder to food for individuals who have difficulty swallowing. Some forms of capsules come with a controlled-release dosage and are used over a defined period of time (sustained-release [SR] or timed-release capsules). These drugs should *never* be crushed or dissolved because this would negate their timed-release action.

SUSTAINED-RELEASE TABLETS AND CAPSULES

Sustained-release drug forms contain several doses of a drug. The doses have special coatings that dissolve at different rates; therefore, the drug is released into the digestive system gradually. Sustained-release drugs are referred to as *delayed release* and *timed release*. An example is diltiazem (Cardizem SR), a calcium channel blocker used in the treatment of angina pectoris and hypertension.

ENTERIC-COATED TABLETS AND CAPSULES

Some tablets and capsules are covered by a special coating that keeps them from dissolving in the stomach, which contains hydrochloric acid. These drugs do not dissolve until they reach the intestine. Therefore, the strength of these drugs remains undiluted as they pass through the stomach, providing a delayed action that is desirable. An example is Ecotrin, a nonnarcotic analgesic used for pain, an antipyretic used for fever, and a nonsteroidal anti-inflammatory used in the treatment of arthritis. Also important is the fact that enteric coatings may prevent nausea and vomiting that some drugs can induce from dissolving in the stomach. Furthermore, enteric coatings prevent decomposition of chemically sensitive drugs (for example, penicillin G and erythromycin) by gastric secretions. These two drugs are examples of substances that are unstable in the acid pH of the stomach.

Focus Point

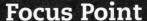

Administering Enteric-coated Tablets

Do not crush or mix enteric-coated tablets or capsules into liquids or foods because it will destroy the enteric coating. This would result in the drug being released into the stomach instead of the small intestine.

CAPLETS

A caplet is shaped like a capsule but has the form of a tablet. The shape and film-coated covering make swallowing easier.

GELCAPS

A *gelcap* is an oil-based medication that is enclosed in a soft gelatin capsule (see Figure 3-4 ■).

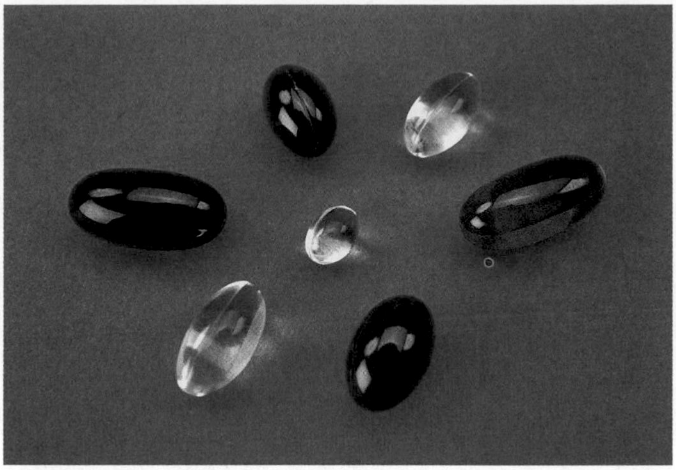

Figure 3-4 ■ Examples of gelcaps.

POWDERS

A drug that is dried and ground into fine particles is called a *powder*. An example is potassium chloride powder (Kato powder).

GRANULES

A small pill, usually accompanied by many others encased within a gelatin capsule, is called a *granule*. In most cases, granules within capsules are specially coated to gradually release medication over an extended period.

TROCHES OR LOZENGES

A hard or semisolid dosage form containing a medication intended for local application in the mouth or throat is called a *troche* or *lozenge*. These are flattened disks. Typically, a troche is placed on the tongue or between the cheek and gum and left in place until it dissolves. The medications most commonly administered by means of troches include cough suppressants and treatments for sore throat.

Liquid Drugs

Liquid preparations include drugs that have been dissolved or suspended. Examples of liquid drugs are syrups, solutions, elixirs, fluidextracts, mixtures and suspensions, tinctures, emulsions, spirits or essences, liniments, gels or jellies, lotions, most aerosols, and magmas.

Focus on Pediatrics

Liquid Drugs

Infants and young children are not able to take solid drug forms such as tablets or capsules. Therefore, they should be given liquid drugs.

SYRUPS AND LINCTUSES

Aqueous solutions containing high concentration of sugars, syrups, and linctuses may or may not have medical substances added (for example, simple syrup and ipecac syrup).

SOLUTIONS

A *solution* is a drug or drugs dissolved in an appropriate solvent. Examples of solutions include elixirs, fluidextracts, spirits, and tinctures, which are highly concentrated forms of drugs.

Elixirs

A drug vehicle that consists of water, alcohol, and sugar is known as an *elixir*. It may or may not be aromatic and may or may not have active medical properties. Their alcohol content makes elixirs convenient liquid dosage forms for many drugs that are only slightly soluble in water. In these cases, the drug is first dissolved in alcohol, and the other elixir components are added. All elixirs contain alcohol (for example, terpin hydrate elixir and phenobarbital elixir). Elixirs differ from tinctures in that they are sweetened. They should be used with caution in patients with diabetes or a history of alcohol abuse. Some pediatric medications retain the name of *elixirs,* although they no longer contain alcohol.

Fluidextracts

A concentrated solution of a drug removed from a plant source by mixing ground parts of the plant with a suitable solvent, usually alcohol, and then separating the plant residue from the solvent is called a *fluidextract.* Typically, 1 mL contains 1 g of the drug. Fluidextracts are not intended to be administered directly to a patient. Instead, they are prescribed to provide a source of drug in the manufacture of final dosage forms. Only vegetable drugs are used (for example, glycyrrhiza fluidextract).

Mixtures and Suspensions

In a *mixture* or a *suspension,* an agent is mixed with a liquid but not dissolved. These preparations must be shaken before being taken by or administered to the patient. Examples include chlorpheniramine/pseudoephedrine (mixture) and betamethasone (suspension).

Tinctures

A *tincture* is an alcoholic preparation of a soluble drug, usually from a plant source. In some cases, the solution may also contain water (for example, digitalis tincture and iodine tincture).

Focus Point

Storing Drugs That Contain Alcohol

Elixirs, spirits, tinctures, and fluidextracts contain alcohol. They must be kept tightly sealed so that the alcohol cannot evaporate. Store them in a dark place as specified on the labels.

EMULSIONS

A pharmaceutical preparation in which two agents that cannot ordinarily be combined or mixed is called an *emulsion.* In the typical emulsion, oil is dispersed inside water. Most creams and lotions are emulsions (for example, Petrogalar Plain).

SPIRITS OR ESSENCES

An alcohol-containing liquid that may be used pharmaceutically as a solvent is called a *spirit* or *essence* (for example, essence of peppermint and camphor spirit).

LINIMENTS

Liniments are liquid suspensions for external application to the skin to relieve pain and swelling.

GELS OR JELLIES

A *gel* is a jellylike, semisolid substance in a nonfatty base that may be used for topical application and contains fine particles. An example is the antacid Altern Gel.

LOTIONS

Lotions are suspensions of drugs in a water base for external use. They are patted onto the skin rather than rubbed in. Lotions tend to settle in their containers and so must be shaken before use. An example is calamine lotion, an antipruritic (anti-itch medication) used to treat exposure to poison ivy.

AEROSOLS

Aerosol medications are frequently delivered by oral inhalers or nebulizers that allow for rapid absorption into the blood circulation. An example is albuterol (Proventil), a bronchodilator used in asthma. Aerosols are generally classified as liquid drugs because they often contain a mist. Those that contain dry powders are considered to be semisolid drugs.

MAGMAS

Magmas contain particles suspended in a liquid, and exhibit a more pasty quality in their consistency than other suspensions. The most popular example of a magma is probably Milk of Magnesia.

INJECTABLE DRUGS

When a rapid response time to medication is desired, or if the patient is not able to take the medication orally, parenteral forms of medication can be selected. Injectable drug forms may be available as powders or solutions. A *powder* consists of dry particles of medications. Because the powder itself cannot be injected, it must be reconstituted to a liquid for injection. A diluent, such as sterile water, is added to the powder and then mixed well. A *solution*, as previously explained, is a mixture of one or more substances that are dissolved in another substance. Most solutions are fluids that form a homogeneous mixture. There are a variety of administration routes for parenteral medications including intra-articular, epidural (into the subarachnoid space), intradermal, subcutaneous, intramuscular (IM), and intravenous (IV).

OTHER FORMS OF MEDICATIONS

There are also other forms of drugs including topical, ophthalmic, otic, nasal, vaginal, and rectal, and drugs that are available in the form of gases.

Topical Drugs

Drugs that are applied to the skin are known as *topical* drugs. They usually provide a local effect. Topical medications include transdermal patches, lotions, ointments, and liniments. Some topical drugs are used to deaden nerves, control itching, or relieve pain and congestion in muscles and joints.

Semisolid Drugs

Semisolid drugs are often used for topical application. These drugs are soft and pliable. Semisolid drugs include creams, ointments, most plasters, and dry-powder aerosols.

CREAMS

A *cream* is a semisolid preparation that is usually white and contains a drug incorporated into both an aqueous and an oily base. Creams may be applied externally or intravaginally. Examples include benzoyl peroxide (Clearasil, to treat acne topically) and terconazole (Terazol, to treat vulvovaginal candidiasis).

OINTMENTS

An *ointment* is a semisolid preparation in an aqueous or oily base for local protective, soothing, astringent, or transdermal application for systemic effects. Ointments can also be used as anti-inflammatory drugs, topical anesthetics, and antibiotics. Examples are zinc oxide ointment and Ben-Gay® ointment.

PLASTERS

A *plaster* is a composition of liquid and powder that hardens when dry. Plasters may be solid but are generally semisolid drugs (for example, salicylic acid plaster used to remove corns).

Transdermal Patches

For a constant, time-released systemic effect, some medications can be absorbed slowly through the skin. Transdermal patches release a very small amount of a drug at a consistent rate, which is absorbed into the skin and then carried off by the capillary blood supply. Examples of drugs used transdermally include nicotine, estrogen, and nitroglycerin.

Gaseous Drugs (Inhalation Drugs)

Pharmaceutical gases include anesthetic agents such as nitrous oxide and halothane. Compressed gases comprise oxygen or carbon dioxide. Most of the oxygen administered in hospitals for therapy is provided from a central source where it is stored as a gas or liquid oxygen. Inhalation medications such as bronchodilators can be administered through metered-dose inhalers (MDIs) or handheld nebulizers (HHNs). Inhalation medications will be discussed in Chapter 25.

Ophthalmic, Otic, and Nasal Drugs

Ophthalmic drugs include drops and ointments that are instilled into the eye for a local effect. They must be sterile and isotonic so that they do not cause infections or burning. Ophthalmic medications may be antibiotic, anesthetic, antiviral, decongestants, or formulations that provide artificial tears. For the ears, otic medications can control localized infections or inflammation, and require very low dosages to be effective. Nasal solutions can treat minor congestion or infection and act locally. They may be in the form of drops or sprays (Figure 3-5 A-C ■).

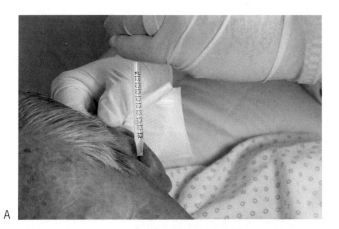

A

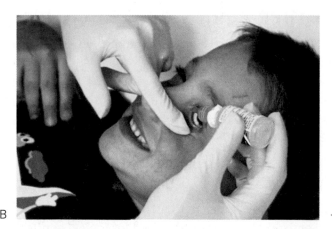

B

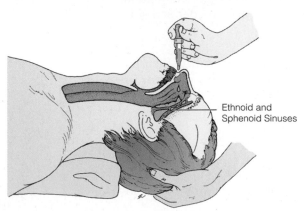

Ethnoid and Sphenoid Sinuses

C

Figure 3-5 ■ Examples of (A) otic, (B) ophthalmic, and (C) nasal drops.

Vaginal Drugs

Vaginal drugs come in a variety of forms including solutions, creams, tablets, and suppositories. Commonly used vaginal drugs include anti-infectives and contraceptives.

Rectal Drugs

Rectal medications are used for patients with nausea or vomiting, constipation, or for those who may be unconscious and, therefore, unable to take drugs by mouth. Rectal medications usually are available as cocoa butter or gelatin-based suppositories, or as enemas. Most rectal drugs offer systemic effects.

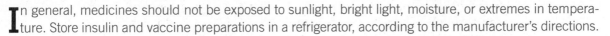

Focus Point

Safe Storage of Drugs

In general, medicines should not be exposed to sunlight, bright light, moisture, or extremes in temperature. Store insulin and vaccine preparations in a refrigerator, according to the manufacturer's directions.

 Apply Your Knowledge 3.4

The following questions focus on what you have just learned about drug forms. *See Appendix E for the correct answers.*

MATCHING
Match the lettered term to the numbered description.

DESCRIPTION

1. _____ A hard or semisolid dosage form containing a medication intended for local application

2. _____ An aqueous solution containing a high concentration of sugars

3. _____ An oil-based medication that is enclosed in a soft specific capsule

4. _____ A small pill, usually accompanied by many others, encased within a gelatin capsule

5. _____ A composition of a liquid and a powder that hardens when it dries

TERM

a. Plaster

b. Gelcap

c. Granule

d. Troche

e. Linctus

MULTIPLE CHOICE
Choose the correct answer from choices a–d.

1. Chewable tablets are commonly used for which of the following compounds?
   a. Antibiotics
   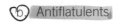 b. Antiflatulents
   c. Antianginals
   d. Antidiarrheals

2. Which of the following is an example of soft gelatin capsules?
    a. Vitamin E
   b. Vitamin C
   c. Vitamin B_{12}
   d. Niacin

(continued)

Apply Your Knowledge 3.4 (continued)

3. A hard or semisolid dosage form containing a drug intended for local application in the mouth is called a(n):

 a. Gelcap

 b. Granule

 c. Lozenge

 d. Enteric-coated tablet

4. Which of the following compound drugs is an example of a plaster?

 a. Zinc oxide to cure wounds

 b. Vitamin A to help vision

 c. Ben-Gay® to relieve pain

 d. Salicylic acid to remove corns

5. A tincture is a soluble drug that contains:

 a. Finer particles

 b. Alcohol

 c. Oil

 d. Magnesium

Dispensing Drugs

There are two methods of dispensing drugs: (1) over the counter (OTC) and (2) by prescription. OTC drugs are available to the public for self-medication without a prescription.

An allied health-care professional who is directly involved in patient care should have an understanding of some basic facts regarding OTC drugs. Today, patients are better informed about their personal health care and want to be active participants in health-care decisions. They need facts to make informed choices when using OTC preparations. Most OTC preparations are safe if used as directed on their packages.

Prescription drugs are issued by a licensed prescriber (medical practitioner, dentist, or veterinary surgeon). In some states, nurse practitioners and even pharmacists can write prescriptions with certain restrictions. According to legal terminology, prescription drugs are those that federal law lists as dangerous, powerful, or habit-forming, and illegal to use except under a prescriber's order. A *prescription* is an order written by an authorized health-care professional for the compounding or dispensing and administration of drugs to a particular patient. A prescription must be signed by a physician or the order cannot be carried out. These drugs have the legend "Caution: Federal Law prohibits dispensing without a prescription" printed on the label. Sometimes, a prescription can be sent by a fax machine, electronically from a physician's computer, or by telephone to the pharmacist. Controlled substances and Schedule I to V drugs were discussed in Chapter 2.

COMPONENTS OF PRESCRIPTIONS

A prescription must be clear, concise, and correct. It has elements that can be correlated with five of the seven nursing rights of medication administration (see Chapter 4 for all seven rights): the patient's name and address (right patient), date written, generic or proprietary drug name (right drug), drug strength and dosage (right dose), route of administration (right route), dosage instruction or frequency of administration (right time), and signature, name, and address of the prescriber (Figure 3-6 ■). Therefore, the component parts of a prescription include:

✻ Name and address of the patient

✻ Address of the prescriber's office

✳ Date

✳ Medication prescribed (*inscription*)

✳ Rx symbol (*superscription*)

✳ Dispensing directions to pharmacist (*subscription*)

✳ Directions for the patient (*signa*)

✳ Refill and special labeling

✳ The prescriber's signature and license or Drug Enforcement Administration (DEA) number

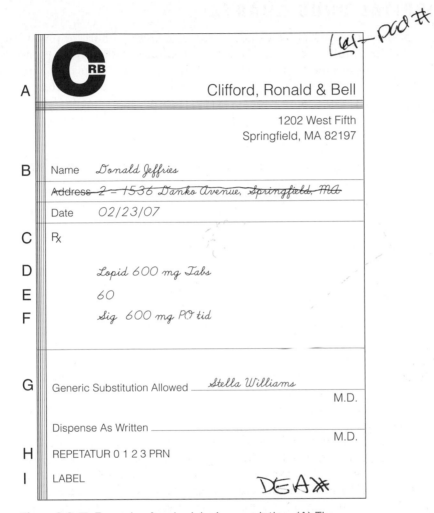

Figure 3-6 ■ Example of a physician's prescription. (A) The health-care provider's name, address, phone number, and registration number; (B) the patient's information and date of prescription; (C) the superscription (Rx); (D) the inscription (names and quantities of ingredients); (E) the subscription (tells pharmacist how to fill the prescription); (F) the signature (Sig) that tells the patient how to use the medication; (G) signature blanks (where physician signs); (H) the repetatur (tells how many refills); and (I) the label (tells pharmacist how to label the medication).

TELEPHONE ORDERS AND STANDING ORDERS

Medications are also sometimes prescribed by physicians who are not present or will not be present when the medication is administered. For example, a physician may telephone a drug prescription (called *telephone orders*) to a pharmacist, who is legally entitled to dispense the prescription, or to a nurse, who is entitled to administer it on oral instructions. In some states, medical assistants are allowed to do this as well. The physician must then, as soon as is practicable, write out the drug order on a prescription pad, sign it, and post or deliver it to the pharmacy, or use the hospital drug chart (see next section of this chapter). A faxed prescription copy can confirm an oral order, but is not legally acceptable because the signature has to be original (that is, in the physician's handwriting); the pharmacist must see the original prescription before releasing the drug to the patient. *Standing orders* are written orders sometimes left by physicians as ongoing prescriptions in a hospital, nursing home, or residential-care setting. These orders have no legal validity unless properly written, dated, and signed, just as is true for any normal prescription.

HOSPITAL DRUG CHARTS

Prescriptions in hospitals are usually written on a drug chart, or physician order sheet, and transcribed onto a medication administration record (MAR; Figure 3-7 ■). These can become quite complicated and may run to many pages in a patient's medical record because patients in hospitals are frequently prescribed 10 to 15 drugs during one stay. In the sample chart, note that the users are instructed:

✳ To use approved names for drugs

✳ Not to alter existing orders

✳ To record all instances when drugs are administered, or when drugs were not administered, giving reasons

✳ To record IV fluid orders on a separate IV orders chart

✳ To have nurse-initiated therapy (for example, mild analgesics, laxatives, antacids) countersigned by a physician

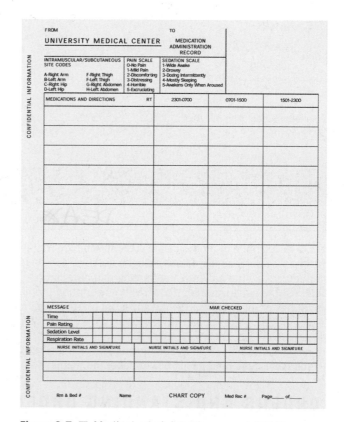

Figure 3-7 ■ Medical administration record (MAR) as used in many hospitals.

Today, the majority of hospitals in the United States (and those in some other countries) are using computer charting.

✳ Apply Your Knowledge 3.5

The following questions focus on what you have just learned about dispensing drugs. *See Appendix E for the correct answers.*

FILL IN THE BLANK
Select terms from your reading to fill in the blanks.

1. OTC drugs are available to the public for self-medication without a _____.
2. "Standing orders" have no legal validity unless they are _____ _____, _____, and _____.
3. Prescriptions in hospitals are usually written on a _____ _____.
4. In the sample chart of patients in the hospital, IV fluid orders are to be recorded on a _____ _____ _____ _____.
5. A prescription must be signed by the _____, or the order cannot be carried out.

MATCHING
Match the lettered term with its numbered description.

DESCRIPTION	TERM
1. _____ Medication prescribed	a. Subscription
2. _____ Rx symbol	b. Signa
3. _____ Legend drug	c. Inscription
4. _____ Dispensing directions to pharmacist	d. Superscription
5. _____ Directions for patient	e. A prescription drug

Chapter Capsule

This section repeats the objectives from the beginning of the chapter and then provides a summary of the most important concepts for that objective. Use this section as a quick review and to check your knowledge.

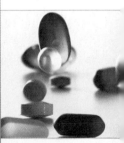

Objective 1: Explain abbreviations used in pharmacology.

- Abbreviations—shortened forms of words representing commonly used medical terms; terms used for writing prescriptions; and terms associated with various measurements
- Use of medical abbreviations by health-care professionals—patients' charts, prescriptions, standing orders, preparation of drugs, drug labels, and dosage instructions

Objective 2: Describe how drugs are named.

- Chemical name—describes the chemical makeup of a drug
- Generic (official, approved, or nonproprietary) name—simpler than the chemical name; not protected by copyright
- Proprietary (brand or trade) name—assigned by manufacturer; protected by copyright

Objective 3: Describe five sources of drug derivation.

- Plants
- Animals (including humans)
- Minerals or mineral products
- Synthetics
- Engineered (investigational) sources

Objective 4: Explain preparations of oral drugs.

- Solid forms—tablets, capsules, powders; disintegration of the solid-dose form must occur before dissolution, a process by which a drug goes into a solution and becomes available for absorption
- Liquid forms—solutions, elixirs, suspensions; more rapidly available for GI absorption than those in solid form

Objective 5: Define solid drug forms.

- Pills—powdered drugs mixed with liquids and rolled into a round or oval shape
- Tablets—powdered drugs compressed with bulk-filling materials under high pressure
- Capsules—drugs contained in an external shell
- Sustained-release tablets and capsules—containing several doses of a drug with special coatings that dissolve at different rates, thereby releasing the drug gradually
- Enteric-coated tablets and capsules—covered by a special coating that keeps the drugs from dissolving in the stomach. These drugs do not dissolve until they reach the intestines.
- Caplets—drugs shaped like capsules but in the form of tablets, with film coatings
- Gelcaps—oil-based medications enclosed in soft gelatin capsules
- Powders—drugs that are dried and ground into fine particles
- Granules—small pills accompanied by many others, encased within gelatin capsules
- Troches or lozenges—flattened disks placed on the tongue or between the cheek and gum, and left in place until they dissolve

Objective 6: Describe topical drugs.

- Semisolid—soft and pliable, and often used for topical applications
- Creams—semisolid preparations that are usually white and contain a drug incorporated into both an aqueous and oily base
- Ointments—semisolid preparations in an aqueous or oily base for local protective, soothing, astringent, or transdermal application for systemic effects
- Plasters—compositions of liquid and powder that harden when dry; may be solid or semisolid
- Transdermal patches—used for a constant, time-released systemic effect as their medications are absorbed slowly through the skin

Objective 7: Explain gaseous drugs.

- Pharmaceutical gases—include anesthetic gases such as nitrous oxide and halothane
- Compressed gases—include therapeutic oxygen or carbon dioxide
- Inhalation medications such as bronchodilators—can be administered through metered-dose inhalers (MDIs) or handheld nebulizers (HHNs)

Objective 8: List seven component parts of a prescription.

- The patient's name and address
- Date written
- Generic or proprietary drug name
- Drug strength and dosage
- Route of administration
- Dosage instruction or frequency of administration
- Signature, name, and address of the prescriber

Objective 9: Define standing orders.

- Orders given by physicians who may not be present at a later time when the medication is needed, or ongoing prescriptions for patients in a hospital, nursing home, or residential-care setting; valid only when written, signed, and dated by the physician or other health-care provider with prescribing authority

Internet Sites of Interest

- Visit the University of California at San Francisco's Drug Product Services Laboratory at: **www.ucsf.edu/dpsl/** and click on Intravenous, Intraspinal, Other Parenteral, Chemotherapy, Oral, Topical, or Rectal to find more information on types of drugs and their routes of administration.
- Information on the parts of a prescription is offered at: **www.mapharm.com/prescr_parts.htm**
- The Institute for Safe Medical Practices provides a list of medical abbreviations, symbols, and dosage designations that are frequently misinterpreted and involved in harmful errors along with their approved substitutions at: **www.ismp.org/Tools/errorproneabbreviations.pdf**
- Search for any medical abbreviation or term at: **www.pharma-lexicon.com**

Chapter 4

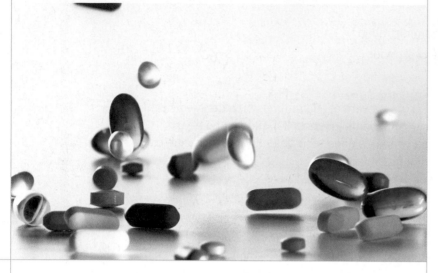

Administration
of Medications

Chapter Objectives

After completing this chapter, you should be able to:

1. Summarize patient assessment factors that have an impact on medication administration.
2. Identify the *seven rights* of drug administration.
3. Discuss some causes of medication errors.
4. Explain the universal policy to be observed if a medication error is detected.
5. Summarize the guidelines for reducing medication errors.
6. List and describe the various routes of medication administration.
7. Identify equipment and supplies required for parenteral administration of medications.
8. Define terms related to needles used in the parenteral administration of medications.
9. Identify sites used for intradermal, subcutaneous, and intramuscular injections.
10. Explain how to administer an intradermal, a subcutaneous, or an intramuscular injection.

Key Terms

Aseptic (a-SEP-tik) (page 70)
Bevel (page 72)
Cannula (KAN-yoo-luh) (page 72)
Gastrostomy tube (gah-STRAW-sto-mee) (page 68)

Gauge (page 72)
Hub (page 72)
Hypodermic (hi-po-DER-mik) (page 71)
Invasive (page 70)

Nasogastric (NG) tube (nay-zoh-GAS-trik) (page 68)
Stat (page 62)
Wheal (page 73)

PRACTICAL SCENARIO

A physician wrote a prescription for ".5 mg IV morphine for postoperative pain" for a 9-month-old infant. The unit secretary recorded the order in the medication administration record (MAR) as "5 mg." An inexperienced nurse followed the directions on the MAR without question and gave the baby 5 mg of IV morphine initially, and another 5-mg dose 2 hours later. About 4 hours after the second dose, the baby stopped breathing and suffered cardiac arrest. If the physician had written "0.5 mg," the unit secretary would probably not have had any misunderstanding of the intended amount, and the nurse would have administered the correct dosage.

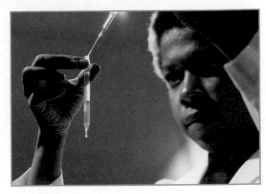

Critical Thinking Questions

1. Although the initial error was not the nurse's, what steps should he or she have taken to avoid this medication error?

2. What measures could the facility implement to curtail future medication errors?

3. Explain how using a standardized written measurement system would have prevented this adverse drug event.

Introduction

It is important to remember that medications have the potential to cause serious harm to the patient. Therefore, the process of dispensing and administering medication orders must always be treated with great care. When you are involved in medication administration, you must be constantly vigilant to prevent errors and deliver quality patient care.

No matter what types of medications are to be administered, the order must come from the physician. If the physician delegates drug administration to the medical assistant, it must be allowable under state laws. Every state has a *medical practice act* that defines whether a medical assistant or other caregiver (besides a nurse) can administer drugs under the supervision of a physician. Some states permit medical assistants to administer only certain types of medications; some prohibit medical assistants from giving injections. To ensure patient safety in drug administration, there are certain procedures that health-care professionals must perform every time a medication is ordered. These procedures are discussed in this chapter.

Principles of Drug Administration

The health-care professionals who may be administering medications should always assess a patient's health status and obtain a medication history prior to giving any medication. The extent of the assessment depends on the patient's illness or current condition, the intended drug, and the route of administration. For example, if a patient has dyspnea, the nurse or medical assistant must assess respirations carefully before administering any medication that might affect breathing. It is important to determine whether the route of administration is suitable. For example, a patient who is nauseated may not be able to tolerate a drug taken orally. In general, the health-care professional assesses the patient prior to administering any medication to obtain baseline data for evaluating the effectiveness of the medication.

The medication history includes information about the drugs the patient is taking currently or has taken recently. This includes prescription drugs; OTC drugs such as antacids, alcohol, and tobacco; and illegal drugs such as marijuana. Sometimes an incompatibility with one or more of these drugs affects the choice of a new medication.

Many patients, especially older adults, often take vitamins, herbs, and food supplements or use folk remedies that they do not list in their medication history. Because many of these have unknown or unpredictable actions and side effects, the health-care professional should always ask about their use and note it in the patient history, with close attention paid to possible incompatibilities with other prescribed medications.

Any problems the patient may have in self-administering a medication must also be identified. A patient with poor eyesight, for example, may require special labels for the medication container; elderly patients with unsteady hands may not be able to hold syringes or inject themselves or another person. Obtaining information about how and where the patient stores medications is also important. If the patient has difficulty opening certain containers, he or she may change containers but leave the old labels on, which increases the risk of medication errors.

Socioeconomic factors need to be considered for all patients, but especially for elderly people. Two common problems are lack of transportation to obtain medications and inadequate finances to purchase medications. If the health-care professional is aware of these problems, proper resources can be obtained for the patient.

THE SEVEN RIGHTS OF DRUG ADMINISTRATION

Safeguarding the patient during drug administration involves using the seven rights of proper drug administration. (The first five rights were introduced in Chapter 3). Two more have been added since the original five were created:

1. **The *right* patient** The easiest way to make sure the drug is being given to the right patient is to ask the patient his or her name, or call the patient by name before administering the medication. You cannot assume that the person to whom you are administering a medication is the correct person without verifying his or her name in this manner. Patients can be confused or anxious and may not hear what you say. Therefore, check the patient's chart.

    Always check for allergies before administering medications. Ask the patient directly, because recent allergic reactions might not be listed in the record. You should explain the medication's name, dosage, desired action, potential effects, and any precautions that need to be taken.

2. **The *right* drug** Determining the right drug begins with clarifying the physician's order, if needed. Each time a drug is dispensed, the medication label must be checked three times during its preparation to confirm the right drug, right dose, and right strength. Compare the physician's written order with the label. The first check is done when the medication is taken from the storage area. The second is performed just before removing the medication from its container. The third check is performed when the medication is returned to the storage area or just before administration.

    Also check the expiration date to ensure that the medication is still effective. If it is expired, dispose of it appropriately. It is appropriate to flush outdated medication into the sewer line. For controlled substances, you must ask someone to witness and document the disposal, referred to as "wasting the medication."

3. **The *right* dose** If the dose ordered does not match the dose available, perform appropriate dosage calculations to determine the accurate dose (see Chapter 5). Remember to have a colleague check your calculations if you doubt the dose accuracy. Many facilities require health-care workers who set up insulin or heparin doses to check them with a coworker. Once you have calculated the amount to be administered, measure it out carefully. Medication errors are significantly reduced by using unit-dose systems because the medications are already in the correct dose.

4. **The *right* route** Check the physician's order to clarify the route of administration for the medication—whether it is oral, topical, or parenteral. Many drugs can be given by a variety of routes. Because the route of administration can affect the medication's absorption, it is important that the drug is given by the correct route. If you are not sure what route is intended, confirm it with the physician.

5. **The *right* time** In the ambulatory care setting, most medications are ordered **stat** (see Chapter 3). However, it is important to check the physician's order to clarify the appropriate time for medications to be administered. Some medications must be

taken on an empty stomach (30 minutes before or 2 hours after a meal), whereas others should be taken with food.

6. **The *right* technique** A health-care professional must be familiar with the proper techniques for all routes of administration. If there are any doubts about the ability to administer a particular drug, always ask for help.

7. **The *right* documentation** Immediately after giving the drug to the patient, document the date and time of administration; the drug's name, strength, dose, and route of administration; any patient reactions to the medication; and details of patient education regarding the drug. If the patient requests a prescription refill, document all pertinent information on the patient chart. The medical record is the legal document recording both the order for the medication and its administration. If the medication ordered was not given, or the patient refused it, the reason must be included in the record. If the patient refuses to take medication you have prepared, do not return it to its original container. Dispose of it, and notify the physician.

✳ Apply Your Knowledge 4.1

The following questions focus on what you have just learned about the seven rights of drug administration. *See Appendix E for the correct answers.*

FILL IN THE BLANK
Select terms from your reading to fill in the blanks.

1. To avoid medication errors, every time a medication is dispensed, check the label _____ times to confirm the right drug and the right _____.

2. Because of the importance of administering medications quickly in the ambulatory care setting, most medications are ordered _____.

3. Immediately after giving the medication to the patient, document the _____ and _____ of administration because the medical record is a legal document recording both the medication's order and its administration.

4. If the patient calls in for a prescription refill, document all _____ _____ on the patient chart to ensure that the medical record is complete and accurate.

5. Patient assessment includes determining whether this is an appropriate _____ for the particular patient.

MULTIPLE CHOICE
Choose the correct answer from choices a–d.

1. In some states, which of the following members of the allied health profession may administer certain medications by injection to patients?
   a. Pharmacy technicians
   b. Surgical technicians
   c. Radiology technicians
   d. Medical assistants

2. How many times should a drug label be checked when medication is dispensed?
   a. 2
   b. 3
   c. 4
   d. 5

(continued)

Apply Your Knowledge 4.1 (continued)

3. Medication errors are significantly reduced by which of the following factors?

   a. The unit-dose system

   b. The knowledge and level of the person administering the drug

   c. The health-care system

   d. The patient's trust

4. In the ambulatory care setting, most medications are ordered:

   a. According to the wishes of the nurse

   b. According to the wishes of the patient

   c. As needed

   d. Stat

5. Which of the following is the most important consideration that should always be checked before administering medications?

   a. Blood pressure

   b. Urine sugar

   c. Allergies

   d. Age of patient

Medication Errors

A *medication error* is the inappropriate or incorrect administration of a drug that should be preventable through effective system controls involving physicians, pharmacists, nurses, risk-management personnel, legal counsel, administrators, and patients. Medication errors can occur because of manufacturing mistakes. Thousands of medication errors occur each year in hospitals throughout the United States. These errors often result in pain, injury, and even death. Major research studies published by the Committee on Quality of Health Care in America reported at least 44,000 deaths and 1.3 million injuries every year as a result of medication errors.

Medication errors usually occur more frequently than they are reported and are the result of either human error or a flawed system within a health-care facility. Errors can occur in three stages within the medication process:

1. The first stage involves prescribing or ordering medication. During this stage, physicians or other persons prescribing the medication may be distracted or interrupted, and as a result, provide incomplete orders—greatly increasing the risk of errors. Medication errors are most prevalent when choosing a medication, its dosage, and the schedule.

2. The second stage is when the medication is dispensed to patients or consumers. Dispensing errors can occur as a result of insufficient or inexperienced staffing and lack of adequate time for patient counseling, and can lead to confusion about how to take the medication or how to assist the patient in taking it. It is an extremely important and effective practice for all health-care professionals to double-check medications against the MAR. This practice helps those who are dispensing the medication to catch errors before medications are dispensed.

3. The third stage is when the medication is administered and monitored for side effects. At this stage, medication administration errors are most commonly attributed to nurses or others who are legally allowed to handle administration. Those who administer medications may be accountable for medication errors that can be attributed to poor communication or misread prescriptions, orders, or drug labels. Other factors

that contribute to errors include similar labeling and packaging of products and medications with similar names (see Appendix C for a list of medications with similar sounding names). After administering medication, health-care professionals must also ensure that the patient does not have a reaction to the medication.

The most common error is dosage; errors also often involve antibiotics and analgesics. For example, a community pharmacist misreads a handwritten prescription for 10 mg of Metadate ER and instead dispenses 10 mg of methadone for a 7-year-old boy. Fortunately, the boy's mother reads the information that accompanies the prescription and realizes the error.

A medication error may occur when dealing with outpatients because of the increasing number of prescriptions in the United States and because pharmacists do not adequately counsel patients. In addition, there is a shortage of pharmacists and pharmacy technicians, which contributes to medication errors. Increased usage of OTC drugs and herbals and the availability of drugs through the Internet also cause medication errors.

A medication error must be reported as soon as it is noticed, and the patient must be monitored to see if any undesirable effect or injury from the medication develops. Medication errors must be documented in the medical record with the signature of the individual who made the error. If allied health professionals who are involved with prescribing, dispensing, or administering medication follow the seven rights of medication administration and adhere to dispensing guidelines, medication errors should not occur.

WHY MEDICATION ERRORS OCCUR

A number of factors cause medication errors, including:

* Use of incorrect abbreviations: Many abbreviations mistaken for different units and different dosages
* Miscommunication: Poor handwriting, similar drug names, dosing unit confusion
* Missing information: Lack of patient information such as allergies, diseases, drug history, laboratory information, and drug information or warnings
* Lack of appropriate labeling: By the manufacturer or the pharmacist
* Environmental factors: Noise, lighting, stress, and fatigue affecting health-care providers
* Poor management: Unhealthy health-care facility culture

Medication errors may occur in inpatient settings such as hospitals and nursing homes or in outpatient settings such as physicians' offices or clinics. They can also happen during the manufacturing process and include errors in formulation, packaging, labeling, and distribution. They may be the result of undiscovered toxicity. Medication errors are preventable and the single largest source of all medical errors.

Medication errors may occur as a result of the following:

* Wrong patient
* Incorrect route
* Incorrect drug
* Incorrect dose
* Incorrect time
* Incorrect technique
* Incorrect information on the patient chart

MANUFACTURING ERRORS

The sulfanilamide disaster of 1937 (see Chapter 2) serves as an example of *formulation* or manufacturing errors. Mislabeling, contamination, wrong drug, wrong concentration, or wrong doses of drugs are other causes of manufacturing errors. Counterfeit drugs and other distribution problems may be involved in medication errors.

Administering Medications

Nurses or medical assistants must be extremely knowledgeable when administering medications in the physician's office. Follow all physician orders exactly as written. If unsure about an order, ask for clarification before proceeding. Administer a medication only after the order is written in the patient's chart. This helps eliminate errors and possible omissions in medication therapy. Always implement the *seven rights* and perform three drug order and label checks when dispensing and administering medications.

REDUCING MEDICATION ERRORS

Medication errors may relate to professional practice, health-care products, procedures, and systems. The following statements are guidelines for communication, education, and policy to assist in decreasing the rate of medication errors. To reduce medication errors, general recommendations include:

✳ Employing an adequate number of allied health staff (nurses, medical assistants, and pharmacy technicians) who are trained to prepare, dispense, and administer medications to patients

✳ Using standardized measurement systems for both inpatients and outpatients

✳ Using prospective error-tracking systems that are run on a consistent basis to target and monitor common patient errors

✳ Clearly defining a system for drug administration, ordering, and dispensing that includes review of original drug orders

✳ Compiling medication profiles for inpatients, outpatients, and ambulatory patients with updated allergy histories in each encounter

✳ Providing suitable work environments for safe, effective drug preparation

Physiologic Changes Impact Medication Effects

The physiologic changes associated with aging include altered memory, less acute vision, decreased renal function, less complete and slower absorption from the GI tract, and decreased liver function. These changes can increase the possibility of cumulative, and possibly toxic, effects of medications.

SAFETY IN DRUG ADMINISTRATION

Every time a medication is ordered, certain procedures must be performed to ensure patient safety. The physician's order must be completely understood and clearly read; any questions about the medication, dose, route of administration, and its strength must be answered by the physician. When questions arise, the drug should be looked up in a pharmacology reference book (such as a drug handbook) to review its possible side effects, precautions, purpose, and recommended dose. Only after all of these steps are taken should the drug be dispensed and administered.

✳ Apply Your Knowledge 4.2

The following questions focus on what you have just learned about medication errors. *See Appendix E for the correct answers.*

FILL IN THE BLANK
Select terms from your reading to fill in the blanks.

1. The sulfanilamide disaster of 1937 is an example of _____ or _____ errors.

2. In America, at least 44,000 deaths occur every year as a result of _____ errors.

3. The most common medication error is _____ of the drug.

4. Medication errors must be documented in the medical record with the _____ of the individual who made the error.

5. The three stages within the medication process during which errors can occur are:

   a. The _____ or _____ of medication

   b. When medication is _____ to patients

   c. When medication is _____ and _____ for side effects

MATCHING
Match the lettered term to the numbered description.

DESCRIPTION

1. _____ One way in which a physician can cause a medication error

2. _____ One way in which a manufacturer or pharmacist can cause a medication error

3. _____ What health-care professionals should double-check medications against

4. _____ A factor that can cause a health-care professional to make a medication error

5. _____ What nurses and other health-care professionals must do after administering medications

TERM

a. Medication administration record (MAR)

b. Monitor for any undesirable effects

c. Use of incorrect abbreviations

d. Lack of complete information on a patient's chart

e. Lack of appropriate labeling

Routes of Drug Administration

Medications may be delivered to the body by different methods. The method of administration depends on the purpose of the medication. Medication may be administered in a variety of ways, but some must be given in specific and limited ways to be effective. Each route has its advantages and disadvantages. Drugs are administered either *enterally* (for absorption through the GI tract) or *parenterally* (by injection) to produce systemic effects. If medications are placed in direct contact with the skin or mucous membranes to be absorbed for a local effect, this is called *percutaneous administration*. When choosing the route and technique of medication administration, the most reliable method of delivery ensures expected results.

ENTERAL ROUTES

The enteral route is the route of drug administration through the GI tract. This method of administration of drugs is safe and convenient for most patients and is relatively economical. Administration of medication through the GI tract may be by the oral, nasogastric or gastrostomy tube, sublingual, or buccal routes.

Oral Route

The oral route is the most common route. It is the easiest and most economical way for a patient to take medication. As long as a patient can swallow and retain the drug in the stomach, this is the route of choice. Medications given by the oral route are absorbed from the stomach and small intestine, traveling first to the liver, where they may be metabolized before they ever reach their target tissues or organs. This process, called *first-pass metabolism*, is discussed in Chapter 1.

Oral medications are contraindicated when a patient is vomiting, has gastric or intestinal suction, or is unconscious and unable to swallow. Generally, oral medications should be taken with enough water to ensure that the drug reaches the stomach. Liquid medications are ideal for children. Solid drugs should not be given to children until they are old enough to safely swallow them without the danger of aspiration.

Focus on Geriatrics

Medications May Stain Teeth and Dentures

Advise elderly patients who have dentures to remove them before taking certain medications. Some oral liquid drugs, such as liquid iron or iodides, may stain the teeth.

Nasogastric and Gastrostomy Routes

For patients who cannot take anything by mouth and have a nasogastric or gastrostomy tube in place, an alternative route for administering medications is through the tube. A **nasogastric (NG) tube** is inserted by way of the nasopharynx (the part of the pharynx that lies above the soft palate and opens into the nasal cavity) and is placed into the patient's stomach for the purpose of feeding the patient or removing gastric secretions. A **gastrostomy tube** is surgically placed directly into the patient's stomach and provides another route for administering medications and nutrition.

Sublingual Route

Medications given via the sublingual route (also known as *percutaneous route*) are held under the tongue until completely dissolved (Figure 4-1 ■). This method is used when rapid action is desired because the mucosa of the oral cavity contains a very rich blood supply, offering fast absorption of certain drugs. Medications administered via the sublingual route are not destroyed by digestive enzymes, and they do not undergo first-pass metabolism in the liver. Examples of medications that can be administered by the sublingual route include nitroglycerin (Nitrostat, Nitrobid) for angina pectoris and ergotamine tartrate (Ergostat) for migraines.

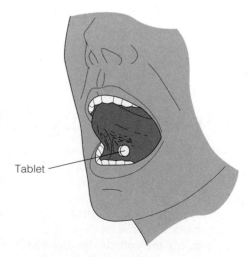

Tablet

Figure 4-1 ■ Medication given via the sublingual route.

Buccal Route

For administration of drugs via the buccal route (a type of percutaneous route), the medication is placed between the gum and cheek and left there until it dissolves (Figure 4-2 ■). Buccal medications are available in the form of tablets, capsules, lozenges, and troches. These medications should not be swallowed. They are absorbed more slowly from the buccal mucosa than the sublingual area. The buccal route is preferred over the sublingual route for sustained-release delivery because of its greater mucosal surface area.

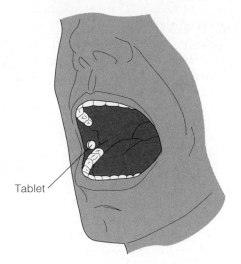

Tablet

Figure 4-2 ■ Administration of drugs via the buccal route.

Focus Point

Buccal and Sublingual Medications

Patients should not drink or eat anything when buccal or sublingual medications are administered until the medication has dissolved completely.

✷ Apply Your Knowledge 4.3

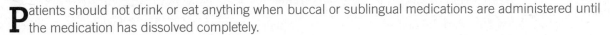

The following questions focus on what you have just learned about enteral routes of drug administration. *See Appendix E for the correct answers.*

MULTIPLE CHOICE
Select the correct answer from choices a–d.

1. Which of the following methods of medication administration is safest?
    a. Intravenous
    b. Intradermal
    c. Intramuscular
    (d) Enteral

2. Which of the following is the most common route by which medications are given?
    a. Oral route
    b. Rectal route
    c. Vaginal route
    d. Intramuscular route

3. The nasogastric tube is inserted through which of the following?
    a. Stomach
    b. Mouth
    c. Nasopharynx
    d. By incision into the trachea

(*continued*)

Apply Your Knowledge 4.3 (continued)

4. Which of the following methods is used when rapid action is desired?

   a. Subcutaneous route

   b. Nasogastric tube

   c. Stomach tube

   d. Sublingual route

5. Which of the following should not be swallowed?

   a. Buccal tablets

   b. Oral liquids

   c. Capsules

   d. Suspensions

MATCHING

Match the lettered term to the numbered description.

DESCRIPTION	TERM
1. _____ Placed between the gum and the cheek	a. Sublingual route
2. _____ The safer route of drug administration for most patients	b. Gastrostomy
	c. Oral route
3. _____ Removal of gastric secretions	d. Nasogastric tube
4. _____ Used for nitroglycerin and ergotamine tartrate	e. Buccal route
5. _____ Placed into the patient's stomach by surgery	

PARENTERAL ROUTES

Parenteral administration, as noted in Chapter 3, refers to the injection of a drug into the body with a needle and syringe. Parenteral administration of medications is a common procedure in medical offices, hospitals, ambulatory centers, home care centers, and other facilities by certain medical workers. Parenteral medications may be given via intradermal, subcutaneous, intramuscular (IM), or intravenous (IV) routes. The intravenous route may be more dangerous than the others because of the possibility of injecting a drug incorrectly into a vein, which may cause serious harm or even death. Because these medications are absorbed more quickly than oral medications and are irretrievable once injected, the allied health worker must prepare and administer them carefully and accurately. The parenteral route is used especially in emergencies when a drug effect is needed immediately. Administering parenteral drugs requires an **invasive** procedure (one that requires insertion of an instrument or device through the skin or a body orifice), and **aseptic** technique must be used (hand washing and other techniques to minimize the risk of infection).

Equipment

Syringes, needles, ampules, and vials are used to administer parenteral medications. Ampules and vials contain medications; syringes and needles are used to withdraw the medication and then administer it to the patients.

SYRINGES

Three parts make up a standard syringe: the barrel (the outside part), which has printed scales used to measure medication amounts; the plunger, which fits inside the barrel; and the tip, which connects with the needle (Figure 4-3 ■). The outside of the barrel and the handle of the plunger may be touched, but no unsterile object should ever come into contact with the tip or inside of the barrel, the plunger's shaft, and the needle's shaft or tip.

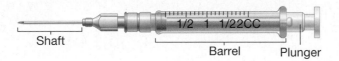

Figure 4-3 ■ The parts of a standard syringe: barrel, plunger, and shaft.

The three most common types of syringes are as follows:

Hypodermic (meaning subcutaneous or under the skin) syringes (available in sizes between 2 mL and 3 mL)—marked in either milliliters or minims

Insulin syringes (available in various sizes)—marked in a specifically designed scale that is used for insulin units; 100-unit syringes are used in North America

Tuberculin syringes (narrow syringes that hold 1 mL or less)—marked in both milliliters and minims

Figure 4-4 ■ shows examples of hypodermic, insulin, and tuberculin syringes.

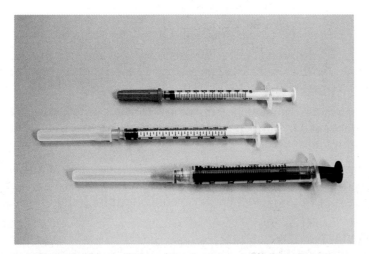

Figure 4-4 ■ (Top to bottom): Tuberculin, insulin, and 3-mL hypodermic syringes.

Injectable medications are often available in disposable prefilled unit-dose systems as follows:

✳ Prefilled syringes, ready to use

✳ Prefilled sterile cartridges and needles that must be attached to a reusable holder (injection system) before use

Examples of prefilled unit-dose systems are shown in Figure 4-5 ■.

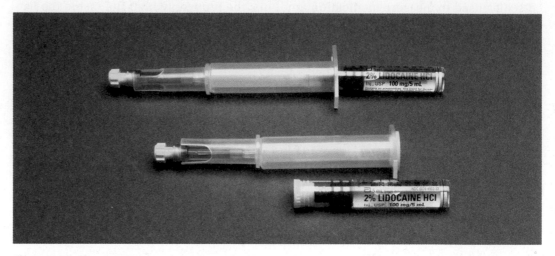

Figure 4-5 ■ Prefilled unit-dose systems.

NEEDLES

Most needles are disposable and are made of stainless steel. Special procedure needles may be reusable and need to be repeatedly sharpened because their points can become dull with use. Dull or damaged needles should never be used.

There are three parts that make up a needle, as follows:

✳ **Bevel**—the slanted part at the needle's tip

✳ **Cannula** or shaft—the actual metal length that makes up the majority of the needle; it is attached to the hub

✳ **Hub**—the part of the needle that fits onto the syringe

There are three variable characteristics in needles used for injections:

✳ **Gauge** (or diameter of the shaft)—the gauge varies from #18 to #28. The larger the gauge, the smaller the shaft's diameter. Larger gauges are required for thicker medications such as penicillin.

✳ Length of the shaft—common lengths range from 1/2 to 2 inches. The correct shaft length is determined by the type of injection, the patient's weight, and the patient's muscle development.

✳ Slant or length of the bevel—longer bevels cause less discomfort and provide the sharpest needles (these are commonly used for intramuscular and subcutaneous injections). Short bevels are used for intravenous or intradermal injections.

AMPULES AND VIALS

Sterile parenteral medications are often packaged in either ampules or vials. An ampule is made of clear glass and usually contains a single dose of a drug. It ranges in size from 1 mL to 10 mL or larger. Ampules have a distinctive neck that is tight or constricted; most ampule necks are prescored to be easily opened and are marked with a colored ink at the point at which they are to be opened.

Ampules are broken open at the constricted neck by using a plastic cap over the top of the ampule (to prevent injury from broken glass) and a cutter within the cap that further scores the neck of the ampule when it is rotated. Once broken open, the medication is aspirated into a syringe by using a filter needle, which prevents aspiration of any glass particles. Figure 4-6 ■ shows an example of drawing medication from an ampule.

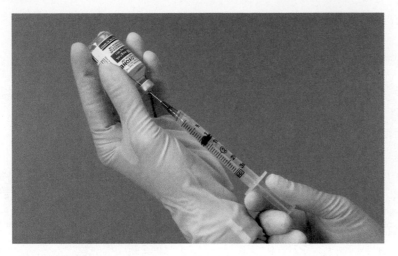

Figure 4-6 ■ Drawing medication from an ampule with a syringe.

A *vial* consists of a small glass bottle that is sealed with a rubber cap and may range from single to multidose sizes. Vials must be pierced with a needle to access the medication. Air is injected into the vial before the medication can be withdrawn from it. The air prevents a vacuum from building up within the vial, allowing easier withdrawal of medication.

Drugs that are dispensed as powders in vials (for reconstitution with solvents, such as sterile water or sterile normal saline, or diluents) include penicillin.

Intradermal Injection

Intradermal (ID) injections are usually given just below the epidermis into the dermis, in the inner forearm or upper back—areas that have little hair growth (Figure 4-7A ■). The intradermal route is commonly used for tuberculin or allergy skin tests, or for administration of local anesthetics. One method of tuberculin screening is the tine test, which is administered with individually packaged disposable sterile stamps with four prongs on the end that have been treated with tuberculin solution. The tine test, however, is not as accurate as the Mantoux (purified protein derivative [PPD]) intradermal screening test. Absorption via this route is slow. A 15-degree angle is used when the needle is inserted between the skin's upper layers (Figure 4-8A ■), and injection of a substance should produce a small **wheal** (a slightly reddened, raised lesion) on the skin's outer surface. With the Mantoux test, a 0.1-mL solution of PPD is injected, using a needle gauge of #26 to #27.

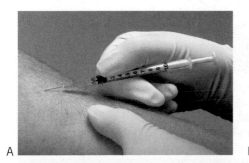
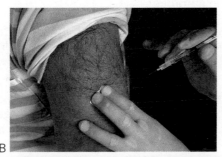
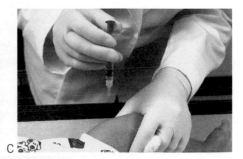

A   B   C

Figure 4-7 ■ (A) Intradermal injection, (B) subcutaneous injection, (C) intramuscular injection.

Subcutaneous Injection

Subcutaneous injections are usually given into subcutaneous tissue below the dermis in the upper arms, upper back, or upper abdomen (see Figure 4-7B ■). The subcutaneous route is commonly used for heparin and insulin injections. Absorption via this

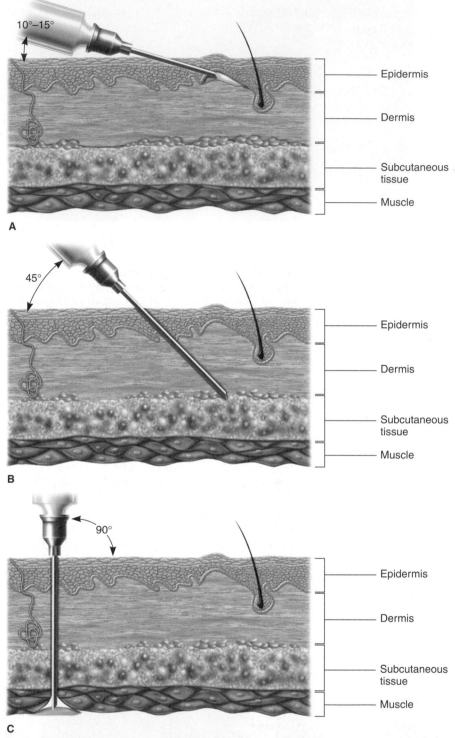

Figure 4-8 ■ Angles and depths of injection for (A) intradermal, (B) subcutaneous, and (C) intramuscular injections.

Focus Point

Heparin Injections

For subcutaneous heparin injections, make sure that 0.1 to 0.2 mL of air is in the syringe to prevent heparin leakage into tissue, thus avoiding localized hemorrhage.

route is slower than via intramuscular injections. A 45-degree angle is usually used, although this depends on the patient's body weight, which also influences the length of needle used (see Figure 4-8B ■). Small volumes of medication (between 0.5 and 1 mL) are given subcutaneously.

Focus Point

Self-administration of Insulin

Teach diabetic patients who must self-administer insulin at home to rotate insulin administration sites.

Intramuscular Injection

IM injections are usually given into the deltoid (upper arm), vastus lateralis (thigh), and ventrogluteal or dorsogluteal (hip) muscles (see Figure 4-7C ■). The IM route is commonly used for drugs that are irritating to subcutaneous tissue. Absorption via this route is more rapid than other methods because of the rich blood supply found in the muscles. A 90-degree angle is used most commonly (see Figure 4-8C ■), although the *Z-track method of IM injection* is used as well. To avoid irritation to the skin and subcutaneous tissues, the Z-track injection method prevents any leakage back from the deep muscle into the upper subcutaneous layers by displacing the upper tissue laterally before the needle is inserted. Larger volumes of medication (1 to 3 mL) can be given at one site using IM injections.

Focus on Pediatrics

Injections in Infants and Young Children

Infants and young children usually require smaller, shorter needles (#22 to #25 gauge, 5/8 to 1 inch long) for IM injection. The gluteal muscles are developed by walking. Therefore, do not use the dorsogluteal site in children younger than 3 years unless the child has been walking for at least 1 year. The vastus lateralis site is recommended as the site of choice for IM injections for infants 7 months or younger.

Focus on Geriatrics

Injections in Older Patients

Older patients may have decreased muscle mass, or muscle *atrophy*. A shorter needle may be needed. Assessment of appropriate injection site is critical. Absorption of medication may occur more quickly than expected.

Intravenous Injection

IV injections are given directly into the veins, most commonly those of the arms. The IV route is used for many varieties of drugs and fluids, and distribution via this route is almost immediate. Drugs given via the IV route may be administered slowly, rapidly (IV push), by piggyback infusions (drugs are mixed with compatible fluids and administered over 30 to 90 minutes), into an existing IV line (the IV port), into an intermittent venous access device such as a heparin lock, or by adding them to an IV solution. IV needles are inserted into veins at short angles (of about 25°) to the skin.

Focus Point

Z-track Technique of Injection Used for Certain Medications

Some specific medications, such as iron, are irritating or may stain the skin. Therefore, use the Z-track technique of injection for these medications.

✳ Apply Your Knowledge 4.4

The following questions focus on what you have just learned about parenteral routes of drug administration. *See Appendix E for the correct answers.*

MULTIPLE CHOICE
Choose the correct answer from choices a–d.

1. A prefilled syringe is known as a:
   a. Flange
   b. Plunger
   c. Vial
   d. Cartridge

2. Which of the following injection methods should be chosen for medications that are irritating or may cause discoloration of the skin?
   a. Intravenous
   b. Z-track
   c. Subcutaneous
   d. Intradermal

3. Hypodermic syringes are commonly used to administer medication by which of the following routes?
   a. Intradermal
   b. Intravenous
   c. Intramuscular
   d. Subcutaneous

4. Which of the following muscles of the body is the preferred injection site for infants?
   a. Gluteus medius
   b. Deltoid
   c. Vastus lateralis
   d. Ventrogluteal

5. The angle of insertion of a needle for intradermal injection is:
   a. 45°
   b. 30°
   c. 15°
   d. 5°

6. Which of the following needle gauges is used for the Mantoux test?
   a. 16–17
   b. 19–20
   c. 23–24
   d. 26–27

MATCHING

Match the lettered term to the numbered description.

DESCRIPTION	TERM
1. ____ Injection of a drug into the body with a needle and syringe is this type of route.	a. Intradermal
2. ____ More dangerous route of administration than others	b. Subcutaneous
3. ____ The tuberculin tine test is an example of this route of administration.	c. Parenteral
4. ____ Route commonly used for insulin and heparin	d. Intramuscular
5. ____ The Z-track method is a commonly used type of this route of administration.	e. Intravenous

OTHER ROUTES OF DRUG ADMINISTRATION

Drugs may be applied to skin and mucous membranes either topically (on the skin's outer layers) or via the eyes (using instillations or irrigations), the ears (using drops of medicated solution), the nose (using drops and sprays), inhalation (drawing breath, vapor, or gas into the lungs), the vagina (using instillations), and the rectum (using suppositories).

Transdermal Applications

Topical skin preparations include creams, ointments, pastes, lotions, powders, sprays, and patches. Transdermal patches allow drugs to be absorbed slowly through the skin to create a constant, time-released systemic effect (Figure 4-9 ■). For example; the nitroglycerin patch is particularly useful for patients with frequent attacks of angina. Other drugs administered via transdermal patches include nicotine (to assist in smoking cessation) and estrogen. The rate of delivery of the drug is controlled and varies with each product (12 hours to 1 week).

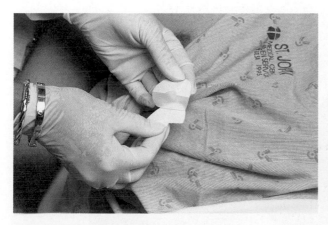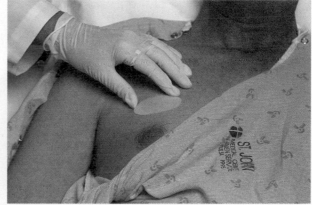

Figure 4-9 ■ Examples of transdermal patches.

Use of Transdermal Patches

Instruct patients to shower with the transdermal patch in place. If the patch is to remain on for 24 hours, a new patch should be applied every day at the same time. Advise patients to rotate sites to prevent skin irritation, and to avoid placing the patch on scars and areas with a large amount of body hair.

Ophthalmic Route

Medications are administered to the eye by using instillations or irrigations in the form of liquids or ointments. Eye drops and ointments are used to administer medication by sterile technique. Prescribed liquids are usually diluted, for example, to less than 1% strength. An eye irrigation is administered to wash out the conjuctival sac to remove secretions or foreign bodies, or to remove chemicals that may injure the eye. Figures 4-10 ■ and 4-11 ■ show the instillation of eye ointments and eye drops into the lower conjunctival sac.

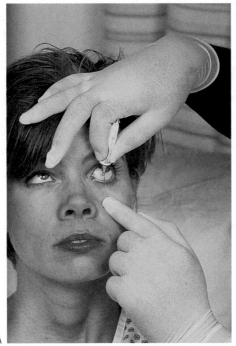
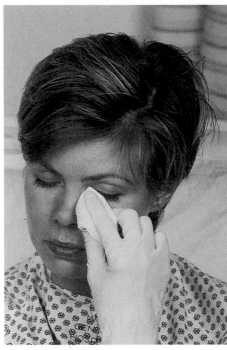

Figure 4-10 ■ Instillation of eye ointments. (A) Eye ointment is instilled into conjunctival sac. (B) Excess is gently wiped away.

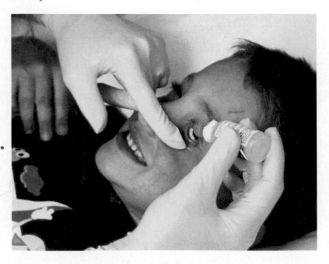

Figure 4-11 ■ Instillation of eye drops.

Otic Route

Localized infection or inflammation of the ear or ears is treated by dropping a small amount of a sterile medicated solution into them. In children younger than 3 years of age, gently pull the earlobe down and back; in adults, gently pull the earlobe up and out (Figure 4-12 ■). The patient must remain lying on his or her opposite side for 5 minutes to allow the medication to run into and coat the surface of the inner ear canal.

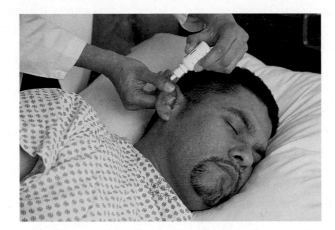

Figure 4-12 ■ Instillation of ear medication.
©Elena Dorfman.

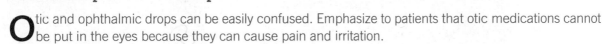

Focus Point

Otic and Ophthalmic Drops

Otic and ophthalmic drops can be easily confused. Emphasize to patients that otic medications cannot be put in the eyes because they can cause pain and irritation.

Nasal Route

Nose drops and sprays generally are used to shrink swollen mucous membranes or to loosen secretions and facilitate drainage. Sometimes, nasal medications are prescribed to treat infections of the nasal cavity or sinuses. Nasal decongestants are the most common nasal instillations. Many of these medications are OTC drugs. The medication should be drawn up into a dropper and held over one nostril at a time. Then, the required number of nose drops are administered. Nasal sprays are usually used with the patient in the supine position with the head tilted back (Figure 4-13 ■).

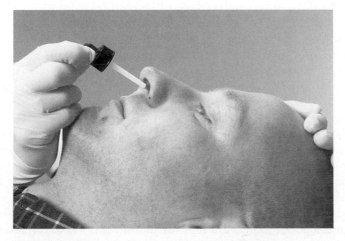

Figure 4-13 ■ Administration of nasal medications.

Self-administration of Medication by Patients

Correct administration of medications by patients at home requires patient education by the health-care professional. Make sure the patient understands the purpose of the drug; the time, frequency, and amount of the dose; any special storage requirements; and the typical side effects that may occur. Emphasize to the patient the possible serious adverse effects of the medication. Advise the patient to report adverse effects to the physician quickly.

Inhalation Route

Inhalation is the act of drawing breath, vapor, or gas into the lungs. Inhalation therapy may involve the administration of medicines, water vapor, and gases such as oxygen, carbon dioxide, and helium. The medication must be inhaled to achieve local effects within the respiratory tract through aerosols (Figure 4-14A–C ■), nebulizers, Spinhalers, or metered-dose inhalers. Some inhaled medications are intended to alter the condition of the mucous membranes (albuterol and anti-inflammatory medications), to alter the character of the secretions in the respiratory system (acetylcysteine), or to treat infections of the respiratory tract (antibiotics like tobramycin).

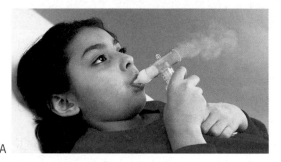
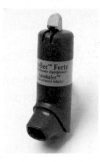
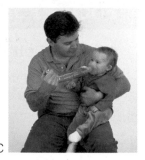

A   B   C

Figure 4-14 ■ (A) A girl breathes mist through a nebulizer with a bite piece in her mouth; (B) A breath-actuated inhaler © *Dorling Kindersley*; (C) Inhaler with face mask *Tim Ridley* © *Dorling Kindersley*.

Oxygen is another medication that is administered by the inhalation route. Because oxygen is a drug, it needs to be prescribed according to the flow rate, concentration, method of delivery, and length of time for administration. Oxygen is prescribed as liters per minute (LPM) and as percentage of oxygen concentration (%). Oxygen toxicity may develop when 100% oxygen is breathed for a prolonged period. A high concentration of inhaled oxygen causes alveolar collapse, intra-alveolar hemorrhage, hyaline membrane formation, disturbance of the central nervous system, and retrolental fibroplasias in newborns.

By far, the predominant use of inhaled medications is for the treatment of asthma or other pulmonary disorders. In treating asthma, a common method of administering medications is by nebulizer (see Figure 4.14A). A nebulizer is used to deliver a fine spray (fog or mist) of medication or moisture to a client. There are two kinds of nebulization: *atomization* and *aerosolization*. In atomization, a device called an *atomizer* produces rather large droplets for inhalation. In aerosolization, the droplets are suspended in a gas, such as oxygen. The smaller the droplets, the further they can be inhaled into the respiratory tract.

The *metered-dose inhaler* (MDI) is a handheld nebulizer (Figure 4-15 ■), which is a pressurized container of medication that the patient can use to release the medication through a nosepiece or mouthpiece.

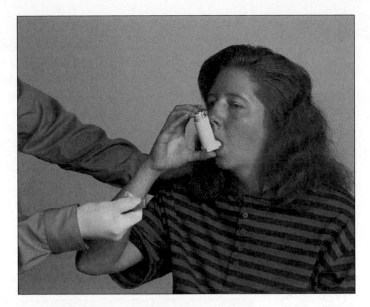

Figure 4-15 ■ Metered-dose inhaler.

Focus Point

Oxygen Precautions

Delivery of oxygen requires specific precautions. Be alert to the flammability of oxygen and make sure no open flames (including lighters, matches, or candles) are being used in the area near the oxygen.

Vaginal Route

Vaginal medications, or instillations, are inserted as creams, jellies, foams, or supposi-tories to treat infections or to relieve vaginal discomfort such as pain or itching. Vagi-nal creams, jellies, and foams are applied by using a tubular applicator with a plunger. Suppositories are designed to melt at body temperature, so they are usually kept in the refrigerator (Figure 4-16A ■). Vaginal suppositories are gelatin or cocoa butter based and are instilled using an applicator (Figure 4-16B ■).

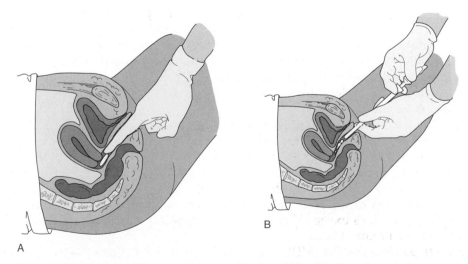

A

B

Figure 4-16 ■ (A) Instilling vaginal suppositories. (B) Instillation of vaginal cream using an applicator.

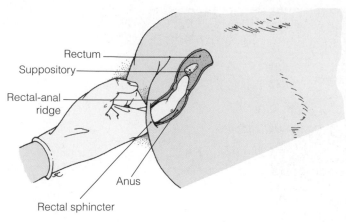

Rectum

Suppository

Rectal-anal ridge

Anus

Rectal sphincter

Figure 4-17 ■ Instillation of rectal medications.

Rectal Route

Rectal medications are commonly given in suppository form. The rectal route is useful if the patient is nauseated, vomiting, or unconscious. Manufacturers supply rectal medications in the form of gelatin- or cocoa butter–based suppositories, which melt in the warmth of the rectum and release the medication, or in the form of enemas as a solution (Figure 4-17 ■).

✳ Apply Your Knowledge 4.5

The following questions focus on what you have just learned about other routes of drug administration. *See Appendix E for the correct answers.*

FILL IN THE BLANK
Select terms from your reading to fill in the blanks.

1. Medication applied in patch form is called _____.

2. Vaginal suppositories are _____ or _____ based.

3. The two forms of nebulization are _____ and _____.

4. When oxygen is breathed for a long time, oxygen _____ may develop.

5. The most common nasal instillation drugs are _____.

6. Nicotine and nitroglycerin are examples of drugs delivered by the _____ route.

7. _____ medications are the most often used drugs for asthma.

8. The metered dose inhaler is a handheld _____.

MATCHING
Match the lettered term to the numbered description. The lettered term may be used more than once.

DESCRIPTION	TERM
1._____ One type of delivery for eye medications	a. Topical
2._____ Route used to wash out the *conjuctival sac* to remove secretions or foreign bodies, or to remove chemicals that may injure the eye	b. Instillation
	c. Irrigation
3._____ Applied locally to the skin or to mucous membranes in areas including the eye, external ear canal, nose, vagina, and rectum	d. Inhalation
	e. Atomization
4._____ Route that may involve the administration of medicines, water vapor, and gases such as oxygen, carbon dioxide, and helium	
5._____ Route that uses large drops of medication for inhalation	

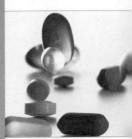

Chapter Capsule

This section repeats the objectives from the beginning of the chapter and then provides a summary of the most important concepts for that objective. Use this section as a quick review and to check your knowledge.

Objective 1: Summarize patient assessment factors that have an impact on medication administration.

■ Depends on patient's illness or current condition, intended drug, and route of administration

■ Includes other factors such as breathing problems, nausea, history of or current medication use, vitamins or food and herbal supplements being taken, and other factors

Objective 2: Identify the seven rights of drug administration.

■ The *right* patient

■ The *right* drug

■ The *right* dose

■ The *right* route

■ The *right* time

■ The *right* technique

■ The *right* documentation

Objective 3: Discuss some causes of medication errors.

■ Miscommunication—due to handwriting, similar names, dosing confusion

■ Missing information—lack of patient, lab, or drug information

■ Lack of appropriate labeling—manufacturer or pharmacist error

■ Environmental factors—noise, lighting, stress, fatigue

■ Poor management—unhealthy culture

Objective 4: Explain the universal policy to be observed if a medication error is detected.

■ Report as soon as possible

■ Monitor patient for adverse effects

■ Document in the medical record

■ Include signature of the individual who made the error in medical record

Objective 5: Summarize the guidelines for reducing medication errors.

■ Sufficient number of trained staff to prepare, dispense, and administer medications

■ Standardized measurement systems for both inpatients and outpatients

■ Consistently used error-tracking system to target and monitor common patient errors

■ Clearly defined system for drug administration, ordering, and dispensing that includes review of original drug orders

■ Medication profiles for inpatients, outpatients, and ambulatory patients with updated allergy histories in each encounter

■ Suitable work environment for safe, effective drug preparation

Objective 6: List and describe the various routes of medication administration.

- Enteral—through the GI tract
  - ❑ Oral—via the mouth
  - ❑ Nasogastric or gastrostomy tube—through the nasopharynx or stomach
  - ❑ Sublingual (percutaneous)—under the tongue
  - ❑ Buccal (percutaneous)—between the gum and cheek
- Parenteral—injected
- Topical (percutaneous)—through the skin
  - ❑ Skin application
  - ❑ Ophthalmic route—eye
  - ❑ Otic route—ear
  - ❑ Nasal route—nose
  - ❑ Inhalation—through the airways
  - ❑ Vaginal—vagina
  - ❑ Rectal—rectum

Objective 7: Identify equipment and supplies required for parenteral administration of medications.

- Syringes, needles, ampules, and vials

Objective 8: Define terms related to needles used in the parenteral administration of medications.

- Bevel—the slanted part at the needle's tip
- Cannula—the metal needle shaft
- Gauge—the needle shaft's diameter
- Hub—the part of the needle that fits onto the syringe

Objective 9: Identify sites used for intradermal, subcutaneous, and intramuscular injections.

- Intradermal—given within the skin layers of the inner forearm or upper back
- Subcutaneous—given into the upper arms, upper back, or upper abdomen
- Intramuscular—given into the upper arm or the thigh or hip

Objective 10: Explain how to administer an intradermal, subcutaneous, or intramuscular injection.

- Intradermal—a 15-degree angle is used; volumes less than 0.1 mL
- Subcutaneous—a 45-degree angle is used; only small volumes of medication
- Intramuscular—a 90-degree angle is used, or the Z-track method; larger volumes of medication

Internet Sites of Interest

- The Institute for Safe Medication Practices provides a list of look-alike or sound-alike drugs that are commonly confused at: **www.ismp.org/Tools/confuseddrugnames.pdf**
- An article about strategies to reduce medication errors is offered by the U.S. Food and Drug Administration at: **www.fda.gov/fdac**. Search "medical errors."

■ About Health & Fitness offers much health and medical information for older adults at: **www.seniorhealth.about.com**. Search for "taking medications."

■ Good teaching information is provided for parents of pediatric patients at: **http://www.fda.gov/fdac**. Search "how to give medicine to children."

■ Prentice Hall's Web site for Drug Guides, at: **www.prenhall.com/drugguides** provides drug updates, administration techniques, a list of common herbal remedies and their interactions, and much more.

■ This Web site, Prescription Drug Info, allows you to search for most drugs by trade name and provides an overview of the drug, its common dosages, the forms in which it is available, its active chemicals, the pharmaceutical company that manufactures it, and the date that it was approved by the FDA: **www.prescriptiondrug-info.com**

■ The Joint Commission provides an index of articles, such as *Using Medication Reconciliation to Prevent Errors, Medication Errors Related to Potentially Dangerous Abbreviations, Infusion Pumps: Preventing Future Adverse Events*, and others at: **www.jointcommission.org/SentinelEvents/SentinelEventAlert**

Checkpoint Review 1

Select the best answer for the following questions.

1. The half-life is the major determinant of which of the following?

   a. The adverse effects of a drug after a single dose
   b. The interaction with another single dose
   c. The duration of elimination of a drug after administration of multiple doses
   d. The duration of action of a drug after a single dose

2. Hypersensitivity is often used synonymously with which of the following terms?

   a. Immunogen
   b. Allergy
   c. Antigen
   d. Allergen

3. Which of the following agencies oversees controlled substances and prosecutes individuals who illegally distribute them?

   a. HIPAA
   b. FDA
   c. DEA
   d. CDC

4. Which of the following federal laws offers a seven-year monopoly on drug sales and tax breaks to induce drug companies to undertake development and manufacturing of such drugs?

   a. Orphan Drug Act of 1983
   b. The Prescription Drug Marketing Act of 1987
   c. The Durham–Humphrey Amendment of 1951
   d. The Comprehensive Drug Abuse Prevention and Control Act of 1970

5. Which of the following is an example of a semisolid drug?

   a. Granules
   b. Caplets
   c. Gelcaps
   d. Gels

6. The angle of insertion for intradermal injections is which of the following degrees?

   a. 30
   b. 90
   c. 15
   d. 45

7. Which of the following is the route of administration of a drug that is placed between the gums and the cheek?

   a. Buccal
   b. Topical
   c. Sublingual
   d. Transdermal

8. Which of the following is the abbreviation for subcutaneous?

   a. SC
   b. Subcutaneous should not be abbreviated to avoid medication errors.
   c. SQ
   d. Sub q

9. The proprietary drug name is also called the:

   a. Chemical name
   b. Generic name
   c. Trade name
   d. None of the above

10. The study of drugs derived from herbal and other natural sources is called:

    a. Pharmacodynamic
    b. Pharmacotherapy
    c. Pharmacognosy
    d. Pharmacology

11. The enteral route is the route of drug administration through which of the following:

    a. Intravenous
    b. Gastrointestinal tract
    c. Intradermal
    d. Topical

12. Which of the following abbreviations means "twice a day"?

    a. bid
    b. qid
    c. qd
    d. tid

13. Administration of corticosteroids may be more effective if administered during what time of the day?

    a. Early morning
    b. Early evening
    c. At noon
    d. At bedtime

14. Which of the following agents is mixed with a liquid but not dissolved?

    a. Elixir
    b. Suspension
    c. Tincture
    d. Fluid extract

15. Bioavailability of a drug means:

    a. The determination of whether two or more drug products release their contents in equal amounts over the same absorption
    b. The degree to which a drug releases itself from its dosage form to become accessible for its intended effect
    c. The process of drug movement into the systemic circulation
    d. The study of the chemical reactions that occur within a living organism

16. The abbreviation qid, as used in prescriptions, means:

    a. Every hour
    b. Every four hours
    c. Every other day
    d. Four times a day

17. The elixir sulfanilamide disaster of 1937 is an example of medication:

    a. Ordering errors
    b. Dispensing errors
    c. Transcribing errors
    d. Formulation errors

18. Which of the following schedule of drugs has the lowest abuse potential of all the controlled substances?

    a. Schedule IV
    b. Schedule III
    c. Schedule V
    d. Schedule II

19. Orphan drugs are used to treat which of the following diseases or conditions?

    a. Shark bite
    b. AIDS
    c. Asthma
    d. Cancer

20. Coal tar is used to treat which of the following disorders?

    a. Rheumatoid arthritis
    b. Scarlet fever
    c. Psoriasis
    d. AIDS

21. Which of the following is the abbreviation for potassium?

    a. Hg
    b. Na
    c. Fe
    d. K

22. Semisolid drugs are most commonly used for:

    a. Topical application
    b. Inhalation
    c. Parental
    d. Oral

23. Which of the following is the most dangerous route of drug administration?

    a. Intradermal
    b. Intramuscular
    c. Intravenous
    d. Subcutaneous

24. Heparin is commonly given by which of the following routes?

    a. Sublingual
    b. Subcutaneous
    c. Intradermal
    d. Rectal

25. Which of the following parts of a prescription is also known as the subscription?

    a. Medication prescribed
    b. Dispensing directions to the pharmacist
    c. Directions for patient
    d. Refill and special labeling

26. Which of the following agents was extensively and legally advertised in newspapers during the nineteenth century when there was virtually no regulation on the sale of drugs in the United States?

    a. Penicillin
    b. Atropine
    c. Barbital
    d. Opium

27. Short needles are used for which of the following routes of drug injections?

    a. Intravenous or intradermal
    b. Intramuscular and subcutaneous
    c. Intradermal and subcutaneous
    d. Intravenous and intramuscular

28. Which of the following is an example of a sublingual tablet?

    a. Insulin
    b. Heparin
    c. Nitroglycerin
    d. Ampicillin

29. Aqueous solutions containing high concentrations of sugar are called what?

    a. Syrups
    b. Spirits
    c. Elixirs
    d. Tinctures

30. All drug administration laws are initiated, implemented, and enforced by which of the following laws?

    a. MSPPA
    b. OSHA
    c. FDA
    d. HIPAA

31. All of the following are examples of the transdermal patch, except:

    a. Estrogen
    b. Testosterone
    c. Nicotine
    d. Nitroglycerin

32. Which of the following part of a word gives the word its central meaning?

    a. Suffix
    b. Prefix
    c. Root
    d. Combining vowel

33. Pancreatin and pepsin come from which of the following sources?

    a. Minerals
    b. Humans and other animals
    c. Synthetic sources
    d. Engineered sources

34. Which of the following medications may stain and irritate the skin, and for which you should use the "Z-track technique" of injection?

    a. Penicillin
    b. Protein plasma
    c. Iodine
    d. Iron

35. Which of the following is an abbreviation meaning "immediately"?

    a. Sig
    b. SOS
    c. Syr
    d. Stat

36. Which of the following agents promotes muscle growth?

    a. Alkylating drugs
    b. Anabolic steroids
    c. Acetylcholine
    d. Acetylcysteine

37. The DEA is a branch of which department that became the nation's sole legal drug-enforcement agency?

    a. U.S. Department of Health
    b. U.S. Department of Labor
    c. U.S. Department of Health and Human Services
    d. U.S. Department of Justice

38. Pharmacy practice regulation is primarily a function of the:

    a. State
    b. Federal government
    c. Board of Pharmacy
    d. U.S. Department of Health

39. Which of the following abbreviations means "by mouth"?

    a. pc
    b. po
    c. prn
    d. pm

40. Which of the following laws was passed to prevent the marketing of new drugs before they had been properly tested for purity, strength, effectiveness, safety, and packaging quality:

    a. The Durham–Humphrey Amendment
    b. Food, Drug, and Cosmetic Act
    c. Safe Medical Devices Act
    d. The Controlled Substances Act

41. The abbreviation *mist* means:

    a. Solution
    b. Liquid
    c. Ointment
    d. A mixture

42. Which of the following syringes are calibrated in units?

    a. Disposable syringes
    b. Needleless syringes
    c. Insulin syringes
    d. Tuberculin syringes

43. A list of officially recognized drug names is known as the:

    a. U.S. Drug Code
    b. National Formulary
    c. National pharmacopeia
    d. International pharmacopeia

44. A wheal occurs on the skin from which of the following injections?

   a. Z-track

   b. Intradermal

   c. Intramuscular

   d. Subcutaneous

45. Which abbreviation means "nothing by mouth"?

   a. Na

   b. NPO

   c. UA

   d. CVA

For questions 46–50, match the lettered drug schedule to the numbered drug.

   DRUG

46. _____ Diphenoloxylate hydrocholide with atropine sulfate (Lomotil®)

47. _____ Certain drugs compounded with small quantities of narcotics

48. _____ Marijuana

49. _____ Diazepam (valium)

50. _____ Morphine

DRUG SCHEDULE

   a. Schedule I

   b. Schedule II

   c. Schedule III

   d. Schedule IV

   e. Schedule V

For questions 51–55, match the lettered abbreviation to the numbered meaning.

   MEANING

51. _____ As directed

52. _____ As needed

53. _____ Four times a day

54. _____ After meals

55. _____ Three times a day

   ABBREVIATION

   a. tid

   b. qid

   c. pc

   d. prn

   e. ud

For questions 56–57, please answer in sentences.

56. A 13-year-old girl is picked up at the medical office by her father. Her parents are divorced, and her mother has legal custody. Her father would like to see the girl's medical records. Can he see the medical records by law? Explain.

   _____

   _____

   _____

   _____

   _____

57. A physician prescribed marijuana for a 35-year-old man who is suffering from advanced AIDS. Before the pharmacy technician dispenses the prescription, a health-care person wants to know in which schedule of drugs the marijuana is. On the Internet, the technician should search under which federal law?

   _____

   _____

   _____

   _____

   _____

Unit 2

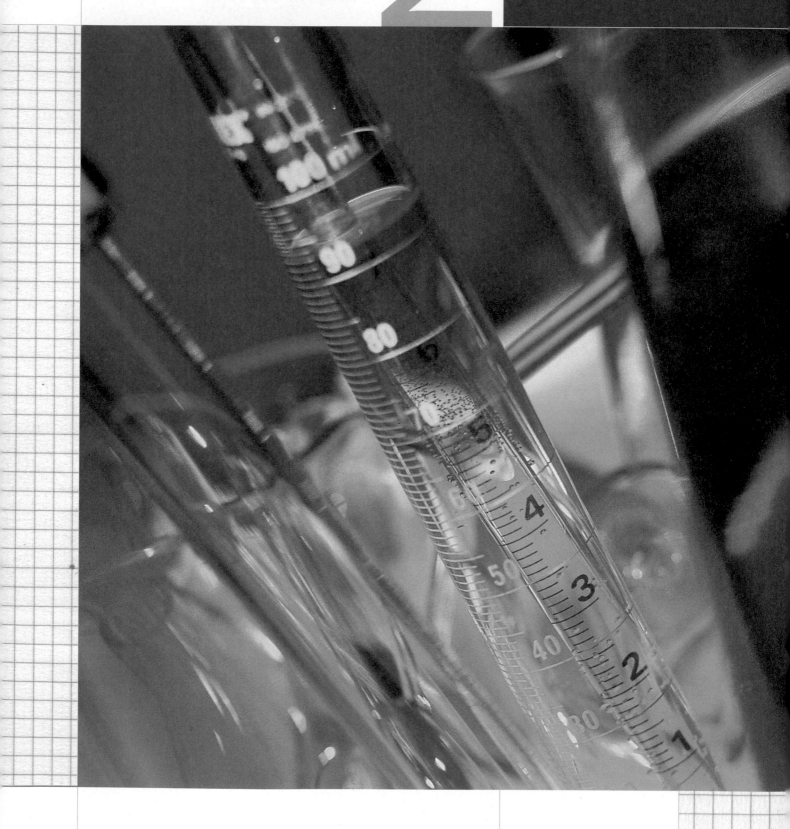

MATHEMATICS AND DOSAGE CALCULATIONS

" It is the health-care professional's responsibiltiy to ensure that the patient receives the proper dose of medication, and to educate the patient about the proper measurement of doses. "

Chapter 5

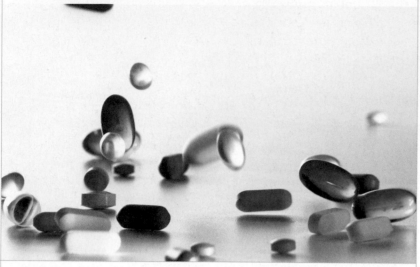

Basic Mathematics

Chapter Objectives

After completing this chapter, you should be able to:

1. Describe the difference between Arabic numbers and Roman numerals.
2. Convert an improper fraction to a mixed fraction.
3. Add fractions having the same denominator.
4. Subtract fractions having the same denominator.
5. Multiply fractions and mixed fractions.
6. Divide fractions and mixed fractions.
7. Add, subtract, multiply, and divide decimals.
8. Define ratios, proportions, and percents.

Key Terms

Arabic number (page 93)
Common fraction (page 96)
Decimals (page 99)
Denominator (dee-NAW-mih-nay-ter) (page 96)
Extremes (page 103)
Fraction (page 95)

Improper fraction (page 96)
Means (page 103)
Minuend (MIN-yoo-end) (page 100)
Mixed fraction (page 96)
Multiplicand (MUL-tih-plih-kand) (page 101)
Multiplier (MUL-tih-ply-er) (page 101)

Numerator (NOO-meh-ray-ter) (page 96)
Percent (page 103)
Ratio (page 102)
Roman numeral (page 93)
Subtrahend (SUB-truh-hend) (page 100)

PRACTICAL SCENARIO

Pharmacy technicians must always be careful when using mathematical equations for compounding. Phil, a pharmacy technician who only recently began working in a pharmacy, is asked by the pharmacist to use a powdered drug and mix it with a solution so that the amount of drug is 3%. Phil converts 3% to a decimal (0.03) so that he can more easily mix the proper amount. He then mixes 0.03 g of the powdered drug into 100 mL of solution. When the pharmacist checks the mixture, he finds that Phil's solution is much too weak.

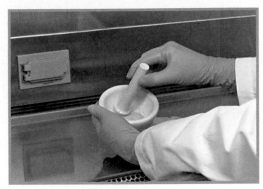

Critical Thinking Questions

1. What miscalculation did Phil make when mixing the solution?
2. When Phil prepares the medication, which rights of administration should he follow?

Introduction

The ability to make accurate dosage calculations requires allied health professionals to have skills in adding, subtracting, multiplying, and dividing whole numbers. It is essential that you have a knowledge of basic mathematics such as Arabic numbers, Roman numerals, fractions, decimals, percents, and ratios to be able to calculate dosages accurately and quickly.

Arabic System and Roman Numeral System

The **Arabic number** system is commonly used in expressing quantity and value, such as 0, 1, 2, 3, 4, 5, 6, 7, 8, and 9. Any number may be represented by combining these numbers. Arabic numbers can be written as whole numbers, decimals (for example, 0.6), and fractions (such as 3/4). The **Roman numeral** system consists of letters that represent number values, most commonly of numbers between 1 and 100. When working with numbers that range from 1 to 30, only three Roman numerals (I [1], V [5], and X [10]) are required, used in various combinations.

Example

$$IV = 4$$
$$XXI = 21$$

Roman numerals are commonly used to express units of the apothecary system of weights and measures in writing prescriptions. The most common Roman numerals and their values are seen in Table 5-1 ■.

READING ROMAN NUMERALS

Roman numerals are read by adding or subtracting the value of the letters. When a letter appears twice in a row, the value of the letter is counted twice, and so on (Example 1). If a lower valued letter follows a larger valued letter, the letters should be added. The letter representing the largest possible number should be used to represent a value. If a lower-valued letter is placed before a higher-valued letter, the lower letter is subtracted from the higher letter (Example 2).

Example 1

$$VII = 5 + 1 + 1 = 7$$
$$III = 1 + 1 + 1 = 3$$
$$XIV = 10 + 4 = 14$$
$$XXI = 10 + 10 + 1 = 21$$
$$XXXIV = 10 + 10 + 10 + 4 = 34$$

Example 2

$$IV = 5 - 1 = 4$$
$$IX = 10 - 1 = 9$$
$$XL = 50 - 10 = 40$$

Table 5-1 ■ The Most Common Roman Numerals and Their Arabic Values

ROMAN NUMERAL	ARABIC VALUE
I	1
II	2
III	3
IV	4
V	5
VI	6
VII	7
VIII	8
IX	9
X	10
XV	15
XX	20
XXV	25
XXX	30
XL	40
L	50
LX	60
LXX	70
LXXV	75
LXXX	80
XC	90
C	100
D	500
M	1000

✳ Apply Your Knowledge 5.1

The following questions focus on what you have just learned about Arabic numbers and Roman numerals. *See Appendix E for the correct answers.*

DO THE MATH
Convert the Roman numerals to Arabic numbers.

1. VIII = _____
2. XXV = _____
3. XV = _____
4. VI = _____
5. XXI = _____

Add or subtract the Roman numerals.

6. VI + VIII = _____
7. XI + IV = _____
8. VII + IX = _____
9. XXI + VI = _____
10. XIX − XII = _____
11. XVII − VI = _____
12. XVIII − XII = _____
13. XXIV − XIV = _____

MATCHING
Match the lettered term to the numbered description. Lettered terms may be used more than once.

DESCRIPTION

1. _____ Commonly used to express units of the apothecary system of weights and measures in prescriptions
2. _____ Read by adding or subtracting the value of letters
3. _____ Commonly used in expressing quantity and value
4. _____ Can be written as whole numbers, decimals, and fractions
5. _____ Only three of these needed to express numbers from 1 to 30

TERM

a. Arabic numbers
b. Roman numerals

Fractions

Health-care workers who deal with administering medications and dispensing drugs need to understand fractions to interpret and act on practitioners' orders, read prescriptions, and understand patients' records. Fractions are used in apothecary and household measures for dosage calculations. A **fraction** is one or more equal parts of a unit. It is written as a divided number, with one portion considered to be a part of the whole amount, such as 1/2 or 3/4 (one part out of a total of two parts; or three parts out of a total of four).

The two parts of a fraction are called the *numerator* and the *denominator*. The **numerator** is the top number of the fraction. The **denominator** is the bottom number and indicates how many equal parts the whole has been divided into. In 3/4 the number "3" is the numerator and the number "4" is the denominator. The numerator shows how many of the parts are used. For example, the fraction 3/4 is read as "three-fourths" and indicates three parts out of the four parts that make up the whole. The fraction bar that separates the numerator and the denominator also means *divided by*. Thus, 3/4 can be read as "three divided by four" or "3 ÷ 4." This definition is important when one changes fractions to decimals.

CLASSIFICATION OF FRACTIONS

Fractions are generally classified into two groups: *common fractions* and *decimal fractions*. A **common fraction** represents equal parts of a whole. A decimal fraction is commonly referred to simply as a *decimal*. Common fractions are subclassified as proper, improper, mixed, and complex.

Proper Fractions

A proper fraction has a numerator that is smaller than the denominator and designates less than one whole unit. For example, 3/4 < 1.

Improper Fractions

An **improper fraction** has a numerator that is greater than or the same as the denominator. The number 5/3 is an improper fraction because the numerator 5 is greater than the denominator 3.

Example

$$5/3 > 1 \quad \text{or} \quad 5/5 = 1$$

Mixed Fractions

A **mixed fraction** is a whole number and a proper fraction combined. The value of the mixed fraction is always greater than 1.

Example

$$5\text{-}2/3 = 5 + 2/3 > 1$$

A mixed fraction can be converted to an improper fraction by converting the whole number to a fraction and adding (see the section "Adding and Subtracting Fractions with Dissimilar Denominators").

Complex Fractions

A complex fraction has the numerator or the denominator or both as a whole number, proper fraction, or mixed fraction. The value may be less than, greater than, or equal to 1.

Example

$$\frac{\frac{3}{5}}{\frac{1}{2}}, \quad \frac{\frac{1}{3}}{50}, \quad \text{and} \quad \frac{25}{\frac{1}{8}}$$

Adding Fractions

If fractions have the same denominator, simply add the numerators and keep the value of the common denominator the same. Then, reduce the numbers to the lowest terms by dividing both the numerator and denominator by the same common divisor (in this case, 2). Remember, by dividing both by 2, you are essentially dividing by 1, because

$$\frac{2}{2} = 1$$

Example

$$\frac{1}{10} + \frac{3}{10} = \frac{4}{10} = \frac{2}{5}$$

Example

$$\frac{4}{18} + \frac{3}{18} + \frac{6}{18} = \frac{13}{18}$$

Subtracting Fractions

If fractions have the same denominator, subtract the smaller numerator from the larger numerator. Keep the denominator the same, and then reduce to the lowest terms to obtain the final answer.

Example

$$\frac{6}{8} - \frac{2}{8} = \frac{4}{8} = \frac{1}{2}$$

Adding and Subtracting Fractions with Dissimilar Denominators

If fractions do not have the same denominator, change the fractions so that they have the smallest common denominator, subtract (or add) the numerators, and leave the denominator the same.

Example

$$\frac{10}{24} - \frac{4}{12} = ?$$

Since 12 is a multiple of 24 (24 ÷ 2 = 12), divide 24 by 2 to reach the smallest common denominator of 12:

$$\frac{10}{24} \div \frac{2}{2} = \frac{5}{12}$$

Then complete the subtraction:

$$\frac{5}{12} - \frac{4}{12} = \frac{1}{12}$$

Sometimes, however, the common denominator is not the smallest number even though both could be divided by 2. In the next example, the numerator 13 cannot be evenly divided by 2. Therefore, multiply the smaller denominator (12) by 2 to get a common denominator of 24. You will also need to multiply the numerator by 2. Remember, by multiplying both the numerator and denominator by 2, you are essentially multiplying by 1.

Example

$$\frac{13}{24} - \frac{2}{12} = ?$$

$$\frac{2}{12} \times \frac{2}{2} = \frac{4}{24}$$

$$\frac{13}{24} - \frac{4}{24} = \frac{9}{24} = \frac{3}{8}$$

As noted in the section on mixed fractions, you can convert a mixed fraction to an improper fraction using the following steps:

Example

$$5\text{-}2/3$$

First convert the whole number to a fraction:

$$5 = \frac{5}{1}$$

Then find a common denominator:

$$\frac{5}{1} + \frac{2}{3} = \frac{15}{3} + \frac{2}{3}$$

And now add the fractions:

$$\frac{15}{3} + \frac{2}{3} = \frac{17}{3}$$

Multiplying Fractions

To multiply fractions, first multiply the numerators; second, multiply the denominators; then place the product of the numerators over the product of the denominators; and finally, reduce to lowest terms.

Example

$$\frac{3}{5} \times \frac{2}{4} = \frac{6}{20} = \frac{3}{10}$$

Dividing Fractions

To divide fractions, first invert (or turn upside down) the divisor, reduce to lowest terms, and then multiply the numerators and divisors.

Example

$$\frac{4}{8} \div \frac{2}{8} = ?$$

Invert the divisor:

$$\frac{4}{8} \times \frac{8}{2} = ?$$

Reduce to lowest terms, and then multiply the numerators and then the denominators:

$$\frac{1}{2} \times \frac{4}{1} = \frac{4}{2} = \frac{2}{1} = 2$$

✳ Apply Your Knowledge 5.2

The following questions focus on what you have just learned about fractions. *See Appendix E for the correct answers.*

FILL IN THE BLANK

Select terms from your reading to fill in the blanks.

1. A proper fraction has a numerator that is _____ than the denominator.

2. The numerator is the _____ of the fraction.

3. A mixed fraction is a whole number and a proper fraction that are _____.

4. If fractions have the same denominator, subtract the _____ numerator from the _____ numerator.

5. To divide fractions, first _____ the divisor and then _____.

6. The numerator in 35/10 is _____.

7. The denominator in 42/100 is _____.

8. The numerator in 88/88 is _____.

9. The denominator in 14/60 is _____.

10. Twelve is the _____ in 12/5.

MULTIPLE CHOICE

Select the correct answer from choices a–d.

1. Determine the proper fraction from the following examples:
   a. 11/11
   b. 32/68
   c. 90/72
   d. 48/38

2. Determine the improper fraction from the following examples:
   a. 14/6
   b. 3/9
   c. 27/45
   d. 17/35

3. Determine the mixed fraction from the following examples:
   a. 2/6
   b. 101/16
   c. 11.238
   d. 6-2/4

DECIMALS

Decimal fractions, or **decimals**, are used with the metric system. Each decimal fraction has a denominator of 10 or a multiple of 10. Instead of writing the denominator, a decimal point is added to the numerator.

Example

$$\frac{3}{4} = \frac{75}{100} = 0.75$$

In writing a decimal fraction, always place a zero to the left of the decimal point, so that the decimal point can readily be seen.

Example

Fraction	Decimal Fraction
$\frac{2}{10}$	0.2
$\frac{19}{100}$	0.19
$\frac{256}{1,000}$	0.256

Decimals increase in value from right to left (Figure 5-1 ■); they decrease in value from left to right. Decimals increase in value in multiples of 10. Each column in a decimal has its own value—it depends on where it is situated in relation to the decimal point.

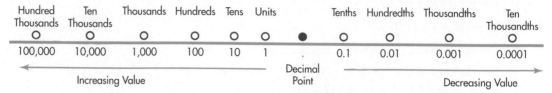

Hundred Thousands	Ten Thousands	Thousands	Hundreds	Tens	Units		Tenths	Hundredths	Thousandths	Ten Thousandths
○	○	○	○	○	○	●	○	○	○	○
100,000	10,000	1,000	100	10	1	.	0.1	0.01	0.001	0.0001

←———————— Increasing Value ————————   Decimal Point   ———————— Decreasing Value ————————→

Figure 5-1 ■ Decimal values as they relate to the location of the decimal point.

Focus Point

Zeros in Decimals

When writing decimals, *eliminate* unnecessary zeros ("trailing" zeros) at the end of a decimal figure (for example, write 2.0 as 2) to avoid confusion, but *always* insert a 0 before the decimal point of numbers less than 0 (for example, 0.25).

Adding and Subtracting Decimal Fractions

To add decimals, write the decimals in a column, placing the decimal points directly under each other. Then add as in the addition of whole numbers, and place the decimal point in the sum directly under the decimal points in the addends.

Example

$$0.2 + 0.5 + 0.7 = 1.4$$

Align the figures as follows:

$$
\begin{array}{r}
0.2 \\
0.5 \\
+0.7 \\
\hline
1.4
\end{array}
$$

To subtract decimals, write the decimals in columns, keeping the decimal points under each other. Then subtract as whole numbers (zeros may be added after the decimal without changing the value), and place the decimal point in the remainder, directly under the decimal point in the **subtrahend** (the number that is deducted) and **minuend** (the number from which another number is deducted).

Example

$$0.525 - 0.30 = 0.225$$

Align the figures as follows:

$$
\begin{array}{rl}
0.525 & \text{(minuend)} \\
-0.30 & \text{(subtrahend)} \\
\hline
0.225 &
\end{array}
$$

Multiplying and Dividing Decimal Fractions

To multiply decimal fractions, multiply the two numbers and count off from right to left as many decimal places in the product (answer) as there were in the **multiplier** (the number that multiplies another number) and **multiplicand** (the number that is multiplied by another number).

Example

$$
\begin{array}{r}
33.86 \quad \text{(multiplicand)} \\
\times\ 5.4 \quad \text{(multiplier)} \\
\hline
182.844 \quad \text{(product)}
\end{array}
$$

Because the multiplicand has two decimal places and the multiplier has one decimal place, you must count off three places from right to left and then insert the decimal point at this spot in the answer.

To divide by a decimal fraction, first move the decimal point in the divisor (the number that divides another number) enough places to the right to make it a whole number. Then move the decimal point in the dividend (the number that is being divided) as many places as it was moved in the divisor. Place the decimal point in the answer directly above the one in the dividend.

Example

$$4.75 \div 0.5 = ?$$

$$\frac{4.75}{0.5} = \frac{\text{dividend}}{\text{divisor}}$$

In this example, 4.75 becomes 475 (the decimal point is moved two places). Therefore, 0.5 becomes 50 (the decimal point is moved two places). Now the problem may be divided as follows:

$$475 \div 50 = 9.5$$

✳ Apply Your Knowledge 5.3

The following questions focus on what you just learned about decimals. *See Appendix E for the correct answers.*

DO THE MATH
Calculate these problems.

1. 0.12 + 5.77 + 9.06 + 18 = _____
2. 9.75 + 4.6 + 0.21 + 43.4 = _____
3. 14.006 − 0.5 = _____
4. 7.192 + 0.077 = _____
5. 28.4 − 0.188 = _____
6. $8.12 − $0.97 = _____
7. $17.52 − $1.93 = _____
8. 6 + 2.93 + 0.63 + 0.009 = _____
9. 5 + 7.2 + 0.07 + 9.33 = _____
10. 600 − 275.97 = _____
11. 3.002 × 0.05 = _____
12. 16.1 × 25.04 = _____
13. 75.1 × 1000.01 = _____
14. 23.2 × 15.025 = _____
15. 1.14 × 0.014 = _____
16. 45 ÷ 0.15 = _____
17. 73 ÷ 13.40 = _____
18. 25.3 ÷ 6.76 = _____
19. 515 ÷ 0.125 = _____
20. 16 ÷ 0.04 = _____

Ratios

A **ratio** is a mathematical expression that compares the relationship of one number to another number, or expresses a part of a whole number. When written, the two quantities are separated by a colon (:). The colon means *division*. The expression 3:4 means there are *three parts to four parts*. Ratios are frequently used to show concentrations of a medication in a solution. They are also used to express measurement equivalents and dosage of medications per unit (such as tablet, or capsule). For example, 1 grain is equal to 15 grams, which in a ratio, would be expressed as 1 grain:15 grams. One tablet containing 500 mg of a medication can be expressed as 1 tablet:500 mg. When measuring insulin, 100 units are contained in 1 mL, which can be written as follows: 100 units:1 mL.

Example

$\frac{2}{5}$ may be expressed as a ratio: 2:5.

✳ Apply Your Knowledge 5.4

The following questions focus on what you have just learned about ratios. *See Appendix E for the correct answers.*

FILL IN THE BLANK

Select terms from your reading to fill in the blanks.

1. The two quantities are separated by a _____ or _____ (symbol).

2. Ratios are frequently used to show concentrations of medication in a _____.

3. A 100-unit insulin syringe contains 100 units in 1 mL, which can be written as a ratio of _____.

4. In administering medications, you can use ratios to express measurement equivalents and dosage of drug per _____.

DO THE MATH

Change the ratios to fractions, and reduce to lowest terms.

1. 0.05:0.15 = _____
2. 6:8 = _____
3. 3:150 = _____
4. 6:10 = _____
5. 4:7 = _____
6. 9:18 = _____

Proportions

A *proportion* is a way of expressing a relationship of equality between two ratios. A proportion may be expressed as:

$$1:4 \ :: \ 3:12$$

or

$$1:4 = 3:12$$

or

$$\frac{1}{4} = \frac{3}{12}$$

The relationship of 1 to 4, in the examples above, is the same as the relationship of 3 to 12. In a proportion, these terms have names. The **means** are the two inside terms, and the **extremes** are the two outside terms. This relationship is shown in Figure 5-2 ■.

In a proportion, the product of the means is equal to the product of the extremes, which in turn equals 1. To prove this, convert the proportion into fractions and then cross-multiply the numerators and denominators.

Example

$$1:5 \; :: \; 2:10$$

Convert to fractions.

$$\frac{1}{5} \quad \frac{2}{10}$$

Cross-multiply the numerators and the denominators of the fraction.

$$\frac{1}{5} \times \frac{2}{10} = \frac{10}{10} = 1$$

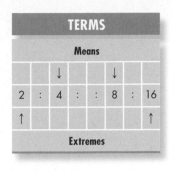

Figure 5-2 ■ The means and extremes of a proportion.

✳ Apply Your Knowledge 5.5

The following questions focus on what you have just learned about means and extremes. *See Appendix E for the correct answers.*

DO THE MATH
Determine the missing means or extremes values.

1. 10:X :: 5:8 = _____

2. 3:12 :: X:36 = _____

3. 33:39 :: 55:X = _____

4. 10:4 :: 20:X = _____

5. 100:X :: 50:2 = _____

6. 21:27 :: X:45 = _____

7. X:15 :: 100:75 = _____

8. 4:25 :: 16:X = _____

Percents

The term **percent**, or the symbol %, means *hundredths*. Thus, a percentage may also be expressed as a fraction, as a decimal fraction, or as a ratio.

Example

40% means *40 parts per hundred* or 40/100

75% means *75 parts per hundred* or 75/100

Example

Percent		Fraction		Decimal		Ratio
60%	=	60/100	=	0.60	=	60:100

Note: To change a percent to a decimal, move the decimal point two places to the left. In the example, the decimal point comes before the whole number 60. To change a fraction to a percent, divide the numerator by the denominator and multiply the results by 100. Then add a percent symbol (%).

Example
To convert 6/10 to a percent:

$$6 \div 10 = 0.6$$
$$0.6 \times 100 = 60\%$$

Example
To convert 1/5 to a percent:

$$1 \div 5 = 0.2$$
$$0.2 \times 100 = 20\%$$

✳ Apply Your Knowledge 5.6

The following questions focus on what you have just learned about percents. *See Appendix E for the correct answers.*

FILL IN THE BLANK
Select terms from your readings to fill in the blanks.

1. To convert a percent to a decimal, the decimal point comes before the _____ _____.

2. The symbol % for *percent* means _____.

3. The _____ 25/100 is equivalent to 25%.

4. To change a fraction to a percent, divide the numerator by the _____ and multiply by 100.

5. To change a _____ to a decimal, move the _____ point two places to the left.

DO THE MATH

Convert the percents to decimals.

1. 2% = _____
2. 18% = _____
3. 40% = _____
4. 106% = _____
5. 0.8% = _____
6. 24-1/2% = _____
7. 150.75% = _____
8. 4.5% = _____

Convert the decimals to percents.

9. 0.08 = _____
10. 32 = _____
11. 0.44 = _____
12. 0.5 = _____
13. 0.019 = _____
14. 5.7 = _____
15. 13 = _____
16. 0.99 = _____

Chapter Capsule

The section repeats the objectives from the beginning of the chapter and then provides a summary of the most important concepts for that objective. Use this section as a quick review and to check your knowledge.

Objective 1: Describe the difference between Arabic numbers and Roman numerals.

■ Arabic—use numbers, decimals, and fractions to express values
■ Roman—use letters that represent number values

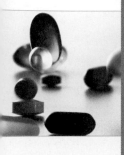

Objective 2: Convert an improper fraction to a mixed fraction.

- 5/3—5 is the numerator and 3 is the denominator
- To convert it to a mixed fraction, divide the numerator by the denominator
- Answers: 1 and 2/3

Objective 3: Add fractions having the same denominator.

- 1/4 + 2/4 = 3/4
- 2/5 + 2/5 = 4/5
- 3/10 + 6/10 = 9/10

Objective 4: Subtract fractions having the same denominator.

- 8/12 − 7/12 = 1/12
- 9/20 − 6/20 = 3/20
- 27/45 − 19/45 = 8/45

Objective 5: Multiply fractions and mixed fractions.

- 1/4 × 1-3/4 = 1/4 × 7/4 = 7/16
- 3/10 × 2-7/10 = 3/10 × 27/10 = 81/100
- 3/7 × 1-2/7 = 3/7 × 9/7 = 27/49

Objective 6: Divide fractions and mixed fractions.

- 1-1/12 ÷ 9/12 = 13/12 × 12/9 = 156/108 = 1-48/108 = 1-4/9
- 2-1/3 ÷ 2/3 = 7/3 × 3/2 = 21/6 = 7/2 = 3-1/2
- 5-1/2 ÷ 1/2 = 11/2 × 2/1 = 22/2 = 11

Objective 7: Add, subtract, multiply, and divide decimals.

- 0.2 + 7.13 + 3.067 = 10.397
- 9.77 − 2.9 − 1.38 = 5.49
- 1.6 × 0.77 × 7.1 = 8.7472
- 12.33 ÷ 3.6 ÷ 1.5 = 2.283333 = (rounds to 2.283)

Objective 8: Define ratios, proportions, and percents.

- Ratios—compare one number to another, or express a part of a whole number; example: 3:4 means *three parts to four parts*
- Proportions—express a relationship of equality between two ratios; example: 1:4 :: 3:12 means the relationship of 1 to 4 is the same as the relationship of 3 to 12
- Percents—mean *hundredths*; may also be expressed as a fraction, a decimal, or a ratio; example: 40% means *40 parts per hundred*, or 40/100

Internet Sites of Interest

- Get online help with math calculations at S.O.S. Math's site: **www.sosmath.com**
- On The Math Page, you can click on a chapter in an online textbook to find instructions and plenty of examples for the arithmetic or algebra problem that is confounding you. Find help at: **www.themathpage.com**
- The hot subjects fractions, decimals, and percents are covered by clicking on the topic at: **www.math.com**

Chapter Objectives

After completing this chapter, you should be able to:

1. Name the basic units of the metric system for weight, volume, and length.
2. Understand metric abbreviations used in the pharmacy and clinical settings.
3. Identify major apothecary and household measurement system units.
4. Discuss milliequivalents and international units.
5. Convert units of measure to equivalent units of measure within the same system of measurement.
6. Recognize the difference between the Celsius and Fahrenheit temperature scales.

Chapter 6

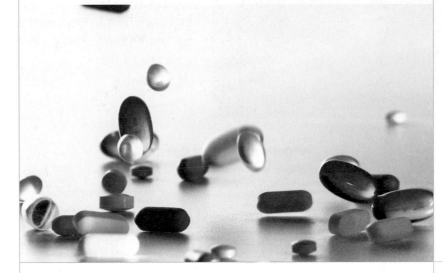

Measurement Systems and Their Equivalents

Key Terms

Apothecary system (ah-PAW-thuh-keh-ree) (page 111)
Drams (page 111)
Grain (page 111)
Gram (page 108)

Household system (page 112)
International Units (page 113)
Liter (LEE-ter) (page 108)
Meter (MEE-ter) (page 108)
Metric system (page 108)

Milliequivalents (mil-lee-KWIH-vuh-lentz) (page 113)
Minims (MIH-numz) (page 111)
Ounces (page 108)
Unit (page 108)

PRACTICAL SCENARIO

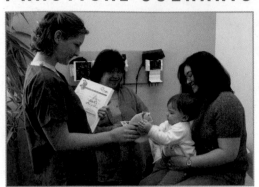

Tara is a 7-month-old girl who is brought to her doctor's office by her mother. Her body temperature is 103.4°F. Her pediatrician orders acetaminophen 7 mL every 4 hours while her fever is above 101°F. You, the medical assistant, advise Tara's mother about carefully following the physician's order. Tara's mother, who grew up in England, asks you if you can convert the temperature of 101°F into Celsius degrees and you agree to do this for her.

Critical Thinking Questions

1. Which formula should you use to convert 101°F into Celsius degrees?
2. What is the answer that you give to Tara's mother?
3. What type of measuring instrument should you instruct Tara's mother to use?

Introduction

Health-care professionals who deal with administration of medications prescribed for patients must ensure the accuracy and correctness of drug dosages. They must have a complete knowledge of the weights and measures used in drug administration for prescribed amounts.

Units of Measure

Three systems of measurement are used in pharmacology and the calculation of drug dosages: (1) metric, (2) apothecary, and (3) household. Today, however, household and apothecary measures such as teaspoons and **ounces** (equivalent to 480 grains or 31.10349 grams) are used less commonly. The most common, most accurate, and safest system of measurement in all countries is the **metric system**, a system based on the decimal system. Medications are administered with three parameters in mind: (1) weight, (2) volume, and (3) length. Weight is the most used parameter and is essential as a dosage **unit** (a unit is defined as a standard of measure, weight, or any other similar quality). Measurement of volume is the next most important parameter and is used for liquids. Length is the least used parameter for dosage calculations.

METRIC SYSTEM

The basic units of weight and volume in the metric system are based on the number "10" as in the decimal system. The metric system uses the basic units of **gram** (g) as the unit of weight (equivalent to 15.432358 grains), **liter** (L) as the unit of volume (equivalent to 1.056688 quarts), and **meter** (m) as the unit of length (equivalent to 39.37007874 inches). In medicine, it is common to use weight for determining medication doses based in kilograms and volume to express liquid amounts. Parts of these basic units are named by adding prefixes that describe multiples or fractions of the standard measures for weight, volume, and length based on units of 10. The prefixes usually relate to Latin and Greek measures. Table 6-1 ■ shows Latin prefixes. Table 6-2 ■ shows Greek prefixes.

Table 6-1 ■ Latin Prefixes

PREFIX*	VALUE	EQUIVALENTS
micro- (mc):	1/1,000,000	= 0.000001
milli- (m):	1/1,000	= 0.001
centi- (c):	1/100	= 0.01
deci- (d):	1/10	= 0.1

*Remember: Latin prefixes denote fractions.

Table 6-2 ■ Greek Prefixes

PREFIX*	VALUE
deca- (da):	10
hecto- (h):	100
kilo- (k):	1,000
mega- (M):	1,000,000

*Remember: Greek prefixes denote multiples.

A system for international standardization of metric units was established throughout the world in 1960 with the introduction of the International System, or SI (from the French *Système International*). Table 6-3 ■ shows SI standardized abbreviation.

Table 6-3 ■ SI Standardized Abbreviations (Metric System)

PARAMETER	UNIT	ABBREVIATION	EQUIVALENTS
Weight	gram (basic unit)	g	1 g = 1,000 mg
	milligram	mg	1 mg = 1,000 mcg = 0.001 g
	microgram	mcg	1 mcg = 0.001 mg = 0.000001 g
	kilogram	kg	1 kg = 1,000 g
Volume	liter (basic unit)	L	1 L = 1,000 mL
	milliliter	mL	1 mL = 1 cc* = 0.001 L
Length	meter (basic unit)	m	1 m = 100 cm = 1,000 mm
	centimeter	cm	1 cm = 0.01 m = 10 mm
	millimeter	mm	1 mm = 0.001 m = 0.1 cm

*Abbreviation should not be used in clinical practice to avoid medication errors.

✳ Apply Your Knowledge 6.1

The following questions focus on what you have just learned about the metric system. *See Appendix E for the correct answers.*

FILL IN THE BLANK

Rewrite the following metric numbers using numerals and abbreviations and fill in the blanks.

1. Twenty-five grams _____

2. Eight milliliters _____

3. Fifty-five hundredths of a milligram _____

4. One hundred micrograms _____

5. Seven and two-tenths micrograms _____

6. Sixteen liters _____

7. Two thousand milliliters _____

8. Four meters _____

9. Nineteen millimeters _____

10. Three and one-half centimeters _____

MULTIPLE CHOICE

Select the correct answer from choices a–d.

1. The metric system is based on which of the following?
   a. Units
   b. Fractions
   c. Decimals
   d. Proportions

2. Which of the following is the least utilized parameter for dosage calculations?
   a. Volume
   b. Length
   c. Unit
   d. Weight

3. In medicine, it is common to use weight for determining medication doses in which of the following increments?
   a. Ounces
   b. Kilograms
   c. Pounds
   d. International Units

4. The abbreviation for the International System is:
   a. INS
   b. IS
   c. SI
   d. SIN

5. The value of the prefix "hecto" is:
   a. 10
   b. 100
   c. 1,000
   d. 1,000,000

APOTHECARY SYSTEM

The **apothecary system** is a very old English system that has slowly been replaced by the metric system. The apothecary system uses **minims** (the basic unit of volume), **drams** (fluidrams—equivalent to 1/8 ounce), ounces (fluidounces), pints, quarts, and gallons to measure volume. It measures weight by grains, drams, ounces, and pounds. The apothecary system also uses Roman numerals to indicate the amount of drug. The basic unit of weight is the **grain**. Today, the apothecary system is used for only a few drugs, such as acetaminophen, aspirin, and phenobarbital. Table 6-4 ■ shows common apothecary equivalents.

Table 6-4 ■ Apothecary System

PARAMETER	UNIT	ABBREVIATION	EQUIVALENTS
Weight	grain	gr	
	dram	dr or ʒ*	
	ounce	oz or ʒ*	1 oz
	pound	lb	1 lb = 16 oz = 7000 (gr)
Volume	minim	M or ɱ*	
	fluidram	fl dr	
	fluidounce	ʒ*	pti = ʒ* 16
	pint	pt	qti = ʒ* 32
	quart	qt	qti = pt ii
	gallon	gal	

*Abbreviation should not be used in clinical practice to avoid medication errors.

Note: There are no essential equivalents of weight or length to learn for this system.

✳ Apply Your Knowledge 6.2

The following questions focus on what you have just learned about the apothecary system of measurements. *See Appendix E for the correct answers.*

FILL IN THE BLANK
Select abbreviations or symbols for the apothecary system to fill in the blanks.

1. fluidounce _____

2. grain _____

3. dram _____

4. quart _____

5. pint _____

6. minim _____

HOUSEHOLD SYSTEM

The **household system** is used in most American homes. This system of measurement is important for a patient at home who has no knowledge of the metric or apothecary systems. However, household measurements, consisting of teaspoons and tablespoons, are not precisely accurate, so they should never be used in the medical setting. The only household units of measurement used to measure drugs are units of volume. These include the drop, teaspoon, tablespoon, ounce (fluid), cup, pint, quart, and gallon. Table 6-5 ■ shows common household units, abbreviations, and equivalents.

Table 6-5 ■ Household Measurements

UNIT	ABBREVIATION	EQUIVALENTS
drop	gtt	15 gtt = 1 mL
teaspoon	t (tsp)	1 tsp = 5 mL
tablespoon	T (or tbs)	1 T = 3t
ounce (fluid)	oz	2 T = 1 oz
cup	cup	1 cup = 8 oz
pint	pt	1 pt = 2 cups
quart	qt	1 qt = 4 cups = 2 pt
gallon	gal	4 qt

Note: Cups, quarts, and gallons are commonly used to measure medications.

✳ Apply Your Knowledge 6.3

The following exercises focus on what you have just learned about conversions among measurement systems. *See Appendix E for the correct answers.*

FILL IN THE BLANK
Select terms from your reading to fill in the blanks.

1. How many cups equal 2 pints? _____
2. Forty-five teaspoons are equivalent to how many tablespoons? _____
3. How many cups are equivalent to 8 ounces? _____
4. How many teaspoons are equivalent to 1 ounce? _____
5. How many drops are equivalent to 2 tablespoons? _____
6. How many tablespoons are equivalent to 1 ounce? _____
7. How many pints are equivalent to 8 cups? _____
8. How many ounces are equivalent to 4 tablespoons? _____
9. A meter is a metric unit that measures _____.
10. A liter is a metric unit that measures _____.
11. A gram is a metric unit that measures _____.
12. 3 cups = _____ oz
13. 220 drops = _____ tsp

MILLIEQUIVALENT MEASURES AND INTERNATIONAL UNITS

Milliequivalents and units are measurements used to indicate the strength of certain drugs. Pharmacists and chemists define *milliequivalent* measures as an expression of the number of grams of equivalent weight of a drug contained in 1 mL of a normal solution. Electrolytes, such as sodium and potassium, are usually measured in milliequivalents (mEq). Examples of drugs that are ordered by prescribers in milliequivalents include potassium chloride, sodium bicarbonate, and sodium chloride. Because the dosage is individualized, there are no calculations involved.

Units mainly measure the potency of heparin, insulin, penicillin, and some vitamins. A unit is the amount of a medication required to produce a specific effect. The size of a unit varies for each drug. Vitamins are measured in standardized units called **International Units**. These International Units show the amount of drug required to produce a certain effect, but they are standardized by international agreement. The International Unit does not measure a medication in terms of its physical weight or volume. Units and milliequivalents cannot be directly converted into the metric, apothecary, or household systems.

Conversion Within and Between Systems

Drug doses are usually ordered in metric system amounts such as grams, milligrams, liters, and milliliters. Sometimes you need to convert drug dosages between the metric, apothecary, and household systems of measurement. First, you must know how the measure of a quantity in one system compares with its measure in another system. For example, you learned the relationships between gram and kilogram; milliliter and liter; and teaspoon and tablespoon. To convert between systems, you may also need to know the relationship between milliliter and teaspoon. For example, 1 tsp = 5 mL, or 1 kg = 1,000 g. Most prescriptions and medication orders are written in the metric system. Medications are usually ordered in a unit of weight measurement such as grams or grains. You must be able to convert between units of measurement within the same system or convert units of measurement from one system to another. Table 6-6 ∎ summarizes equivalent measures for volume in three different systems.

Table 6-6 ∎ Approximate Equivalents for Volume and Weight

	METRIC	APOTHECARY	HOUSEHOLD
Volume	5 mL	1 dr	1 tsp
	15 mL	3 or 4 dr	1 T
	30 mL	1 oz	2 T = 1 oz
	240 mL	8 oz	8 oz = 1 cup
	480 mL	16 oz	2 cups = 1 pt
	960 mL	32 oz	2 pt = 1 qt
Weight	1 mg	gr 1/60	
	15 mg	gr 1/4	
	30 mg	gr ss (1/2 grain)	
	60 mg	gr i (1 grain)	
	0.5 g	gr vii ss (7-1/2 grains)	
	1 g (1,000 mg)	2.2 lb, gr xv, 15 grains	
	1 kg	220 lbs	

✱ Apply Your Knowledge 6.4

The following questions focus on what you have just learned about conversion between different systems for volume and weight. *See Appendix E for the correct answers.*

FILL IN THE BLANK
Convert the following amounts and fill in the blanks.

1. 5 L = _____ oz
2. 0.25 L = _____ oz
3. 20 oz = _____ L
4. 12 oz = _____ L
5. 4 oz = _____ mL
6. 8-1/2 oz = _____ mL
7. 1/2 oz = _____ mL
8. 60 mL = _____ oz
9. 150 mL = _____ oz
10. 15 mL = _____ oz
11. 5 g = _____ gr

12. 0.5 g = _____ gr
13. 0.1 g = _____ gr
14. 3 gr = _____ g
15. 1-1/2 gr = _____ g
16. 4 gr = _____ mg
17. 1-1/2 gr = _____ mg
18. 7-1/2 gr = _____ mg
19. 150 mg = _____ gr
20. 30 mg = _____ gr
21. 15 mg = _____ gr

TEMPERATURE CONVERSION

Two common scales of temperature are used throughout the world: Celsius (Centigrade) and Fahrenheit scales. The Fahrenheit scale is still used in the United States; the Celsius scale is used in most other parts of the world. The abbreviation used in the Fahrenheit scale is an "F", and in the Celsius scale, it is a "C."

Water freezes at 32°F and at 0°C. This difference of 32° is used in converting temperature from one scale to the other. It can also be determined that water boils at 212°F and at 100°C.

There is a 180° difference between the freezing and boiling points on the Fahrenheit scale and a 100° difference between these two points on the Celsius scale. The difference between the boiling point and the freezing point on the Fahrenheit scale and the Celsius scale can be set as a ratio of each Celsius degree being 9/5 times greater than each Fahrenheit degree, as seen in the following formula:

$$180:100 = \frac{180}{100} = \frac{9}{5}$$

If the fraction 9/5 is expressed as a decimal, it can be stated that each Celsius degree is 1.8 times greater than each Fahrenheit degree. To convert a given temperature from one scale to the other, you may use one of the following formulas:

$$°F = 1.8°C + 32$$

$$°F = 9/5°C + 32$$

Example: Convert 100°C to Fahrenheit:

°F = 1.8 × 100°C + 32	°F = 9/5 × 100°C + 32
°F = 180 + 32	°F = 180 + 32
°F = 212	°F = 212

Example: Convert 212°F to Celsius:
(Note: Subtract 32 from both sides of the equation.)

$$212°F = 1.8°C + 32$$
$$212°F - 32 = 1.8°C + 32 - 32$$
$$180°F = 1.8°C$$
$$°C = 100$$

or

$$212°F = 9/5°C + 32$$
$$212°F - 32 = 9/5°C + 32 - 32$$
$$180°F = 9/5°C$$
$$°C = 180°F ÷ 9/5$$
$$°C = 180°F × 5/9$$
$$°C = 100°F$$

Figure 6-1 ■ indicates that water freezes at 32°F and at 0°C.

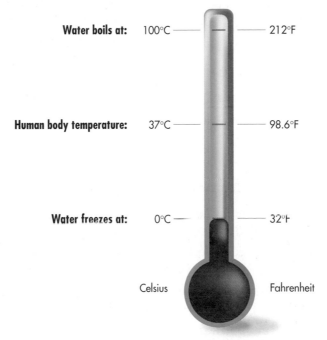

Water boils at: 100°C ———— 212°F

Human body temperature: 37°C ———— 98.6°F

Water freezes at: 0°C ———— 32°F

Celsius   Fahrenheit

Figure 6-1 ■ Thermometer showing the temperatures at which water freezes (0°C and 32°F).

✳ Apply Your Knowledge 6.5

The following questions focus on what you have just learned about temperature conversions. *See Appendix E for the correct answers.*

FILL IN THE BLANK
Convert to the Celsius or Fahrenheit scale and fill in the blanks.

1. 13°C _____
2. 21°C _____
3. 34°C _____
4. 45°C _____
5. 67°C _____
6. 97°C _____
7. 99.9°C _____

8. 106°C _____
9. 38°F _____
10. 52°F _____
11. 76°F _____
12. 98°F _____
13. 104°F _____
14. −16°F _____

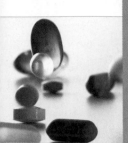

Chapter Capsule

This section repeats the objectives from the beginning of the chapter and then provides a summary of the most important concepts for that objective. Use this section as a quick review and to check your knowledge.

Objective 1: Name the basic units of the metric system for weight, volume, and length.

- Weight—gram (g)
- Volume—liter (L)
- Length—meter (m)

Objective 2: Understand metric abbreviations used in the pharmacy and clinical settings.

- Grams (g)
- Milligrams (mg)
- Micrograms (mcg)
- Kilograms (kg)
- Liters (L)
- Milliliters (mL)

Objective 3: Identify major apothecary and household measurement system units.

- Apothecary—minims, drams (fluidrams), ounces (fluidounces), pints, quarts, gallons, grains, drams, pounds
- Household—drops, teaspoons, tablespoons, ounces (fluid), cups, pints, quarts, gallons

Objective 4: Discuss milliequivalents and international units.

- Milliequivalents and units are measurements used to indicate the strength of certain drugs.
- Milliequivalent measures are defined as expressions of the number of grams of equivalent weight of a drug contained in 1 mL of a normal solution.
- Electrolytes, such as sodium and potassium, are usually measured in milliequivalents.
- Other drugs ordered in milliequivalents include potassium chloride, sodium bicarbonate, and sodium chloride.
- Units mainly measure the potency of heparin, insulin, penicillin, and some vitamins.
- A unit is the amount of a medication required to produce a specific effect, and the size of a unit varies for each drug.
- Vitamins are measured in standardized units (per international agreement) called International Units.
- International Units do not measure a medication in terms of its physical weight or volume.

Objective 5: Convert units of measure to equivalent units of measure within the same system of measurement.

- For example: 1 kg = 1,000 g; 1 g = 1,000 mg; 1 mg = 1,000 mcg
- 1 L = 1,000 mL
- 1 m = 1,000 mm; 1 cm = 10 mm
- 1 lb = 16 oz = 7,000 gr
- 1 pt = 16 fluidounces
- 2 pt = 1 qt
- 1 T = 3 tsp

- 2 T = 1 oz
- 1 cup = 8 oz

Objective 6: Recognize the difference between the Celsius and Fahrenheit temperature scales.

- Celsius—used in most parts of the world besides the United States; abbreviation for Celsius is C; water freezes at 0°C; water boils at 100°C

- Fahrenheit—used in the United States; abbreviation for Fahrenheit is F; water freezes at 32°F; water boils at 212°F; °F = 1.8°C + 32; or °F = 9/5°C + 32

Internet Sites of Interest

- A conversion calculator for length, weight, pressure, volume, and temperature can be found at this Web site: **www.worldwidemetric.com/Measurements.html**

- For a quick check of common weights and measures used by pharmacy technicians and other medical professionals, visit: **http://www.rxtrek.net/weights.htm**

- Click on the appropriate calculator at: **www.sciencelab.com/data/conversion.shtml** and convert between different units of measure for weight and mass, metric weight, temperature, length, distance, volume, speed, pressure, area, force, energy, frequency, power, torque, and astronomical units.

Chapter 7

Dosage Calculations

Key Terms

PRACTICAL SCENARIO

A physician orders a medication in the amount of 250 mg per 5 mL for a patient's upper respiratory tract infection. Prior to dispensing, the medical assistant calculated the amount of medication required as 125 mg/mL. This would have meant the patient might have received 625 mg/5 mL instead of what the physician ordered. A second person in the medical office checked the calculation and found the error prior to administration. Therefore, it is essential for allied health-care professionals to accurately calculate dosage calculations, and always consult another coworker or physician to verify accuracy.

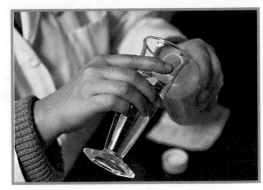

PhotoDisc/GettyImages

Critical Thinking Questions

1. What information did the medical assistant need to know before doing her calculation?
2. What is the formula the medical assistant should have used to calculate the proper dosage?
3. Besides checking that the dosage calculation was right, what other "rights" does the assistant need to check?

Introduction

The ability to accurately calculate drug dosages is an essential skill in health care. Serious harm to patients may result from a mathematical error during a calculation and the subsequent administration of a drug dosage. It is the responsibility of those administering drugs to carry out medical orders precisely and efficiently.

General Dosage Calculations

The *dose* of a drug is the amount a patient takes for the intended therapeutic effect, and the *dosage regimen* is the schedule of dosing for a drug. Many factors contribute to determining the dose and dosage regimen, including potency of the drug and route of administration, as well as patient factors such as weight, disease state, and tolerance. A *loading dose* may be required for some drugs to produce an adequate blood level that yields the desired therapeutic effect; this dose then would be followed by smaller *maintenance doses* to maintain an adequate blood level. A *prophylactic dose* of a drug may be given to prevent a disease, but a *therapeutic dose*, which is usually higher than the prophylactic dose, is given to treat an ongoing disease. The dose for most drugs is given in units of weight (for example, 500 mg), but the dose for some drugs, such as biologics, is given based on activity.

The doses for many drugs, such as antihypertensives, are general and usually not patient-specific. However, the doses for some drugs require patient data such as body surface area, clinical laboratory values, or pharmacokinetic parameters.

It is the health-care professional's responsibility to ensure that the patient receives the proper dose of medication, and to educate the patient about the proper measurement of doses. For solid-dosage forms, the correct dose is easily administered in premeasured tablets or capsules. If the drug is a liquid, however, the dose is usually a volume that must be accurately measured using a standardized 5-mL teaspoon, **calibrated** dropper (a dropper that is marked with graduated measurements), or syringe. If the pharmacist compounds a specific product for a patient, it is also his or her responsibility to ensure that the correct amount of drug is delivered in each dose.

As a health-care professional, you must also be familiar with the following terms to understand dosage calculations:

✳ Amount to administer—The volume of a medication that contains the desired dose; the number of tablets (or milliliters of a solution) administered once to provide the desired amount of a drug.

✳ **Desired dose**—The amount to be administered at one time. It must be in the same unit of measurement as the dosage unit.

✳ Dosage ordered—The total amount of ordered drug, along with the frequency it is to be administered. Its measurement units may not be the same as the dosage unit.

✳ Dosage strength—The dose on hand, per the dosage unit. If the dose on hand is 100 mg per capsule and the dosage unit is 1 capsule, the dosage strength is 100 mg/capsule.

✳ Dosage unit—The volume of medication that contains a quantity of drug as listed on the drug label. If a drug contains 50 mg of drug per capsule, the dosage unit is 1 capsule.

✳ Dose on hand—The amount of drug in a dosage unit. If a drug has 150 mg of drug per capsule, the dose on hand is 150 mg.

Calculating Dosages

The first step in computing medication dosage, regardless of the method used, is to make certain the strength of the drug ordered and the strength of the drug available are in the same unit of measure. If necessary, **conversion** (changing) to a single unit must be carried out. Once this is done, the problem can be set up using the formula:

$$\frac{D}{H} \times Q = X$$

The answer is most commonly signified by the letter X. In this formula, D represents the desired dosage of the drug to be administered. H represents the dosage of the drug available. D and H must always be in the same unit of measure. Q represents the number of tablets, capsules, milliliters, minims, and so forth that contains the available dosage. X represents the number of tablets, capsules, milliliters, minims, and so on of the desired dose (the amount to be administered). Q and X must always be in the same unit of measure. Make certain that all the terms in the formula are labeled with the correct units of measure.

Several formulas can be used to calculate drug dosages. One formula uses ratios:

$$\frac{\text{Dose on hand } (H)}{\text{Quantity on hand } (Q)} = \frac{\text{Desired dose } (D)}{\text{Quantity desired } (X)}$$

Example

Amoxil 500 mg is ordered. It is supplied in a liquid form containing 250 mg in 5 mL. To calculate the dosage, use the formula:

$$\frac{250 \text{ mg } (H)}{5 \text{ mL } (Q)} = \frac{500 \text{ mg } (D)}{X}$$

Then, cross-multiply:

$$250 X = 5 \text{ mL} \times 500 \text{ mg}$$

$$X = \frac{5 \times 500}{250}$$

Therefore, the dose ordered is 10 mL.

You can also use the formula above to calculate dosages:

$$\text{Amount to administer } (X) = \frac{\text{Desired dose } (D)}{\text{Dose on hand } (H)} \times \text{Quantity on hand } (Q)$$

Example

Heparin, an anticoagulant, is often distributed in vials, in prepared **dilutions** (less concentrated mixtures) of 10,000 units/mL. If the order calls for 2,500 units, you can use the previous formula to calculate, as follows:

$$X = \frac{2,500 \text{ units}}{10,000 \text{ units/mL}} \times 1$$

$$X = 0.25 \text{ or } 1/4 \text{ mL}$$

✵ Apply Your Knowledge 7.1

The following questions focus on what you have just learned about general dosage calculations. *See Appendix E for the correct answers.*

MATCHING

Match the lettered terms to the numbered descriptions. The lettered terms may be used more than once.

DESCRIPTION	TERM
1. _____ The amount to be administered at one time	a. Dosage unit
2. _____ The amount of drug in a dosage unit	b. Dosage strength
3. _____ The volume of medication that contains a quantity of drug	c. Dosage ordered
	d. Desired dose
4. _____ The volume of a medication that contains the desired dose	e. Dose on hand
	f. Amount to administer
5. _____ The total amount of ordered drug, along with the frequency it is to be administered	
6. _____ The dose on hand per the dosage unit	

DRUG DOSAGE CALCULATIONS

Calculate the drug dosages.

1. Ordered: cimetidine (Tagamet) 0.2 g PO qid

   On hand: Tagamet 400 mg is available

   How many tablet(s) would you administer per dose? _____

2. Ordered: methyldopa (Aldomet) 150 mg PO tid

   On hand: Aldomet 250 mg/5 mL is available

   How many milliliters would you administer per dose? _____

3. Ordered: lorazepam (Ativan) 1 mg PO tid

   On hand: Ativan 0.5 mg is available

   How many tablet(s) would you administer? _____

4. Ordered: clarithromycin (Biaxin) 100 mg PO qid

   On hand: Biaxin 125 mg/5 mL is available

   How many milliliters (mL) should the patient receive per dose? _____

Calculating Oral Dosages

Oral medications are divided into solid types (such as tablets and capsules) and liquids. The *tablet* is the most common form of solid oral medication. Certain tablets are specially designed to be administered sublingually (under the tongue), or buccally (between the cheek and gum). Some tablets are chewable; others dissolve in water to make a liquid that the patient can drink. Always check the drug label to find out how a tablet is meant to be administered. *Capsules* are usually oval-shaped gelatin shells that contain medication in powder or granule form.

SOLID DOSES

Tablets may be broken into parts only if they are **scored** (notched), and they must be broken only along the line of the scoring. Unscored tablets must *not* be broken into parts.

Before administering medication to a patient, you need to determine how many tablets or capsules will deliver the *desired dose*. If necessary, convert the *dosage ordered* to the *desired dose*, using the same unit of measurement as the dose on hand. Then, you can calculate the *amount to administer* by using the fraction proportion method.

$$\frac{\text{Dose on hand } (H)}{\text{Dosage unit } (Q)} = \frac{\text{Desired dose } (D)}{\text{Amount to administer}}$$

or

$$\text{Desired dose } (D) \times \frac{\text{Dosage unit } (Q)}{\text{Dose on hand } (H)} = \text{Amount to administer}$$

Example 1

Ordered: Zocor 40 mg bid

On hand: Zocor 20 mg tablets

The dosage ordered is 40 mg, the dose on hand is 20 mg, and the dosage unit is 1 tablet. The units of the dosage ordered and the dose on hand are the same, so no conversion is needed. The desired dose is 40 mg.

Use the formula:

$$D \times \frac{Q}{H} = X$$

$$40 \text{ mg} \times \frac{1 \text{ tablet}}{20 \text{ mg}} = X$$

$$X = 2 \text{ tablets}$$

Example 2

Ordered: Cardura 8 mg PO daily

The label is shown in Figure 7-1 ■. How many capsules will you administer to the patient?

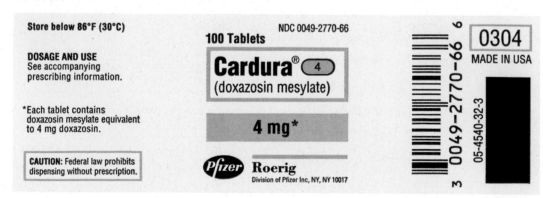

Figure 7-1 ■ Drug label for Cardura.

Reproduced with permission of Pfizer Inc. All rights reserved.

Use the formula:

$$D \times \frac{Q}{H} = X$$

$$8 \text{ mg} \times \frac{1 \text{ tablet}}{4 \text{ mg}} = 2 \text{ tablet}$$

Example 3
Ordered: Norvasc 5 mg PO daily
The label is shown in Figure 7-2 ▪. How many tablets will you administer to the patient?

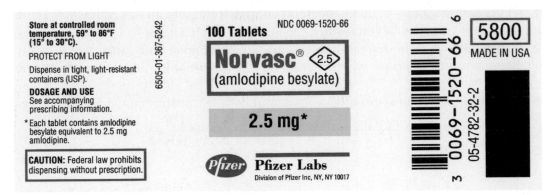

Figure 7-2 ▪ Drug label for Norvasc.
Reproduced with permission of Pfizer Inc. All rights reserved.

Use the formula:

$$D \times \frac{Q}{H} = X$$

$$5 \text{ mg} \times \frac{1}{2.5 \text{ mg}} = X$$

$$\frac{5}{2.5} = 2 \text{ tablets}$$

Focus on Pediatrics

Administering Medicine to Young Children

Dosage cups are convenient for children who know how to drink from a cup without spilling, but for children who can't drink from a cup, the following options are available:

- ▪ *Syringes* are convenient for infants who cannot drink from a cup. A parent can squirt the medicine into the back of the child's mouth, where it is less likely to spill out, or can measure out a dosage for a babysitter to use with the child later.

- ▪ *Droppers* are safe and easy to use with pediatric patients, but must be measured at eye level and administered quickly to avoid losing any of the medication.

- ▪ *Cylindrical dosing spoons* have long handles that can be held easily by small children with small cups that fit easily into their mouths.

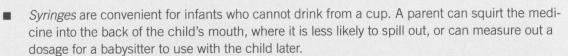

Liquid Doses

Liquid medications can be measured in small units of volume. Therefore, a greater range of dosages can be ordered and administered. They are commonly used for children and elderly patients. Liquid medications can also be given via feeding tubes. Many medications are given as liquids, which are supplied initially as powders. Liquid preparations are drugs that have been dissolved or suspended. Examples of liquid drugs are syrups, spirits, elixirs, suspensions, and so on. Liquid drugs can be administered systemically by mouth or by injection throughout the body.

Three measuring devices used in the administration of oral medications are:

1. The measuring cup—calibrated in fluid ounces, fluidrams, cubic centimeters, milliliters, teaspoons, or tablespoons.

2. The medicine dropper/oral syringe—medicine droppers are calibrated in milliliters, minims, or drops, whereas oral syringes are usually calibrated in cubic centimeters.

3. The calibrated spoon—usually calibrated in both teaspoons and cubic centimeters.

To calculate oral liquid doses, this formula can be used:

$$D \times \frac{H}{Q} = X$$

Example 1

The physician orders 400 mg of the antibiotic cefdinir (Omnicef). Figure 7-3 ■ shows the availability of the drug. Calculate how many milliliters you will administer.

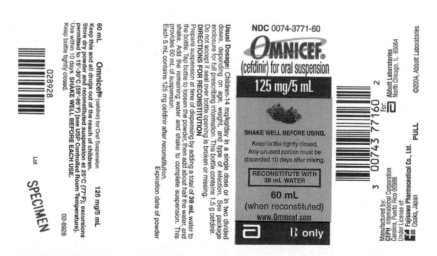

Figure 7-3 ■ Drug label for Omnicef.
Reproduced with permission of Abbott Laboratories.

The label on the bottle indicates that 5 mL contains 125 mg of cefdinir. Therefore,

$$\frac{5 \text{ mL}}{125 \text{ mg}}$$

$$400 \times \frac{5}{125} = \frac{2,000}{125} = 16 \text{ mL}$$

Example 2

The pediatrician orders EryPed 200 (erythromycin) 375 mg. Figure 7-4 ■ shows the availability of this drug. Calculate how many milliliters you will administer.

Figure 7-4 ■ Drug label for EryPed 200.
Reproduced with permission of Abbott Laboratories.

$$375 \times \frac{5 \text{ mL}}{200} = \frac{1,875}{200} = 9.375 \text{ mL} = 9.4 \text{ mL}$$

Focus on Geriatrics

New Medication-Dispensing Systems Help Elderly Patients

Advances in communication and artificial intelligence are examples of the ways that medication-dispensing systems are improving care for elderly patients. Some systems help to manage home administration of complex, multiple drug regimens by offering "smart" bottles arranged on a tray that alert the patient when it is time to take a medication. The bottles release the correct amount of medication dosages and offer a self-locking feature to prevent accidental overdose. When supplies get low, the system alerts the pharmacist or caregiver. A complete record of all medications dispensed is retained by the system for future reference.

✳ Apply Your Knowledge 7.2

The following questions assess your knowledge about calculating oral drug doses. *See Appendix E for the correct answers.*

LABELING
Calculate the drug dosages using the labels shown.

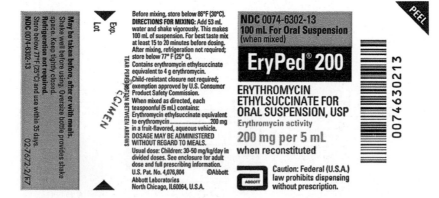

Reproduced with permission of Abbott laboratories.

1. Erythromycin (EryPed 200) 245 mg = _____ mL

(continued)

Apply Your Knowledge 7.2 (continued)

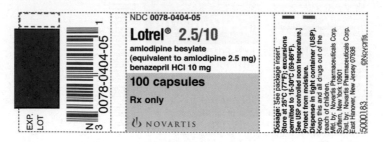

Copyright Novartis Pharmaceuticals Corporation. Reprinted with permission.

2. Amlodipine (Lotrel) 7.5 mg = _____ cap

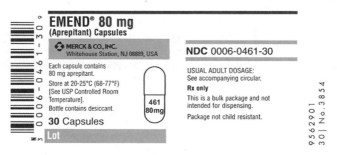

The label for the product Emend 80 mg is reproduced with permission of Merck & Co., Inc., copyright owner.

3. Aprepitant (Emend) 240 mg = _____ cap

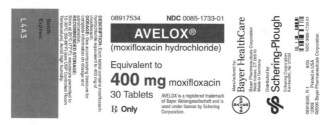

Reproduced with Permission from Bayer

4. Moxifloxacin (Avelox) 0.08 g = _____ tab

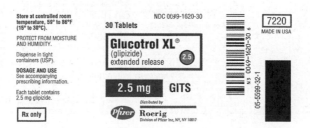

Reproduced with permission of Pfizer Inc. All rights reserved.

5. Glipizide (Glucotrol XL) 0.01 g = _____ tab

DRUG DOSAGE CALCULATIONS

Calculate the solid or liquid doses to be administered.

1. Ordered: nifedipine (Procardia) 20 mg PO tid

   On hand: Procardia 10 mg is available

   How many capsule(s) would you administer? _____

2. Ordered: levothyroxine (Synthroid) 0.3 mg PO daily

   On hand: Synthroid 0.15 mg is available

   How many tablet(s) would you administer? _____

3. Ordered: Keflex 500 mg PO bid

   On hand: Keflex 250 mg/5 mL

   How many milliliters would you administer per dose? _____

4. Ordered: Augmentin 1 g PO bid

   On hand: Augmentin 400 mg/5 mL is available

   How many milliliters would you administer per dose? _____

5. Ordered: Singulair 5 mg PO daily

   On hand: Singulair 5 mg is available

   How many tablet(s) would you administer per dose? _____

Calculating Parenteral Medications

Injections are mixtures that contain the drug dissolved in an appropriate liquid. Medication can be administered by injection intradermally (within the skin), subcutaneously (into fatty tissue under the skin), intramuscularly (IM, into the muscle), and intravenously (IV, into the vein). Such **injectable** medications are prescribed in grams, milligrams, micrograms, grains, or units. The injectable drugs can be prepared in packages as solvents (diluents or solutions) or in powdered form. Drug solutions for injection are commercially premixed and stored in vials and ampules for immediate use.

INTRADERMAL INJECTION

An intradermal injection is usually used for skin testing to diagnose the cause of an allergy or to determine the presence of a microorganism. The common syringe that is used for intradermal testing is the tuberculin syringe with a 25-gauge needle.

The inner portion of the forearm is usually used for diagnostic testing because there is less hair in the area, and the test results are more visible. The upper back may also be used as a testing site. Test results are read 48 to 72 hours after the intradermal injection. A reddened or raised area is a positive reaction.

SUBCUTANEOUS INJECTION

Drugs injected into the subcutaneous tissue are absorbed slowly because there are fewer blood vessels in fatty tissue. The amount of drug solution administered subcutaneously is generally 0.5 to 1 mL at a 45-degree angle.

The two types of syringes used for subcutaneous injections are the tuberculin syringe (1 mL), calibrated in 0.1-mL and 0.01-mL increments, and the 3-mL syringe, calibrated in 0.1-mL increments. To calculate dosages for subcutaneous or IM injections, use the basic formula of $D/H \times V$, or the ratio and proportion method. Heparin is a drug commonly administered subcutaneously.

Medications given by IM injection are absorbed more rapidly than those given by subcutaneous injection. The volume of solution for IM injections is 0.5 to 3.0 mL. For calculating intramuscular dosages, the following example can be used:

Example 1
Ordered: gentamicin 60 mg IM
On hand: gentamicin is available 80 mg/2 mL in a vial
To calculate, the following formula is used:

$$\frac{D}{H} \times V = \frac{60}{80} \times 2 = \frac{120}{80} = 1.5 \text{ mL}$$

Or

$$H : V :: D : X$$

$$80 \text{ mg} : 2 \text{ mL} :: 60 \text{ mg} : X \text{ mL}$$

$$80\,X = 120$$

$$X = \frac{120}{80} = 1.5 \text{ mL}$$

Example 2
Ordered: atropine 0.2 mg subcutaneously Stat
On hand: atropine 400 mcg/mL (0.4 mg/mL)
By using the same formula, you can calculate the amount of atropine to be given.

$$\frac{D}{H} \times V = \frac{0.2 \text{ mg}}{0.4 \text{ mg}} \times 1 \text{ mL} = \frac{0.2}{0.4} \times 1 = 0.5 \text{ mL}$$

INSULIN INJECTION

Insulin is a pancreatic hormone that stimulates glucose metabolism. Patients who have insulin-dependent diabetes often need regular injections of insulin to keep their blood glucose from rising to levels that could be life threatening. These regular injections must be rotated to various sites of the body to prevent scarring of the tissue at a single injection site. Different forms of insulin are available, and it may be administered several ways, depending on the form. These ways include subcutaneous injections, intravenous administration, and continuous administration through an insulin pump.

There are four types of insulin: (1) quick-onset, short-duration, (2) intermediate-acting, (3) long-acting, and (4) ultra-long-acting (see Chapter 22 for complete information on insulins). Insulin is packaged in two ways: (1) vials containing 10 mL of solution with 100 units of insulin per mL and (2) prepackaged syringes that contain smaller amounts of insulin. In the United States, insulin is usually standardized to 100 units/mL. Insulin vials can combine NPH (Humulin N, Iletin II) and regular insulin (Humulin R, Novolin R) in one solution. The most common is 70/30, but 50/50 is also available (Figure 7-5 ■).

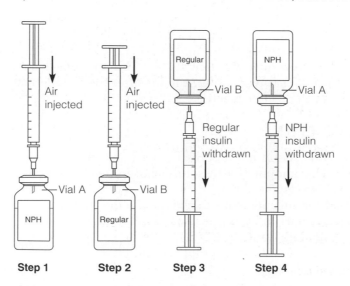

Figure 7-5 ■ Mixing regular and NPH insulins in one syringe.

Step 1   Step 2   Step 3   Step 4

The three types of insulin syringes are:

1. 100-unit syringes
2. 50-unit syringes
3. 30-unit syringes (Figure 7-6 ■)

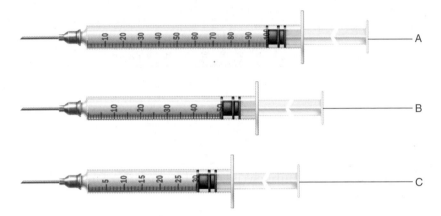

Figure 7-6 ■ (A) 100-unit, (B) 50-unit, and (C) 30-unit insulin syringes.

Focus Point

Preparing Insulin Injections

For more accurate measurements, use a 30-unit insulin syringe for insulin doses less than 30 units, and a 50-unit insulin syringe for insulin doses less than 50 units if a standard 100-unit syringe is not available. To successfully remove insulin from a vial for injection, first inject the same quantity of air as the ordered insulin volume before withdrawing the appropriate insulin quantity. If the physician orders two types of insulins to be administered, the insulins may be combined in one syringe to allow for one injection. Draw up the shorter-acting insulin first.

The size of the syringe depends on the size of the dose to be administered. For example, if you needed to give 18 units of regular insulin and 11 units of NPH insulin, you would select a 30-unit syringe. Similarly, if you needed 35 units of regular and 40 units of NPH, you would select a 100-unit syringe to administer these larger unit sizes. The smallest size syringe that will contain the number of units required is best because it is easier to see the unit markings on the syringe.

Example 1
Find how much liquid is in the tuberculin syringe in Figure 7-7 ■.

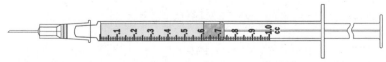

Figure 7-7 ■ Tuberculin syringe.

You can see that the top ring of the plunger is even with one line above 0.60 mL. Each marking line represents 0.01 mL, so the amount of liquid in this syringe is 0.61 mL.

Example 2

Figure 7-8 ■ shows a 100-unit insulin syringe. In this type of syringe, 100 units is equivalent to 1 mL. Each measurement line on the syringe measures 2 units, or 0.02 mL.

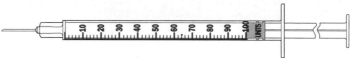

Figure 7-8 ■ 100-unit insulin syringe.

Example 3

Figure 7-9 ■ shows a 50-unit insulin syringe. In this type of syringe, each measurement line only measures 1 unit, or 0.01 mL.

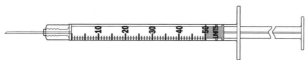

Figure 7-9 ■ 50-Unit insulin syringe.

Example 4

Figure 7-10 ■ shows a 30-unit insulin syringe, also known as a Lo-Dose® syringe. In this type of syringe, the measurement lines are the same as in the 50-unit insulin syringe, measuring just 1 unit, or 0.01 mL.

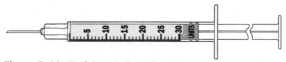

Figure 7-10 ■ 30-unit insulin syringe.

Example 5

Figure 7-11 ■ shows a partially filled 50-unit insulin syringe. You can see that the top ring of the plunger is even with 3 lines above the number 25. Because each line represents 1 unit, this syringe contains 28 units of liquid.

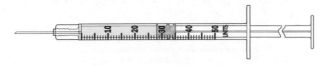

Figure 7-11 ■ A partially filled 50-unit insulin syringe.

Example 6

Figure 7-12 ■ shows a partially filled 100-unit insulin syringe. You can see that the top ring of the plunger is even with 1 line above 70. Because each line represents 2 units, this syringe contains 72 units of liquid.

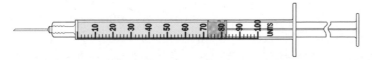

Figure 7-12 ■ A partially filled 100-unit insulin syringe.

Focus Point

Safe Insulin Practices

Avoid keeping insulin on top of medication carts or counters, or under pharmacy compounding hoods because it could be confused with heparin (which is also measured in units). Immediately return insulin to a proper storage area after use. If insulin concentration is not 100 units/mL, apply *bold warning labels* to alert the user about the concentration. Always use single standard concentration for all adult IV insulin infusions. Prescribers should order insulin cartridges for outpatients to help ensure correct dispensing.

HEPARIN CALCULATION

The anticoagulant heparin is measured in USP (United States Pharmacopeia) units. It is given to patients to reduce or prevent the blood from clotting. Heparin can be administered to a patient by subcutaneous injection or intravenous injection.

The abbreviation U should be avoided in practice to prevent medication errors. Vials of heparin are prepared by the manufacturer in a variety of strengths. The vials come in 1,000-unit, 5,000-unit, 20,000-unit, and 40,000-unit sizes. Ampules are supplied in 1,000-unit, 5,000-unit, and 10,000-unit sizes.

Heparin is also available in premixed intravenous solutions—for example, 12,500 units in 250 mL of 5% dextrose in water (D_5W); or 25,000 units in 500 mL of 0.45% saline solution. With a premixed parenteral solution, you have to convert the physician's order to the volume of solution that contains the amount of heparin ordered.

Example 1

Ordered: heparin 5,000 units subcutaneously q8h
On hand: heparin is available as 10,000 units/mL.
You need to convert units to milliliters.

$$10,000 \text{ units} = 1 \text{ mL} = 5,000 \text{ units}:X \text{ mL}$$

$$10,000 \, X = 5,000$$

$$X = \frac{5,000}{10,000} = \frac{1}{2} = 0.5 \text{ mL}$$

Example 2
Ordered: 1,000 mL of D$_5$W containing 20,000 units of heparin, which is to be infused at 30 mL/h
How much heparin should be given to the patient per hour?

$$20,000 \text{ units}:1,000 \text{ mL} = X \text{ units}:30 \text{ mL}$$

$$1,000\,X = 20,000 \times 30$$

$$\frac{1,000\,X}{1,000} = \frac{60,000}{1,000}$$

$$X = 600 \text{ units/h}$$

INTRAVENOUS CALCULATION

Intravenous (IV) fluid therapy is used to administer fluids that contain water, dextrose, vitamins, electrolytes, and drugs. Medications for IV administration are usually available in small-volume vials that are mixed in a large-volume solution by the pharmacist before administration to the patient. The drug added to a parenteral solution is often available in a solution. Therefore, the additive amount is calculated in terms of volume, usually in milliliters.

The amount of drug in a parenteral solution is clearly stated on the label, but the pharmacist must be careful to notice whether the amount is given in terms of concentration (for example, 5 mg/mL) or amount of drug in the vial (for example, 80 mg in a 2-mL vial). The concentration is used to calculate the correct volume to be mixed with a parenteral diluent to produce the prescribed dose.

Intravenous fluids and drugs may be administered by intermittent or continuous IV infusion. Intermittent IV infusion, such as IV piggyback and IV push infusions, are used for IV administration of drugs and supplement fluids. Continuous IV infusions are used to replace fluid or to help maintain fluid levels and electrolyte balance and to serve as vehicles for drug administration. Detailed discussions of IV solutions, equipment, and calculations are not suitable for this pharmacology book. Therefore, for more detail, it would be advisable to refer to a pharmaceutical calculations textbook.

✳ Apply Your Knowledge 7.3

The following questions assess your knowledge of calculating doses of parenteral medications. *See Appendix E for the correct answers.*

LABELING
Answer the drug labeling questions using the labels depicted below.

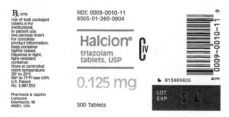

1. How many milligrams are contained in the Halcion bottle? _____

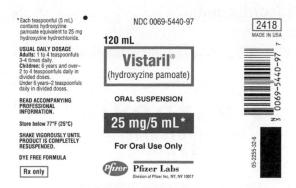

2. What is the usual daily adult dose of Vistaril? _____

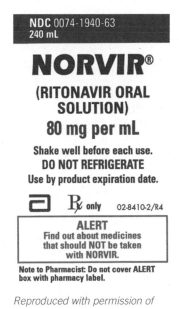

3. How many milligrams of Norvir are contained in this package? _____

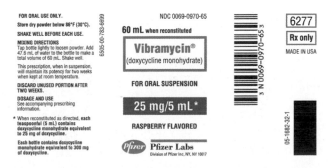

4. How many milligrams of Vibramycin are there in 2.5 mL of solution? _____

(*continued*)

Apply Your Knowledge 7.3 (continued)

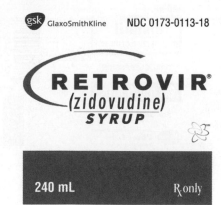

Each 5 mL (1 teaspoonful) contains zidovudine 50 mg and sodium benzoate 0.2% added as a preservative.

See package insert for Dosage and Administration.

Store at 15° to 25°C (59° to 77°F).

GlaxoSmithKline
Research Triangle Park, NC 27709
Made in Canada

4153827   A000747   Rev. 3/03

gsk GlaxoSmithKline   NDC 0173-0113-18

RETROVIR®
(zidovudine)
SYRUP

240 mL   R only

LOT   EXP

A 0 0 0 7 4 7

Reproduced with permission of GlaxoSmithKline.

5. How many milliliters of Retrovir are needed for a 150-mg dose of zidovudine? _____

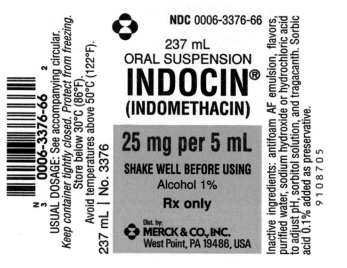

The label for the product Indocin 25 mg per 5 mL is reproduced with permission of Merck & Co., Inc., copyright.

6. If only half the Indocin suspension was used, how many milliliters would be left? _____

DRUG DOSAGE CALCULATIONS

Calculate the amount of medications that you should administer.

1. Ordered: Humulin R U-500 insulin in 80 units

   Administer: _____

2. Ordered: 150 units Humulin R, IV Stat

   Administer: _____

3. Ordered: Heparin sodium 5,000 units subcutaneously q8h

   On hand: Heparin 10,000 units/mL is available

   Administer: _____

4. Ordered: Valium 10 IM

   On hand: Valium 5 mg/mL is available

   Administer: _____

5. Ordered: Lidocaine 25 mg subcutaneously

   On hand: Lidocaine 5% solution

   Administer: _____

6. Ordered: Lanoxin 300 mcg IM Stat

   On hand: Lanoxin (digoxin) 500 mcg in 2 mL

   Administer: _____

7. Ordered: Zantac 50 mg IM qid

   On hand: Zantac 25 mg/mL

   Administer: _____

Dosage Calculation in Pediatrics

The pediatrician must determine the proper kind and amount of medication for a child. Dosages for infants and children are usually less than the adult dosages for the same medication. The body mass in children is smaller, and their metabolism is different from that of adults. Therefore, dosage calculations for pediatric patients (infants or children) must be precise.

For many years, pediatric dosage calculations used pediatric formulas such as Clark's Rule, Young's Rule, and Fried's Rule (see pages 137–138). These formulas are based on the weight of the child in pounds or on the age of the child in months, and aid in determining how much medication should be prescribed for a particular child.

Today, the most accurate methods of determining an appropriate pediatric dose are by weight and body area. You must know whether the amount of a prescribed pediatric dosage is the safe or appropriate amount for a particular patient. If this information is not on the drug label, it can be found on the package insert, in the *Physician's Desk Reference* (*PDR*), on a hospital formulary, in the *United States Pharmacopoeia*, or in pharmacology texts.

Focus Point

Questions to Ask When a Child Is Prescribed Medication

Encourage parent or caregivers of children to ask their physician the following questions:

- What is the drug and what is it used for?
- Will it cause a problem with other drugs my child is taking?
- How often and for how many days or weeks should I give my child this medicine?
- What if I miss giving my child a dose?
- How soon will the drug start working?
- What side effects does it have, and what should I do if my child has any of these side effects?
- Should I stop giving the medicine when my child gets better?
- Is there a less expensive generic version that I can use?

DRUG DOSAGE CALCULATION BY BODY SURFACE AREA

Body surface area (BSA) is determined by using a **nomogram** (a numerical relationship chart), and the child's height and weight. This is considered to be the most accurate method of calculating a child's dose. Standard nomograms give a child's body surface area according to weight and height (Figure 7-13 ■).

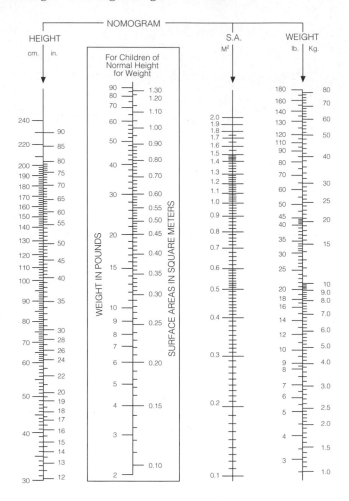

Figure 7-13 ■ Pediatric nomogram used for determining body surface area.

The calculation formula is the ratio of the child's body surface area to the surface area of an average adult (1.7 square meters, or 1.7 m^2), multiplied by the normal adult dose of the drug:

Example 1

$$\text{child's dose} = \frac{\text{surface area of child (m}^2)}{1.7 \text{ m}^2} \times \text{normal adult dose}$$

A child who weighs 12 kg and is 60 cm tall has a body surface area of 0.4 m^2. Therefore, a child's dose of ampicillin that corresponds to an adult dose of 250 mg would be as follows:

$$\text{child's dose} = \frac{0.4 \text{ m}^2}{1.7 \text{ m}^2} \times 250 \text{ mg} = 0.23 \times 250 = 58.32 \text{ mg}$$

Example 2
The pediatrician ordered: digoxin 0.64 mg/m^2 PO daily
The child's BSA is 0.9 square meters. How many milligrams would you administer to this child as a loading dose?

First, you need to convert body surface area to dose in milligrams:

$$0.9 \text{ m}^2 = X \text{ mg}$$

$$0.9 \text{ m}^2 \times \frac{? \text{ mg}}{? \text{ m}^2} = X \text{ mg}$$

Because 0.64 mg = 1 m², the equivalent fraction is:

$$\frac{0.64 \text{ mg}}{1 \text{ m}^2}$$

You then cancel the square meters and obtain the dose in milligrams.

$$0.9 \text{ m}^2 \times \frac{0.64 \text{ mg}}{1 \text{ m}^2} = 0.576 \text{ mg or } 0.58 \text{ mg}$$

Therefore, the child should receive 0.58 mg of digoxin.

DRUG DOSAGE CALCULATION BY BODY WEIGHT

Drug manufacturers sometimes recommend a dosage based on the weight of the child. This method uses a specific number of milligrams, micrograms, or units for each kilogram of body weight: mg/kg, mcg/kg, units/kg. Usually, drug data for pediatric dosage (mg/kg) is supplied by manufacturers in a drug information insert.

Example

Ordered: amoxicillin 60 mg PO tid

On hand: 125 mg/5 mL
Child's weight: 12-1/2 lb

To calculate, first change pounds to kilograms.

$$\frac{12.5 \text{ lb}}{2.2 \text{ kg}} = 5.7 \text{ kg}$$

Second: The pediatric dosage for a child who weighs 20 kg is 20–40 mg/kg/day in three equal doses.

$$20 \text{ mg/kg/day} \times 5.7 \text{ kg} = 114 \text{ mg/day}$$

$$40 \text{ mg/kg/day} \times 5.7 \text{ kg} = 228 \text{ mg/day}$$

$$60 \text{ mg} \times 3 = 180 \text{ mg}$$

Because 180 mg falls within the recommended daily dose range for amoxicillin, it is considered a safe dose.

Clark's Rule

Clark's Rule is based on the weight of the child, which is much more accurate than Young's or Fried's rules. Clark's Rule uses average adult weight (usually considered to be 150 lb or 70 kg), and assumes that the child's dose is proportionately less. To calculate pediatric dose by Clark's Rule, you should use the following formula:

Example

Calculate the dose of cortisone for a 42-lb child (adult dose = 100 mg).

$$\text{pediatric dose} = \frac{\text{child's weight in lb}}{150 \text{ lb}} \times \text{adult dose}$$

$$\frac{42 \text{ lb}}{150 \text{ lb}} \times 100 \text{ mg} = 28 \text{ mg}$$

Young's Rule

Young's Rule is used for children older than 1 year of age.

Example

$$\text{pediatric dose} = \frac{\text{child's age in years}}{\text{child's age in years} + 12} \times \text{adult dose}$$

Calculate the dose of Tylenol for a 5-year-old child (adult dose + 1,000 mg):

$$\frac{5 \text{ years}}{5 \text{ years} + 12} \times 1{,}000 \text{ mg} = 294 \text{ mg}$$

Fried's Rule

Fried's Rule is a method of estimating the dose of medication for infants younger than 1 year of age.

$$\frac{\text{child's age in months}}{150 \text{ lb}} \times \text{average adult dose}$$

Example

Calculate the dose of phenobarbital for an 8-month-old infant (adult dose = 400 mg).

$$\frac{8 \text{ mo}}{150 \text{ lb}} \times 400 \text{ mg} = 21 \text{ mg}$$

✳ Apply Your Knowledge 7.4

The following questions focus on what you have just learned about dosage calculations for pediatric patients. *See Appendix E for the correct answers.*

MULTIPLE CHOICE

Choose the correct answer from choices a–d.

1. The most accurate methods of determining an appropriate pediatric dose are:

   a. Clark's rule and Young's rule

   b. Young's rule and Fried's rule

   c. By weight and body area

   d. By weight and Clark's rule

2. If safe pediatric dosage is not on the drug label, it can also be found on the package insert or in:

   a. Nursing literature

   b. The *Physician's Desk Reference*

   c. The patient's record

   d. The MAR

3. Body surface area is determined by using the child's height and weight and a:

   a. Nomogram

   b. Sonogram

   c. Child's dose of a similar medication

   d. Loading dose

4. Drug manufacturers sometimes recommend a dosage based on the:

   a. Height of the child

   b. Weight of the child's parents

   c. Usual daily dosage

   d. Weight of the child

5. Which of the following dosage calculation methods is the most accurate?

   a. Clark's Rule

   b. Young's Rule

   c. Fried's Rule

   d. The child's height

DO THE MATH
Convert the weights (in pounds) to kilograms.

1. 55 lb   =   _____

2. 11 lb   =   _____

3. 157 lb   =   _____

4. 18 lb   =   _____

5. 209 lb   =   _____

6. 27 lb   =   _____

7. 93 lb   =   _____

8. 135 lb   =   _____

Chapter Capsule

This section repeats the objectives from the beginning of the chapter and then provides a summary of the most important concepts for that objective. Use this section as a quick review and to check your knowledge.

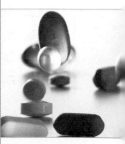

Objective 1: Discuss the differences between dosage ordered, desired dose, and dose on hand.

- Dosage ordered: total amount ordered and its frequency of administration
- Desired dose: amount to be administered at one time
- Dose on hand: amount of drug in a dosage unit

Objective 2: Explain how to use the formula $D/H \times Q = X$ to calculate drug dosages.

- D = desired dosage
- H = dosage available
- D and H: must always be in the same unit of measure
- Q = number of tablets, milliliters, or other units that contain H
- X = number of capsules, minims, or other units that D will be contained in (also known as the "amount to be administered")

Objective 3: Describe the proper use of scored and unscored tablets.

- Scored tablets: must be broken only along the line of the scoring
- Unscored tablets: must not be broken into parts

Objective 4: List the measuring devices used in the administration of oral medications.

- Measuring cups
- Medicine droppers/oral syringes
- Calibrated spoons

Objective 5: Calculate intramuscular dosages.

- $D \times H \times V = X$
- Or: $H{:}V :: D{:}X$

Objective 6: Name the most common types of insulin used in the United States.

- Quick-onset, short-duration insulin
- Intermediate-acting insulin
- Long-acting insulin
- Ultra-long-acting insulin

Objective 7: Explain the steps required for the proper injection of insulin.

- Step 1: Inject the same quantity of air as the ordered insulin volume into the vial
- Step 2: Withdraw the appropriate quantity of insulin
- Step 3: Draw up the shorter-acting insulin first, if using two types of insulin
- Step 4: Inject the insulin per the physician's instructions

Objective 8: Convert physician orders of heparin to the volume of solution that contains the amount of heparin ordered.

- If required, convert units to milliliters: 10,000 units = 1 mL
- Then use the formula: X mL = ordered units/available units
- Or: 10,000 units:1 mL :: ordered units:X mL

Objective 9: Calculate whether the amount of a prescribed pediatric dosage is the safe or appropriate amount for a particular patient.

- For the calculation: use either the child's weight or body area
- To find safe pediatric dosages, check: drug labels, package inserts, the *Physician's Desk Reference*, hospital formularies, the *U.S. Pharmacopoeia (USP)*, or pharmacology texts

Objective 10: Define the most accurate method of calculating a child's dose, and perform correct calculations using this method.

- Most accurate method: the body surface area (BSA) method
  - To find the child's body surface area: use a nomogram, which compares the child's weight and height
- Use this formula:
  Child's dose = m^2 (child's BSA) ÷ 1.7 m^2 × normal adult dose

Internet Sites of Interest

- *Diabetes Health* magazine presents an article at: **www.diabeteshealth.com** that discusses errors in calculation of insulin dosage by adolescents and the impact of utilizing an insulin dosage calculator (IDC). Search "insulin dosage calculator adolescents."

- Med Calc for Nurses offers information about dosage calculations, a variety of common medication calculations, and quizzes to assess your skills at: **http://home.sc.rr.com/nurdosagecal/**

- Targeted to medical assistants' needs, **www.mapharm.com/dosage_calc.htm** provides an overview of dosage calculations.

- The National Association of Chain Drug Stores (NACDS) explains why insurance companies are fostering pill-splitting and the dangers. Search for *Pill-Splitting is a Patient-Safety Concern* at: **www.nacds.org/**

- Prescription Drug Info at: **www.prescriptiondrug-info.com/Drugs/Regular_Insulin.asp** offers dosages for regular insulin.

- Click on many topics for pediatric patients, such as medication administration methods, calculating safe dosages, and safety issues, at: **www.accd.edu/sac/nursing/math/pedsmath.html**

Checkpoint Review 2

1. Circle the *improper* fraction(s).

$$\frac{3}{4} \qquad 2\text{-}\frac{5}{8} \qquad \frac{4}{4} \qquad \frac{9}{7} \qquad \frac{18}{19} \qquad \frac{1\frac{5}{2}}{3}$$

2. Circle the *complex* fraction(s).

$$\frac{3}{5} \qquad 1\text{-}\frac{3}{4} \qquad \frac{6}{6} \qquad \frac{7}{6} \qquad \frac{8}{9} \qquad \frac{\frac{1}{100}}{\frac{1}{160}}$$

3. Circle the *proper* fraction(s).

$$\frac{1}{3} \qquad \frac{1}{12} \qquad \frac{12}{1} \qquad \frac{16}{16} \qquad \frac{132}{12}$$

4. Circle the *mixed* number(s) *reduced to lowest terms*.

$$\frac{2}{5} \qquad 1\text{-}\frac{1}{6} \qquad \frac{5}{7} \qquad 1\text{-}\frac{2}{9} \qquad \frac{2}{3} \qquad 7\text{-}\frac{7}{9}$$

Change the following proper or improper fractions to fractions, whole numbers, or mixed numbers, and reduce to lowest terms.

5. $\frac{12}{16}$ = _____

6. $\frac{4}{4}$ = _____

7. $\frac{30}{9}$ = _____

8. $\frac{44}{16}$ = _____

9. $\frac{100}{75}$ = _____

Change the following mixed numbers to improper fractions.

10. $6\text{-}\frac{1}{2}$ = _____

11. $7\text{-}\frac{5}{6}$ = _____

12. $1\text{-}\frac{1}{5}$ = _____

13. $10\text{-}\frac{2}{3}$ = _____

14. $102\text{-}\frac{3}{4}$ = _____

Circle the correct answer.

15. Which is smaller? $\frac{1}{100}$ or $\frac{1}{1,000}$

16. Which is larger? $\frac{1}{15}$ or $\frac{1}{10}$

17. Which is smaller? $\frac{3}{10}$ or $\frac{5}{10}$

18. Which is larger? $\frac{2}{9}$ or $\frac{5}{9}$

Add and then reduce your answers to lowest terms.

19. $\frac{3}{4} + \frac{2}{3}$ = _____

20. $\frac{3}{4} + \frac{1}{8} + \frac{1}{6}$ = _____

21. $\frac{1}{7} + \frac{2}{3} + \frac{11}{21}$ = _____

22. $\frac{1}{4} + \frac{5}{33}$ = _____

23. $\frac{12}{17} + 5\text{-}\frac{2}{7}$ = _____

24. $7\text{-}\frac{4}{5} + \frac{2}{3}$ = _____

Multiply and then reduce your answers to lowest terms.

25. $\frac{3}{10} \times \frac{1}{12}$ = _____

26. $\frac{1}{100} \times 3$ = _____

27. $\frac{3}{4} \times \frac{2}{3}$ = _____

28. $\frac{5}{8} \times 1\text{-}\frac{1}{6}$ = _____

29. $\frac{3}{4} \times \frac{1}{8}$ = _____

30. $12\text{-}\frac{1}{2} \times 20\text{-}\frac{1}{3}$ = _____

Divide and then reduce your answers to lowest terms.

31. $\dfrac{1}{60} \div \dfrac{1}{2}$ = _____

32. $\dfrac{1}{8} \div \dfrac{7}{12}$ = _____

33. $2\dfrac{1}{2} \div \dfrac{3}{4}$ = _____

34. $\dfrac{1}{150} \div \dfrac{1}{50}$ = _____

Select terms from your reading to fill in the blanks.

35. Liters and milliliters are metric units that measure _____.

36. 1 mg is _____ of a gram.

37. 1 liter = _____ mL.

38. 1,000 mcg = _____ mg.

39. There are _____ mL in a liter.

40. Which is smallest: a kilogram, gram, or milligram? _____

41. Which is largest: a kilogram, gram, or milligram? _____

42. Milligrams are metric units that measure _____.

Circle the correct metric notation.

43. 4 kg   4.0 kg   kg 04   4 kG   4 KG

44. .6 g   0.6 Gm   0.6 g   .6 Gm   0.60 g

45. 2.5 mm   2-1/2 mm   2.5 Mm   2.50 MM   2-1/2 MM

46. mg 20   20 mG   20.0 mg   20 mg   20 MG

Write out the term for these abbreviations.

47. g _____

48. mm _____

49. cm _____

50. kg _____

51. mcg _____

52. mL _____

Write out the terms for these abbreviations and symbols.

53. qt _____

54. gr _____

55. ℳ _____

56. ℨ _____

Write out the terms for these equivalencies.

57. 16 oz = pt _____

58. qt i = oz _____

Write the following apothecary quantities using abbreviations and proper notation.

59. ten grains _____

60. two pints _____

61. one-half ounce _____

62. sixteen pints _____

63. four ounces _____

64. three grains _____

Write these measurements using abbreviations.

65. 3 tablespoons _____

66. 10 teaspoons _____

67. 6 drops _____

68. 25 milliequivalents _____

Convert these measurements to the units shown.

69. 1 oz = _____ T

70. 16 oz = _____ lb

71. 4 T = _____ oz

72. 24 oz = _____ cups

Write out the terms for these abbreviations.

73. 20 mEq _____

74. 15 lb _____

75. 50 gtt _____

76. 8 T _____

Calculate the amounts to administer and write in the blank spaces.

77. Order: *Lanoxin 0.125 mg PO daily*
    On hand: Lanoxin 0.25 mg tablets
    Administer: _____ tablet(s)

78. Order: *Duricef 1 g PO bid*
    On hand: Duricef 500 mg capsules
    Administer: _____ capsule(s)

79. Order: *Synthroid 0.1 mg PO daily*
    On hand: Synthroid 50 mcg tablets
    Administer: _____ tablet(s)

80. Order: *Diabinese 0.1 g PO daily*
    On hand: Diabinese 100 mg tablets
    Administer: _____ tablet(s)

81. Order: *amoxicillin 100 mg PO qid*
    On hand: 80 mL bottle of Amoxil (amoxicillin)
                 Oral pediatric suspension 125 mg for 5 mL
    Administer: _____ mL

82. Order: *Septra-DS suspension 200 mg PO bid*
    On hand: Septra-DS suspension 400 mg for 5 mL
    Administer: _____ mL

83. Order: *Esidrix solution 100 mg PO bid*
    On hand: Esidrix solution 50 mg for 5 mL
    Administer: _____ t

84. Order: *digoxin elixir 0.25 mg PO daily*
    On hand: digoxin elixir 50 mcg / mL
    Administer: _____ mL

85. Order: *Tylenol 0.5 g PO q4h PRN pain*
    On hand: Tylenol 500 mg for 5 mL
    Administer: _____ t

86. Order: *Pathocil 125 mg PO q6h*
    On hand: Pathocil suspension 62.5 mg for 5 mL
    Administer: _____ t

87. Order: *erythromycin 1.2 g PO q8h*
    On hand: erythromycin 400 mg per 5 mL
    Administer: _____ mL

88. Order: *cephalexin 375 mg PO tid*
    On hand: cephalexin 250 mg per 5 mL
    Administer: _____ t

89. Order: *Demerol syrup 75 mg PO q4h PRN pain*
    On hand: Demerol syrup 50 mg for 5 mL
    Administer: _____ mL

90. Order: *Coumadin 7.5 mg PO daily*
    On hand: Coumadin 2.5 mg tablets
    Administer: _____ tablet(s)

91. Order: *Urecholine 50 mg PO tid*
    On hand: Urecholine 25 mg tablets
    Administer: _____ tablet(s)

92. Order: *V-Cillin K 300,000 units PO qid*
    On hand: V-Cillin K 200,000 units for 5 mL
    Administer: _____ mL

93. Order: *codeine gr 1/4 PO daily*
    On hand: codeine 30 mg tablets
    Administer: _____ tablet(s)

94. Order: *Orinase 250 mg PO bid*
    On hand: Orinase 0.5 g tablets
    Administer: _____ tablet(s)

95. Order: *Ceclor suspension 225 mg PO bid*
    On hand: Ceclor suspension 375 mg for 5 mL
    Administer: _____ mL

96. Order: *Aspirin gr v PO daily*
    On hand: Aspirin 325 mg tablets
    Administer: _____ tablet(s)

97. Order: *Levaquin 0.5 g PO daily*
    On hand: Levaquin 500 mg tablets
    Administer: _____ tablet(s)

98. Order: *atropine gr 1/100 IM on call to OR*
    On hand: atropine 0.4 mg / mL
    Administer: _____ mL

99. Order: *lidocaine 50 mg IV Stat*
    On hand: lidocaine 2%
    Administer: _____ mL

100. Order: *heparin 3,500 units subcutaneous q12h*
    On hand: heparin 5,000 units / mL
    Administer: _____ mL

101. Order: *Lasix 60 mg IV Stat*
    On hand: Lasix 20 mg for 2 mL ampule
    Administer: _____ mL

Using the formula $D \times Q/H = X$, answer the following:

102. (*D*) represents _____.

103. (*Q*) represents _____.

104. (*H*) represents _____.

105. (*X*) represents _____.

Select terms from your reading to fill in the blanks.

106. The common syringe that is used for intradermal testing is the _____.

107. The volume of solution for IM injection is 0.5 to _____ mL.

108. The most common insulin combining NPH and regular insulin is _____, but 50/50 insulin is also available.

109. The anticoagulant heparin is measured in _____ units.

110. Intravenous fluids and drugs may be administered by intermittent or _____ IV infusion.

111. Body surface area (BSA) is determined by using a _____ and the child's height and weight.

112. Dosage calculations use pediatric formulas such as Clark's rule, _____ rule, and _____ rule.

113. Clark's rule is based on the _____ of the child.

114. _____ rule is used for children older than 1 year of age.

115. _____ rule is a method of estimating the dose of medication for infants younger than 1 year of age.

Unit 3

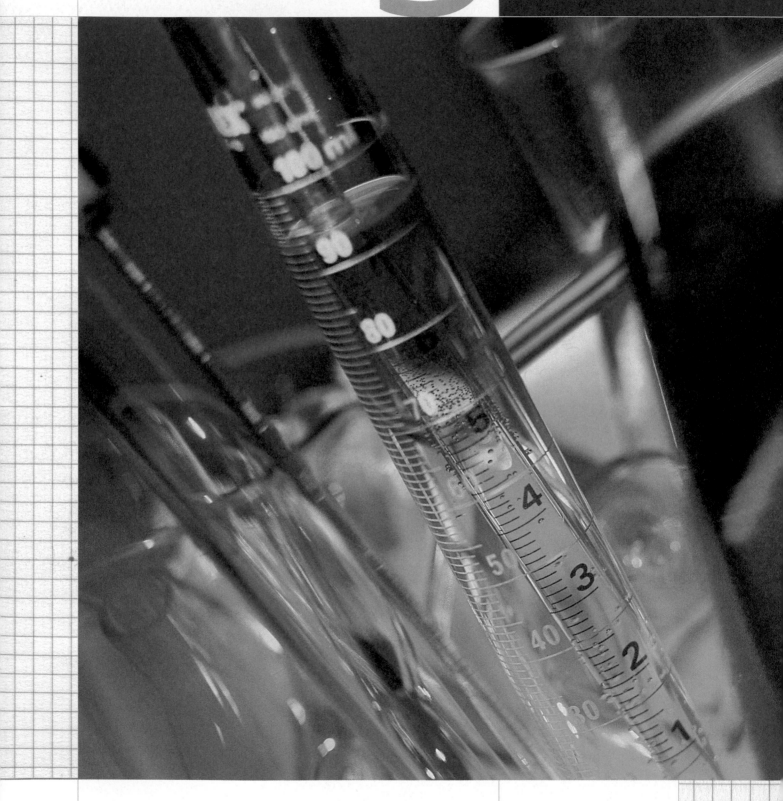

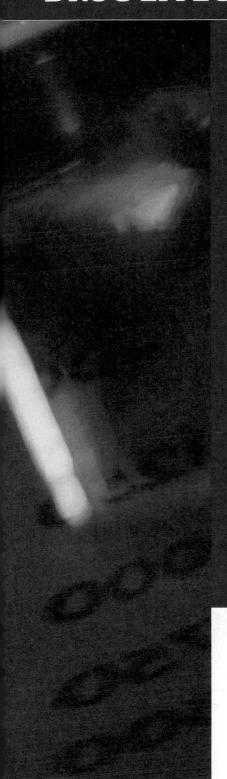

DRUG EFFECTS ON MULTIPLE SYSTEMS

"Antibiotic use has had a tremendous impact on the way microorganisms respond to various agents. Subtherapeutic doses or overuse can affect microorganism resistance."

Chapter 8

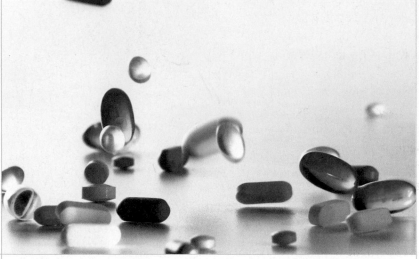

Nutritional Aspects of Pharmacology

Chapter Objectives

After completing this chapter, you should be able to:

1. Identify the seven basic food components and their major functions.
2. Differentiate the classifications of nutrients.
3. Explain the role of calories in the diet.
4. Define the role of essential fatty acids in optimal health.
5. List the water-soluble vitamins.
6. Discuss the toxicity of vitamin A.
7. Indicate the significance of vitamin E deficiency in infants.
8. List the five essential trace minerals and the symptoms of their toxicity.
9. Explain general indications for total parenteral nutrition (TPN).
10. Describe the benefits of food additives.

Key Terms

Alpha tocopherol (AL-fa toh-KAW-fer-rol) (page 157)

Additives (page 169)

Anemia (uh-NEE-mee-uh) (page 156)

Antioxidant (page 159)

Ascorbic acid (as-SCOR-bik) (page 153)

Beri-beri (BEH-ree BEH-ree) (page 154)

Calciferol (kal-SIH-fuh-rol) (page 158)

Calcitonin (kal-sih-TOE-nin) (page 158)

Calcitriol (kal-SIH-tree-ol) (page 158)

Carotene (KAH-roh-teen) (page 158)

Cholecalciferol (koh-luh-kal-SIH-feh-rol) (page 157)

Cholesterol (koh-LES-teh-rol) (page 151)

Cobalamin (koh-BAL-luh-min) (page 156)

Cretinism (KREE-tin-izim) (page 163)

Fiber (page 151)

Goiter (GOY-ter) (page 163)

Hypervitaminosis (hy-per-vy-tuh-mih-NOH-sis) (page 158)

Macrominerals (mak-ro-MIH-neh-ruls) (page 150)

Major minerals (page 161)

Pellagra (peh-LEH-gruh) (page 155)

Phylloquinone (fil-loh-KWIH-nohen) (page 157)

Rickets (page 158)

Spina bifida (SPY-nuh BIFF-ih-duh) (page 156)

PRACTICAL SCENARIO

Kate, an abnormally thin 15-year-old girl, is taken to the emergency department (ED) by her mother who reports that the girl is dizzy and shaky, complaining of a pounding heartbeat, and has been having crying spells for the last 2 weeks. Medical records indicate that Kate was diagnosed at age 12 with bulimia nervosa (BN), an eating disorder associated with emotional distress that is characterized by frequent episodes of binge eating (eating an amount of food within 1 hour that is significantly larger than normal for most people) and purging (self-induced vomiting and abuse of diuretics or laxatives). For the last 6 months, Kate has been eating small quantities of only a few foods and exercising excessively because she believes she is still too fat. Her mother fears that Kate's illness has evolved into anorexia

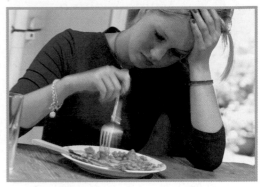

Trish Grant © Dorling Kindersley

nervosa (AN), a common progression. The medical examination finds that Kate has lost 30% of her body weight in 1 year, her electrolytes are seriously imbalanced, and she is hypoglycemic and suffering from protein energy malnutrition. She is admitted to the hospital for immediate treatment.

Critical Thinking Questions

1. Assuming Kate's gastrointestinal (GI) tract is functional, what would be the most efficient method of reversing her physiologic and nutritional starvation?

2. Which of Kate's nutritional deficits is the probable cause of her cardiac arrhythmia?

Introduction

Nutrition is the process of how the body takes in and uses food and other sources of nutrients for growth and repair of tissues. It is a five-part process that includes intake, digestion, absorption, metabolism, and elimination. This chapter gives you an understanding of how a well-planned diet can lead to optimal health and well-being for your patients, and it provides important information about food and drug interactions.

Nutrients

The human body needs a variety of nutrients for energy, growth, repair, and basic processes. Seven basic food components provide these nutrients and work together to help keep the body healthy:

1. Proteins
2. Fatty acids (also called *lipids* or *fats*)
3. Carbohydrates
4. Fiber
5. Vitamins
6. Minerals
7. Water

Only proteins, fats, and carbohydrates contain calories and provide the body with energy. The remaining four food components perform a variety of other essential functions. The nutritional sciences study the nature and distribution of nutrients in food, their metabolic effects, and the consequences of inadequate food intake.

A nutrient is any element or compound from the diet that supports normal metabolism, growth, reproduction, or other normal body functioning. Some nutrients are called *essential* because they are needed by the body for normal functioning. Essential nutrients cannot be synthesized by the body and, thus, must be derived from the diet. Essential nutrients include vitamins, minerals, amino acids, fatty acids, and some carbohydrates. On the other hand, *nonessential* nutrients are those that the body can synthesize from other compounds, although they may also be derived from the diet. Another way that nutrients are subdivided is into *macronutrients* and *micronutrients*.

Macronutrients

Macronutrients are needed by the body in relatively large amounts and constitute the bulk of the diet. They supply energy as well as essential nutrients needed for growth, maintenance, and activity. Carbohydrates, fats (including essential fatty acids), proteins, **macrominerals** (dietary minerals needed by the human body in high quantities), and water are macronutrients. Carbohydrates are converted to glucose (a simple sugar) and other monosaccharides (carbohydrates that cannot form any simple sugar); fats are converted to fatty acids and glycerol; and proteins are converted to peptides and amino acids. These macronutrients are interchangeable as sources of energy; fats yield 9 kilocalories of energy per 1 g consumed (9 kcal/g); proteins and carbohydrates yield 4 kcal/g.

The macrominerals, such as sodium, chloride, potassium, calcium, phosphorus, and magnesium, are required by humans in relatively large quantities (that is, grams) per day. Water is also considered a macronutrient because it is required in the amount of 1 mL/kcal of energy expended, or about 2,500 mL/day.

ESSENTIAL AMINO ACIDS

Essential amino acids are those components of proteins that cannot be synthesized by the body and must be provided by the diet. Of the 20 amino acids in proteins, 9 are essential. The requirement for dietary protein correlates with the growth rate, which varies at different times in the life cycle. The amino acid composition of proteins varies widely.

ESSENTIAL FATTY ACIDS

Essential fatty acids (such as linoleic acid and linolenic acid) are required in amounts equaling 6% to 10% of fat intake (5–10 g/day). These fatty acids must be provided by the diet; for example, vegetable oils provide linoleic acid and linolenic acid. Essential fatty acids are required for the formation of prostaglandins (hormone-like substances) and thromboxanes (biochemically related to the prostaglandins). Fatty acids, particularly omega-3 fatty acids, appear to play a role in decreasing the risk of coronary artery disease. Research has shown that consumption of omega-3 fatty acids decreases triglyceride levels and the growth rate of atherosclerotic plaque, slightly lowers blood pressure, and decreases the risk of arrhythmias.

Fatty acids can be either saturated or unsaturated. The chemical structure of a *saturated* fatty acid contains all the hydrogen possible and therefore is dense, heavy, and solid at room temperature. Examples of saturated fats are the fats found in dairy products and meats.

Unsaturated fatty acids can take on more hydrogen and are less heavy and less dense. Unsaturated fats are usually liquid at room temperature. If fatty acids have one unfilled hydrogen bond, the fat is called *monounsaturated*. Olives, olive oil, and peanut oil contain monounsaturated fats. *Polyunsaturated* fats, such as corn, safflower, and soy oils, have two or more unfilled hydrogen bonds. All essential fatty acids are polyunsaturated fatty acids, but not all polyunsaturated fatty acids are essential fatty acids.

Cholesterol, a natural lipid found in cell membranes, is found in highest concentrations in animal muscles and organ cells. Cholesterol does not exist in plants. It is essential for certain cell structures; however, excess cholesterol can deposit in blood vessels, form atherosclerotic plaque, and lead to cardiovascular disease.

CARBOHYDRATES

Carbohydrates in food provide about two thirds of an individual's fuel for daily energy needs. They aid in fat metabolism and help reserve protein for uses other than supplying energy, such as repairing and building our bodies. The daily requirement for carbohydrates is 50% to 60% of total caloric intake. Carbohydrate deficiency leads to weight loss, protein loss, and fatigue.

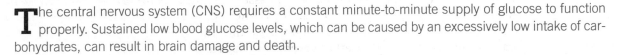

Focus Point

Blood Glucose Levels

The central nervous system (CNS) requires a constant minute-to-minute supply of glucose to function properly. Sustained low blood glucose levels, which can be caused by an excessively low intake of carbohydrates, can result in brain damage and death.

There are two basic types of carbohydrates: *simple sugars*, which are found in fruits, some vegetables, milk, and table sugar; and *complex carbohydrates*, which are found in grain foods such as pastas, breads, and rice, and fruits and vegetables such as potatoes, broccoli, corn, apples, and pears. The two types of carbohydrates have a function in health and consist of many variations. With the exception of fibers, carbohydrates are easily digested and absorbed into the body. Simple sugars are quickly absorbed, whereas complex carbohydrates must be processed before they can be absorbed in the intestinal tract. A small amount of glucose is stored in the liver and muscles as glycogen (starch). This stored glucose is available to supplement dietary supplies of carbohydrates. Excess amounts of carbohydrates are stored in the body as fat or *adipose* tissue. Carbohydrates are also needed to regulate protein and fat metabolism.

Focus on Pediatrics

Lactose Sensitivity

Lactose is the sugar contained in human and animal milk. It must be broken down in the body by the enzyme lactase to enable the body to digest dairy products. Many infants and children have trouble digesting foods that contain lactose and must eliminate those foods from their diets. Children who are especially sensitive to dietary lactose are often referred to as being *lactose intolerant*. Generally, removing milk products from the diet is recommended for lactose-intolerant children. Lactose-free milk can be substituted, as can sources of calcium such as yogurt, buttermilk, and cheese, which contain less lactose than milk.

FIBER

Fiber is a type of complex carbohydrate that does not supply energy or heat to the body. Fiber is the tough, stringy part of vegetables and grains. It can be classified as soluble or insoluble. *Soluble fiber*, found in foods such as oats, dry beans, barley, and some fruits and vegetables, tends to absorb fluid and swell when eaten. Water-soluble fiber helps to lower blood cholesterol levels. It also may stabilize blood sugar levels in the body by slowing the absorption of carbohydrates into the blood. *Insoluble fiber*, which is found in the bran of whole wheat and brown rice, primarily promotes regular bowel movements by contributing to stool bulk, which stimulates peristalsis. It also helps to prevent colon cancer (the stool bulk scours the intestines of waste matter as it passes through) and seems to reduce the risk of heart attack. Although insoluble fiber is not absorbed by the body, it serves to increase and soften the bulk of the stool, promoting normal defecation. Therapeutically, insoluble fiber can help treat and prevent constipation, diverticular disease, and irritable bowel syndrome (IBS). It is linked to reduction in gallstone formation and risks of certain types of cancer, especially colon cancer, and other diseases.

The recommended amount of daily dietary fiber intake for adults is 25 to 40 g/1,000 kcal. Because fiber works with other substances and nutrients, it is advisable to get dietary fiber from a variety of food sources. Adequate water intake is especially important for fiber to work properly. Without adequate water intake, constipation and bloating may occur. Water also stimulates peristalsis in the intestine.

✳ Apply Your Knowledge 8.1

The following questions focus on what you have just learned about macronutrients and their role in health. *See Appendix E for the correct answers.*

MATCHING
Match the lettered term to the numbered description.

DESCRIPTION

1. _____ Include(s) vitamins, minerals, amino acids, fatty acids, carbohydrates

2. _____ Include(s) essential amino acids and essential fatty acids

3. _____ Include(s) linoleic and linolenic acids

4. _____ Provide(s) about two-thirds of daily energy needs

5. _____ Is(are) linked to reduction of blood cholesterol levels

TERM

a. Essential fatty acids

b. Fiber

c. Essential nutrient

d. Macronutrients

e. Carbohydrates

FILL IN THE BLANK
Select terms from your reading to fill in the blanks.

1. Saturated fatty acids are _____ at room temperature; unsaturated fatty acids are _____ at room temperature.

2. Cholesterol is found in high concentrations in _____ and _____.

3. Carbohydrate deficiency contributes to _____, _____, and _____.

4. Carbohydrates found in fruits, table sugar, and milk are called _____; carbohydrates found in grains, rice, and some vegetables are called _____.

5. Fiber is classified as either _____ or _____.

Micronutrients

Vitamins and essential trace minerals comprise *micronutrients*, a group of nutrients that are required in very small amounts by the human body for normal functioning. Foods contain small amounts of these micronutrients. However, if any of these micronutrients is lacking in the diet, biochemical alterations—such as changes in the structure and function of tissues and organs—result and possibly cause deficiency or diseases.

VITAMINS

Vitamins are organic compounds required for normal human growth, development, and maintenance of normal body function—however, the amount needed by the body is very small. The total volume of vitamins that a healthy individual normally requires per day would barely fill a teaspoon! Thus, vitamin requirements are measured in milligrams or micrograms—exceedingly small and difficult units to visualize. Deficiencies of vitamins occur when a special condition or disorder creates an increased need in a particular person at a particular time.

Vitamins are classified by their solubility: they are soluble in either water or fat. This difference has importance in bodily storage of vitamins and in vitamin deficiency or toxicity.

Water-Soluble Vitamins (B and C Vitamins)

Water-soluble vitamins include eight members of the vitamin B group (see Table 8-1 ■) and vitamin C (**ascorbic acid**). All members of the B-vitamin group act as coenzymes (organic chemicals that must combine with an enzyme in order for the enzyme to function), usually after being processed. The coenzymes are frequently grouped together because many are found in similar foodstuffs.

Table 8-1 ■ Water-Soluble Vitamins

GENERIC NAME	TRADE NAME	FUNCTIONS	HYPOVITAMINOSIS (*DEFICIENT INTAKE*)	HYPERVITAMINOSIS (*EXCESSIVE INTAKE*)
B₁ (thiamine)	Betalins, Bewon, Biamine	Metabolic reactions coenzyme	Anorexia, depression, dyspnea, loss of muscle strength, memory loss, and peripheral neuritis	Very little toxicity; in extreme overdosage, symptoms include hypotension, neuromuscular or ganglionic blockage, and respiratory depression
B₂ (riboflavin)	Riboflavin	Metabolic reactions coenzyme	Anemia, dermatitis of face, sore throat and mouth, and swollen tongue	Low toxicity levels, but in extreme overdosage, symptoms include dark urine, nausea, and vomiting
B₃ (nicotinamide, niacin, or nicotinic acid)	Niac, Nicobid, Novoniacin	Metabolic reactions coenzyme	Dementia, diarrhea, dizziness, headache, impaired memory, insomnia, skin eruptions, and sore mouth	Diarrhea, dizziness, dry skin, dysrhythmias, flushing, muscle pain, nausea, pruritus, and vomiting
B₅ (pantothenic acid)	None	Metabolic reactions coenzyme	Induced in humans via a metabolic antagonist; symptoms include cardiac instability, depression, frequent infections, and neurologic disorders	None, except in unusually high doses: diarrhea
B₆ (pyridoxine)	Beesix, hexa Betalin, Nestrex	Amino-acid metabolic coenzyme	Peripheral neuritis, seborrheic-like skin lesions, seizures, and sore mouth	Low toxicity (except in chronic overuse; then, neurotoxicity including clumsiness, lack of muscle coordination, and numbness)

(*continued*)

Table 8-1 ■ **Water-Soluble Vitamins** (*continued*)

GENERIC NAME	TRADE NAME	FUNCTIONS	HYPOVITAMINOSIS (*DEFICIENT INTAKE*)	HYPERVITAMINOSIS (*EXCESSIVE INTAKE*)
B₇ (biotin)	None	Metabolic reactions coenzyme	Anorexia, depression, dry skin, fine and brittle hair, fungal infections, hair loss, muscle pain, nausea and vomiting, rashes, and seborrheic dermatitis	No documented cases of overdosage
B₉ (folate, folic acid, or pteroylglutamic acid)	Apo-Folic, Folacin, Folvite	Amino acid and nucleic acid metabolic coenzyme	Megaloblastic anemia	Allergic reactions, fever, pruritus, rashes, and redness of skin
B₁₂ (cobalamin, cyanocobalamin, or hydroxocobalamin)	Hydrobexan, Hydroxo-12, LA-12	Nucleic acid metabolic coenzyme	Abnormal blood cell production, confusion, dementia, memory loss, and nervous system damage	No toxic effects; overdosage is extremely rare, but may cause a deficiency of the other B vitamins
choline	None	Metabolic reactions coenzyme	Liver damage in adults, alterations in memory, and increased fetal brain-cell death	None listed for choline alone, but when used in combination preparations, symptoms of overdosage include confusion, diarrhea, dizziness, drowsiness, headache, hearing impairment, respiratory changes, sweating, and vomiting
C (ascorbic acid)	Apo-C, Ascorbicap, Cebid	Coenzyme and antioxidant	Anemia, gingivitis, and scurvy	Dizziness, kidney stones; in high doses, diarrhea, nausea and vomiting, and redness of skin

THIAMINE (VITAMIN B₁)

Also called *vitamin B₁*, thiamine is converted into a pyrophosphate, which functions as a coenzyme in some important carbohydrate metabolic processes. For example, the metabolism of alcohol depends on thiamine pyrophosphate. Alcoholics frequently suffer from thiamine deficiency because heavy consumption of alcohol interferes with the body's ability to absorb the vitamin from food.

The main natural dietary sources of thiamine are whole grains (especially wheat germ), lean meats, fish, soybeans, and other beans. Processed foods are often fortified with thiamine.

Deficiency of thiamine leads to the disease **beri-beri**, which is characterized by edema, cardiovascular abnormalities, and neurologic symptoms.

RIBOFLAVIN (VITAMIN B₂)

Riboflavin—also called *vitamin B₂*—is important in the metabolism of fats, carbohydrates, and proteins. The main dietary sources of riboflavin are dairy products, yeast products, and liver. Almonds are also a good source, and many other plant products contain reasonable amounts.

A deficiency of riboflavin causes cheilosis (fissures on the lips) and stomatitis (cracks in the angles of the mouth). Glossitis (inflammation of the tongue) and seborrhoeic dermatitis—mainly of the face and scrotum—can occur, as well as a decreased resistance to infections. There is no known danger of excessive consumption of riboflavin. However, patients using riboflavin supplements should be warned that their urine may be bright yellow.

Riboflavin is sensitive to light and other foods; therefore, vitamin supplements containing riboflavin should be kept out of direct sunlight.

NICOTINAMIDE (VITAMIN B₃)

Nicotinamide is also known as *niacin*. Humans can actually make some of this vitamin from the amino acid tryptophan. The main food sources of nicotinamide are liver, yeast products, peanuts, whole grain cereals, and fish (tuna is exceptionally high in this vitamin). Deficiency of nicotinamide causes **pellagra**, a condition marked by "the four Ds": dementia, dermatitis, diarrhea, and death.

Nicotinamide is therefore used chiefly in the treatment of pellagra. It also has been found to be useful with thiamine and riboflavin in the treatment of nutritional deficiency in chronic alcoholism because these patients are also suffering from deficiencies of thiamine and riboflavin. Large doses lower cholesterol, triglycerides, and free fatty acids. Therefore, nicotinamide is used in the treatment of hypercholesterolemia (high blood cholesterol level), mostly in combination with the cholesterol-lowering drugs cholestyramine, colestipol, or clofibrate (see Chapter 19). Toxicity associated with high doses of niacin includes hepatic impairment, severe hypotension, and various skin conditions.

Focus Point

Pharmacologic Doses of Niacin

At high doses, niacin decreases blood levels of low-density lipoprotein (LDL) cholesterol (the bad cholesterol) and triglyceride levels, both of which are linked with cardiovascular disease. In addition, pharmacologic doses of niacin improve high-density lipoprotein (HDL) cholesterol (the good cholesterol) levels. When niacin is used in this sense, it functions more as a drug than a vitamin and should be used only under medical supervision.

PANTOTHENIC ACID (VITAMIN B₅)

The term *pantothenic* derives from the Greek, meaning "all over the place." This vitamin is needed for the formation of the important coenzyme A, which is required for numerous biochemical processes. A deficiency syndrome has been experimentally induced in human volunteers and results in vomiting, cramps, abdominal pains, and personality changes. Pantothenic acid is readily available in many plant and animal sources. It is very difficult for individuals to have a deficiency of this vitamin.

PYRIDOXINE (VITAMIN B₆)

Vitamin B₆ does not denote a single substance, but rather is a collective term for a group of naturally occurring pyridines that are metabolically and functionally interrelated: pyridoxine, pyridoxal, and pyridoxamine. The various forms of pyridoxine are widely distributed in animal and plant products, making deficiency rare.

Vitamin B₆ reputedly has several therapeutic uses. It is used routinely in patients on isoniazid therapy to prevent neuritis. Pyridoxine is also prescribed to treat hyperemesis gravidarum (nausea during pregnancy), particularly when given parenterally, and to suppress lactation when given orally.

BIOTIN

Biotin is widely available in the foods we eat, and deficiency is almost unknown. It is also made by the natural flora of the intestine. Biotin does not seem to produce any toxicity if taken in excess, and abuse of this vitamin does not seem to be common.

FOLATE

The name *folate* comes from the Latin word *falium*, meaning "leaf." The name was given to this vitamin because a major source is from dark green, leafy vegetables. *Folate* is now used as the common, generic name for this vitamin that exists in many chemical forms. The most stable form of folate is folic acid, which is rarely found in food but is the form usually used in vitamin supplements and fortified food products. In its basic coenzyme role, folate is essential to the formation of all body cells because it takes part in the creation of DNA, the important cell nucleus material that transmits genetic characteristics. Folate is also essential to the formation of hemoglobin and synthesis of amino acids.

A direct deficiency of folate causes a special type of **anemia** (a deficiency of hemoglobin, red blood cell number, or red blood cell volume) called *megaloblastic anemia*, which is a particular risk during pregnancy because of increased fetal growth demands for folate. Rapidly growing adolescents—especially those following fad diets—and those who smoke develop low levels of folate in the blood, risking anemia.

The role of adequate folate in reducing the serious public health problem of neural defects during pregnancy has received increasing study and public awareness in recent years. Neural tube defects, such as **spina bifida** (a condition wherein the spinal column is imperfectly closed, resulting in protrusion of the meninges or spinal cord) and anencephaly (the congenital absence of most of the brain and spinal cord), are the most common birth defects involving the brain and spinal cord. Therefore, increased folic acid intake is recommended for all women who are capable of becoming pregnant. Adverse effects of excess consumption of folate from foods have not been observed.

COBALAMIN (VITAMIN B₁₂)

Vitamin B_{12} is also known as **cobalamin**, which promotes normal function of all cells, especially normal blood formation. It is also necessary for proper nervous system function.

Although it is essential, the amount of dietary vitamin B_{12} needed for normal human metabolism is very small. Vitamin B_{12} deficiency is responsible for pernicious anemia. A component of the digestive gastric secretions called *intrinsic factor* is necessary for absorption of vitamin B_{12} into the bloodstream. Gastrointestinal (GI) disorders that destroy the cell lining can disrupt the secretion of intrinsic factor and thus inhibit vitamin B_{12} absorption. If the vitamin cannot be absorbed to make hemoglobin, pernicious anemia occurs. In such cases, vitamin B_{12} must be given by injection to bypass the absorption defect. Deficiency is much more common in elderly individuals because of lack of either intrinsic factor or hydrochloric acid in the stomach, not because of insufficient dietary intake.

Although small amounts of vitamin B_{12} are stored in the liver, excess intake of vitamin B_{12} does not produce adverse effects in healthy individuals; therefore, no toxicity has been established. This vitamin is naturally found only in animal products (it is originally made by bacteria in the intestine of herbivores), such as fish, meat, poultry, eggs, milk, and milk products; breakfast cereals often are fortified with vitamin B_{12}.

VITAMIN B FACTORS (CHOLINE)

Choline is a water-soluble nutrient associated with the B-complex vitamins. Although it is synthesized in the human body, choline plays an important role as a structural component of cell membranes. Choline is an essential component in the production of acetylcholine, which is a neurotransmitter involved in memory storage, muscle control, and many other functions. A deficiency of choline from food sources appears to be associated with liver damage. This occurs because very-low-density lipoproteins (VLDL) cannot be synthesized, causing fat to accumulate in the liver and resulting in liver damage. Choline deficiency can affect healthy nerve function and may play a role in the development of Huntington's chorea, Parkinson's disease, and Alzheimer's disease.

Choline is found naturally in a wide variety of foods, especially milk, eggs, liver, and peanuts.

Excess choline rarely causes toxicity. Adverse effects have only been observed in cases in which choline intake was several times greater than normal intake from food. Very high doses of choline have been associated with lowered blood pressure, fishy body odor, sweating, excessive salivation, and reduced growth rate.

ASCORBIC ACID (VITAMIN C)

Vitamin C (ascorbic acid) is required for building and maintaining strong tissues for wound healing, resistance to infection, and enhanced iron absorption. Vitamin C has several critical functions in the body. It acts as a protective agent (antioxidant) and plays a role in many metabolic and immunologic activities—perhaps as a preventative agent in many cancers and cardiovascular disease. Ascorbic acid is thought to lower the incidence of atherosclerosis by aiding the conversion of cholesterol to bile acids. It enhances iron bioavailability, promotes calcium absorption, and aids in wound healing and tissue repair. Ascorbic acid is also essential for the body's constant production of collagen in connective tissue as part of normal tissue turnover.

A deficiency of ascorbic acid can result in scurvy—a serious and severe disease caused by the degeneration of connective tissue. Scurvy is marked by anemia, edema of the gums, and bleeding into the skin and mucous membranes.

The two best sources of vitamin C are capsicums and guavas—not citrus fruits, as is commonly believed. Kiwi fruit is also very high in asorbic acid. If large doses of ascorbic acid are used, plenty of water should be taken at the same time to avoid the formation of kidney stones. Diarrhea and gastritis can occur with large doses.

Focus on Geriatrics

Vitamin C and Cataracts

Vitamin C may be protective against the development of cataracts. The body concentrates vitamin C in the lenses of the eyes in higher levels than what is present in the blood plasma. The use of vitamin C supplements for 10 or more years is associated with 77 to 83% lower prevalence of early to moderate lens opacities (cataracts).

Fat-Soluble Vitamins

dissolve in fat, w/meal.

Fat-soluble vitamins include retinol (vitamin A), **cholecalciferol** (vitamin D₃), ergocalciferol (vitamin D₂), **alpha tocopherol** (vitamin E), and **phylloquinone** (vitamin K₁) and menaquinone (vitamin K₂). Unlike water-soluble vitamins, the fat-soluble vitamins are stored in the body. This storage can create an excess of these vitamins and may lead to toxicities. Excess amounts of vitamin A, in particular, can cause toxicity.

RETINOL (VITAMIN A)

The major function of vitamin A, or retinol, is in the retina of the eye. Retinol is an essential part of rhodopsin, which is a pigment in the eye commonly known as visual purple. A mild deficiency of vitamin A may cause night blindness, slow adaptation to darkness, or glare blindness. Adequate intake of retinol prevents two eye conditions, xerophthalmia (blindness) and xerosis (burning and itching).

Focus on Pediatrics

Vitamin A Deficiency

Dietary vitamin A deficiency is the number one cause of blindness in children worldwide.

Retinol also maintains healthy epithelial tissue (the vital outside layer of protective cells covering open surfaces of the body) such as skin and the inner mucous membranes in the nose, throat, eyes, GI tract, and genitourinary tract. These tissues provide our primary barrier to infection. Retinol is essential to the growth of skeletal and soft tissues and influences the stability of cell membranes and protein synthesis. Vitamin A is also important in the production of immune cells responsible for fighting bacterial, parasitic, and viral attacks.

Fish-liver oils, butter, egg yolk, liver, and cream are sources of natural vitamin A. Although vitamin A only occurs naturally in the fat part of milk, the FDA requires that all milk—including nonfat milk—be fortified with vitamin A. **Carotene** is found in dark green and yellow vegetables and fruits. Beta-carotene (one of three carotenes: alpha, beta, and gamma) is important to human nutrition because the body can convert it to vitamin A, thus making it a primary source of the vitamin. Some good sources of beta-carotene are turnip greens, spinach, carrots, sweet potatoes, mangos, pumpkins, and apricots.

The liver can store large amounts of retinol. In healthy individuals, the storage efficiency in the liver of ingested retinol is more than 50%, and the liver contains about 90% of the body's total store. Thus, large amounts of supplemental retinol added to normal dietary sources can cause toxicity. Excess vitamin A intake is called **hypervitaminosis** A. Symptoms of this toxicity include loss of hair, jaundice, joint pain, and thickening of long bones. Liver injury and ascites (fluid accumulation in the abdominal cavity) may occur.

Focus Point

Overconsumption of a Vitamin or Mineral

Nutrition experts suggest that individuals who suspect they have been taking too much of a vitamin (or mineral) should not stop taking it completely, but rather should cut back to about half the current dosage. This is because the body has adjusted itself to the overly large dose, and stopping it altogether could trigger a deficiency. Individuals should consult their doctors or a registered dietician in these cases, especially if they have diabetes or high blood pressure.

CHOLECALCIFEROL (VITAMIN D)

Vitamin D is not actually a true vitamin because it is made in our own bodies with the help of the sun's ultraviolet rays. Today we know that the compound made in our skin by sunlight is actually a prohormone (an intraglandular chemical substance that can be processed to become a hormone). This compound, when distributed in the skin, has been given the name cholecalciferol, often shortened to **calciferol** (vitamin D_3), which controls calcium metabolism in bone building. The initial compound produced in the skin by sunlight is a cholesterol base. Calciferol is activated by cholesterol in the liver, and then in the kidney, becoming the active vitamin D hormone called **calcitriol**.

Calcitriol acts physiologically with two other hormones, the parathyroid hormone (PTH), which is critical to calcium and phosphorus balance, and **calcitonin**, a thyroid hormone that lowers blood levels of calcium and phosphate and promotes bone formation. In balance with these two hormones, vitamin D stimulates absorption of calcium and phosphorus in the small intestine. A deficiency of calcitriol causes **rickets**, a condition characterized by malformation of skeletal tissue in growing children. Children with rickets have soft long bones that bend under their own weight.

Only yeast and fish-liver oils are natural sources of vitamin D. Therefore, the only regular food sources of vitamin D are those that have been fortified with the vitamin.

Excess intake of vitamin D, especially in infants, can be toxic. Symptoms of toxicity, or hypervitaminosis D, include calcification of soft tissue, such as in the kidneys, lungs, and fragile bones. A deficiency of vitamin D leads to rickets, osteomalacia, and osteoporosis. Hypoparathyroidism may also occur, because calcium cannot be absorbed for use by the body without vitamin D. (For a discussion of osteoporosis, see Chapter 22; for hypoparathyroidism, see Chapter 23.)

TOCOPHEROL (VITAMIN E)

Early vitamin studies identified a substance necessary for animal reproduction that was chemically an alcohol. This substance was named *tocopherol*. The most vital function of tocopherol is its action as an antioxidant. An **antioxidant** is an agent that prevents cellular structure from being broken down by oxygen. Vitamin E can protect fragile red blood cell walls (mainly in premature infants) from breaking down—a condition that is termed *hemolytic anemia*.

A deficiency of vitamin E in young infants, especially premature infants who miss the final 1 to 2 months of gestation when tocopherol stores are normally built up, are particularly vulnerable to hemolytic anemia. In older children and adults, a deficiency of tocopherol disrupts normal synthesis of myelin (the protective fat covering of nerve cells that helps them pass messages along specific tissue such as spinal cord fibers) and affects physical activity such as walking and vision.

The richest sources of tocopherol are vegetable oils (wheat germ, soybean, and safflower oil), nuts, fortified cereals, and avocado.

Tocopherol from food sources has no known toxic effect in humans. Supplemental intake of tocopherol that exceeds the normal dose may interfere with vitamin K activity and blood clotting.

VITAMIN K

Vitamin K is composed of a group of substances with similar biologic activity in blood clotting. The major form found in plants and initially isolated from alfalfa is phylloquinone, or vitamin K_1, because of its chemical structure. Phylloquinone is our dietary form of vitamin K, whereas menaquinone, or vitamin K_2, is synthesized by intestinal bacteria.

Vitamin K is known to have two metabolic functions in the body: blood clotting and bone development. Vitamin K is essential for maintaining normal levels of some blood-clotting factors, particularly the factor prothrombin. Phylloquinone can serve as an antidote for the excess effects of anticoagulant drugs such as warfarin (Coumadin). Phylloquinone is often used in the control and prevention of certain types of hemorrhages.

Because intestinal bacteria synthesize menaquinone, a constant supply is normally available to back up dietary sources. Therefore, deficiency of vitamin K is not usually found in humans. Only some clinical conditions related to blood clotting, malabsorption, or lack of intestinal bacteria to synthesize the vitamin lead to deficiency. Green leafy vegetables are clearly the best dietary sources of vitamin K. Small amounts of phylloquinone are found in milk and dairy products, meats, fortified cereals, fruits, and vegetables.

Toxicity from vitamin K—even when large amounts are taken over extended periods—has not been observed.

Focus on Pediatrics

Vitamin K

Because the intestinal tract of a newborn is sterile, phylloquinone is routinely given to prevent hemorrhage when the umbilical cord is cut. The "vitamin K shot" given at birth has the trade names of *AquaMephyton, Mephyton,* or *Phytonadione.*

Focus on Natural Products

Mineral and Vitamin Interactions

Caution patients to adhere to the following guidelines when taking vitamins and mineral supplements:

- Insufficient vitamin D intake hinders the uptake of calcium.
- High amounts of supplemental vitamin C reduce copper levels in the body.
- Vitamin C can increase iron absorption as much as 30%.
- Excessive amounts of vitamin E interfere with iron absorption.
- Vitamin B_6 is required to metabolize magnesium and zinc.

*Apply Your Knowledge 8.2

The following questions focus on what you have just learned about vitamins and their role in health. *See Appendix E for the correct answers.*

FILL IN THE BLANK
Select terms from your reading to fill in the blanks.

1. Water-soluble vitamins include _____ and eight members of the _____ group.

2. Deficiency of thiamine leads to the disease _____.

3. Nicotinamide is also known as _____ and _____.

4. A direct deficiency of folate causes a special type of anemia called _____.

5. Scurvy is caused by a deficiency of _____.

6. Adequate intake of vitamin A (retinol) prevents xerophthalmia, which is _____, and xerosis, which is _____.

7. Blood clotting and bone development are two metabolic functions attributed to _____.

8. _____ accelerates the absorption of iron from the small intestine.

MATCHING
Match the lettered term to the numbered description.

DESCRIPTION	TERM
1. _____ Acts as an antioxidant.	a. Vitamin D
2. _____ Stimulates absorption of calcium and phosphorus in the small intestine.	b. Vitamin K
3. _____ Causes xerosis and xerophthalmia when taken in excess.	c. Vitamin A
4. _____ Is involved with bone development and blood clotting.	d. Vitamin E

Focus Point

Proper Dosage of Vitamins

A nurse or medical assistant should advise patients about vitamins to prevent deficiency or toxicity. Patients should be told that vitamins are noncaloric essential nutrients, found in a wide variety of foods, which are needed in very small amounts for specific metabolic control and disease prevention. They should be warned that certain health problems are related to inadequate or excessive vitamin intake.

MINERALS

The body requires stores of minerals in varying amounts. For example, the body stores relatively large quantities of calcium, mostly in bone tissues: adults who weigh 150 pounds have about 3 pounds of calcium in their bodies. On the other hand, about 3 grams of iron are stored in adults of similar weight. In both cases, the amount of each mineral is essential for its specific task.

Major Minerals

Elements called **major minerals,** such as calcium, occur in large amounts in the body. The daily requirements of the major minerals—including calcium, phosphorus, sodium, potassium, magnesium, and chlorine—are more than 100 mg/day.

CALCIUM

Calcium and phosphorus deficiencies are usually due to metabolic rather than nutritional deficits. Calcium acts in bone formation, impulse conduction, myocardial and skeletal muscle contractions, and blood-clotting. The major sources of calcium are milk, cheese, salmon, green leafy vegetables, and whole grains.

Calcium absorption is dependent on vitamin D, the amount of phosphorus in the blood, and parathyroid hormone. Bone deformities such as rickets, osteomalacia, and osteoporosis occur with calcium deficiency. Excess amounts of calcium in the blood, or hypercalcemia, may cause constipation, hypotension, nausea, vomiting, kidney stones, and cardiac arrhythmias.

PHOSPHORUS

Phosphorus is also needed for bone formation, as well as tooth formation and energy. Fat storage and metabolism of other nutrients depend on this mineral. The best sources of phosphorus are milk, cheese, legumes, beef, fish, and pork.

Phosphorus supplements may cause electrolyte imbalances, GI upsets, and bone or joint pain. Phosphorus deficiency can cause anemia, bone brittleness, confusion, and weakness. The toxic effects of excessive phosphorus may cause hypocalcemia and kidney stones.

SODIUM

Sodium is the major electrolyte in the extracellular fluid. It helps body fluid balance and acid–base balance. Sodium also regulates nerve transmission and cell membrane irritability. The primary source of sodium is table salt. Other sources include meat, milk, celery, and carrots.

Deficiency of sodium may cause headache, confusion, nausea, weakness, anxiety, muscle spasms, and hypotension. Sodium toxicity produces hypertension and edema.

POTASSIUM

Potassium is a major electrolyte of intracellular fluid. It is found in blood, nerve tissue, and muscle fibers. Potassium is necessary for normal cardiac and muscle function. The best sources for potassium are oranges, bananas, red meats, vegetables, yams, milk products, and coffee.

Potassium deficiency can cause loss of muscle tone, weakness, paralysis, cardiac arrhythmias, and digitalis toxicity. Excessive potassium may produce muscle weakness, diarrhea, severe dehydration, abdominal pain, hypotension, and cardiac arrest.

MAGNESIUM

Magnesium is required to form proteins. It stimulates muscle contraction and nerve transmission, activates enzymes, and aids in bone formation. Good sources of magnesium include green leafy vegetables, whole grains, and legumes.

An excess or deficit in magnesium may cause tetany, convulsions, or muscle spasms.

CHLORINE

Chlorine is a major electrolyte, along with sodium, in the extracellular fluid. It is a component of gastric hydrochloric acid. Its sources include table salt, meat, milk, and processed foods. A deficiency in chlorine is rare, and toxic levels do not occur.

Essential Trace Minerals

Essential trace minerals, also called *microminerals*, are defined as those having a required intake of less than 100 mg/day. They are not less important than major minerals; rather, they are needed in smaller amounts. These minerals include iron, iodine, fluoride, zinc, chromium, selenium, manganese, molybdenum, and copper. Fluoride forms a compound with calcium (CaF_2) that stabilizes the binding substances in bones and teeth and prevents tooth decay. Except for deficiencies of iron and zinc, other deficiencies of microminerals are uncommon in clinical practice in industrialized countries. Therefore, in the following section, only iron, zinc, fluoride, and copper are discussed.

IRON

Although essential for life, iron is toxic in excess. Thus, the body has developed systems for balancing iron intake and excretion and for efficiently transporting iron into and out of cells to maintain health. Iron functions in the synthesis of hemoglobin and in the body's general metabolism. The human body contains about 45 mg of iron per kilogram of body weight.

Iron is widely distributed in the U.S. food supply, mainly in meat, eggs, vegetables, and cereals. The body absorbs iron more readily when it is ingested with vitamin C.

The major condition caused by iron deficiency is anemia. Iron-deficiency anemia is the most prevalent nutritional problem in the world today. Women and children are affected more than others. Iron deficiency may result from several causes, including:

✳ Inadequate supply of dietary iron

✳ Excessive blood loss

✳ Inability to form hemoglobin because of the absence of other necessary factors such as vitamin B_{12} (for example, pernicious anemia)

✳ Lack of gastric hydrochloric acid necessary to help liberate iron for absorption

On the other hand, iron toxicity can occur from a single large dose (20 to 60 mg/kg) and can be fatal.

Focus on Pediatrics

Iron Toxicity

In the United States, iron overdose from supplements is the leading cause of poisoning among young children. Symptoms include nausea, vomiting, and diarrhea. If not treated immediately, several organ systems may be adversely affected, such as the brain, kidneys, liver, and heart.

IODINE

In humans, the basic function of iodine is to participate in the thyroid gland's synthesis of the hormone thyroxine, which in turn controls the body's basal metabolic rate. After thyroxine is used to stimulate metabolic processes in cells, it is broken down in the liver, and the iodine portion is excreted in bile as inorganic iodine. The average adult body contains only 20 to 50 mg of iodine.

Seafood provides a good amount of iodine, although the major reliable source is iodized table salt.

A lack of iodine in the diet contributes to several deficiency diseases such as **goiter** (a swelling of the thyroid gland), **cretinism** (a condition of extreme hypothyroidism characterized by physical deformity, dwarfism, and mental retardation), and myxedema (a life-threatening complication of hypothyroidism, marked by coma, hypothermia, and respiratory depression). Goiter is a classic condition that often occurs in areas where the water and soil contain little iodine.

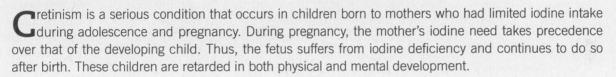

Focus on Pediatrics

Cretinism

Cretinism is a serious condition that occurs in children born to mothers who had limited iodine intake during adolescence and pregnancy. During pregnancy, the mother's iodine need takes precedence over that of the developing child. Thus, the fetus suffers from iodine deficiency and continues to do so after birth. These children are retarded in both physical and mental development.

Intake of iodine through supplementation may result in toxicity for some individuals. Excess iodine may result in acne-like skin lesions or may worsen the preexisting acne of adolescents or young adults.

ZINC

Zinc is an essential trace element with wide clinical significance. It is especially important during growth periods such as pregnancy, lactation, infancy, childhood, and adolescence. Zinc is more abudant in the adult body than any of the other microminerals—about 1.5 g in women and 2.5 g in men. Zinc is present in minute quantities in all body organs, tissues, fluids, and secretions.

Zinc is very important during periods of rapid tissue growth, such as childhood and adolescence. Retarded physical growth (such as dwarfism) and retarded sexual maturation (especially in men) have been observed in some populations in whom dietary intake of zinc is low. Zinc deficiency commonly causes poor wound healing, hair loss, diarrhea, and skin irritation. Impaired taste and smell are improved with increased zinc intake if previous dietary intake has been inadequate.

The greatest source of dietary zinc in the United States is meat, which supplies about 70% of the zinc consumed. Seafood, particularly oysters, is another excellent source of zinc.

Zinc toxicity from food sources is uncommon. However, prolonged supplementation in excess of recommendations can cause adverse effects such as nausea, vomiting, and decreased immune function. Excess zinc inhibits the absorption of copper, thus resulting in copper deficiency.

FLUORIDE

Fluoride forms a strong bond with calcium, which means that fluoride accumulates in calcified body tissues, such as bones and teeth. Fluoride's main function in human nutrition is to prevent dental caries. Fluoride strengthens the ability of the tooth structure to withstand the erosive effect of bacterial acids. The continuous intake of fluoride throughout life maximizes the protective effect of fluoride on teeth and maintains an adequate level of fluoride in tooth enamel. Fish products and tea contain the highest concentration of fluoride in foods.

Because fluoride stimulates new bone formation, it has become an experimental drug in the treatment of osteoporosis. Presently, no evidence supports fluoride's ability to prevent osteoporosis. There is also no recommendation to increase fluoride intake during pregnancy and lactation.

Focus on Pediatrics

Fluoride

Fluoridated toothpaste and other tooth products containing fluoride should not be swallowed; therefore, children younger than 6 years of age should not use these products because they are unable to avoid swallowing them.

COPPER

This trace element has frequently been called the "iron twin" because the two are metabolized in much the same way and share functions as components of cell enzymes. Both are also related to energy production and hemoglobin synthesis. Severe copper deficiency is rare. However, copper depletion that causes low blood levels, has been observed during total parenteral nutrition (TPN) and in cases of anemia. An increase in copper intake is recommended for pregnant or lactating women to meet increased needs.

The richest food sources of copper are organ meats, especially liver, followed by seafood, nuts, seeds, legumes, and grains.

Wilson's disease is a genetic disorder causing excess storage of copper in the body. Without treatment, Wilson's disease can result in liver and nerve damage.

✳ Apply Your Knowledge 8.3

The following questions focus on what you have just learned about essential trace minerals and their role in health. *See Appendix E for the correct answers.*

MULTIPLE CHOICE

Choose the correct answers from choices a–d.

1. Which of the following single large doses of iron can cause fatal toxicity?

   a. 2 to 6 mg/kg

   b. 6 to 12 mg/kg

   c. 12 to 18 mg/kg

   d. 20 to 30 mg/kg

2. Which of the following is the most serious condition that occurs as a result of iodine deficiency in the diet?

   a. Cretinism

   b. Pernicious anemia

   c. Goiter

   d. Wilson's disease

3. Which of the following trace elements has commonly been called the "iron twin"?

   a. Fluoride

   b. Copper

   c. Zinc

   d. Iodine

TOTAL PARENTERAL NUTRITION

TPN supplies all of the patient's daily nutritional requirements. A peripheral vein may be used for short periods, but when concentrated solutions are used for prolonged periods, thrombosis can occur. Therefore, central venous access is usually required. TPN is used not only in the hospital for long-term administration, but also at home, enabling many persons who have lost small-intestine function to lead useful lives.

✸ Apply Your Knowledge 8.4

The following questions focus on what you have just learned about nutrition. *See Appendix E for the correct answers.*

MULTIPLE CHOICE
Choose the correct answer from choices a–d.

1. What is the result if a person's energy intake is less than his or her energy expenditure?
   a. Body weight stays the same
   b. Body weight increases
   c. Body weight decreases
   d. Obesity

2. Which of the following is the preferred route for supplemental nutrition when the integrity of the GI tract is preserved?
   a. Total parenteral nutrition
   b. Enteral nutrition
   c. Consistency diets
   d. Modified consistency diets

3. How is parenteral nutrition administered?
   a. Subcutaneously
   b. Intramuscularly
   c. Intravenously
   d. Intradermally

4. If a patient has lost small-intestine function, which of the following may be implemented?
   a. Total parenteral nutrition
   b. Enteral nutrition
   c. Bowel preparation
   d. Modified consistency diet

5. Enteral nutrition contains foods rich in which of the following?
   a. Water
   b. Protein
   c. Fat
   d. Vitamins

FILL IN THE BLANK
Select terms from your reading to fill in the blanks.

1. RDA stands for _____.

2. Diets that provide food in physically altered form (chopped, ground, pureed) are called _____.

3. To use enteral nutrition, the patient must have a functioning _____.

4. Hospitalized patients often receive _____ or _____ solutions through parenteral nutrition.

5. To be used for long periods, total parenteral nutrition requires _____ access.

Nutrient–Drug Interactions

The concept of drug interaction is often extended to include situations in which food or certain dietary items influence the activity of a drug. For example, drug interactions with foods, herbs, or other natural substances may alter the activity of a drug.

Foods can influence the absorption of a number of drugs. In some situations, absorption may be delayed, but not reduced. In other circumstances, the total amount of drug absorption may be the result of slowed gastric emptying. However, food also may affect absorption by binding with a drug, decreasing the access of drugs to sites of absorption, altering the dissolution rate of drugs, or altering the pH of the GI contents.

The presence of food in the GI tract reduces the absorption of many anti-infective agents. However, there are some exceptions, such as penicillin V (Pen-Vee-K), amoxicillin (Amoxil), doxycycline (Doryx, Vibramycin), and minocycline (Dynacin, Minocin). With these drugs it is generally recommended that they be given at least 1 hour before or 2 hours after meals to achieve optimum absorption.

There have been reports of serious reactions (hypertensive crises) occurring in people being treated with monoamine oxidase inhibitors (MAOIs) such as phenelzine (Nardil) and isocarboxazid (Marplan) following ingestion of certain foods containing a high amount of tyramine.

Tyramine is metabolized by MAOIs; normally, enzymes in the intestinal wall and in the liver protect against the pressor actions of amines in foods. However, when these enzymes are inhibited, large quantities of unmetabolized tyramine can accumulate and act to release norepinephrine from adrenergic neurons. Among the foods having the highest tyramine content are aged cheeses (e.g., cheddar; in contrast, cottage and cream cheeses contain little or no tyramine and need not be restricted). Other foods with very high amounts of tyramine include certain alcoholic beverages (e.g., Chianti wine), pickled fish (e.g., herring), concentrated yeast extracts, and broad-bean pods.

The consumption of grapefruit juice has been reported to increase the serum concentration and activity of a number of medications, such as certain calcium channel blockers (e.g., amlodipine [Norvasc], nisoldipine [Nisocor] and cyclosporine [Neoral]. The bioavailability of most of these agents is generally low, primarily as a result of extensive first-pass metabolism. It has been suggested that components of grapefruit juice reduce the activity of the cytochrome P-450 enzymes (a group of enzymes involved in the metabolism of many drugs).

Certain drugs, such as laxatives, colchicine, cholestyramine (Questran), and colestipol (Colestid), have been reported to cause malabsorption problems that result in decreased absorption of vitamins and nutrients from the GI tract. It should be recognized that these agents also can alter absorption of other drugs that are administered simultaneously.

Many drugs affect appetite, which in turn can lead to deficiencies of certain nutrients. Drugs also may affect absorption and tissue metabolism (Table 8-2 ■).

Certain drugs affect mineral metabolism. Diuretics, especially thiazide diuretics, and corticosteroids, such as prednisone, hydrocortisone, methylprednisolone, and others, can cause potassium depletion, which increases the risk of digitalis-induced cardiac arrhythmias. Potassium depletion may also result from the regular use of purgatives (agents that promote bowel movements). Corticosteroids and aldosterone cause marked sodium and water retention. Sodium and water retention also occur with estrogen-progestin oral contraceptives (Ortho-Novum, Norinyl) and phenylbutazone (Alka Butazolidin, Azolid). Sulfonylureas (used to treat type 2 diabetes), phenylbutazone, and lithium (Eskalith) can impair the uptake or release of iodine by the thyroid gland; oral contraceptives can lower plasma zinc levels and elevate copper levels. Prolonged use of corticosteroids, which reduces the work of the construction cells in the bone causing bone loss, can lead to osteoporosis (see Chapters 22 and 26 for more information about osteoporosis).

Vitamin metabolism is also affected by some drugs. Ethanol alcohol impairs thiamine absorption, and isoniazid (INH) is a pyridoxine (vitamin B_6) antagonist. Ethanol

Table 8-2 ■ Drugs That Affect Appetite, Absorption, and Tissue Metabolism

DRUGS OR DRUG CLASSIFICATIONS	DRUG EFFECTS
Alcohol, antihistamines, insulin, some psychoactive drugs, steroids, sulfonylureas, thyroid hormone	Increased appetite
Bulk agents (guar gum, methylcellulose), cyclophosphamide, digitalis, glucagon, indomethacin, morphine	Decreased appetite
Chlortetracycline, indomethacin, kanamycin, methotrexate, neomycin, p-aminosalicylic acid, phenindione	Malabsorption
Coumarin, narcotic analgesics, phenothiazines, phenytoin, probenecid, thiazide diuretics	Hyperglycemia
Aspirin, barbiturates, beta-blockers, monoamine oxidase inhibitors, phenacetin, phenylbutazone, sulfonamides	Hypoglycemia
Aspirin and p-aminosalicylic acid, chlortetracycline, colchicine, dextrans, fenfluramine, glucagon, L-asparaginase, phenindione, sulfinpyrazone, trifluperidol	Reduced plasma lipids
Adrenal corticosteroids, chlorpromazine, ethanol, growth hormone, oral contraceptives (estrogen–progesterone type), thiouracil, vitamin D	Increased plasma lipids
Chloramphenicol, tetracycline	Decreased protein metabolism

and oral contraceptives inhibit folic-acid absorption. Anticonvulsant-induced vitamin D deficiency is well recognized. Vitamin B_{12} malabsorption has been reported with salicylic acid, potassium iodide (Lugol's solution, Thyro-block), colchicine, ethanol, and oral contraceptive use.

Food Additives and Contaminants

The addition of chemicals to foods to facilitate their processing and preservation, to enhance their restorative or stimulating properties, and to control natural contaminants, is stringently regulated. Only food **additives** that have passed exacting laboratory testing are permitted to be used at specific levels.

Reported health problems suspected to be caused by some food additives have been trivial and largely anecdotal. Adverse health effects of approved additives and contaminants in the long-term have not been established.

The benefits of additives, including reducing waste and providing the public with a greater variety of attractive foods than would otherwise be possible, must be weighed against known risks. The issues involved are frequently complex. The use of nitrite in cured meats is an example. Nitrite inhibits the growth of *Clostridium botulinum* and imparts a desired flavor. However, there is evidence that nitrite is converted in the body to nitrosamines, which are known carcinogens in animals. On the other hand, the amount of nitrite added to cured meat is small compared with the amount that may be ingested from naturally occurring good nitrates that are converted to nitrite by the salivary glands. In addition, dietary vitamin C can reduce nitrite formation in the GI tract.

Patients need to know about the role of nutrition in helping to prevent specific medical conditions. Health-care professionals should emphasize to patients that careful reading of food package is a good habit, and that nutrient–drug interactions can create adverse effects. Therefore, patients should always tell their health-care providers what nutrient supplements they are taking on a regular basis and also ask about nutrient–drug interactions when prescribed a new medication.

✳ Apply Your Knowledge 8.5

The following questions focus on what you have just learned about nutrient–drug interactions. *See Appendix E for the correct answers.*

MATCHING
Match the lettered term to the numbered description.

DESCRIPTION

1. _____ Induce(s) vitamin D deficiency
2. _____ Can lead to osteoporosis
3. _____ Can cause potassium depletion
4. _____ Impair(s) thiamine absorption
5. _____ Inhibit(s) folic acid absorption

TERM

a. Thiazide diuretics
b. Oral contraceptives
c. Corticosteroids (prolonged use)
d. Ethanol
e. Anticonvulsant agents

FILL IN THE BLANK
Answer the following questions about the sample product label.

1. How many calories are in two servings? _____
2. Is the quantity of sodium or carbohydrate greater? _____
3. Which substance has the highest percentage of daily value? _____
4. How many calories are in each cracker? _____
5. How many calories from fat are in each cracker? _____

Nutrition Facts

Serving Size 19 crackers (31g)
Servings Per Container   about 8

Amount Per Serving

Calories 140   Calories From Fat 35

% Daily Value*

Total Fat	4 g	**6%**
Saturated Fat	1 g	**4%**
Polyunsaturated Fat	1.5 g	
Monounsaturated Fat	1.5 g	
Cholesterol	0 mg	**0%**
Sodium	220 mg	**9%**
Total Carbohydrate	22 g	**7%**
Dietary Fiber	2 g	**7%**
Sugars	4 g	
Protein	3 g	

Vitamin A 0% • Vitamin C 0%
Calcium   0% • Iron   6%

*Percent Daily Values are based on a 2,000 calorie diet. Your daily values may be higher or lower depending on your calorie needs:

		Calories:	2,000	2,500
Total Fat	Less than		65 g	80 g
Sat. Fat	Less than		20 g	25 g
Cholesterol	Less than		300 mg	300 mg
Sodium	Less than		2,400 mg	2,400 mg
Total Carbohydrate			300 g	375 g
Dietary Fiber			25 g	30 g

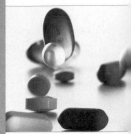

Chapter Capsule

This section repeats the objectives from the beginning of the chapter and then provides a summary of the most important concepts for that objective. Use this section as a quick review and to check your knowledge.

Objective 1: Identify the seven basic food components and explain their major functions.

- Proteins, lipids (fats), carbohydrates, fiber, vitamins, minerals, and water
- Provide energy, promote growth and repair of the body, and ensure the basic processes for life by keeping the body healthy

Objective 2: Differentiate the classifications of nutrients.

- Generally classified as macronutrients and micronutrients
- Macronutrients (needed by the body in relatively large amounts): carbohydrates, fats, proteins, macrominerals, and water
- Micronutrients (required by the body in small amounts): vitamins and essential trace minerals

Objective 3: Explain the role of calories in the diet.

- Supply the body with energy
- About two-thirds of total calories come from carbohydrates

Objective 4: Define the role of essential fatty acids in optimal health.

- Linoleic and linolenic acid (provided by vegetable oils); required for the formation of prostaglandins (hormone-like substances) and thromboxanes (biochemically related to the prostaglandins)

Objective 5: List the water-soluble vitamins.

- B and C vitamins

Objective 6: Discuss the toxicity of vitamin A.

- Called *hypervitaminosis A*
- Marked by loss of hair, jaundice, joint pain, and thickening of long bones
- May also cause liver injury and fluid accumulation in the abdominal cavity (ascites)

Objective 7: Indicate the significance of vitamin E deficiency in infants.

- Causes infants to be particularly vulnerable to hemolytic anemia

Objective 8: List the five essential trace minerals and the symptoms of their toxicity.

- Iron: nausea, vomiting, and diarrhea
- Iodine: acne-like skin lesions, worsening of preexisting acne
- Zinc: nausea, vomiting, and decreased immune function
- Fluoride: discolored teeth, brittle tooth enamel and bones, brain damage, heartburn, and pain in the extremities
- Copper: liver and nerve damage

Objective 9: Explain general indications for total parenteral nutrition (TPN).

- Inability to use the oral route
- Coma or depressed mental state
- Severe burns or serious illness with high metabolic requirements
- Severe protein-energy malnutrition

Objective 10: Describe the benefits of food additives.

■ Reduce waste

■ Provide greater variety of attractive foods

■ Inhibit bacterial growth

■ Impart desired flavor

■ Enhance restorative or stimulating properties

■ Control natural contaminants

 Internet Sites of Interest

■ Medline Plus, a service of the U.S. National Library of Medicine and the National Institutes of Health (NIH), provides information about the latest vitamin- and mineral-related studies at: **www.nlm.nih.gov/medlineplus/vitamins.html**

■ For general information and resources regarding dietary supplements, search the Food and Nutrition Information Center at the Web site of the U.S. Department of Agriculture: **www.nal.usda.gov/**

■ The American Dietetic Association provides a wealth of nutrition fact sheets at: **www.eatright.org/**

■ Nutritional tips for pregnant women are available at the Web site of the Weight-control Information Network (WIN), a service of the National Institute of Diabetes and Digestive and Kidney Diseases (NIDDK): **http://win.niddk.nih.gov/publications/two.htm**

■ The National Heart, Lung, and Blood Institute (NHLBI) provides a tipsheet for reading food labels at: **www.nhlbi.nih.gov/**. Search for "food labels."

■ Guidelines for good nutrition for older adults is available at the Web site of the National Institute on Aging: **www.niapublications.org**. Search for "nutrition."

■ The Office of Dietary supplements of the NIH offers information on dietary supplement decision making, claims and labeling, research, consumer safety, and nutritional recommendations at: **http://ods.od.nih.gov/Health_Information/Health_Information.aspx**

Chapter Objectives

After completing the chapter, you should be able to:

1. Identify the major types of antibiotics by drug class.

2. Describe the principal mechanisms of action of cephalosporins, vancomycin, and isoniazid.

3. Outline the main adverse effects of macrolides, aminoglycosides, and chloramphenicol.

4. Contrast bactericidal and bacteriostatic actions.

5. List the first-line antituberculosis agents and two characteristic adverse effects of each drug.

6. Explain the classifications of cephalosporins.

7. Discuss contraindications, precautions, and interactions of the penicillins and tetracyclines.

8. List three antiviral drugs for HIV and AIDS-related secondary viral infections, and explain their mechanisms of action.

Chapter 9

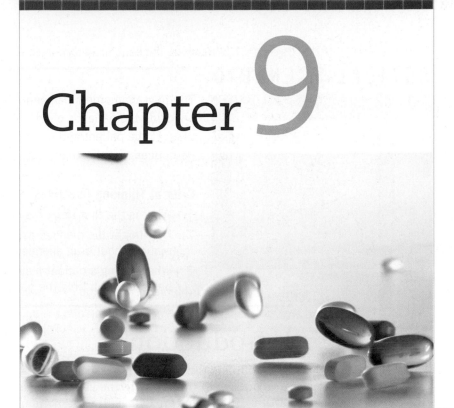

Antibacterial and Antiviral Agents

Key Terms

Antibacterial spectrum (an-tie-bak-TEE-ree-ul SPEK-trum) (page 182)

Antibiotics (an-tie-by-AW-tiks) (page 175)

Antimicrobial (an-tie-my-KRO-bee-ul) (page 177)

Bacteria (page 176)

Bactericidal (bak-tee-ree-SY-dul) (page 177)

Bacteriostatic (bak-tee-ree-oh-STAH-tik) (page 177)

Broad-spectrum (page 185)

Candidiasis (kan-dih-DIE-uh-sis) (page 190)

Fungi (FUNG-guy) (page 176)

Gram-negative (page 182)

Gram-positive (page 180)

Immunocompromised (im-myoo-no-KOM-pro-miezd) (page 203)

Nucleoside (NEW-clee-oh-sied) (page 203)

Parasites (PAH-rah-syts) (page 176)

Pathogenic (pah-thoh-JEH-nik) (page 174)

Serum sickness (page 180)

Subtherapeutic doses (page 175)

Viruses (page 176)

PRACTICAL SCENARIO

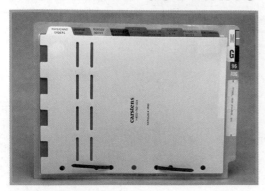

The physician orders penicillin for a 15-year-old patient without closely checking the patient's chart. While the medical assistant prepares to explain to the patient and her mother how she should take the medication, he notices that the chart indicates the patient has an allergy to penicillin.

Critical Thinking Questions

1. What is the first thing the medical assistant should do?
2. How might the medical assistant ensure that the physician sees information about drug allergies in a patient's chart?
3. When taking a patient history, what important question should *always* be asked each time the patient is seen in the office or clinic?

Introduction

Infection is the most common cause of death for many people afflicted with a chronic or critical illness, with the very young and the very old being particularly susceptible. Infections are caused by microorganisms that gain entry into the body. Once a microorganism invades the human body, the signs and symptoms generally associated with infection are generated, including fever and an elevated white blood cell (WBC) count. The microorganisms that cause infection and disease are called *pathogens*, and the major types of microorganisms that can cause infection include bacteria, viruses, fungi, and parasites, which will be defined further in this chapter.

Different pathogens inhabit various environments such as hospitals, the food supply, water, and animals or humans. Globalization of the world's population and faster air travel to nearly every spot on the Earth have major implications for the worldwide spread of infectious agents. Rapidly spreading infections may be particularly dangerous to populations when infected individuals are asymptomatic for long periods or the infection itself is difficult to identify for other reasons.

Infection with **pathogenic** (disease-causing) microorganisms has become a tool of war and terrorism throughout the world. "Weapons of mass destruction" may be nuclear, chemical, or biological in nature. Whether the situation involves anthrax spores sent through the mail or the threat of smallpox being introduced to a nonimmunized population, the various methods of preventing infections have key roles in the defense of humanity. Health-care professionals play a vital part in the prevention, early detection, and management of infections.

Transmission of Infection

Transmission of disease requires a chain of events that must occur unbroken to allow one human to infect another. The pathogenic organism must live and reproduce in a reservoir (Figure 9-1 ■). The reservoir may be a human being, as with the influenza virus; an animal, as in bats with rabies; or soil, as in enterobiasis (pinworm infection).

The pathogen must have a portal of exit, with a mode of transmission from the reservoir to a susceptible victim. For example, *Neisseria gonorrhoeae*, the organism that is responsible for gonorrhea, usually resides in the urethra of the male and the vaginal canal of the female. The microorganism is transmitted by sexual contact.

Control of infectious disease occurrence depends on breaking this chain of transmission in one or more places (Figure 9-2 ■). A pathogen can be vulnerable in one or more links of the transmission chain. Some pathogens, such as bacteria, are susceptible to direct attack with antibiotics. Antibiotics are designed to directly kill the pathogen or hold it in check so that the body's defenses can eradicate it. Some microorganisms

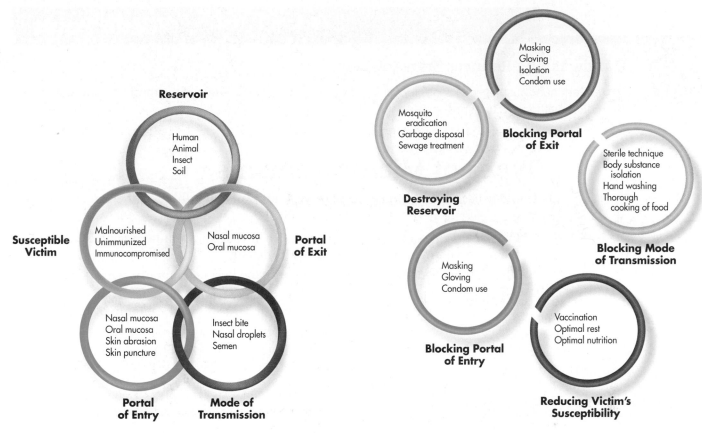

Figure 9-1 ■ Chain of transmission of microorganisms from host to victim.

Figure 9-2 ■ Breaking the chain of transmission of microorganisms from host to victim.

have developed resistance to **antibiotics** (substances produced by microorganisms that, in low concentrations, are able to inhibit or kill other microorganisms) through repeated exposure to **subtherapeutic doses** (doses that are below the level used to treat diseases) and use of antibiotics for nonbacterial infections. This *antibiotic resistance* is a major threat to the success of management of bacterial infections.

Destroying nonhuman reservoirs and vectors of the pathogen can also break the chain of transmission. For example, controlling the number of mosquitoes with insecticides is a method used to curb the spread of malaria and West Nile virus (see Chapter 10). Blocking the portal of exit can also block transmission of the pathogen. Having patients with tuberculosis wear masks as they move through the hospital, and implementing respiratory isolation techniques to stop droplet transmission, are interventions aimed at blocking the portal of exit.

Finally, host susceptibility is an important aspect of the transmission of a pathogen. Factors such as age, gender, ethnic group, and genetic makeup affect the susceptibility of the host. Although these factors cannot be changed, improving the host's immune system by improving his or her nutritional status, decreasing stress, and limiting fatigue can decrease the host's susceptibility to infection. Immunization of the host also has a key role in blocking the transmission of infection and provides active immunity, thus allowing the creation of host antibodies to help prevent future infections. In contrast, immunoglobulin given to the host can provide passive immunity to some infections, allowing for short-term prevention of disease transmission or infection.

Antibiotic use has had a tremendous impact on the way microorganisms respond to various agents. Using subtherapeutic doses of or overusing antibiotics can affect the resistance that microorganisms have to them. Resistance may be altered because of mutation (a change in gene chemistry that continues in subsequent cell divisions) or by the continuous exposure of a microbe to an antibiotic.

Focus Point

Handwashing Reduces Transmission

Frequent handwashing with soap, friction, and warm running water is one of the most effective ways to reduce pathogenic transmission.

Types of Microorganisms

The four basic types of microorganisms that can be helpful or pathogenic to the host are:

1. **Bacteria:** single-celled organisms with a cell wall and cellular organelles that allow them to live independently in the environment
2. **Viruses:** tiny genetic parasites that require the host cell to replicate and spread
3. **Fungi:** nonphotosynthetic, eukaryotic single or multicellular organisms that are found throughout the environment; fungi have a cell wall containing sterol
4. **Parasites:** protozoa, roundworms, flatworms, and arthropods

✳ Apply Your Knowledge 9.1

The following questions test your understanding of transmission of infection and types of microorganisms. *See Appendix E for the correct answers.*

MATCHING

Match the lettered term with the numbered description.

DESCRIPTION	TERM
1. _____ Reservoir	a. Viruses
2. _____ Transmitted by mosquitoes	b. Droplet transmission
3. _____ Single-celled organisms living independently	c. Weapons of mass destruction
4. _____ Bats can carry this disease	d. Sexually transmitted disease
5. _____ May be chemical or biological in nature	e. Bacteria
6. _____ Tiny genetic parasites	f. West Nile virus
7. _____ Gonorrhea	g. Rabies
8. _____ Tuberculosis	h. Humans, animals, soil

MULTIPLE CHOICE

Choose the correct answers from choices a–d.

1. Which of the following factors is a major threat to the successful treatment of bacterial infections?

   a. Globalization of the world's population

   b. Weapons of mass destruction

   c. Antibiotic resistance

   d. Doses for severe bacteremia that are greater than therapeutically necessary

2. Immunoglobulin given to the host may provide:

   a. Passive immunity

   b. Active immunity

   c. Antibiotic resistance

   d. Hepatitis

3. Weapons of mass destruction may include all of the following, except:

   a. Those that are biological

   b. Nonpathogen microbes

   c. Chemicals

   d. Nuclear weapons

4. Which of the following is the most important factor to control infections?

   a. Wearing masks

   b. Using gloves

   c. Coughing into the hands

   d. Handwashing

Antibacterial Agents

There is little distinction today between the terms *antibiotic* and **antimicrobial** (referring to an agent that tends to destroy microbes, prevent their multiplication or growth, or prevent their pathogenic action). The most common sources of natural antibiotics are molds and bacteria. Antibiotics are produced by one microorganism and inhibit the growth of others. However, many antibiotics are now partially or wholly synthesized in commercial laboratories. Included in this group are the penicillins, cephalosporins, aminoglycosides, tetracyclines, and macrolides. Important synthetic antibacterial agents, including nitrofurantoin and the quinolones, are also used clinically.

Antibiotics inhibit the growth of, or kill, microorganisms when given in sufficient concentrations—ideally low enough to exert their effect but remain harmless to the host. Systemic antibacterial agents can be **bactericidal** (capable of killing microbes) or **bacteriostatic** (capable of inhibiting microbial growth), but also rely on host defenses to aid in eliminating bacterial pathogens.

Antibiotics were discovered in 1928 when Sir Alexander Fleming was performing research on influenza. One year later, he found penicillin by culturing the mold *Penicillium notatum*. In 1938, British researchers studied the effects of natural penicillins on infectious disease. In 1941, natural penicillins were used clinically for the treatment of infections.

Factors to consider when selecting antibiotics for therapy in patients should include identification of:

✳ Likely or specific microorganisms

✳ Antimicrobial susceptibility

✳ Bactericidal versus bacteriostatic properties

✳ Host status, such as allergy history, age, pharmacokinetic factors, renal and hepatic function, pregnancy status, anatomic site of infection, and host defenses

Sulfonamides

Sulfanilamide's (sulfa drugs) are antibacterial agents that were first synthesized in 1908, but it was many years before their therapeutic value was discovered. In 1937, researchers in England synthesized sulfapyridine, which was the first sulfonamide used with great success in combating pneumonia. After that, a large number of other sulfonamides, such as sulfathiazole and sulfadiazine, were synthesized. Today, sulfamethoxazole is the most commonly used sulfonamide and is usually combined with trimethoprim and abbreviated SMZ/TMP.

The sulfonamides and trimethoprim act by inhibiting the folic-acid synthesis that most bacteria require. Although humans rely on dietary sources for the folic acid they need, most bacteria must synthesize it on their own. Sulfonamides were the first antimicrobial agents, but their clinical use has been greatly restricted as a result of the development of resistant bacteria, their significant side effects, and the availability of other drugs. The sulfonamides are no longer preferred for the treatment of urinary tract infections (UTIs), but are still important and effective for some infections. This is particularly true for new sulfa drugs. Table 9-1 ■ lists the various sulfa drugs.

How do they work?

The mechanism of the antimicrobial action of the sulfonamides has been analyzed extensively. These agents block a specific step in the biosynthetic pathway of folic acid. They are primarily bacteriostatic, meaning that they slow the multiplication of bacteria. Bacteria cannot absorb folic acid; therefore, it is made from precursors, specifically para-aminobenzoic acid (PABA). The sulfonamides interfere with PABA and folic-acid formation, thereby destroying the bacteria. The efficacy of sulfonamides generally is enhanced when the drugs are used in combination with trimethoprim, which inhibits conversion of dihydrofolate to folinic acid.

How are they used?

Sulfonamide therapy alone has a minor place in the treatment of infectious diseases. Major advantages of sulfonamides are their low cost and ease of administration. The combination of trimethoprim with sulfamethoxazole is the treatment of choice for most UTIs, otitis media (especially in children), sinusitis, some lower respiratory infections, and ulcerative colitis.

What are the adverse effects?

Major disadvantages of sulfonamides are their untoward effects (blood dyscrasias, crystalluria, hematuria, and life-threatening hepatitis). However, the new sulfa drugs in use today cause fewer allergic reactions than do the older drugs. Sulfonamides may cause several adverse effects, such as aplastic anemia, leukopenia, thrombocytopenia, and even agranulocytosis. Loss of appetite is a common mild adverse effect, with nausea, vomiting, diarrhea, fever, stomatitis (inflammation of the mouth), and photosensitivity also being seen. Crystalluria may occur during use of older sulfonamides, but may be helped by increased fluid intake on the part of patients throughout therapy.

What are the contraindications and interactions?

Sulfonamides must be avoided in patients with known hypersensitivity, during lactation, and in children younger than 2 years of age. These drugs are contraindicated near the end of pregnancy.

Sulfonamides may interact with oral anticoagulants and cause increased anticoagulant effects. Sulfonamides accompanied by methotrexate may increase the risk of bone marrow suppression. These agents may prevent the metabolism of oral hypoglycemic drugs, resulting in an increase of hypoglycemic reaction. When a sulfonamide is administered with a hydantoin, the serum hydantoin level may be increased.

What are the important points patients should know?

Instruct patients to take sulfonamide drugs on an empty stomach either 1 hour before or 2 hours after a meal with a full glass of water (at least eight to ten 8-ounce glasses of water should be consumed every day). Instruct patients to complete the full course of therapy and avoid prolonged exposure to sunlight, which may result in a skin reaction that is similar to severe sunburn.

cause skin Rash.

Table 9-1 ■ Various Sulfa Drugs

GENERIC NAME	TRADE NAME	AVERAGE DOSAGE IN ADULTS	ROUTE OF ADMINISTRATION
mafenide	Sulfamylon	Apply to burned area 1–2 times/d	Topical
silver sulfadiazine	Silvadene, Thermazene, SSD (cream)	Apply to burned area 1–2 times/d	Topical
sulfadiazine	Sulfadiazine	Loading dose: 2–4 g; maintenance dose: 2–4 g/d in 4–6 divided doses	PO
sulfamethizole	Thiosulfil Forte	0.5–1 g tid–qid	PO
sulfamethoxazole	Gantanol	Initial dose: 2 g; maintenance dose: 1 g bid–tid	PO
sulfasalazine	Azulfidine	Initial therapy: 1–4 g/d in divided doses; maintenance therapy: 2 g/d in evenly spaced doses of 500 mg qid	PO
sulfisoxazole	Gantrisin	Loading dose: 2–4 g; maintenance dose: 4–8 g/d in 4–6 divided doses	PO
trimethoprim (TMP) and sulfamethoxazole (SMZ)	Bactrim, Septra	160 mg TMP/800 mg SMZ q12h	PO
		8–10 mg/kg/d (based on TMP) in 2–4 divided doses	IV

Penicillins

The name *penicillin* now designates a number of antibiotic substances produced by the growth of various *Penicillium* species, or by other means. The penicillins are listed in Table 9-2 ■.

How do they work?

Penicillin interferes with the synthesis of peptidoglycans, important building blocks of bacterial cell walls. The penicillins may be bactericidal or bacteriostatic. There are four classes of penicillins: (1) natural penicillins, (2) penicillinase-resistant penicillins, (3) aminopenicillins, and (4) extended-spectrum penicillins.

How are they used?

Although penicillin G is the original penicillin, it remains the drug of choice for the treatment of almost all infections caused by nonpenicillinase-producing and nonmethicillin-resistant **gram-positive** bacteria (those that have the ability to resist de-colorization with alcohol after being treated with Gram's crystal violet stain that imparts a violent color to the bacterium when viewed by microscope). Penicillin is the drug of choice against infections by gram-positive, nonpenicillinase-producing *cocci*, such as *Staphylococcus aureus* or *S. epidermidis*, and *Streptococcus* group B. Therefore, penicillins can be used for UTIs, gonorrhea, syphilis, septicemia, meningitis, pneumonia, and other respiratory infections. Due to penicillanse-producing organisms, many skin or other types of infections must be treated with an extended-spectrum penicillin, sometimes along with another drug.

What are the adverse effects?

Penicillin is a very safe drug in most cases, with low toxicity. However, hypersensitivity reactions may occur in a low percentage of patients. The most common manifestation of this allergic response is a raised itchy skin rash, **serum sickness** (a reaction to a foreign serum), angioedema and difficulty breathing, and nephropathy.

Side effects of oral administration of penicillins are nausea, vomiting, diarrhea, and black "hairy" tongue (temporary overgrowth of harmless bacteria or yeast in the mouth). A nonallergic and harmless rash may also occur during amoxicillin therapy and is differentiated from a true hypersensitivity reaction based on the absence of raised or itchy rash. Very high concentrations of penicillin are neurotoxic, and nerve damage has resulted from intramuscular administration.

[handwritten margin note: Anaphylactic → Shock]

What are the contraindications and interactions?

Penicillins are contraindicated in patients with a history of hypersensitivity to penicillin or the cephalosporins. The drugs should be used cautiously in patients with renal disease or during pregnancy and lactation. Some penicillins, such as penicillin V and ampicillin, may interfere with the effectiveness of birth control pills that contain estrogen. The effectiveness of penicillin decreases when it is used with the tetracyclines because penicillin is bactericidal and requires actively producing bacteria for full effect (while the tetracyclines are bacteriostatic). Absorption of most penicillins is affected by food. They should be given 1 hour before or 2 hours after meals.

What are the important points patients should know?

Advise patients to take penicillin on an empty stomach (1 hour before or 2 hours after meals) to facilitate absorption. Note that amoxicillin may be taken with meals to decrease gastric upsets. Hypersensitivity may occur after oral administration of penicillin, so advise the patient to discontinue the medication and immediately contact his or her physician.

Table 9-2 ■ Penicillins

GENERIC NAME	TRADE NAME	AVERAGE DOSAGE IN ADULTS	ROUTE OF ADMINISTRATION
Natural Penicillins			
penicillin G (aqueous)	Pfizerpen	Up to 20–30 million units/d; dosage may also be based on weight	IV or IM
penicillin G benzathine	Bicillin L-A	Up to 2.4 million units/d	IM
penicillin G procaine, IM	Wycillin	600,000–2.4 million units/d	IM
penicillin V	Beepen VK, Pen-Vee-K	125–500 mg q6h or q8h	PO

Table 9-2 ■ Penicillins

GENERIC NAME	TRADE NAME	AVERAGE DOSAGE IN ADULTS	ROUTE OF ADMINISTRATION
Semisynthetic Penicillins, Penicillinase-Resistant Penicillins			
cloxacillin sodium	Cloxapen, Tegopen	250–500 mg q6h	PO
dicloxacillin sodium	Dynapen, Dycill, Pathocil	125–250 mg q6h	PO
nafcillin	Unipen, Nallpen	250 mg–1 g/d	PO
		500 mg q4–6h	IM
		3–6 g/d for 24–48 hours only	IV
oxacillin sodium	Bactocill	500 mg–1 g q4–6h	PO
		250 mg–1 g q4–6h	IM, IV
Aminopenicillins			
amoxicillin	Amoxil, Trimox, Wymox	250–500 mg q8h or 875 mg bid	PO
amoxicillin and clavulanate acid	Augmentin	250–500 mg q8h or 875 mg q12h	PO
ampicillin (oral)	Omnipen, Principen, Totacillin	250–500 mg q6h	PO
ampicillin sodium (parenteral)	Omnipen-N	1–12 g/d in divided doses q4–6h	IM, IV
ampicillin / sulbactam	Unasyn	0.5–1 g sulbactam with 1–2 g ampicillin q6–8h	IM, IV
bacampicillin	Spectrobid	400–800 mg q12h; dosage may also be based on weight	PO
Extended-Spectrum Penicillins			
mezlocillin sodium	Mezlin	200–300 mg/kg/d in 4–6 divided doses; up to 350 mg/kg/d	IM, IV
piperacillin sodium and tazobactam sodium	Zosyn	12 mg/1.5 g given as 3.375 g q6h	IV
piperacillin sodium	Pipracil	3–4 g q4–6h; maximum dosage 25 g/d	IM, IV
ticarcillin disodium	Ticar	150–300 mg/kg/d q3h, q4h, or q6h; maximum dosage 24 g/d	IM
		150–300 mg/kg/d q3h, q4h, or q6h; maximum dosage 2 g/d	IV
ticarcillin and clavulanate potassium	Timentin	3.1 g q4–6h or 200–300 mg/kg/d in divided doses q4–6h	IV

Focus Point

Penicillin Allergy

Allergic reaction to penicillin is an immediate life-threatening systemic reaction that typically occurs after exposure to penicillin injection. The patient must be closely observed for this reaction after injection.

Cephalosporins

The cephalosporins are a group of antibiotics closely related to the penicillins. Currently, they are classified into four generations, based on their **gram-negative** spectrum and stability in the presence of beta-lactamases (agents that retard action of enzymes). Gram-negative bacteria cannot resist decolorization with alcohol after being treated with Gram's crystal violet. Following decolorization, they can be readily counterstained with safranin, which gives them a pink or red color when viewed under a microscope. However, this classification scheme is becoming less reliable because newer agents have led to more exceptions and less precise criteria for differences in the **antibacterial spectrum** (the range of bacteria against which an agent is effective). Those with a broad spectrum are effective against many different kinds of bacteria, while those with a narrow spectrum may be effective against only a single type, or a few (Table 9-3 ■).

The different generations of cephalosporins are explained below:

✳ First-generation: Exhibit highest activity against gram-positive bacteria and lowest activity against gram-negative bacteria

✳ Second-generation: Are more active against gram-negative bacteria and less active against gram-positive bacteria than the first-generation cephalosporins

✳ Third-generation: Are considerably less active than first-generation agents against gram-positive bacteria (especially staphylococci), have a much expanded spectrum of activity against gram-negative organisms, are more resistant to gram-negative beta-lactamases

✳ Fourth-generation: Have improved gram-positive spectrum, and expanded gram-negative activity of third-generation cephalosporins

How do they work?

The cephalosporins have a mechanism of action that is very similar to that of the penicillins. They affect the bacterial cell wall and are bactericidal, resulting in the destruction of bacteria.

How are they used?

The cephalosporins are effective in a wide variety of infections because they have a broad spectrum. The first- and second-generation cephalosporins are used frequently for prophylaxis during certain surgical procedures to reduce the risk of postoperative wound infections. Cefazolin is preferred because it has a higher serum concentration and longer elimination half-life. A number of second- and third-generation cephalosporins are effective alternatives as prophylactic agents for various surgical procedures. Cephalosporins are generally not the first drugs of choice for any bacterial infections because equally effective and less expensive alternatives are available.

What are the adverse effects?

Hypersensitivity occurs in about 5 to 10% of patients taking cephalosporins; manifestations are drug fever, skin rash, urticaria (hives), serum sickness, anaphylaxis, neutropenia, and nephritis. Other adverse effects of cephalosporins include pain, sterile abscess, nausea, vomiting, glossitis, diarrhea, and abdominal pain. Cephalosporins have a 5 to 10% cross-sensitivity with penicillins.

What are the contraindications and interactions?

Cephalosporins should not be used in combination with other antibiotics that cause nephrotoxicity or ototoxicity. Diuretics such as furosemide and ethacrynic acid also enhance nephrotoxicity and make certain cephalosporins ototoxic. Estrogen-containing oral contraceptives and cephalosporins taken concurrently may result in therapeutic failure.

What are the important points patients should know?

Instruct patients to take cephalosporins on an empty stomach. If gastric irritation occurs, patients may take these drugs with food.

Table 9-3 ■ Cephalosporins

GENERIC NAME	TRADE NAME	AVERAGE DOSAGE IN ADULTS	ROUTE OF ADMINISTRATION
First-generation			
cefadroxil	Duricef	500 mg–1 g/d	PO
cefazolin	Ancef, Kefzol, Zolicef	250 mg–1 g/d	IM or IV
cephalexin	Keflex	25 mg–1 g/d	PO
cephalothin	Cephalonia	50 mg–2 g/d	IV
cephapirin	Cefadyl	25 mg–4 g/d	PO
cephradine	Velosef	250 mg/d	PO, IM, or IV
Second-generation			
cefaclor	Ceclor	125–500 mg/d	PO
cefonicid	Monocid	50 mg–12 g/d	IM or IV
cefoxitin	Mefoxin	2 g/d	IV
cefuroxime	Ceftin	125–500 mg/d	PO
Third-generation			
cefixime	Suprax	100–400 mg/d	PO
cefoperazone	Cefobid	1–6 g/d	IM or IV
cefotaxime moxalactam	Claforan	75 mg–4 g/d	IV
cefprozil	Cefzil	250–500 mg/d	PO
ceftriaxone	Rocephin	1–2 g/d	IV
Fourth-generation			
cefepime	Maxipime	500 mg–2 g/d	IM or IV

Superinfections

Superinfections may be caused by a disruption of the nonpathogenic microorganisms within the human body (also known as *normal flora*) that is often attributed to the use of antibiotics. When antibiotics destroy large numbers of normal flora, the chemical environment of the body is altered and a new infection is "superimposed" on an original infection (hence the term *superinfection*). The altered chemical environment allows for the uncontrolled growth of microorganisms (fungal or bacterial) that are not affected by the antibiotic in use. Superinfections may occur with any antibiotic and most often when antibiotics are used for long periods or over repeated therapy courses.

Superinfections can develop rapidly and become very serious or even life-threatening. Oral penicillins and cephalosporins often cause bacterial superinfections in the bowel, characterized by diarrhea (or bloody diarrhea), abdominal cramping, fever, and rectal bleeding. A common bacterial superinfection is *pseudomembranous colitis*. Both penicillins and cephalosporins are commonly associated with vaginal yeast infections.

Focus on Geriatrics

The Risk of Superinfection Among Elderly Patients

Older patients taking penicillin over a long period or those who are chronically ill or debilitated are more likely to contract a superinfection such as pseudomembranous colitis. This condition is potentially life threatening and produces a toxin that affects the lining of the colon. Signs and symptoms include abdominal cramping and severe diarrhea containing visible blood and mucus. Use of antibiotics should be discontinued, and severe cases may require treatment with intravenous fluids and electrolytes, oral vancomycin, and protein supplements.

✳ Apply Your Knowledge 9.2

The following questions focus on what you have just learned about sulfonamides, penicillins, and cephalosporins. *See Appendix E for the correct answers.*

FILL IN THE BLANK
Select terms from your reading to fill in the blanks.

1. The sulfonamides act by inhibiting _____, which most bacteria must synthesize, whereas humans can rely on dietary sources.
2. The cephalosporins are a group of antibiotics closely related to the _____.
3. Penicillins and cephalosporins may interfere with the effectiveness of birth control pills that contain _____.
4. The cephalosporins affect the bacterial cell wall and are described as _____.
5. _____ were the first antimicrobial agents discovered.
6. The first-generation cephalosporins have the highest activity against _____ and the lowest against _____ bacteria.

MULTIPLE CHOICE
Choose the correct answers from choices a–d.

1. The most common source of natural antibiotics is:
   a. Viruses
   b. Bacteria
   c. Molds
   d. Both b and c
2. Which of the following is the mechanism of action of the sulfonamides?
   a. Interfering with synthesis of peptidoglycans
   b. Interfering with DNA synthesis
   c. Inhibiting folic acid synthesis
   d. Terminating cell replication

3. Which of the following is the original penicillin?
   a. Nafcillin
   b. Penicillin G
   c. Penicillin V
   d. Oxacillin sodium

4. Absorption of the majority of penicillin is affected by which of the following factors?
   a. Food
   b. Fever
   c. Female chromosomes
   d. Male chromosomes

5. The mechanism of action of the cephalosporins is very similar to that of which of the following antibiotics?
   a. Tetracyclines
   b. Fluoroquinolones
   c. Aminoglycosides
   d. Penicillins

Aminoglycosides

Aminoglycosides have been very important antibiotics for the treatment of infections caused by gram-negative bacilli. They are **broad-spectrum** antibiotics (effective against a wide range of organisms). The clinically important aminoglycosides are amikacin (Amikin), gentamicin (Garamycin), kanamycin (Kantrex), neomycin (Mycifradin), netilmicin (Netromycin), streptomycin (Streptomycin), and tobramycin (Nebcin). Table 9-4 ■ lists various aminoglycosides.

How do they work?
The aminoglycosides combine with bacterial (not human) ribosomes to arrest protein synthesis. This interference prevents cell reproduction, resulting in death of the bacteria.

How are they used?
Large doses of aminoglycosides are given orally before abdominal surgery to reduce the number of intestinal bacteria. The usual route of administration for systemic effects is either intramuscular (IM) or intravenous (IV). Aminoglycosides are also commonly administered via the ophthalmic or otic route in the form of eye or ear drops to treat localized infections.

What are the adverse effects?
The serious adverse effects of aminoglycosides include ototoxicity and nephrotoxicity. Nephrotoxicity may occur, depending on renal function, age of the patient, and drug dose. Careful drug dosing is very important with younger and older patients. Prolonged use of aminoglycosides may cause a superinfection.

What are the contraindications and interactions?
Aminoglycosides should not be used during pregnancy because they may cause fetal harm—in particular, hearing loss and deafness in newborn babies. When aminoglycosides are used concurrently with penicillins, the desired effects of the aminoglycosides may be greatly decreased. Still, these drugs are often used in combination, especially in the treatment of bacterial endocarditis. These drugs should be given several hours apart. The drug action of warfarin (an oral anticoagulant) can increase if taken simultaneously with aminoglycosides. The risk of ototoxicity increases when ethacrynic acid and aminoglycosides are given.

What are the important points patients should know?

Instruct patients to increase fluid intake while taking aminoglycosides. This measure assists in preventing renal failure from nephrotoxicity. To minimize toxicity problems, short treatment periods (7–10 days) and once-daily administration should be used.

Table 9-4 ■ Aminoglycosides

GENERIC NAME	TRADE NAME	AVERAGE DOSAGE IN ADULTS	ROUTE OF ADMINISTRATION
amikacin	Amikin	15 mg/kg/d in 2–3 divided doses	IV or IM
gentamicin	Garamycin	3–5 mg/kg/d (standard dose)	IM
		6–7 mg/kg/d (once daily)	IV PO
kanamycin	Kantrex	15 mg/kg q8–12h	PO, IM, or IV
neomycin sulfate	Mycifradin	50–100 mg/kg/d	PO
		10–15 mg/d	Topical
netilmicin	Netromycin	3–6 mg/kg/d	IV or IM
streptomycin	Streptomycin	0.5–1 g q12–24h	IM
tobramycin	Nebcin	3–5 mg/kg/d (standard dose)	IV, IM, or ophthalmic
vancomycin	Vancocin	6–7 mg/kg/d (once daily)	PO or IV

Macrolides

The term *macrolide* refers to the large chemical ring structure characteristic of these antibiotics. The macrolides include erythromycin (E-mycin, others), azithromycin (Zithromax), clarithromycin (Biaxin), troleandomycin (Tao), and dirithromycin (Dynabac). Erythromycin is produced by *Streptomyces erythreus*. Macrolides are bacteriostatic at normal doses and bactericidal at higher doses. They are also commonly used as alternative drugs in patients who are allergic to penicillin because they are effective against many of the same organisms. Table 9-5 ■ lists common macrolides. The macrolides are active against gram-positive and gram-negative aerobic bacteria and atypical organisms including chlamydiae, mycoplasmae, legionellae, rickettsia, and spirochetes.

How do they work?

The mechanism of action of the macrolides is inhibition of bacterial protein synthesis by binding to the bacterial ribosome, which stops bacterial growth. Macrolides bind equally to ribosomes from gram-positive and gram-negative bacteria.

How are they used?

Macrolides are indicated for treatment of bacterial-related exacerbations of chronic obstructive pulmonary disease (COPD), skin structure infections, pharyngitis, tonsillitis, sinusitis, bronchitis, and other respiratory tract infections, pneumonia, acute otitis media, duodenal ulcers, pelvic inflammatory disease, intestinal amebiasis, rheumatic fever, soft-tissue infections, urethritis, syphilis, Legionnaires' disease, and urinary tract or rectal infections.

What are the adverse effects?

The macrolides, in general, are considered safe agents. Gastrointestinal effects, such as abdominal pain, nausea, and vomiting, are the most common adverse effects. The newer macrolides cause fewer GI side effects. Hepatotoxicity related to the macrolides is rare but may be serious. Extremely high doses of IV erythromycin and oral clarithromycin have been associated with ototoxicity. Phlebitis may occur with intravenous administration of the macrolides.

What are the contraindications and interactions?

Macrolides are contraindicated in patients with hypersensitivity to them. They must be avoided in individuals who have a history of erythromycin-associated hepatitis or liver dysfunction. Erythromycin inhibits the hepatic metabolism of theophylline. It may interfere with the metabolism of digoxin, corticosteroids, and cyclosporine. In fact, drug interaction between macrolides and cyclosporine, and the resulting toxicity, has led to the removal of several drugs from the market in the United States.

What are the important points patients should know?

Instruct patients to take oral macrolides with a full glass of water on an empty stomach (1 hour before or 2 hours after meals) to get the maximum effect. Enteric-coated, sustained-release preparations can be administered with food and are often prescribed for patients with a GI intolerance.

Table 9-5 ■ Commonly Used Macrolides

Upper Respiratory infection (handwritten annotation pointing to Zithromax)

GENERIC NAME	TRADE NAME	AVERAGE DOSAGE IN ADULTS	ROUTE OF ADMINISTRATION
azithromycin	Zithromax	5–2000 mg	PO
clarithromycin	Biaxin	7.5–500 mg	PO
dirithromycin	Dynabac	250 mg	PO
erythromycin base	Eryc, E-mycin	250 mg	PO
erythromycin estolate	Ilosone	30 mg–1 g	IM, IV, or PO
erythromycin stearate	Erythrocin	30 mg–1 g	IV or PO
troleandomycin	Tao	125–500 mg	PO

✳ Apply Your Knowledge 9.3

The following questions focus on generic and trade names of antibacterial and antiviral drugs. *See Appendix E for the correct answers.*

MATCHING

Match the letter trade name to the numbered generic drug name.

GENERIC NAME	TRADE NAME
1. _____ kanamycin	a. Garamycin
2. _____ clindamycin	b. Zithromax
3. _____ tobramycin	c. Biaxin
4. _____ erythromycin estolate	d. Amikin
5. _____ azithromycin	e. Nebcin
6. _____ gentamicin	f. Dynabac
7. _____ dirithromycin	g. Vancocin
8. _____ vancomycin	h. Ilosone
9. _____ amikacin	i. Cleocin
10. _____ clarithromycin	j. Kantrex

(continued)

Apply Your Knowledge 9.3 (continued)

MULTIPLE CHOICE

Choose the correct answers from choices a–d.

1. All of the following are in the class of aminoglycosides, except:

   a. Neomycin

   b. Streptomycin

   c. Clindamycin

   d. Amikacin

2. The usual route of administration for systemic effects of aminoglycosides is:

   a. Intradermal

   b. Subcutaneous

   c. Intramuscular

   d. Intramuscular or intravenous

3. Which of the following is a serious adverse effect of aminoglycosides?

   a. Voice alteration

   b. Ototoxicity

   c. Toothache

   d. Postural hypotension

4. Which of the following is NOT a macrolide antibiotic?

   a. Clarithromycin

   b. Vibromycin

   c. Troleandomycin

   d. Azithromycin

5. Extremely high doses of IV erythromycin have been associated with which of the following adverse effects?

   a. Nephrotoxicity

   b. Hepatotoxicity

   c. Ototoxicity

   d. Granulocytopenia

Fluoroquinolones

The antibacterial drugs known as quinolones have been in use since 1964 when nalidixic acid was released. Since 1990, the fluoroquinolones have become a dominant class of bactericidal antimicrobial agents.

In general, the fluoroquinolones possess activity against gram-positive, gram-negative, and atypical organisms. The older fluoroquinolones (ciprofloxacin [Cipro], norfloxacin [Noroxin], and ofloxacin [Floxin]) are highly active against gram-negative pathogens, but their activity against gram-positive pathogens is limited. The newer fluoroquinolones have enhanced activity against the gram-positive pathogens, while maintaining similar gram-negative activity (Table 9-6 ■).

How do they work?

The fluoroquinolones exert their bactericidal effect by interfering with an enzyme (DNA gyrase) that is required by bacteria for the synthesis of DNA. This action inhibits cell reproduction, resulting in the death of the bacteria.

How are they used?

The fluoroquinolones have a broad spectrum of antimicrobial activity. They are used to treat UTIs, prostatitis, gonorrhea, anthrax, pneumonia and other respiratory tract infections, and infections of bones and joints.

What are the adverse effects?

Adverse effects are usually mild and transient. They include nausea, vomiting, diarrhea, flatulence, abdominal discomfort, skin rashes, photosensitivity (especially severe with sparfloxacin), and some nephrotoxicity. Rare but severe reactions that have also been reported include neuropsychiatric effects, cardiac abnormalities, and liver dysfunction. In children, fluoroquinolones may damage developing cartilage.

What are the contraindications and interactions?

Fluoroquinolones should be avoided in children younger than 18 years and in pregnant or lactating women. When used with caffeine, symptoms such as insomnia and hyperactivity may occur. Antacids decrease the absorption of the drug and should not be given for 2 hours following the administration of the antibiotic.

What are the important points patients should know?

Advise patients that fluoroquinolones should not be taken with milk or other dairy products, antacids, magnesium laxatives, and iron supplements. Advise patients to drink adequate fluids to maintain a high urine output, thereby preventing crystalluria. Instruct patients to report visual disturbances, dizziness, light-headedness, or depression that may indicate potential early CNS toxicity. If these manifestations occur, advise patients to avoid driving and operating heavy machinery and report the effects immediately. Alcohol may worsen these effects and should be avoided.

Table 9-6 ■ Fluoroquinolones

GENERIC NAME	TRADE NAME	AVERAGE DOSAGE IN ADULTS	ROUTE OF ADMINISTRATION
Classical Fluoroquinolones			
ciprofloxacin	Cipro	500–750 mg q12h (oral) 400 mg q12h (IV)	PO, IV
enoxacin	Penetrex	200–400 mg q12h for 1–2 wk	IV PO
levofloxacin	Levaquin	250–500 mg/d (both)	PO, IV
lomefloxacin	Maxaquin	400 mg/d for 2 wk	PO
nalidixic acid	NegGram	500 mg and 300 mg/5 mL	PO
norfloxacin	Noroxin	400 mg q12h for 3 d (both)	PO, ophthalmic
ofloxacin	Floxin	200–400 mg q12h (both)	PO, IV
Newest Fluoroquinolones			
gatifloxacin	Tequin	400 mg/d for 7–14 d (both)	PO, IV
moxifloxacin	Avelox	400 mg/d for 5–10 d	PO
sparfloxacin	Zagam	Loading dose: 400 mg Day 1; then 200 mg/d for 10 d	PO
trovafloxacin	Trovan	100 mg	PO

Avoid Fluoroquinolones in Children

Fluoroquinolones should be avoided in children because studies in young animals have documented erosion of cartilage. However, these agents have been used safely in children with cystic fibrosis without harm.

Tetracyclines

The tetracyclines are all very much alike with respect to their antimicrobial spectra and the untoward effects they elicit. They differ mainly in their absorption, duration of action, and suitability for parenteral administration (Table 9-7 ■).

How do they work?

The tetracyclines are broad-spectrum antibiotics and are mainly bacteriostatic. They bind to the bacterial ribosomes and prevent protein synthesis. The tetracyclines have activities against both gram-positive and gram-negative bacteria, mycobacteria, rickettsia, and chlamydiae.

How are they used?

The tetracyclines are used in the treatment of infections caused by a wide range of microorganisms. They are effective against *Rickettsia* (Rocky Mountain spotted fever and typhus fever). These drugs are also indicated for therapy of chlamydial infections, cholera, brucellosis, tularemia, and amebiasis. Tetracyclines are prescribed as an alternative to penicillin for the treatment of gonorrhea, syphilis, Lyme disease, anthrax, and *Haemophilus influenzae* respiratory infections. Doxycycline (Vibramycin) is highly effective in the prophylaxis of "traveler's diarrhea."

What are the adverse effects?

The tetracyclines cause a number of untoward effects. GI toxicity is common with oral use; it is probably due to the combined effect of local irritation and alteration of the intestinal flora. Manifestations are heartburn, nausea, vomiting, and diarrhea. They are also associated with photosensitivity reactions, predisposing patients to severe sunburn.

The broad-spectrum antibacterial activity of the tetracyclines may cause superinfections as can that of penicillins, cephalosporins, and sulfa drugs. This occurs most commonly in the bowel, but it also may occur readily in the mouth, lungs, and vagina. The most common superinfection is **candidiasis**, which is an infection or disease caused by *Candida*, especially *Candida albicans*—usually resulting from debilitation, physiologic change, prolonged administration of antibiotics, and barrier breakage. Overgrowth from staphylococci may also occur. Staphylococcal enteric superinfections are frequently fatal.

Various hypersensitivity reactions or hepatotoxicity may occur. Tetracyclines may cause a darker pigment (graying) in developing teeth in children younger than 8 years and may impair bone growth.

What are the contraindications and interactions?

The tetracyclines should be avoided in patients with hypersensitivity, liver diseases, and in children younger than 8 years. These drugs are also contraindicated in pregnant and lactating women.

Certain foods (such as dairy products) and drugs (such as laxatives, antacids that contain aluminum and calcium, and iron preparations) may reduce the absorption of tetracyclines. Therefore, it is recommended that tetracyclines be taken on an empty stomach. Phenytoin and barbiturates can decrease the effectiveness of tetracyclines.

What are the important points patients should know?

Instruct patients that tetracyclines should be taken on an empty stomach (1 hour before or 2 hours after meals) to facilitate absorption. The absorption of tetracyclines is strongly influenced by the presence of food and other drugs. Advise patients that because tetracyclines can cause photosensitivity reactions they should avoid the sun during the warmest time of day (10 A.M. to 2 P.M.), use a sunblock, and wear a hat as well as protective clothing. Tetracyclines should be stored away from light and extreme heat because the effects of light and heat cause tetracyclines to decompose and produce toxic breakdown products. Expired tetracyclines should be disposed of immediately.

Table 9-7 ■ Tetracyclines *Alternative to penicillin for gonorrhea, syphilis, chlamydial infec.; infected Acne*

GENERIC NAME	TRADE NAME	AVERAGE DOSAGE IN ADULTS	ROUTE OF ADMINISTRATION
chlortetracycline	Aureomycin	250–500 mg q6h	PO
demeclocycline	Declomycin	150 mg q6h	PO
doxycycline	Vibramycin	100–200 mg initially; then 100 mg bid	PO
minocycline	Minocin	200 mg initially; then 100 mg bid (both)	PO, IV
oxytetracycline	Terramycin	250 mg/d	PO
tetracycline	Achromycin, Sumycin Panmycin, Steclin	250–500 mg q6h; 100 mg bid–tid	PO, IM

✳ Apply Your Knowledge 9.4

The following questions focus on what you have just learned about fluoroquinolones and tetracyclines. *See Appendix E for the correct answers.*

MULTIPLE CHOICE

Choose the correct answers from choices a–e.

1. The fluoroquinolones are used to treat which of the following illnesses?

    a. Tuberculosis

    b. Gonorrhea

    c. Pancreatitis

    d. Hematoma

    e. West Nile disease

2. Ciprofloxacin is contraindicated in children younger than age:

    a. 1 month

    b. 12 months

    c. 18 months

    d. 12 years

    e. 18 years

(continued)

Apply Your Knowledge 9.4 (continued)

3. The most common superinfection occurring from the use of tetracyclines is:

 a. Candidiasis

 b. Gonorrhea

 c. Tuberculosis

 d. Meningitis

 e. None of the above

4. Ciprofloxacin should not be taken with which of the following?

 a. Laxatives

 b. Iron supplements

 c. Milk

 d. Antacids

 e. All of the above

5. The drug(s) of choice for Lyme disease is/are:

 a. Penicillins

 b. Clindamycin

 c. Tetracyclines

 d. Spectomycin

 e. Vancomycin

LABELING

In Questions 1–5, refer to the following drug label and fill in the specific drug information needed.

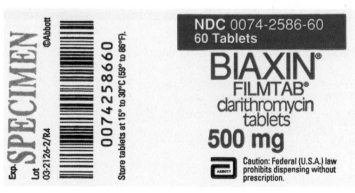

Copyright Abbott Laboratories. Reprinted with permission.

1. What is the generic name of the drug?

   _____

2. What is the name of the manufacturer of the drug?

   _____

3. What is the brand name of the drug?

   _____

4. What is the form of the drug?

   _____

5. What is the lot number of the drug?

   _____

In Questions 6–10, refer to the following drug label to fill in the specific drug information needed.

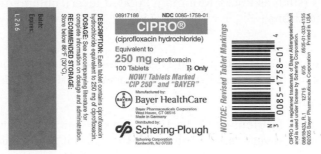

Reproduced with Permission from Bayer

6. What is the strength of the tablets?

_____

7. What is the brand name of the drug?

_____

8. What is the generic name of the drug?

_____

9. What is new about the drug?

_____

10. What is the manufacturer's name?

_____

MISCELLANEOUS ANTIBACTERIAL AGENTS

These antibacterial agents are principally second-line drugs because of emerging resistance, concerns with toxicity, or special activity against selected organisms. Discussion of chloramphenicol, clindamycin, streptogramin, rifampin, vancomycin, and other miscellaneous antibacterial agents follows (Table 9-8 ■).

Table 9-8 ■ Miscellaneous Antibacterial Agents

GENERIC NAME	TRADE NAME	AVERAGE DOSAGE IN ADULTS	ROUTE OF ADMINISTRATION
chloramphenicol	Chloromycetin, others	12.5 mg/kg qid	PO
clindamycin	Cleocin	500 mg–2 g/d in 3–4 divided doses	IV
		500 mg q6h	PO
		8–20 mg/kg/d in 3–4 equal doses	IM
		15–40 mg/kg/d in 3–4 equal doses	Topical
linezolid	Zyvox	600 mg bid	PO
spectinomycin	Trobicin	2 g as single dose	IM
vancomycin	Vancocin	500 mg qid–1 g bid	IV

CHLORAMPHENICOL

Chloramphenicol (Chloromycetin, others) is highly effective against rickettsial diseases (such as Rocky Mountain spotted fever), chlamydial diseases, and many bacterial infections.

How does it work?

Chloramphenicol is primarily bacteriostatic and a secondary bactericidal medication against a few bacterial strains. This agent interferes with protein synthesis.

How is it used?

Because of serious toxic reactions, the systemic use of chloramphenicol should be limited only to very serious infections that cannot be managed by other drugs. It is still the drug of choice for typhoid fever.

What are the adverse effects?

Bone-marrow injury is the major toxic effect of chloramphenicol. Thrombocytopenia, granulocytopenia, and aplastic anemia are the most serious blood cell formation disturbances observed and have resulted in a number of fatalities. In neonates, its use may cause *gray-baby syndrome*.

What are the contraindications and interactions?

Chloramphenicol must be avoided in patients with known hypersensitivity to the drug. It must be used cautiously in patients with severe liver or kidney disease, in elderly patients, and during pregnancy or lactation.

Chloramphenicol may inhibit the metabolism of dicoumarol, tolbutamide, and phenytoin, leading to prolonged action and increased effects of these drugs. Phenobarbital can reduce the effect of chloramphenicol levels and may cause toxicity.

What are the important points patients should know?

Advise patients to take oral chloramphenicol with a full glass of water on an empty stomach and to avoid driving or operating heavy machinery if confusion or visual disturbances occur. Instruct patients to report any manifestation of blood dyscrasias, such as sore throat, weakness, unexplained bruising or bleeding, and fever, to their physician promptly.

Focus on Pediatrics

Gray-baby Syndrome

Gray-baby syndrome is a fatal cyanosis. Its symptoms include vomiting, abdominal distension, and loose, green stools owing to the inability of infants to metabolize the drug.

CLINDAMYCIN

Clindamycin (Cleocin) is an antibacterial agent used as an alternate drug for treating infections caused by penicillin-resistant *Staphylococci aureus*.

How does it work?

Clindamycin is bacteriostatic and inhibits bacterial protein synthesis. This agent is active against most gram-positive and many anaerobic organisms.

How is it used?

Clindamycin is the drug of choice for treatment of GI infections caused by *Bacteroides fragilis*. It is perhaps the best drug for the topical treatment of acne vulgaris. Lincomycin has marked toxicity. It is used only against infections for which it has been determined to be the most effective drug, including joint, bone, abdominal, and female genitourinary tract infections.

What are the adverse effects?

Clindamycin may cause abdominal pain, nausea, vomiting, and diarrhea. It may also result in antibiotic-associated (pseudomembranous) colitis.

What are the contraindications and interactions?

The contraindications include previous hypersensitivity to lincomycin and clindamycin, or impaired liver function. This agent should be avoided in newborn babies. It is not safe for use in pregnant or lactating women. Clindamycin must be used cautiously in patients with impaired kidney function, history of GI disease (particularly colitis), history of liver disease, or asthma. It may potentiate the effects of neuromuscular blocking agents.

What are the important points patients should know?

Advise patients to take lincomycin with a full glass of water on an empty stomach. Because the medicine works best when the dose is constant, remind patients to take doses as scheduled.

SPECTINOMYCIN

Spectinomycin (Trobicin) is an antibiotic produced by *Streptomyces spectabilis*. This agent is bacteriostatic. It has variable activity against a wide variety of gram-negative and gram-positive organisms.

How does it work?

Spectinomycin suppresses protein synthesis in gram-negative bacteria, especially *Neisseria gonorrhoeae*.

How is it used?

Spectinomycin is used only for the treatment of uncomplicated gonorrhea in patients sensitized or resistant to penicillin.

What are the adverse effects?

The common adverse effects of spectinomycin include headache, dizziness, chills, fever, insomnia, nervousness, nausea, and vomiting. It also causes pain and soreness at the injection site.

What are the contraindications and interactions?

The safety of spectinomycin during pregnancy, lactation, and in infants or children is not established. This drug is also contraindicated in known cases of hypersensitivity to spectinomycin. No significant drug or food interactions for this agent are known.

What are the important points patients should know?

Advise patients to use condoms to prevent transmission of gonorrheal infection. It may be necessary to treat patients' partners to prevent reinfection. Instruct patients to avoid driving or operating heavy machinery if dizziness occurs after administration.

VANCOMYCIN

Vancomycin (Vancocin) is the drug of choice for severe infections caused by drug-resistant *Staphylococcus* and *Clostridium* infections.

How does it work?

Vancomycin suppresses cell-wall synthesis and is bactericidal. This drug is eliminated, unchanged, by the kidneys.

How is it used?

Vancomycin is usually reserved for serious infections, especially those caused by methicillin-resistant staphylococci. It is useful in patients who are allergic to penicillin or cephalosporins. Typical uses include osteomyelitis, endocarditis, and staphylococcal pneumonia. When given orally, vancomycin is useful in the treatment of pseudomembranous colitis.

What are the adverse effects?

The most serious side effects of vancomycin are ototoxicity and nephrotoxicity. Additional adverse effects include chills, fever, nausea, skin rashes, and urticaria. Local pain and phlebitis at the site of intravenous injection have been reported, as well as a flushing sensation that can occur if the agent is infused too rapidly.

What are the contraindications and interactions?

Vancomycin must be avoided in patients with known hypersensitivity to this drug. It is also contraindicated in patients with previous hearing loss. Vancomycin should be administered with caution in neonates, children, older adults, pregnant women, and in patients with impaired kidney function or renal failure. Vancomycin increases neuromuscular blockade of the muscle relaxants atracurium, pancuronium, tubocurarine, and vecuronium.

What are the important points patients should know?

Advise patients to notify their health-care providers if they experience ringing in the ears while taking this medicine.

Focus Point

Red-Man Syndrome and Vancomycin

Vancomycin may cause "red-man syndrome," a condition that is manifested by facial flushing and hypotension due to very rapid infusion of the drug. A 1-g dose should be infused over at least 60 minutes.

LINEZOLID

Linezolid (Zyvox) is an oxazolidinone, a class of totally synthetic antibiotics first investigated in the late 1980s as antidepressant drugs. Later, these agents were discovered to have excellent antibacterial activity. The main reason for their development has been the increased resistance of gram-positive pathogens. The FDA approved the first agent of this class in April 2000. The initial drug was linezolid (Zyvox), which is the only oxazolidinone commercially available to date.

How does it work?

Linezolid is a protein–synthesis inhibiting compound that usually produces a bacteriostatic effect. The principal activity is against gram-positive aerobic organisms, including staphylococci, streptococci, and enterococci.

How is it used?

Linezolid is used for gram-positive drug-resistant microorganisms that are highly virulent.

What are the adverse effects?

In general, linezolid is well tolerated. The most common adverse effects are nausea, vomiting, diarrhea, and leukopenia.

What are the contraindications and interactions?

Linezolid is contraindicated in patients hypersensitive to the drug or its components. Use of linezolid with adrenergic drugs such as dopamine, epinephrine, or pseudoephedrine may cause hypertension. Blood pressure and heart rate should be monitored. Other items that may cause interactions include serotoninergic drugs and foods and beverages high in tyramine (including aged cheeses, air-dried meats, chocolate, fish, sauerkraut, red wines, tap beers, and soy sauce).

What are the important points patients should know?

Advise patients to avoid foods that contain tyramine while taking oxazolidinones.

✳ Apply Your Knowledge 9.5

The following questions focus on what you have just learned about the miscellaneous antibacterial agents. *See Appendix E for the correct answers.*

MATCHING
Match the lettered drug to the numbered item that corresponds to the drug's adverse effect, use, or other descriptor.

ADVERSE EFFECT, USE, DESCRIPTOR

1. _____ Pseudomembranous colitis
2. _____ The initial drug was linezolid
3. _____ Gray-baby syndrome
4. _____ Used only for uncomplicated gonorrhea
5. _____ Red-man syndrome

DRUG

a. Chloramphenicol
b. Vancomycin
c. Spectinomycin
d. Oxazolidinones
e. Lincomycin

FILL IN THE BLANK
Select terms from your reading to fill in the blanks.

1. Chloramphenicol is still the drug of choice for _____.
2. An alternative drug for treating infections caused by penicillin-resistant *Staphylococci aureus* is _____.
3. Spectinomycin suppresses protein synthesis in gram-negative bacteria, especially _____.
4. The drug of choice for treatment of GI infections caused by *Bacteroides fragilis* is _____.
5. Chloramphenicol, in neonates, may cause _____.

ANTITUBERCULOSIS AGENTS

Tuberculosis (TB) is a worldwide disease caused by *Mycobacterium tuberculosis*, an acid-fast aerobic bacillus. Any organ system can be affected by the disease, but the most common sites are the lungs and lymph nodes.

Worldwide, 3 million people die of tuberculosis each year. There are an estimated 10 to 15 million people in the United States with tuberculosis. Ninety percent of cases involve reactivation of prior infection; the remainder of cases are new infections. The majority of new cases occur in malnourished individuals, those living in overcrowded conditions, immunosuppressed individuals, incarcerated persons, immigrants, and elderly persons.

The twentieth century was characterized by a decline in the incidence of tuberculosis in most developed countries. This was largely due to antibiotic drugs, active immunization, screening of people and livestock, and better living conditions. More recently, a disturbing rise in occurrence of this infection has been seen. This increase appears to be due to immigration patterns, drug-resistant strains of TB, and a prevalence of conditions that impair immunity (for example, HIV/AIDS and organ transplant therapy).

As many as four different drug combinations may be required to treat TB. These combinations are divided into the first- and second-line antituberculotics, on the basis of their efficacy, activity, and adverse effects. Therapy is usually started with ethambutol (myambutol), isoniazid (INH), rifampin (Rifadin, Rimactane), and pyrazinamide (PZA) for the first 2 months, followed by isoniazid and rifampin for a further minimum of 4 months. This regimen is suitable if bacteriology shows fully sensitive acid-fast bacilli (which may include *Mycobacteria* or *Nocardia*) on culture (Table 9-9 ■).

Table 9-9 ■ Most Commonly Used Antituberculotics

GENERIC NAME	BRAND NAME	AVERAGE DOSAGE IN ADULTS	ROUTE OF ADMINISTRATION
capreomycin	Capastat	1 g/d	IM
ciprofloxacin	Cipro	100–750 mg q12h	PO
		200–400 mg 8–q12h	IV
cycloserine	Seromycin	250 mg q12h	PO
ethambutol	Myambutol	400 mg/d	PO
ethionamide	Trecator-SC	500–750 mg/d	PO
isoniazid (INH)	Laniazid, Nydrazid	5–10 mg/kg/d (up to 300 mg/d)	PO, IM
isoniazid-pyrazinamide-rifampin	Rifater	300 mg/d	PO, IV
ofloxacin	Floxin	200–400 mg q12h	PO
pyrazinamide	PZA	15–35 mg/kg/d in 3–4 divided doses (up to 2 g/d)	PO
rifampin	Rifadin, Rimactane	600 mg/d with other antituberculars	PO, IV
rifapentine	Priftin	600 mg twice weekly for 2 mo; then 600 mg/wk for 4 mo	PO
streptomycin sulfate	Streptomycin	15 mg/kg (up to 1 g) as a single dose	IM

ISONIAZID

Isoniazid (INH) is the most potent and selective of the known tuberculostatic antibacterial agents. It is tuberculocidal to growing bacteria and the most effective agent in the therapy of tuberculosis. The drug is never used alone because of the rapid emergence of resistance.

How does it work?

Isoniazid acts by interfering with the biosynthesis of bacterial proteins, nucleic acid, and lipids.

How is it used?

Isoniazid is used in the treatment of all forms of active tuberculosis caused by susceptible organisms and as a preventative in high-risk persons, such as household members and persons with positive tuberculin skin test reactions.

What are the adverse effects?

The common adverse effects include restlessness, insomnia, convulsions, optic neuritis, and psychoses. The drug also may cause nausea, vomiting, aplastic anemia, fever, and skin rashes.

What are the contraindications and interactions?

History of isoniazid-associated hypersensitivity reactions, liver damage, and pregnancy are contraindications for its use. This drug should be used cautiously in patients with chronic liver disease, renal dysfunction, history of convulsive disorders, and chronic alcoholism.

What are the important points patients should know?

Advise patients that isoniazid is absorbed better on an empty stomach. Instruct patients to avoid driving or operating heavy machinery if dizziness or drowsiness occurs and to contact their physician if tinnitus (ringing in the ears), visual changes, dizziness, or ataxia (an inability to coordinate muscle activity) occur. Patients must notify their physician if symptoms of hepatotoxicity occur, including fever, liver tenderness, loss of appetite, malaise, or jaundice.

Focus on Geriatrics

Risk of Fatal Hepatitis with Isoniazid Therapy

Older patients taking isoniazid are very susceptible to a potentially fatal hepatitis, especially if they regularly drink alcohol. Careful monitoring for signs of liver impairment is necessary. Good patient observation alerts the caregiver to the warning signs, which include increased serum alanine transferase and increased serum aspartate transaminase (liver enzymes), increased serum bilirubin (a substance released into the blood when red blood cells break down), and jaundice. Liver dysfunction in older adults may also be caused by the antitubercular drugs pyrazinamide and rifampin.

ETHAMBUTOL

Ethambutol (myambutol) is a tuberculostatic drug that is effective against tubercle bacilli that are resistant to isoniazid (INH) or streptomycin (Streptomycin).

How does it work?

Ethambutol's mechanism of action is not completely understood, but it appears to inhibit RNA synthesis and arrest multiplication of tubercle bacilli. The emergence of resistant TB strains is delayed by administering ethambutol in combination with other antituberculosis drugs.

How is it used?

Ethambutol can be used in conjunction with at least one other antituberculotic in the treatment of pulmonary tuberculosis.

What are the adverse effects?

Ethambutol occasionally causes optic neuritis, with blurred vision and diminished visual acuity to green light. Although these effects disappear on discontinuation, the drug should be discontinued at the first indication of a loss in visual acuity. Eye tests should be made before and at monthly intervals after the onset of therapy.

Other adverse effects include pruritus, anorexia, nausea, vomiting, abdominal pain, headache, vertigo, fever, hallucinations, and abnormal liver function.

What are the contraindications and interactions?

Ethambutol is contraindicated in patients with optic neuritis or history of hypersensitivity to the drug. It is also contraindicated in children younger than 6 years. Ethambutol should be used cautiously in patients with renal impairment, hepatic disease, gout, cataracts, diabetic retinopathy, and in those who are pregnant or lactating. Ethambutol absorption is decreased with aluminum salts.

What are the important points patients should know?

Instruct patients about the importance of regular eye examinations while taking ethambutol. If the patient experiences problems with vision, the drug should be stopped immediately.

Advise patients to take ethambutol with meals to lessen gastric irritation and to avoid driving or operating heavy machinery if drowsiness or dizziness occurs.

RIFAMPIN

Rifampin (Rifadin, Rimactane) is a broad-spectrum antibiotic, effective against most gram-positive bacteria, and variably active against gram-negative organisms. *Mycobacterium tuberculosis* is very susceptible to this drug.

How does it work?

Rifampin inhibits the activity of DNA-dependent RNA polymerase (an enzyme responsible for creating different RNA molecules) in susceptible bacterial cells, thereby suppressing RNA synthesis.

How is it used?

Rifampin is used primarily with other antituberculosis agents for the initial treatment and retreatment of clinical tuberculosis and as short-term therapy to eliminate meningococci from the nasopharynx of an asymptomatic carrier of *N. meningitides* when the risk of meningococcal meningitis is high.

What are the adverse effects?

Fatigue, drowsiness, headache, confusion, dizziness, nausea, vomiting, heartburn, skin rashes, and renal insufficiency may be observed with rifampin administration. This drug may also cause a reddish-orange discoloration of body fluids such as tears, urine, sweat, and saliva.

What are the contraindications and interactions?

Rifampin must be avoided in patients with a history of hypersensitivity to the drug. It should be used with caution in patients with hepatic disease or a history of alcoholism, and in those who are pregnant or lactating.

Rifampin decreases concentrations of alfentanil (Alfenta; an opioid analgesic), alosetron (Lotronex; used to treat irritable bowel syndrome), barbiturates, benzodiazepines, and many other drugs. The use of rifampin with oral anticoagulants or oral hypoglycemics may decrease the effects of these drugs.

What are the important points patients should know?

Inform patients that rifampin may cause urine, feces, saliva, sputum, sweat, and tears to develop a red-orange appearance. This effect is harmless. Advise patients not to wear soft contact lenses because they may become permanently stained. Instruct patients to take rifampin on an empty stomach and to avoid driving or operating heavy machinery if drowsiness or dizziness occurs. Instruct patients to notify their physician if manifestations of hepatotoxicity, including fever, loss of appetite, liver tenderness, malaise, or jaundice, occur.

PYRAZINAMIDE

Pyrazinamide (PZA) is an antituberculosis drug used for initial treatment in combination with isoniazid and rifampin. It generally is administered with isoniazid (INH), which it potentiates. However, it is quite toxic and should be held in reserve until other therapy fails.

How does it work?

Pyrazinamide is bacteriostatic against *M. tuberculosis*. When employed alone, resistance may develop in 6 to 7 weeks. Therefore, administration with other effective agents is recommended.

How is it used?

Pyrazinamide is used for short-term therapy of advanced tuberculosis before surgery and to treat patients unresponsive to primary agents such as isoniazid (INH) and streptomycin (Streptomycin).

What are the adverse effects?

Hepatotoxicity is the principal adverse effect reported with pyrazinamide use. Other adverse effects include nausea, vomiting, diarrhea, skin rashes, and myalgia.

What are the contraindications and interactions?

Pyrazinamide should be avoided in patients with a history of hypersensitivity to the drug. It is contraindicated in patients who have severe liver damage, or who are pregnant or lactating. Pyrazinamide must be used cautiously in patients with gout or diabetes mellitus, history of peptic ulcer, and impaired kidney function. Pyrazinamide decreases the effects of allopurinol, colchicine, and probenecid. This drug increases liver toxicity when used with rifampin.

What are the important points patients should know?

Instruct patients to notify their physician if manifestations of hepatotoxicity, including fever, liver tenderness, loss of appetite, malaise, or jaundice, occur.

✳ Apply Your Knowledge 9.6

The following questions focus on what you have just learned about the antituberculosis agents. *See Appendix E for the correct answers.*

FILL IN THE BLANK

Select terms from your reading to fill in the blanks.

1. _____ is the most potent and selective of the known antituberculosis agents.

2. Ethambutol can be used in _____ with at least one other antituberculosis drug.

3. The most common sites affected by tuberculosis are the _____ and _____ _____.

4. A reddish-orange discoloration of body fluids (tears, urine, sweat, saliva) may be caused by _____.

5. Because of its toxicity _____ should be used only after other therapy has failed.

MATCHING

Match the letter trade name to its numbered generic drug name.

GENERIC NAME	TRADE NAME
1. _____ rifampin	a. Trecator-SC
2. _____ isoniazid (INH)	b. Rifater
3. _____ isoniazid-rifampin	c. Nydrazid
4. _____ ethambutol	d. Myambutol
5. _____ ethionamide	e. Priftin

Antiviral Agents

Viruses cause much of the morbidity and mortality in populations worldwide, but the number of drugs available to treat such viruses is still quite low. Antiviral drug development has become very active in the last decade, especially with the challenges of the AIDS epidemic.

Only a few antiviral drugs have been successfully used in the United States. However, several viral diseases, including measles, mumps, rubella, polio, chickenpox, smallpox, and rabies are prevented by vaccines. The antiviral agents reviewed here are acyclovir (Zovirax), amantadine (Symmetrol), didanosine, ribavirin (Virazole), zanamivir (Relenza), ganciclovir (Cytovene), and zidovudine (AZT, Retrovir). Table 9-10 ■ shows classification of various antiviral drugs.

Table 9-10 ■ Antiviral Drugs

GENERIC NAME	TRADE NAME	AVERAGE DOSAGE IN ADULTS	ROUTE OF ADMINISTRATION
acyclovir	Zovirax	5–10 mg/kg over 1h q8h for up to 7 d	IV
		200–800 mg q4–8h for 5–10 d	PO
amantadine hydrochloride	Symmetrel	200 mg/d single dose or 100 mg/d bid	PO
cidofovir	Vistide	5 mg/kg over 1 h/wk for 2 consecutive wk; then once every 2 wk	IV
didanosine	Videx, Videx EC	125–300 mg bid	PO
famciclovir	Famvir	125–500 mg q8–12h for 5–7 d	PO
foscarnet sodium	Foscavir	Initial: 40–90 mg/kg over 1h q8–12h for 2–3 wk	IV
		Maintenance: 90–120 mg/kg/d	
ganciclovir	Cytovene	Induction: 5 mg/kg q12h for 7–21 d	IV
		Maintenance: 5–6 mg/kg/d for 5–7 d	
		Maintenance: 1000 mg tid with food or 500 mg q3h while awake up to 6 times/d	PO
oseltamivir phosphate	Tamiflu	75 mg daily for 5 d–6 wk	PO
rimantadine hydrochloride	Flumadine	100 mg bid (usually for 1 wk)	PO
ribavirin	Virazole	(For infants and children with RSV): solution 20 mg/mL delivered in mist at 12.5 L/min for 12–18 h, 3–7 d	Inhalation
tenofovir disoproxil fumarate	Viread	300 mg/d with a meal	PO
valacyclovir hydrochloride	Valtrex	500 mg–2 g/d, bid–tid for 3–10 d	PO
valganciclovir	Valcyte	900 mg bid with food for 21 d; maintenance: 900 mg/d with food	PO
zanamivir	Relenza	5 mg blister bid via Diskhaler	Inhaler
zidovudine	AZT, Retravir	200 mg q4h × 1 mo, then 100 mg q4h	PO

HIV INFECTIONS

Human immunodeficency virus (HIV), which results in aquired immunodeficiency syndrom (AIDS), is caused mainly by two viruses (HIV-1 and HIV-2). HIV-1 is found worldwide, whereas HIV-2 infections are most common in parts of Africa and India. The antiviral drugs used to suppres HIV are effective mostly against the HIV-1 strain.

The virus infects a group of helper T lymphocytes, which are called *CD4 cells*. This results in the AIDS patient becoming more susceptible to other infections, such as bacteria, fungi, protozoans, and other viruses. Most AIDS patients die from these secondary infections. It is important to remember that not all individuals infected with HIV develop AIDS, but they continue to be carriers of the virus.

Antiviral drugs are used alone or in combinations for the treatment of HIV infection. Highly active antiretroviral therapy (HAART) has been shown to reduce viral load, increase CD4 lymphocyte counts in individuals infected with HIV, delay the onset of AIDS, and prolong survival of patients with AIDS. Both the incidence of and mortality from AIDS have declined substantially since 1996 due to HAART. The benefits of HAART, which involve the combination of three to four drugs effective against HIV, have been widely publicized. Two distinct categories of drugs are combined: **nucleoside** analogues (derived from nucleic acid) and protease inhibitors.

The use of HAART presents formidable challenges, including harsh side effects and the potential for rapid development of drug resistance. Protease inhibitors do not work as well with a third category of HIV drugs, the nonnucleoside analogues, which should not be taken alone. Presently, because of the limited number of HAART medications available in the United States, only a few drug combinations are possible. HAART regimens can also fail because of lack of viral load response (the body's reaction to antiviral agents), or the patient's poor adherence to treatment. Missing a single dose of HAART even twice a week can cause the development of drug-resistant HIV. This is a real danger because adherence to the drug regimen is difficult. The simplification of HIV antiretroviral therapy regimens has been shown to improve adherence. One combination antiviral agent approved for the treatment of HIV infection and AIDS is 2',3'-dideoxycytidine (ddC, also called *zalcitabine*), which is to be used only with the popular drug zidovudine (AZT, Retrovir).

ACYCLOVIR

Acyclovir (Zovirax) is an antiviral agent used for initial and recurrent mucosal and cutaneous herpes simplex virus types 1 and 2. It is also used for herpes zoster infections in **immunocompromised** (weakened immune system) patients. Valacyclovir (Valtrex), which is a chemically modified version of acyclovir, is used for the suppression and treatment of mucosal herpes infections.

How does it work?
Acyclovir interferes with DNA synthesis and inhibits viral multiplication.

How is it used?
Acyclovir is also used to treat herpes simplex, herpes simplex encephalitis in patients older than 6 months, acute herpes zoster (shingles), and chickenpox.

What are the adverse effects?
Adverse effects of acyclovir include vertigo, headache, tremors, depression, hair loss, and phlebitis at injection sites. It may also cause nausea, vomiting, anorexia, or diarrhea.

What are the contraindications and interactions?
Acyclovir is contraindicated in patients allergic to this agent. It should not be used in patients with renal disease or seizures or during lactation.

What are the important points patients should know?
Instruct patients to report adverse effects of therapy, including decreased urination, CNS changes (such as confusion, anxiety, or depression), and gastric irritation.

AMANTADINE

Amantadine (Symmetrel) is used to prevent or treat symptoms of influenza A viral infections (also known as the *flu* or *grippe*) as well as respiratory tract illnesses.

How does it work?

Amantadine inhibits replication of the influenza A virus by interfering with viral attachment and by the uncoating (disassembly or disintegration) of the virus.

How is it used?

Amantadine is used to treat a wide variety of patients of all ages who have symptoms of influenza, but it may also be used to treat some patients with parkinsonism.

What are the adverse effects?

The most pronounced adverse effects of amantadine are insomnia, nightmares, confusion, ataxia (loss of muscular control), headache, dizziness, dyspnea, hypotension, edema, urine retention, constipation, nausea, and dry mouth.

What are the contraindications and interactions?

Amantadine is contraindicated in patients with hypersensitivity to the drug, and should be used cautiously in elderly patients and patients with seizure disorders, peripheral edema, heart failure, hepatic disease, eczema-type rash, mental illness, orthostatic hypotension, renal impairment, and cardiovascular disease. Amantadine interacts with anticholinergics and CNS stimulants. It also should not be used with the herb known as jimsonweed or with alcohol.

What are the important points patients should know?

Advise patients to report adverse effects of therapy, including CNS changes (such as confusion, insomnia, nightmares), and urine retention. Instruct patients to rise slowly from a sitting or lying position to avoid experiencing dizziness caused by postural hypotension.

DIDANOSINE

Didanosine (Videx, Videx EC) is an antiretroviral and nucleoside reverse transcriptase inhibitor (NRTI).

How does it work?

Didanosine can inhibit the replication of the HIV virus that has become resistant to zidovudine (AZT). Its mechanism of action is similar to that of zidovudine.

How is it used?

Didanosine is used in advanced HIV infection in patients who are intolerant to AZT or who demonstrate significant clinical or immunological deterioration during zidovudine therapy.

What are the adverse effects?

The major adverse effects of didanosine are peripheral neuropathies and pancreatitis, which may be fatal. These effects are more likely in high doses of the drug. This drug is minimally toxic to bone marrow. Common adverse effects include headache, dizziness, insomnia, seizures, abdominal pain, nausea, vomiting, diarrhea, constipation, and dry mouth.

What are the contraindications and interactions?

Contraindications for didanosine include hypersensitivity to the drug and pregnancy or lactation. It must be administered cautiously to individuals with peripheral vascular disease, history of neuropathy, chronic pancreatitis, renal impairment, or liver disease.

Aluminum and magnesium-containing antacids may increase the aluminum- and magnesium-associated adverse effects. The effectiveness of dapsone may be reduced by didanosine. Absorption of didanosine is significantly decreased by food.

What are the important points patients should know?
Instruct patients to maintain an adequate fluid intake to increase urine output, thereby preventing renal problems.

RIBAVIRIN

Ribavirin (Virazole) is a synthetic nucleoside analogue with broad-spectrum antiviral activity against both DNA and RNA viruses.

How does it work?
Its exact mechanism of action is not fully understood, but it is believed to involve multiple mechanisms, including selective interference with viral ribonucleic protein synthesis.

How is it used?
Ribavirin given by aerosol into an infant oxygen hood has been effective for the treatment of respiratory syncytial virus pneumonia.

What are the adverse effects?
The adverse effects of ribavirin include abdominal cramps, jaundice, anemia, and hypotension.

What are the contraindications and interactions?
Ribavirin is contraindicated in patients with severe cardiovascular disease, congestive heart failure, angina, pancreatitis, and hepatitis. It is also contraindicated in patients with renal failure, sickle-cell disease, pregnancy, and lactation. No specific drug interactions have been identified, but clinical experience with the systemic administration of ribavirin is limited.

What are the important points patients should know?
Advise patients to report adverse effects of hepatotoxicity, including fever, liver tenderness, loss of appetite, and jaundice.

GANCICLOVIR

Ganciclovir (Cytovene) is a synthetic purine (crystalline, organic base) nucleoside analogue that is approved for the treatment of cytomegalovirus (CMV) infections, but not for HIV itself.

How does it work?
After conversion to ganciclovir triphosphate, ganciclovir is incorporated into viral DNA and inhibits viral DNA polymerase. By this action, it can terminate viral replication.

How is it used?
Ganciclovir is used for prophylaxis and treatment of systemic CMV infections in immunocompromised patients, including HIV-positive and transplant patients. It is also prescribed for CMV retinitis.

What are the adverse effects?
Ganciclovir's black box warnings include increased potential for dose-limited neutropenia, thrombocytopenia, and anemia. Other adverse effects are fever, headache, disorientation, ataxia, confusion, tremor, edema, and phlebitis.

What are the contraindications and interactions?
Ganciclovir is contraindicated in patients with hypersensitivity to the drug or to acyclovir (Zovirax). It must be avoided in lactating women. Ganciclovir should be used cautiously in patients with renal impairment, older adults, and pregnant women. Its safety and efficacy in children are not established. No specific drug interactions have been identified.

What are the important points patients should know?
Instruct patients to report adverse effects of therapy, including CNS changes such as confusion, depression, ataxia, and tremor.

ZIDOVUDINE

Zidovudine (AZT, Retrovir) is often known by the abbreviation AZT, which stands for *azidothymidine* (its simplified chemical name).

How does it work?

Zidovudine is a major nucleoside in DNA. On entering host cells, this drug is converted to a triphosphate by endogenous (grown from within) cellular enzymes. It appears to act by being incorporated into growing DNA chains by viral reverse transcriptase, thereby terminating viral replication.

How is it used?

Zidovudine is used for patients who have asymptomatic HIV infection and early or late symptomatic HIV disease. It can also be prescribed for prevention of perinatal transfer of HIV during pregnancy.

What are the adverse effects?

Common adverse effects of zidovudine include fever, dyspnea, malaise, weakness, myalgia, and myopathy. In some patients, headache, insomnia, dizziness, anxiety, or bone marrow depression may be seen.

What are the contraindications and interactions?

Acetaminophen (Tylenol), ganciclovir (Cytoven), and interferon alfa-2A(Roferon-A) may enhance bone marrow suppression. Interaction of aspirin, dapsone (DDS), indomethacin (Indocin), methadone (Dolophine, Methadone), vincristine (Oncovin, VCR), and valproic acid (Depakene) may increase the risk of AZT toxicity.

Zidovudine is contraindicated in patients hypersensitive to the drug, in severe bone marrow depression, hepatomegaly, hepatitis, or other liver disease risk factors, and in those with renal insufficiency. It interacts with a wide variety of drugs, including atovaquone (Malarone), fluconazole (Diflucan), probenecid (Benemid, others), doxorubicin (Adriamycin, Rubex), ribavirin, stavudine (Zerit), and phenytoin (Dilantin).

What are the important points patients should know?

Advise patients to avoid taking nonsteroidal anti-inflammatory drugs (NSAIDs) such as aspirin or indomethacin or paracetamol while taking zidovudine. These drugs may inhibit the metabolism of zidovudine, therefore increasing the possibility of toxicity.

✳ Apply Your Knowledge 9.7

The following questions focus on what you have just learned about antiviral agents and HIV infections. *See Appendix E for the correct answers.*

MATCHING

Match the lettered drug to its numbered therapeutic use.

THERAPEUTIC USE

1. _____ Treatment of respiratory syncytial virus pneumonia
2. _____ Treatment of cytomegalovirus infections
3. _____ Treatment of herpes simplex encephalitis
4. _____ Treatment of asymptomatic HIV infection
5. _____ Treatment of symptoms of influenza

DRUG

a. zidovudine
b. amantadine
c. ribavirin
d. acyclovir
e. ganciclovir

MULTIPLE CHOICE

Choose the correct answers from choices a–d.

1. HIV-2 infections are most common in:
   a. China
   b. The United States
   c. Africa
   d. Worldwide

2. Both the incidence of and mortality from AIDS have declined substantially because of which of the following?
   a. Vaccine against the virus
   b. Immunoglobulin
   c. AZT
   d. HAART

3. Which of the following drugs is used to treat herpes simplex encephalitis in patients older than 6 months?
   a. Ribavirin
   b. Acyclovir
   c. Amantadine
   d. Ganciclovir

4. Which of the following is the trade name of cidofovir?
   a. Vistide
   b. Zovirax
   c. Symmetrel
   d. Relenza

5. The generic name of Virazole is:
   a. ganciclovir
   b. acyclovir
   c. ribavirin
   d. zanamivir

Chapter Capsule

This section repeats the objectives from the beginning of the chapter and then provides a summary of the most important concepts for that objective. Use this section as a quick review and to check your knowledge.

Objective 1: Identify the major types of antibiotics by drug class.

■ Sulfa drugs, penicillins, cephalosporins, aminoglycosides, tetracyclines, macrolides, synthetic antibacterial agents (such as nitrofurantoin and the quinolones)

Objective 2: Describe the principal mechanisms of action of cephalosporins, vancomycin, and isoniazid.

■ Cephalosporins—bactericidal, affecting the bacterial cell wall
■ Vancomycin—bactericidal, suppressing cell-wall synthesis
■ Isoniazid—interfering with biosynthesis of bacterial proteins, nucleic acid, and lipids

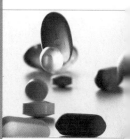

Objective 3: Outline the main adverse effects of macrolides, aminoglycosides, and chloramphenicol.

- Macrolides—abdominal pain, nausea, and vomiting
- Aminoglycosides—ototoxicity and nephrotoxicity
- Chloramphenicol—bone-marrow injury, blood-cell formation disturbances, and gray-baby syndrome

Objective 4: Contrast bactericidal and bacteriostatic actions.

- Bactericidal—kills bacteria
- Bacteriostatic—inhibits growth of bacteria

Objective 5: List the first-line antituberculosis agents and two characteristic adverse effects of each drug.

- Isoniazid—restlessness, insomnia
- Ethambutol—optic neuritis, blurred vision
- Rifampin—fatigue, drowsiness
- Pyrazinamide—hepatotoxicity, nausea

Objective 6: Explain the classifications of cephalosporins.

- First-generation: highest activity against gram-positive bacteria and lowest activity against gram-negative bacteria
- Second-generation: more active against gram-negative bacteria and less active against gram-positive bacteria than the first-generation cephalosporins
- Third-generation: considerably less active than first-generation agents against gram-positive bacteria; much expanded spectrum of activity against gram-negative organisms
- Fourth-generation: improved gram-positive spectrum of activity; expanded gram-negative activity of third-generation cephalosporins

Objective 7: Discuss contraindications, precautions, and interactions of the penicillins and tetracyclines.

- Penicillins—contraindications: hypersensitivity, renal disease, pregnancy, lactation; precautions: give 1 hour before or 2 hours after meals; interactions: estrogen-containing birth control pills, tetracyclines
- Tetracyclines—contraindications: hypersensitivity, liver diseases, children younger than 8 years, pregnancy, lactation; precautions: take tetracyclines on an empty stomach; interactions: dairy products, laxatives, antacids containing aluminum and calcium, iron preparations, phenytoin, barbiturates

Objective 8: List three antiviral drugs for HIV or AIDS-related secondary viral infections and explain their mechanisms of action.

- Didanosine—enters host cells and is incorporated into growing DNA chains by viral reverse transcriptase, thereby terminating viral replication
- Ganciclovir—after conversion to ganciclovir triphosphate, incorporated into viral DNA, inhibiting viral DNA polymerase and then terminating viral replication
- Zidovudine—mechanism of action similar to didanosine

Internet Sites of Interest

- AIDSLINE® contains abstracts on AIDS topics compiled by the U.S. National Library of Medicine. Abstracts are arranged by year at: **www.aegis.com/aidsline**

- A wealth of information on treatments for infectious diseases is available at the Web site of the National Foundation for Infectious Diseases at: **www.nfid.org/publications**

- The appropriate use of antibiotics is a topic of great concern for the public and health-care providers. See the Web site of the Alliance for the Prudent Use of Antibiotics (APUA) at: **www.tufts.edu/med/apua** for consumer and professional information on the topic.

- Reports and news articles on HIV/AIDS in children around the world is available on the UNICEF Web site at: **www.unicef.org/aids**

Chapter 10

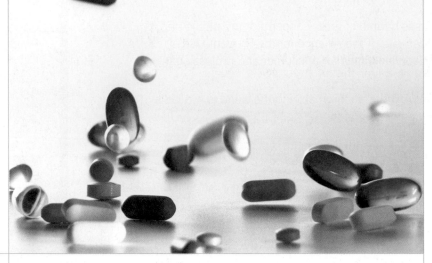

Antifungal, Antimalarial, and Antiprotozoal Agents

Chapter Objectives

After completing this chapter, you should be able to:

1. Identify the risk factors that will most likely cause patients to acquire systemic and serious fungal infections.
2. List four different pharmacotherapies for the treatment of systemic and superficial fungal infections.
3. Explain how fungi and protozoans may gain access to a human host.
4. Describe the general drug actions, uses, and contraindications of antifungal agents.
5. Describe the general drug indications of antimalarial agents.
6. Identify the three common protozoans that cause dysentery, trichomoniasis, and giardiasis.
7. Explain the drugs most frequently used in treatment of intestinal amebiasis and their contraindications.
8. Discuss drugs used to treat protozoal infections.

Key Terms

Fungicidal (fun-jih-SY-dul) (page 216)
Mycoses (my-KOH-seez) (page 211)
Porphyria (por-FEE-ree-uh) (page 216)
Protozoan (pro-toh-ZO-un) (page 211)
Radical cure (page 217)
Thrush (page 212)

PRACTICAL SCENARIO

A 62-year-old woman with lung cancer is also exhibiting symptoms of an infection. She is admitted to her local hospital, and after testing, her physician diagnoses her as having aspergillosis, a fungal disease of the lungs. He prescribes amphotericin B by intravenous injection.

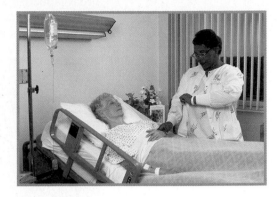

Critical Thinking Questions

1. The patient asks the nurse what adverse effects she can expect from the drug. What would be the appropriate answer for the nurse to give the patient?

2. Can you think of any adverse reactions the nurse needs to monitor this patient for?

3. What patient education should the nurse provide to this patient?

Introduction

Most healthy human beings are resistant to fungal infections but may become infected when overwhelming numbers of fungi infiltrate their systems. Fungi may enter the body in routes that include the skin, mucous membranes, and respiratory tract. Because of the common use of antibiotics and drugs such as oral contraceptives, more and more patients are at risk for fungal infections.

Malaria is a serious disease that is caused by a **protozoan**, a single-celled highly mobile microorganism. *Plasmodium* protozoans, which cause malaria, are transmitted to humans by mosquitoes. Malaria can become a long-term condition and can kill affected persons because of its severity.

Other infections caused by protozoans include dysentery, amebiasis, and a sexually transmitted disease known as *trichomoniasis*. The number of severe protozoan infections is large, and many of these infections do not exhibit specific symptoms.

Fungal Infections

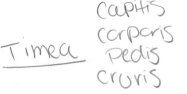

Molds and yeasts are so widely distributed in air, dust, contaminated objects, and normal flora that humans are constantly being exposed to them. More than one million species of fungi have been identified. Only about 20 of these are associated with systemic infections and cause opportunistic infections. Normal healthy individuals are resistant to most fungal infections, called **mycoses**, and are infected only when faced with overwhelming numbers of the fungi. In other cases opportunistic pathogens may invade an individual whose natural resistance is low because of other illnesses or even some medications.

Mycoses involve complex interactions among the portal of entry into the human body, the number of infecting organisms generally required to cause disease, the virulence of the fungus, and the host's resistance. Fungi enter the body mainly via respiratory, mucous, and cutaneous routes. In general, the agents of primary mycoses have a respiratory portal (spores inhaled from the air). Subcutaneous agents enter through compromised skin, and cutaneous and superficial agents enter through contamination of the skin surface. Spores and yeasts can all be infectious, but spores are most often involved because of their durability and abundance.

The human body is extremely resistant to fungi. Among its numerous antifungal defenses are the normal integrity of the skin, mucous membranes, and respiratory cilia; but the most important defenses are cell-mediated immunity, phagocytosis (a process in which cells, called *phagocytes*, consume foreign material), and the inflammatory reaction.

A common opportunistic infection is candidiasis (also called *moniliasis* or *thrush*). **Thrush** is a yeast infection in the mouth caused by *Candida albicans*, a normal resident of the GI tract and vagina (Figure 10-1 ■). Thrush can occur during the use of broad-spectrum antibiotics or by alteration of the environmental conditions in the female reproductive system due to pregnancy or oral contraceptive use. This disease usually results from debilitation (immunosuppression, especially AIDS).

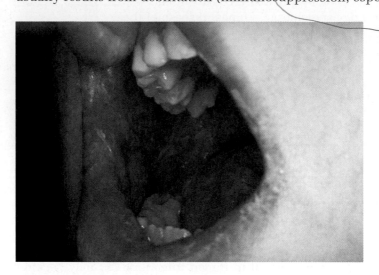

Figure 10-1 ■ Oral *Candida albicans*. *Courtesy of Charles J. Kirkpatrick, M.D. President, Innovative, Therapeutics, Inc.*

The incidence of human fungal infections has increased in recent years because more patients are now at risk for these pathogens. Causes include increased exposure resulting from more frequent surgeries, use of broad-spectrum antimicrobials, immunosuppressive drug therapy for cancer and organ transplantation patients, and HIV.

Antifungal Agents

Antifungal drugs are classified into three categories:

1. Drugs for systemic mycoses
2. Oral drugs for mucocutaneous infections
3. Topical drugs for mucocutaneous infections (Table 10-1 ■)

Table 10-1 ■ Antifungal Agents

GENERIC NAME	TRADE NAME	AVERAGE DOSAGE IN ADULTS	ROUTE OF ADMINISTRATION
Systemic Antifungal Drugs			
amphotericin B	Amphocin	0.25–1.5 mg/kg/d	IV
caspofungin	Cancidas	70 mg on day 1; then 50 mg/d; infuse doses over 1 h	IV
fluconazole	Diflucan	100–200 mg/d	PO, IV
flucytosine	Ancobon	12.5–37.5 mg/kg q6h	PO
griseofulvin	Fulvicin, Grifulvin V	500 mg/d	PO
itraconazole	Sporanox	200 mg/d	PO
✱ ketoconazole	Nizoral	200–400 mg/d	PO
✱ nystatin	Mycostatin (suspension)	400,000–600,000 mg qid	PO
	Nilstat (tablets)	1,000,000 mg bid	PO

Table 10-1 ■ Antifungal Agents

GENERIC NAME	TRADE NAME	AVERAGE DOSAGE IN ADULTS	ROUTE OF ADMINISTRATION
Topical Antifungal Drugs			
amphotericin B	Fungizone	Apply to lesions 2–4 times/d for 1–4 wk	Topical
ciclopirox	Loprox, Penlac	Massage cream into affected area and surrounding skin in morning and evening	Topical
clotrimazole	Lotrimin	Apply small amount to affected areas in morning and evening	Topical
✳econazole	Spectazole	Apply sufficient amount to affected areas in morning and evening	Topical
haloprogin	Halotex	Apply liberally to affected area bid for 2–3 wk	Topical
naftifine	Naftin	Apply cream once daily, or apply gel twice daily; may use up to 4 wk	Topical
oxiconazole	Oxistat	Apply to affected area once daily in evening	Topical

The major drugs for systemic mycoses include amphotericin B (Amphocin), flucytosine (Ancobon), ketoconazole (Nizoral), and griseofulvin (Fulvicin, Grifulvin V). Nystatin (Mycostatin) and fluconazole (Diflucan) are used for local *C. albicans* infections of the skin and mucous membranes.

Focus on Pediatrics

Thrush in Babies

In babies, thrush causes difficulty in breastfeeding and chronic diaper rash (which may appear as slightly raised ulcers or skin lesions of a creamy white color). Oral thrush (white patches in the mouth or throat) in babies may infect the nipples of the mother, causing drying or cracking.

AMPHOTERICIN B

Amphotericin B (Amphocin) has the widest spectrum of antifungal activity of any systemic antifungal drug.

How does it work?

Most antifungal drugs act by interfering with the synthesis of ergosterol, a chemical found in fungal cell membranes. This results in a change in the permeability of the fungal cell membrane, and either slowed growth or destruction of the fungal organism.

How is it used?

Administration of amphotericin B by the IV route is extremely useful for therapy of systemic fungus diseases. It is also used by nasal spray in the prophylaxis of aspergillosis in immunocompromised patients, and orally for treatment of oral candidiasis.

What are the adverse effects?

Amphotericin B may induce chills and fever, nausea and vomiting, diarrhea, abdominal cramps, dyspepsia, headache, vertigo, thrombophlebitis, anemia, cardiac arrest, and skin rashes. The most serious adverse effect of amphotericin B is renal damage. This drug is also able to cause blood dyscrasias and loss of hearing.

What are the contraindications and interactions?

Amphotericin B is contraindicated in patients hypersensitive to the drug and should be used cautiously in patients with impaired renal function. It interacts with many other drugs, including antineoplastics, cardiac glycosides, corticosteroids, nephrotoxic drugs (including antibiotics and pentamidine), thiazides, and flucytosine (Ancobon); it should not be used with leukocyte transfusions.

What are the important points patients should know?

Inform patients that when given intravenously (IV), this drug may cause fever, chills, headache, and nausea in the first few hours of therapy, but these adverse reactions usually decrease as therapy continues. Advise patients to notify their physician if improvement does not occur within 1 to 2 weeks and to report loss of hearing, dizziness, cloudy or pink urine, or greatly increased urination. Treatment of cutaneous infections, such as nail infections, usually requires several months or longer of therapy. Advise patients to wash towels and clothing that were in contact with affected areas after each treatment. Topical cream slightly discolors the skin when rubbed in, and nail lesions may be stained. Instruct patients to drink plenty of fluids.

Focus on Geriatrics

Amphotericin B and Kidney Damage

Amphotericin B (Amphocin) is a very toxic agent that, in most cases, should be administered intravenously. Elderly patients who use this drug must be very careful because kidney damage is the most serious toxic effect of amphotericin B. Elderly patients who have renal impairment must be tested for creatinine clearance.

Focus on Natural Products

Interactions Between Gossypol and Amphotericin B

The herb gossypol, which is derived from cottonseed oil, may be used to treat endometriosis in women. It may also be used by both men and women to prevent pregnancy. Gossypol used with amphotericin B (Amphocin) may increase risk of renal toxicity.

FLUCYTOSINE

Flucytosine (Ancobon) is an antifungal agent used for a wide variety of severe fungal infections.

How does it work?

Flucytosine is converted in the fungus to 5-fluorouracil, which is incorporated into ribonucleic acid (RNA) and interferes with normal protein synthesis.

How is it used?

Certain fungal organisms are more sensitive to interference from the drug than are human cells, so flucytosine is useful in the treatment of some fungal infections. It is the drug of choice to treat chromomycosis and of second choice to treat systemic candidiasis. It may be combined with amphotericin B (Amphocin) for first-choice treatment of aspergillosis or cryptococcosis (a fungal disease of the lungs), especially in patients with meningitis.

What are the adverse effects?
Flucytosine, commonly causes nausea, vomiting, diarrhea, and skin rashes. Bone marrow suppression, manifest by anemia, leukopenia, and thrombocytopenia, has been reported. Sedation, confusion, hallucinations, headache, and vertigo occur infrequently.

What are the contraindications and interactions?
Flucytosine is contraindicated in patients hypersensitive to the drug and should be used with extreme caution in patients who have impaired hepatic or renal function or who have bone marrow suppression. It interacts with amphotericin B, causing synergistic effects and increasing toxicity.

What are the important points patients should know?
Instruct patients to report fever, sore mouth or throat, and a tendency for unusual bleeding or bruising to their physician. They must be aware that the general duration of therapy is 4 to 6 weeks, but it may need to be continued for several months. Instruct patients not to breast feed while taking this drug without consulting their physician.

KETOCONAZOLE
Ketoconazole (Nizoral) is an antifungal used to treat many varieties of candidiasis infections, as well as coccidioidomycosis, blastomycosis, histoplasmosis, chromomycosis, paracoccidioidomycosis, and severe cutaneous dermatophyte infections that resist griseofulvin (Fulvicin, Grifulvin V) therapy.

How does it work?
Ketoconazole blocks the fungal synthesis of ergosterol, which is essential to the integrity of the cell membranes of nearly all pathogenic fungi.

How is it used?
Ketoconazole has a broad spectrum of antifungal activity. This drug, or amphotericin B, is the drug of choice for the treatment of blastomycosis, coccidioidosis, and histoplasmosis. It is an alternative drug for candidiasis. Successful treatment sometimes requires months.

What are the adverse effects?
The most common adverse effects of ketoconazole include nausea and vomiting, diarrhea, pruritus (severe itching), abdominal cramps, headache, photophobia, fever, and impotence.

What are the contraindications and interactions?
Ketoconazole should not be used in patients with hypersensitivity to this drug or in patients with chronic alcoholism or fungal meningitis. Safety during pregnancy and lactation and in children younger than 2 years has not been established. Ketoconazole should be used cautiously in patients with a history of liver disease or with HIV infection.

Cimetidine (Tagamet) inhibits and rifampin (Rifadin) induces the metabolism of ketoconazole. Rifadin decreases the biosynthesis of androgens and estrogens.

What are the important points patients should know?
Instruct patients to promptly report the signs and symptoms of hepatotoxicity to their physician. Advise them to avoid over-the-counter (OTC) drugs for gastric distress (such as Rolaids, Tums, and Alka-Seltzer), and to check with their physicians before taking any other nonprescription medications. Tell patients to not alter the dose or dose interval before consulting their physicians.

GRISEOFULVIN

Griseofulvin (Fulvicin, Grifulvin V) is an effective agent in the treatment of superficial fungal infections.

How does it work?

Griseofulvin is fungistatic and not **fungicidal** (having a killing action on fungi). Its action involves deposition in newly formed skin and nail beds, where it binds to keratin, protecting these sites from new infection.

How is it used?

Griseofulvin is used systemically and is highly effective in the management of dermatophyte infections of the skin, hair, and nails. Because it does not kill but only arrests reproduction of the organism, it is necessary to continue medication long enough for the entire epidermis to be replaced, thereby removing reinfecting organisms.

What are the adverse effects?

Griseofulvin may cause hypersensitivity, skin rashes, pruritus, serum sickness, severe headache, insomnia, fatigue, mental confusion, psychotic symptoms, and vertigo. This agent also causes heartburn, nausea, vomiting, diarrhea, flatulence, dry mouth, and unpleasant taste sensations. Nephrotoxicity and hepatotoxicity may occur.

What are the contraindications and interactions?

Griseofulvin is contraindicated in patients with **porphyria** (a group of diseases affecting heme, the oxygen-binding portion of hemoglobin) or liver disease. Safe use of this drug during pregnancy, lactation, or in children younger than 2 years has not been established.

Griseofulvin with alcohol may cause flushing and tachycardia. Barbiturates may decrease hypoprothrombinemic effects of oral anticoagulants. Griseofulvin may increase estrogen metabolism and decrease contraceptive efficacy of oral contraceptives.

What are the important points patients should know?

Advise patients to continue treatment as prescribed to prevent relapse. Instruct them to avoid exposure to intense natural or artificial sunlight because photosensitivity reactions may occur. Advise women to not breast feed while taking this drug without consulting their physician.

✳ Apply Your Knowledge 10.1

The following exercises focus on what you have just learned about antifungal agents. *See Appendix E for the correct answers.*

MULTIPLE CHOICE

Choose the correct answers from choices a–d.

1. Which of the following antifungal drugs must be injected intravenously for systemic fungal diseases?
   a. Flucytosine
   b. Amphotericin B
   c. Griseofulvin
   d. Ketoconazole

2. *Plasmodium* protozoans cause which of the following?
   a. Malaria
   b. Dysentery
   c. Amebiasis
   d. Trichomoniasis

3. Fungal infections of the nails are often effectively treated with which of the following?

a. Quinidine

b. Metronidazole

c. Griseofulvin

d. Chloroquine

4. Which of the following should not be used in patients with fungal meningitis?

a. Primaquine

b. Ketoconazole

c. Griseofulvin

d. Chloroquine

5. Which of the following is the drug of choice to treat chromomycosis, and the drug of second choice to treat systemic candidiasis?

a. Ketoconazole

b. Quinine

c. Hydroxychloroquine

d. Flucytosine

MATCHING

Match the numbered contraindication (or cautioned use) to the lettered drug. Lettered drugs may be used more than once, and some contraindications may have more than one answer.

CONTRAINDICATION/CAUTIONED USE	DRUG
1. _____ Impaired renal function	a. Flucytosine
2. _____ Children younger than 2 years	b. Ketoconazole
3. _____ Bone-marrow suppression	c. Amphotericin B
4. _____ Chronic alcoholism	d. Griseofulvin
5. _____ Porphyria	
6. _____ Fungal meningitis	
7. _____ Pregnancy and lactation	
8. _____ Concurrent antineoplastics	

Malarial Infections

Malaria is caused by several species of the protozoan *Plasmodium*, of which *Plasmodium vivax* and *P. falciparum* are the most common. The most serious infections involve *P. falciparum*, which causes a higher incidence of complications and deaths. These protozoans all have complex life cycles involving both the anopheles mosquito and the red blood cells of the human host. The infection caused by *P. vivax* is a persisting tissue phase that continues to infect the blood at intervals for many years. Thus, the ideal drug to combat malarial infections should eradicate the *microzoan* from not only the blood, but from the tissue as well, to effect what is termed a **radical cure**.

Antimalarial Agents

Several antimalarials differ in their point of interruption of the cycle of the parasite (an organism that lives on or in another and draws its nourishment therefrom) and in the type of malaria affected. In addition, parasite resistance (especially that of *P. falciparum*) to these drugs is an important therapeutic problem.

Antimalarial drugs include chloroquine (Aralen), primaquine (Primaquine), quinine (Quinamm), and hydroxychloroquine (Plaquenil). Some agents are used for the actual prevention of malaria. They include mefloquine (Lariam), quinacrine (Mepacrine), and folic-acid antagonists, such as pyrimethamine (Daraprim) (Table 10-2 ■).

Table 10-2 ■ Antimalarial Drugs

GENERIC NAME	TRADE NAME	AVERAGE DOSAGE IN ADULTS	ROUTE OF ADMINISTRATION
chloroquine	Aralen	300–700 mg/wk, 2 wk prior to exposure, and for up to 4 wk after leaving endemic area	PO
doxycycline (tetracycline)	Vibramycin	100 mg daily 1–2 days before, continuously during, and 4 wk after travel	PO
hydroxychloroquine	Plaquenil	400 mg/wk	PO
mefloquine	Lariam	5 tablets with water as single oral dose; then 250 mg/wk and then every other wk	PO
primaquine	Primaquine	15 mg/d for 14 d	PO
pyrimethamine	Daraprim	25 mg once/wk up to 10 wk	PO
quinine	Quinamm	260–650 mg q8h for 6–12 d	PO

CHLOROQUINE

Chloroquine (Aralen) is one of the most commonly used drugs for both prophylaxis and treatment of acute malarial attacks that are caused by *P. vivax, P. malariae, P. ovale*, and susceptible strains of *P. falciparum*.

How does it work?

Chloroquine is a protozoacidal drug. The agent destroys *Plasmodia* by interfering with the microorganism's metabolism or inhibiting normal replication of the protozoan.

How is it used?

Chloroquine is used for control of acute attacks of vivax malaria and for suppression against all plasmodia except chloroquine-resistant *P. falciparum*. The drug is neither a prophylactic nor a radical curative agent in vivax malaria. In regions where *P. falciparum* is generally sensitive to chloroquine, it is markedly effective in terminating acute attacks of nonresistant falciparum malaria and usually brings about a complete cure in this type of malaria.

Chloroquine is the drug of choice for the oral treatment of all malaria except that caused by resistant *P. falciparum*.

What are the adverse effects?

The adverse effects include pigmentation of the skin and nail beds, pruritus, fatigue, toxic psychosis, and ototoxicity. Chloroquine may also cause corneal opacities (clouding of the corneas of the eyes) and retinopathy.

What are the contraindications and interactions?

Chloroquine is contraindicated in patients with liver disease, hypersensitivity to 4-aminoquinolines, psoriasis, porphyria, and renal disease. This drug also should not be used in children or in pregnant or lactating women.

Certain antacids and laxatives decrease chloroquine absorption, and chloroquine may interfere with response to rabies vaccine.

What are the important points patients should know?

Advise patients to promptly report visual or hearing disturbances, muscle weakness, loss of balance, and symptoms of blood dyscrasia (fever, sore mouth or throat, unexplained fatigue, easy bruising, or bleeding). Instruct them to wear dark glasses in sunlight or bright light (because of photophobia) to reduce the risk of ocular damage and to avoid driving or other potentially hazardous activities until reaction to the drug is known. Inform patients that this drug may cause rusty yellow or brown discoloration of the urine.

PRIMAQUINE

Primaquine (Primaquine) is an antimalarial agent that is very important for the radical cure of relapsing vivax or ovale malaria. It is not employed for suppressive therapy or for control of the acute clinical attacks of the disease.

How does it work?

Primaquine acts directly on the preformed nucleic acid deoxyribonucleic acid (DNA) in the microorganisms. It is also gametocidal against the four human malaria species. The mechanism of antimalarial action is unknown.

How is it used?

Primaquine is indicated for cure of relapsing vivax malaria. It eliminates symptoms and the infection as well as prevents relapse.

What are the adverse effects?

Primaquine in recommended doses is generally well tolerated. It infrequently causes nausea, vomiting, abdominal cramps, and headache. More serious (but rare) adverse effects include leukopenia, agranulocytosis, and cardiac arrhythmias.

What are the contraindications and interactions?

Primaquine is contraindicated in patients with rheumatoid arthritis and lupus erythematosus. Primaquine should be avoided in pregnancy.

What are the important points patients should know?

Instruct patients to examine their urine after each voiding and report darkening or red tinge or decrease in urine volume. Advise them to report chills, fever, pain in the region of the diaphragm, and cyanosis (all of which suggest a hemolytic reaction). Instruct patients to not breast feed while taking this drug.

QUININE

Quinine (Quinamm) remains the first-line therapy for falciparum malaria, especially severe disease. A chemically related drug, quinidine gluconate (Quinaglute Duratabs), is an antidysrhythmic drug that is used off-label to treat severe malaria via IV administration.

How does it work?

Quinine is an agent that is destructive to *gametes*, or germ cells, and acts rapidly against all *Plasmodium* malaria except *P. falciparum*. The actual mechanism of action of quinine is unknown.

How is it used?

Quinine is the treatment of choice for severe *P. falciparum*. It is not generally used in chemoprophylaxis owing to its toxicity.

What are the adverse effects?

The adverse effects of quinine include visual and hearing disturbances, fever, headache, flushing, syncope (fainting), and cardiovascular collapse. It can also cause vomiting, diarrhea, and abdominal pain.

What are the contraindications and interactions?

Quinine should be discontinued if signs of hypersensitivity occur. It should be avoided in those with visual or auditory problems. It must be used with great caution in those with underlying cardiac abnormalities. Aluminum-containing antacids may block absorption. Quinine can raise plasma levels of warfarin and digoxin. Dosage must be reduced in renal insufficiency.

What are the important points patients should know?

Instruct patients to report feelings of faintness to their physician and to eat a balanced diet with no excesses in fruit juices or milk. Advise patients to not self-medicate with OTC drugs without advice from their physician and to not increase, decrease, skip, or discontinue doses without consulting their physician.

HYDROXYCHLOROQUINE

Hydroxychloroquine (Plaquenil) suppresses malaria attacks that are caused by *P. vivax, P. malariae, P. ovale*, and susceptible strains of *P. falciparum*.

How does it work?

The mechanism of action of hydroxychloroquine is based on its ability to form complexes with the DNA of parasites, thereby inhibiting replication and transcription to RNA and DNA synthesis of the parasites.

How is it used?

Hydroxychloroquine is a suppressive prophylaxis agent that is also used for the treatment of acute malarial attacks due to all forms of susceptible malaria. This drug is used adjunctively with primaquine (Primaquine) for the eradication of *P. vivax* and *P. malariae*. Hydroxychloroquine is commonly prescribed for the treatment of rheumatoid arthritis and lupus erythematosus.

What are the adverse effects?

Hydroxychloroquine may cause nausea, vomiting, anorexia, diarrhea, abdominal cramps, and weight loss. This agent may also produce fatigue, vertigo, headache, anxiety, retinopathy, blurred vision, and mood changes. The serious adverse effects (which are rare) include aplastic anemia, agranulocytosis, thrombocytopenia, and alopecia.

What are the contraindications and interactions?

Hydroxychloroquine should be avoided in patients with known hypersensitivity to the drug, or in patients with visual field changes associated with quinoline compounds. It is also contraindicated in patients who have psoriasis or porphyria. Safe use of hydroxychloroquine for juvenile arthritis or in lactating women is not established. It must be used cautiously in patients with liver disease, alcoholism, and impaired renal function.

Aluminum- and magnesium-containing antacids and laxatives decrease hydroxychloroquine absorption. This agent may interfere with response to rabies vaccine.

What are the important points patients should know?

Inform patients about adverse effects and related symptoms when receiving prolonged therapy with this drug. Advise them to follow the drug regimen exactly as prescribed by their physician and to keep this drug out of the reach of children. Instruct women to not breast feed while taking this drug without first consulting their physician.

Focus on Pediatrics

Antimalarial Drugs and Children

Children who will be traveling to countries that require antimalarial vaccinations should be vaccinated 4 to 6 weeks prior to embarking to ensure full protection. Also, for antimalarial prescription drugs, infants' and children's dosages usually must be specially prepared; thus, adequate time needs to be allowed for this as well. Guidelines must be followed exactly because *overdosage can be fatal*. One agent in particular, hydroxychloroquine (Plaquenil), is particularly toxic to infants and children, and extra care must be taken in administration. As few as 3 to 4 tablets (250–mg strength) of chloroquine (Aralen), which is similar to hydroxychloroquine, has resulted in death in small children.

✳ Apply Your Knowledge 10.2

The following questions focus on what you have just learned about antimalarials. *See Appendix E for the correct answers.*

FILL IN THE BLANK
Select terms from your reading to fill in the blanks.

1. Chloroquine is one of the most commonly used drugs for both prophylaxis and treatment of acute _____, which is caused by *Plasmodium* _____, _____, or _____.

2. Primaquine acts directly on _____ in the microorganisms.

3. Quinine is the first-choice therapy for _____ malaria.

4. Aluminum-containing antacids and laxatives _____ hydroxychloroquine absorption. These agents may interfere with the response to _____ vaccine.

5. The most serious infections of malaria involve *Plasmodium* _____, which causes a higher incidence of complications and _____.

MATCHING
Match the lettered trade name to its numbered generic drug name.

GENERIC NAME	TRADE NAME
1. _____ quinine	a. Aralen
2. _____ hydroxychloroquine	b. Quinamm
3. _____ chloroquine	c. Primaquine
4. _____ mefloquine	d. Plaquenil
5. _____ primaquine	e. Lariam

Protozoal Infections

Although protozoal infections are very common, they are actually caused by only a small number of species often restricted geographically to the tropics and subtropics. Two protozoal organisms, *Entamoeba histolytica* and *Giardia lamblia*, are frequently responsible for causing dysentery (an inflammatory disease of the lower intestinal tract) in humans. Infection caused by the protozoan *E. histolytica* is also called *amebic dysentery* or *amebiasis*, and is relatively rare in the United States. The third important protozoal infection is *Trichomonas vaginalis* (*T. vaginalis*), which causes a sexually transmitted disease (common in the United States) called *trichomoniasis* (Figure 10-2 ■).

Amebic infections generally remain confined to the intestines, where they may give rise to dysentery, or they may locate elsewhere, especially in the liver. The chemotherapy of amebiasis must provide drugs to treat both the intestinal and extraintestinal forms of the disease and be capable of eliminating amebic cysts from the intestine.

The most commonly reported intestinal protozoal infection in the United States is giardiasis, caused by the flagellated protozoan *G. lamblia*. Most patients are asymptomatic. However, these organisms cause a diarrhea that can be transient or persistent. Infection results from ingestion of *G. lamblia* cysts, which may exist in water that is contaminated with fecal matter.

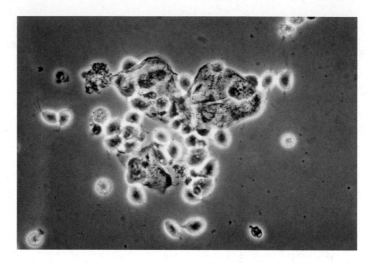

Figure 10-2 ■ Vaginal discharge with microorganisms due to trichomoniasis.

Antiprotozoal Agents

Drugs that are used for the treatment of *E. histolytica* include metronidazole (Flagyl), iodoquinol (Yodoxin), tetracyclines, and paromomycin (Humatin). No safe drug exists that will eradicate all the motile forms, cysts, and extraintestinal amoebas in amebic infections, but combination drug therapy can eliminate parasites from all sites. Chemotherapy with metronidazole is usually successful in cases of giardiasis (Table 10-3 ■).

Table 10-3 ■ Antiprotozoal Agents

GENERIC NAME	TRADE NAME	AVERAGE DOSAGE IN ADULTS	ROUTE OF ADMINISTRATION
iodoquinol	Yodoxin	630–650 mg tid for 20 d; may repeat after a 2–3 wk drug-free interval;	PO
		For trichomoniasis, giardiasis: 2 g once or 250 mg tid for 7 d	PO
		For amebiasis: 500–750 mg tid	PO
metronidazole	Flagyl	1 dose of 2 g, or 500 mg bid for 7 d	PO, IV
paromomycin	Humatin	25–35 mg/kg divided in 3 doses for 5–10 d	PO

METRONIDAZOLE

Metronidazole (Flagyl) is an amebicide that is used to treat liver abscess, intestinal amebiasis, trichomoniasis, anaerobic infections, vaginosis, diarrhea, colitis, and pelvic inflammatory disease (PID), and prevent postoperative infection following colorectal surgery.

How does it work?

Metronidazole is a direct-acting trichomonacide and amebicide that works at both intestinal and extraintestinal sites. It apparently enters cells of microorganisms that contain the enzyme nitroreductase, forming unstable compounds that bind to DNA, inhibiting synthesis and causing cell death.

How is it used?

Metronidazole is prescribed for asymptomatic and symptomatic trichomoniasis in female and male patients. It is also used for acute intestinal amebiasis and amebic liver abscess. Metronidazole usually is indicated for preoperative prophylaxis in colorectal surgery, elective hysterectomy or vaginal repair, and emergency appendectomy.

What are the adverse effects?

The adverse effects of metronidazole include nausea, vomiting, anorexia, abdominal cramps, metallic or bitter taste, skin rashes, pruritus, flushing, fever, vertigo, headache, confusion, depression, restlessness, and insomnia. The urine sometimes turns a dark color.

What are the contraindications and interactions?

Metronidazole should not be used in patients with diseases of the central nervous system. The drug has been found to be carcinogenic in mice and rats. It has been used in pregnancy without consequence, but it is advisable to withhold it during pregnancy, if possible. Metronidazole interacts with cimetidine, disulfiram, lithium, oral anticoagulants, phenobarbital, phenytoin, and alcohol.

What are the important points patients should know?

Instruct patients to adhere closely to the established regimen without schedule interruptions or dose change. They must refrain from intercourse during therapy for trichomoniasis unless a condom is used to prevent reinfection. Inform patients that sexual partners should receive concurrent treatment. Asymptomatic trichomoniasis in men is a frequent source of reinfection in their female partners. Also instruct patients to avoid alcohol while taking this drug.

Focus Point

Fungal Superinfections

Usually occurring in the anal and genital areas or in the vagina or mouth, fungal superinfections cause anal or vaginal itching, vaginal discharge, and lesions of the tongue or mouth. A common type of fungal superinfection is known as *candidiasis* or *moniliasis*. This superinfection may occur because of an overgrowth of yeast-like fungi in the vagina. Normally, multiplication of these microorganisms is controlled because of a strain of vaginal bacteria known as *Doderlein bacillus*. Penicillin therapy may destroy these bacteria, causing the fungi to multiply at a rapid rate. Symptoms include vaginal discharge and itching.

IODOQUINOL

Iodoquinol (Diquinol, Yodoxin) is an anti-infective, antiamebicide, and antiprotozoal agent.

How does it work?

Iodoquinol is a direct-acting amebicide that works in the intestinal lumen. When it enters the cells of protozoa, it affects the DNA, inhibiting synthesis and causing cell death.

How is it used?

Iodoquinol is used only as a luminal amebicide and has no effect against extraintestinal amebic infections. It is commonly prescribed either concurrently or in alternating courses with another intestinal amebicide.

What are the adverse effects?

Infrequent adverse effects of iodoquinol include diarrhea—which usually stops after several days—nausea, vomiting, abdominal pain, anorexia, headache, rash, and pruritus. Iodoquinol can cause blurred vision, optic atrophy, permanent loss of vision, and thyroid hypertrophy.

What are the contraindications and interactions?

Iodoquinol is contraindicated in patients with hypersensitivity to any iodine-containing preparations or foods, and those with hepatic or renal damage. Safe use during pregnancy or lactation is not established.

What are the important points patients should know?

Instruct patients to report skin rash and symptoms of a sudden drop in their leukocyte count, such as chills, fever, weakness, and fatigue, and to complete the full course of treatment. Their stools need to be examined at 1, 3, and 6 months after termination of treatment to ensure the infection has not returned.

✳ Apply Your Knowledge 10.3

The following questions focus on what you have just learned about antiprotozoal infections and agents. *See Appendix E for the correct answers.*

MULTIPLE CHOICE

Choose the correct answer from choices a–d.

1. Metronidazole is prescribed for which of the following asymptomatic and symptomatic infections?

    a. Cryptococcosis

    b. Candidiasis

    c. Trichomoniasis

    d. *Plasmodium falciparum*

2. Which of the following drugs has been found to be carcinogenic in mice and rats?

    a. Metronidazole

    b. Rifampin

    c. Vancomycin

    d. Erythromycin

3. In the United States, endemic amebiasis is relatively:

    a. Common in the Northeastern states

    b. Common in the Southwestern states

    c. Rare in the Southern states

    d. Rare in all 50 states

4. A metallic or bitter taste is reported during use of which of the following agents?

    a. Rifampin

    b. Metronidazole

    c. Quinacrine

    d. Phenytoin

5. Iodoquinol is used in which of the following conditions?

    a. Hepatic abscess

    b. Thyroid hypertrophy

    c. Optic atrophy

    d. Amebic intestinal infections

FILL IN THE BLANK

Select terms from your reading to fill in the blanks.

1. An inflammatory disease of the lower intestinal tract is known as _____.

2. A common sexually transmitted disease in the United States, which is caused by a protozoal infection, is _____.

3. The most commonly reported intestinal protozoal infection in the United States is _____.

4. The drug of choice to eradicate *T. vaginalis* is _____.

5. Iodoquinol is contraindicated in patients with hypersensitivity to any preparations or foods that contain _____.

Chapter Capsule

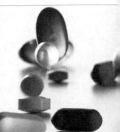

This section repeats the objectives from the beginning of the chapter and then provides a summary of the most important concepts for that objective. Use this section as a quick review and to check your knowledge.

Objective 1: Identify the risk factors that will most likely cause patients to acquire systemic and serious fungal infections.

- Constant exposure to systemic-causing infections present in the air, dust, fomites, and even among the normal flora in the environment of humans
- Exposure to overwhelming numbers of fungi
- Immunosuppression (especially HIV and AIDS) and immunosuppressive drug therapies (including those used for cancer and organ transplantation patients)
- Frequent surgeries
- Use of broad-spectrum antimicrobials

Objective 2: List four different pharmacotherapies for the treatment of systemic and superficial fungal infections.

- Amphotericin B (Amphocin)
- Flucytosine (Ancobon)
- Ketoconazole (Nizoral)
- Griseofulvin (Fulvicin, Grifulvin V)

Objective 3: Explain how fungi and protozoans may gain access to a human host.

- Fungi: via respiratory, mucous, and cutaneous routes
- Protozoans: via creatures such as mosquitoes that attack the red blood cells; other protozoans are transmitted by sexual activity or consumption of contaminated foods or water

Objective 4: Describe the general drug actions, uses, and contraindications of antifungal agents.

■ Actions: interference with the synthesis of ergosterol, a chemical found in fungal cell membranes

■ Uses: systemic fungal diseases; superficial moniliasis infections; in the prophylaxis of aspergillosis in immunocompromised patients; cryptococcosis (a fungal disease of the lungs often occurring in patients with meningitis); blastomycosis; histoplasmosis; candidiasis; dermatophyte infections of the skin, hair, and nails

■ Contraindications: hypersensitive patients, those with impaired hepatic or renal function, bone marrow suppression, chronic alcoholism, and porphyria; ketoconazole (Nizoral) should not be used for patients with fungal meningitis or HIV infection; the safety of use for both ketoconazole and griseofulvin (Fulvicin, Grifulvin V) during pregnancy or lactation, and in children younger than 2 years old, has not been established

Objective 5: Describe the general drug indications of antimalarial agents.

■ Chloroquine (Aralen): control of acute attacks of vivax malaria; suppression against all Plasmodia except chloroquine-resistant *P. falciparum*; oral treatment of all malaria except that caused by resistant *P. falciparum*

■ Primaquine (Primaquine): cure of relapsing vivax malaria

■ Quinine (Quinamm): treatment of severe *P. falciparum*

■ Hydroxychloroquine (Plaquenil): suppressive prophylaxis agent; treatment of acute malarial attacks due to all forms of susceptible malaria; used adjunctively with primaquine for the eradication of *P. vivax* and *P. malariae*

Objective 6: Identify the three common protozoans that cause dysentery, trichomoniasis, and giardiasis.

■ Dysentery: *Entamoeba histolytica* and *Giardia lamblia*

■ Trichomoniasis: *Trichomonas vaginalis*

■ Giardiasis: *Giardia lamblia*

Objective 7: Explain the drugs most frequently used in treatment of intestinal amebiasis and their contraindications.

■ Metronidazole (Flagyl)—a direct-acting trichomonacide and amebicide that works at both intestinal and extraintestinal sites; contraindicated in patients with CNS diseases and should be withheld during pregnancy

■ Iodoquinol (Yodoxin)—a direct-acting amebicide that works in the intestinal lumen; contraindicated in patients with hypersensitivity to any iodine-containing preparations or foods, and those with hepatic or renal damage; safe use during pregnancy or lactation is not established

Objective 8: Discuss drugs used to treat protozoal infections.

■ Metronidazole (Flagyl): for *E. histolytica*, amebiasis, and trichomoniasis

■ Other drugs that treat *E. histolytica* are iodoquinal (Yodoxin), tetracyclines, and paromomycin (Humatin)

■ Adverse effects: nausea, vomiting, anorexia, abdominal cramps, metallic or bitter taste, skin rashes, pruritus, flushing, fever, vertigo, headache, confusion, depression, restlessness, insomnia, darkening of urine; found to be carcinogenic in mice and rats

Internet Sites of Interest

- For information on nail fungus, including diagnosis and treatments, check out the Mayo Clinic Web site at: **http://www.mayoclinic.com/**. Search "nail fungus."

- Patients with HIV and those who are immunocompromised are more susceptible to fungal infections than healthy individuals. Information on opportunistic fungal infections in HIV-positive individuals can be found at: **http://www.thebodypro.com/treat/candida.html**, a Web site provided by the HIV/AIDS Resources for Healthcare Professionals.

- The Centers for Disease Control and Prevention (CDC) offers tips for travelers who may visit areas where malaria is a concern at: **http://www.cdc.gov/malaria/travel/index.htm**

- At **http://healthresources.caremark.com/topic/protodrugs** you can find information provided by Caremark on protozoal infections and the drugs used to treat them, including patient education tips.

- A fact sheet on trichomoniasis is provided by the CDC at: **http://www.cdc.gov/std/Trichomonas/STDFact-Trichomoniasis.htm** and contains reliable patient education information.

Chapter 11

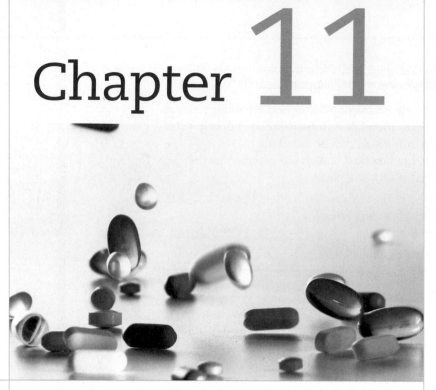

Vaccines and Immunoglobulins

Key Terms

Active immunity (ih-MYOO-nih-tee) (page 232)

Antibodies (AN-tih-bah-deez) (page 229)

Antigens (AN-tih-jenz) (page 231)

Asplenia (as-PLEN-ee-yuh) (page 239)

Attenuated (ah-TEN-yoo-ay-ted) (page 233)

Booster (page 238)

Cell-mediated immunity (page 230)

Globulins (GLOB-yoo-linz) (page 241)

Humoral (HYOO-moh-rul) **immunity** (page 231)

Immune response (page 229)

Immunity (page 229)

Immunogen (ih-MYOO-no-jen) (page 232)

Immunoglobulins (ih-myoon-o-GLOB-yoo-linz) (page 232)

Isotypes (EYE-so-typz) (page 241)

Lymph (limf) (page 229)

Lymphatic (lim-FAH-tik) **vessels** (page 229)

Lymphocytes (LIM-foh-sites) (page 229)

Lymphoid (LIM-foyd) **organs** (page 229)

Macrophages (MAK-ro-fah-jez) (page 231)

Passive immunity (page 232)

Pathogens (PAH-tho-jenz) (page 229)

Toxin (TOKS-in) (page 233)

Toxoids (TOX-oyds) (page 233)

Vaccination (vak-sih-NAY-shun) (page 232)

Vaccine (vak-SEEN) (page 233)

PRACTICAL SCENARIO

A young mother of a newborn is seen at the pediatrician's office for the child's first visit. While you are taking a history of the infant, the mother confides that she does not want her infant to receive any vaccinations because she has heard that immunizations cause autism and seizures. She asks you why her infant needs to be vaccinated.

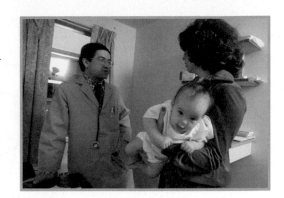

Critical Thinking Questions

1. What would you tell her is the purpose of vaccinations?
2. Are there reasons why her child should not be vaccinated?
3. What questions would you suggest she ask the pediatrician to allay her concerns?

Introduction

Immunizing agents and allergenic extracts are two of the main groups of drugs that are classified as *biologics* by the Food and Drug Administration (FDA). Biologics are chemical agents that produce biological responses in the body. As a group, particularly the active immunizing agents, biologics possibly have prevented more morbidity and mortality than all other drugs combined. *Vaccina vaccine* may be considered the most effective drug to date because it has virtually eradicated smallpox from our world. A similar success for the *poliomyelitis virus vaccines* appears imminent.

The Immune System

The human immune system is a truly amazing constellation of responses to attacks from outside the body. The immune system is part of the lymphatic system, which is composed of the lymph vessels, lymph nodes, and other organs such as the thymus gland, spleen, and tonsils. This system rids foreign substances from the blood and lymph, combats infectious diseases, maintains tissue fluid balance, and absorbs fats.

When microorganisms or foreign substances invade the body, the body responds by producing more white blood cells, or **lymphocytes**. The body continues to fight the invaders by forming special proteins manufactured by the lymphocytes, called **antibodies**. The dominant cells of the lymphatic system, lymphocytes are vital to our ability to resist or overcome infection and disease. They respond to the presence of (1) invading **pathogens**, such as bacteria or viruses; (2) abnormal body cells, such as cancer cells; and (3) foreign proteins, such as the toxins released by some bacteria. Lymphocytes attempt to eliminate these threats or render them harmless by a combination of physical and chemical attack.

Lymphocytes respond to specific threats, such as a bacterial invasion of a tissue, by organizing a defense against that specific type of bacterium. Such a *specific defense* of the body is known as an **immune response**. **Immunity** is the ability to resist infection and disease through the activation of specific defenses.

The lymphatic system, shown in Figure 11-1 ■, includes the following three components:

1. Vessels: A network of **lymphatic vessels** begins in peripheral tissues and ends at connections to the venous system.
2. Fluid: A fluid called **lymph** flows through the lymphatic vessels.
3. Lymphoid organs: **Lymphoid organs** are connected to the lymphatic vessels and contain large numbers of lymphocytes. Examples of the organs are the lymph nodes, the spleen, and the thymus.

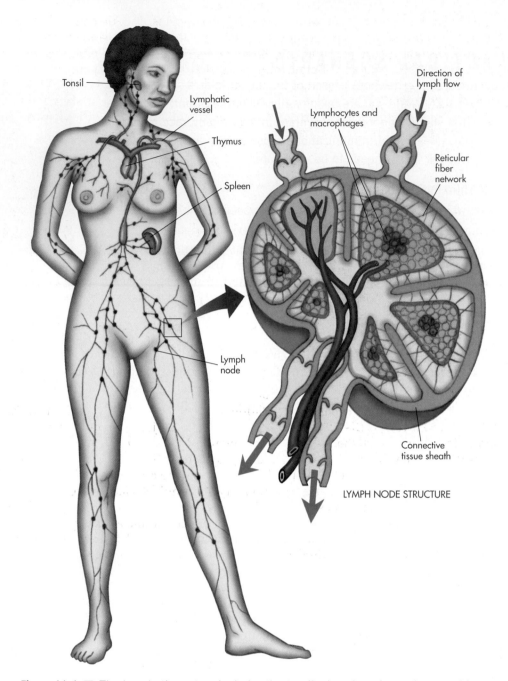

Figure 11-1 ■ The lymphatic system includes the tonsils, lymph nodes, spleen, and lymphatic vessels. Within the lymph nodes are the macrophages and lymphocytes.

The blood contains three classes of lymphocytes:

1. T cells (thymus-dependent)
2. B cells (bone marrow–derived)
3. NK cells (natural killers)

T cells comprise approximately 80% of circulating lymphocytes. *Cytotoxic* T cells directly attack foreign cells or body cells infected by viruses. These lymphocytes are the primary cells that provide **cell-mediated immunity**.

B cells constitute 10 to 15% of circulating lymphocytes. B cells can differentiate into *plasma cells*, which are responsible for the production and secretion of *antibodies*. Antibodies are globular proteins that are often called *immunoglobulins*. Antibodies react with specific chemical targets called **antigens**. Antigens are usually pathogens, parts or products of pathogens, or other foreign compounds.

NK (natural killer) cells make up the remaining 5 to 10% of circulating lymphocytes. These lymphocytes attack foreign cells, normal cells infected with viruses, and cancer cells that appear in normal tissues.

Cell-Mediated Immunity and Humoral Immunity

Cell-mediated immunity depends on the functions of the T cells, which are responsible for a delayed type of immune response. The T lymphocyte becomes sensitized by the first contact with a specific antigen. T cells and **macrophages** (immune cells derived from monocytes) work together in cell-mediated immunity to destroy the antigen. T cells attack the antigens directly, rather than producing antibodies. Cell-mediated immunity may also occur without macrophages. T cells defend the body against viral, fungal, and some bacterial infections. If cell-mediated immunity is lost, as in the case of acquired immunodeficiency syndrome (AIDS), the body is unable to protect itself against many viral, bacterial, and fungal infections.

Humoral immunity is based on the antigen–antibody response. B cells, which are responsible for humoral immunity, produce circulating antibodies to act against an antigen. B cells arise from a separate population of stem cells of the bone marrow than that which produces T cells. These cells undergo multiplication and processing in lymphoid tissue elsewhere than in the thymus gland. B cells, like T cells, have surface receptors that enable them to recognize the appropriate antigen; but unlike T cells, B cells do not themselves interact to neutralize or destroy the antigen. On recognition of the antigen, they take up residence in secondary lymphoid tissue and proliferate to form daughter lymphocytes. These B cells then develop into plasma cells. The plasma cells produce antibodies and release them into the circulation at the lymph nodes. Some of the activated B cells do not become plasma cells. Instead, they turn into memory cells, which continue to produce small amounts of the antibody long after the infection has been overcome.

✴ Apply Your Knowledge 11.1 ▬▬▬▬▬

The following questions focus on what you have just learned about white blood cells and immunity. *See Appendix E for the correct answers.*

FILL IN THE BLANK
Select terms from your reading to fill in the blanks.

1. _____ is the ability to resist infection and disease through the activation of specific defenses.

2. The blood contains three classes of lymphocytes: NK cells, B cells, and _____.

3. B cells can differentiate into plasma cells, which are responsible for the production and secretion of _____.

4. In _____, B cells produce circulating antibodies to act against an antigen.

5. _____, the dominant cells of the lymphatic system, are vital to our ability to resist or overcome infection and disease.

(continued)

Apply Your Knowledge 11.1 (continued)

MATCHING

Match the lettered term to the numbered description.

DESCRIPTION

1. _____ Includes the immune system
2. _____ Manufacture special proteins called antibodies
3. _____ Comprise bacteria and viruses
4. _____ Examples are the spleen and tonsils
5. _____ Constitute 80% of the circulation
6. _____ Derived from bone marrow

TERM

a. Pathogens

b. Lymphoid organs

c. Lymphocytes

d. T cells

e. Lymphatic system

f. B cells

Immunity

Immunity is the state or condition of being resistant to invading microorganisms. It is normally acquired either by contracting a disease and then developing immunity to it, or by being vaccinated with proteins from the causative agent. For example, a person with a normal immune system who contracts rubella (German measles) develops a life-long immunity to the disease. Alternatively, a person may be vaccinated with dead rubella viruses to acquire immunity. In each case, the immune system responds to proteins in the virus and develops a *memory* for it. The next time the person is exposed to the live virus, the immune system *remembers* its past exposure and attacks and kills the virus before it can cause an infection.

Immunizing agents are broadly classified on the basis of the type of immunity they induce. Knowing the properties of the different types of immunity is fundamental to understanding immunizing agents and their applications. There are two main types of immunity—active and passive.

Active immunity is a form of acquired immunity that develops in an individual in response to an **immunogen** (antigen). This may be naturally acquired by exposure to an infectious disease or artificially acquired by receiving active immunizing agents (*vaccines*). The term **vaccination** is used as a synonym for active immunization.

Passive immunity involves the transfer of the effectors of immunity, which are called **immunoglobulins** or antibodies, from an immune individual to another. This occurs naturally by the active transport across the placental barrier of immunoglobulin G (IgG) antibodies from mother to fetus and, to a lesser extent, by the transfer of IgA antibodies in the mother's milk to the nursing infant. The onset of passive immunity is much quicker than that of active immunity, but the duration is much shorter because there is no active immune response to the immunogen (see Figure 11-2 ■).

know definitions →

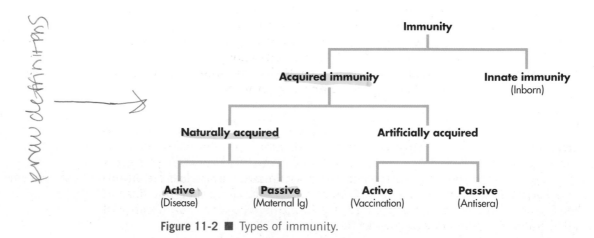

Figure 11-2 ■ Types of immunity.

IMMUNIZING AGENTS

Immunizing agents are among the oldest of modern drugs and can be traced to the beginning of immunology in 1798 when Edward Jenner introduced his vaccine for smallpox. A **vaccine** is a preparation of killed microorganisms, living **attenuated** (their virulence has been reduced) organisms, or living virulent organisms that are administered to produce or artificially increase immunity to a particular disease. They are the most successful and powerful drugs yet developed. Active immunizing agents have the following advantages:

✳ Their main action is to *prevent* rather than to treat disease; most of the commonly used vaccines are highly effective.

✳ They have been proven to be remarkably *safe* in actual practice.

✳ Active immunizing agents are generally available at a relatively *low cost*.

Active immunizing agents are immunogenic drugs that are usually administered to patients prior to their being exposed to diseases to provide long-term, even permanent, protection against the diseases. Active immunization, perhaps, will one day be used for a variety of conditions, ranging from cancer to drug abuse.

Passive immunizing agents date to the early part of the twentieth century following the discovery of immunoglobulins (antibodies). Various antitoxins derived from animals held an important place in therapy prior to the development of antibiotics, but these products, in contrast to the vaccines, had a number of problems with respect to both efficacy and safety.

Focus on Pediatrics

Routine Immunization Reduces Disease

Immunization for diphtheria, tetanus, and pertussis (DTP) has been routinely given in the United States since the late 1940s, resulting in dramatic reductions in the incidence of all these diseases.

Vaccines

Most vaccines consist of entire microorganisms that may be either *inactivated* (killed) or *attenuated* (live). One way to attenuate a virus is through laboratory manipulation, in which a bacterium is developed that lacks a **toxin** (a chemical produced by a microorganism that can be harmful), an enzyme, or some other normal constituent that causes symptoms of disease. The bacterium's virulence is thereby lessened.

Most bacterial vaccines contain killed bacteria or their components. It is important to understand that the live vaccines contain less immunogen than the killed vaccines, and must actually cause an infection within the patient in order to induce a protective immune response.

Another type of vaccine contains **toxoids,** which are protein toxins that have been modified to reduce their hazardous properties without significantly altering their antigenic properties. The oldest and best-known active immunizing agents are diphtheria toxoid and tetanus toxoid, which protect against the bacteria exotoxine.

A *simple vaccine* is one that protects against a single disease, whereas a *combined vaccine* is a combination product that protects against two or more diseases.

How do they work?

The principle underlying vaccination is that exposure to an antigen (a virus or bacterium) in a relatively harmless form sensitizes immune cells for a possible subsequent exposure to the organism. On reexposure, the memory of the previous challenge triggers an immune response more quickly. As the person's own immune processes are stimulated by this agent, this is a form of active immunity. Usually, more than one dose of the vaccine is required to trigger a rapid and full immune response. The number of doses needed reflects the potency of the vaccine.

How are they used?

The indications and recommendations for the use of vaccines depend on several factors, such as safety and efficacy, as with other drugs. The FDA approves the indications for each licensed product. Vaccines are used against a range of bacterial infections, which includes diphtheria, tetanus, pertussis, pneumonia, tuberculosis, typhoid, cholera, meningitis, plague, and Q fever. Vaccines are also available against viral infections such as measles, mumps, rubella (MMR), poliomyelitis, hepatitis A and B, influenza, rabies, and yellow fever (see Tables 11-1 ■ and 11-2 ■).

What are the adverse effects?

The most common adverse effects associated with vaccinations include localized inflammation at the site of injection, a mild fever, headache, malaise, nausea, and dizziness. Convulsions resulting in permanent brain damage have been reported after administration of pertussis vaccine, but these reactions are rare. In some individuals, allergic reaction may occur immediately after vaccination. The recipient should be observed for a short time after the vaccine is administered, and adrenaline should always be available in case anaphylaxis occurs.

What are the contraindications and interactions?

Immunizations are contraindicated in people with acute febrile illness, during pregnancy, and lactation, and in those who are known to have developed anaphylactoid reactions with previous vaccines.

When several vaccines are given at the same time, the potential for drug interaction is increased. An example of this situation would be when typhoid, cholera, and plague vaccines are administered together.

What are the important points patients should know?

Instruct patients to monitor the injection site for reactions. Advise women to avoid breastfeeding until checking with their physician.

Table 11-1 ■ Bacterial Vaccines

VACCINE	ROUTES OF ADMINISTRATION
Live Attenuated Vaccines	
Bacillus Calmette Guérin (BCG) vaccine	Percutaneously (PC)
Typhoid vaccine	PO or subcutaneously
Inactivated Vaccines	
Anthrax vaccine, adsorbed	Subcutaneously
Cholera vaccine	Intradermally, subcutaneously, IM
Hemophilus influenzae type b (Hib)	IM
Lyme disease vaccine	IM
Meningococcal polysaccharide vaccine	Subcutaneously
Pertussis vaccine, adsorbed	IM
Pneumococcal conjugate vaccine	Subcutaneously or IM
Tetanus toxoid, adsorbed	IM

Table 11-2 ■ Inactivated Virus Vaccines

VACCINE	ROUTES OF ADMINISTRATION
Hepatitis A vaccine	IM
Hepatitis B vaccine	IM
Influenza virus vaccine (types A & B)	IM
Poliovirus vaccine, inactivated	Subcutaneously
Rabies virus vaccine	IM

✳ Apply Your Knowledge 11.2

The following exercise focuses on what you have just learned about various types of immunities, vaccines, and toxoids. *See Appendix E for the correct answers.*

FILL IN THE BLANK

Select terms from your reading to fill in the blanks.

1. Immunity is the state or condition of being resistant to invading _____.

2. An immunogen is another word for an _____.

3. Passive immunity involves the transfer of the effectors of immunity, which are called _____ or _____, from an immune individual to another.

4. Edward Jenner introduced a vaccine for _____ in 1798.

5. _____ immunizing agents are usually administered prior to a patient being exposed to a disease.

6. Bacterial vaccines contain _____ bacteria, _____ living bacteria, or _____ bacteria.

7. Toxoids are _____ toxins that have been modified to reduce toxicity without significantly altering antigenic properties.

8. Exposure to an antigen in a relatively harmless form sensitizes immune cells for a possible subsequent exposure to the organism. This is the principle underlying how _____ work.

9. When several vaccines are given at the same time, the potential for drug interaction is _____.

10. The number of vaccine doses needed reflects the _____ of the drug.

Standards for Childhood Immunization

The Advisory Committee on Immunization Practices (ACIP) currently recommends that children be immunized against eight infectious diseases, as well as against hepatitis A in areas of high incidence (see Table 11-3 ■). Childhood immunization remains one of the most important public health measures in the United States.

Hemophilus influenzae type b (Hib) was the leading cause of invasive bacterial disease (e.g., meningitis) among children until pediatric immunization was introduced in 1988. The vaccine contains inactivated bacteria (HibTiter, PedvaxHIB).

The *Salk* inactivated vaccine (IPV, IPOL; 1954) and the Sabin live vaccine (1961) are two types of polio immunizations that have been very effective against poliomyelitis. There has been no poliomyelitis in the Americas in recent years, except for vaccine-associated disease, and a few importation cases.

Table 11-3 ■ Childhood Immunization Schedule

DEPARTMENT OF HEALTH AND HUMAN SERVICES • CENTERS FOR DISEASE CONTROL AND PREVENTION

Recommended Childhood and Adolescent Immunization Schedule UNITED STATES • 2006

Vaccine ▼ Age ▶	Birth	1 month	2 months	4 months	6 months	12 months	15 months	18 months	24 months	4–6 years	11–12 years	13–14 years	15 years	16–18 years
Hepatitis B[1]	HepB	HepB		HepB[1]		HepB					HepB Series			
Diphtheria, Tetanus, Pertussis[2]			DTaP	DTaP	DTaP		DTaP			DTaP	Tdap	Tdap		
Hemophilus influenzae type b[3]			Hib	Hib	Hib[3]	Hib								
Inactivated Poliovirus			IPV	IPV		IPV				IPV				
Measles, Mumps, Rubella[4]						MMR				MMR		MMR		
Varicella[5]						Varicella					Varicella			
Meningococcal[6]											MCV4		MCV4	
										MPSV4			MCV4	
Pneumococcal[7]			PCV	PCV	PCV	PCV				PCV	PPV			
Influenza[8]						Influenza (Yearly)				Influenza (Yearly)				
Hepatitis A[9]						HepA Series								

This schedule indicates the recommended ages for routine administration of currently licensed childhood vaccines, as of December 1, 2005, for children through age 18 years. Any dose not administered at the recommended age should be administered at any subsequent visit when indicated and feasible. ▮ Indicates age groups that warrant special effort to administer those vaccines not previously administered. Additional vaccines may be licensed and recommended during the year. Licensed combination vaccines may be used whenever any components of the combination are indicated and other components of the vaccine are not contraindicated and if approved by the Food and Drug Administration for that dose of the series. Providers should consult the respective ACIP statement for detailed recommendations. Clinically significant adverse events that follow immunization should be reported to the Vaccine Adverse Event Reporting System (VAERS). Guidance about how to obtain and complete a VAERS form is available at www.vaers.hhs.gov or by telephone, 800-822-7967.

▮ Range of recommended ages   ▮ Catch-up immunization   ▮ 11–12 year old assessment

Courtesy of Centers for Disease Control and Prevention, National Immunization Program http://www.cdc.gov/Nip/. These recommendations must be read along with the footnotes, which can be found in Appendix D.

Measles, mumps, and rubella (German measles) are three important viral diseases that can potentially be eradicated by mass active immunization. The combined vaccine (MMR) was licensed in 1971 and has been recommended for routine immunizations since 1977.

Hepatitis B infection is a major worldwide health problem with many facets, including acute and chronic disease, liver failure and cirrhosis, hepatic carcinoma, and chronic carriers. Neonates born to mothers who are positive for hepatitis B should be immunized immediately both with the vaccine (Energix B, Heptava B) and hepatitis B immunoglobulin.

Varicella (*chickenpox*) is a highly communicable disease that is generally benign, but that also causes herpes and sometimes may be accompanied by serious complications, such as encephalitis and bacterial superinfection. Varicella is more serious in adults and particularly in the immunodeficient, where it can cause devastating disease. The varicella vaccine (Varivax) was licensed in 1995 and appears to be very effective in protecting against chickenpox, but it is much too early to completely evaluate the impact of the immunization program on the epidemiology of varicella-zoster.

The ACIP recommends hepatitis A vaccination (Havrix, VAQTA) for children residing in communities where the incidence of hepatitis A is high and common.

In June of 2006, the FDA licensed the first vaccine developed to prevent cancer (and other diseases) in women that are caused by certain types of the genital human papillomavirus (HPV). This vaccine (trade name, Gardasil), protects against four HPV types (6, 11, 16, and 18) that are responsible for cervical cancer and 90% of genital warts. This vaccine is recommended for females between the ages of 9 and 26 years.

✳ **Apply Your Knowledge 11.3** ▬▬▬▬▬▬▬▬▬▬▬

The following questions focus on what you have just learned about the various childhood immunizations. *See Appendix E for the correct answers.*

FILL IN THE BLANK

Select terms from your reading to fill in the blanks.

1. Immunization for _____, _____, and _____ (DTP) has been routine in the United States since the late 1940s.

2. _____ _____ was the leading cause of invasive bacterial disease among children until pediatric immunization was introduced in 1988.

3. Three important viral diseases that potentially can be eradicated by mass active immunization are _____, _____, and _____.

4. Varicella-zoster is known to be causative for herpes zoster, but also for the common, highly communicable disease known as _____.

5. _____ immunization remains one of the most important public health measures in the United States.

MATCHING

Match the lettered virus to the numbered vaccine that is used to prevent it.

VACCINE	VIRUS
1. _____ HibTiter and PedvaxHIB	a. Poliomyelitis
2. _____ IPV, IPOL	b. Measles, mumps, and rubella
3. _____ MMR	c. Hepatitis B
4. _____ Energix B and Heptava B	d. *Hemophilus influenzae* type b
5. _____ Varivax	e. Hepatitis A
6. _____ Havrix and VAQTA	f. Chickenpox

The best time for females to receive this vaccine is ages 10 to 11 (this age group is utilized because ideally, the vaccine should be administered before onset of sexual activity). The recommendations for HPV vaccine are as follows: three intramuscular injections over a six-month period, with the second dose given 2 months after the first dose, and the third dose given 6 months after the first dose.

The HPV vaccine has been tested in more than 11,000 women in many countries throughout the world, including the United States. It has been found to be safe with no serious side effects. The vaccine appears to be effective for at least five years. Efficacy studies for this vaccine in men are ongoing, but currently no data supports its use in men.

Standards of Immunization for Adults Younger than Age 65

Pertussis vaccine is not recommended for adults, but the other nine vaccines (see Table 11-3) are commonly indicated under certain circumstances if there is not evidence of immunity, such as a reliable history of having the disease or positive serological tests. Three circumstances in which it is particularly important that the pediatric immunizations are up to date are as follows:

1. Individuals who travel internationally, since some of these diseases remain prevalent in other parts of the world

2. Women of childbearing age who may become pregnant, since the immunity (such as IgG) that women transfer to the fetus depends on their immune status

3. Individuals with chronic illnesses, since they may be more susceptible to a disease or its adverse effects

The only routine immunization recommended for all normal adults between the ages of 18 and 65 years is a **booster** dose (a dose given to increase the effectiveness of the original medication) of adult diphtheria and tetanus toxoid every 10 years. Unfortunately, many adults in this country do not comply with this recommendation and may not even be aware of it. Sometimes, patients with traumatic injury are given a tetanus booster in the emergency department or physician's office at the time of injury.

Annual influenza immunization (Fluzone, FluShield) is recommended for those at high-risk for influenza complications, as well as those capable of *nosocomial* (hospital) transmission of influenza to high-risk patients—for example, physicians, nurses, pharmacists, and others who provide inpatient, outpatient, and home health-care services, as well as nonprofessional caregivers.

Pneumococcal vaccine (Pneumovax 23, Pnu-Immune 23) should be administered to people with any major immunosuppression condition, such as human immunodeficiency virus (HIV) infection, organ transplant, and some cancers. This vaccine also should be administered to patients with pulmonary or cardiovascular diseases, chronic hepatic or renal disorders, and diabetes mellitus. Meningococcal vaccine (Menomune A/C/Y/W) is recommended for some travelers and some closed populations in which outbreaks may occur.

The only disease for which an *International Certificate of Vaccination* may still be required is yellow fever. Travelers to underdeveloped countries (and some developed countries) may find other vaccines recommended. Hepatitis A vaccine (Havrix, VAQTA) is most likely, though cholera, typhoid, and plague vaccines may occasionally be suggested.

Hepatitis B vaccine (Energix B, Heptavax B) is essential for health-care workers with exposure to human blood and tissues, and a number of other immunizations are recommended for those in high-risk occupations.

Bacillus Calmette Guérin (BCG) vaccine is recommended only in extremely high-risk individuals in whom other controls are impractical. BCG vaccine is commonly used to treat bladder cancer by direct instillation into the bladder. This is sometimes called non-specific immunotherapy, but the precise mechanism is unknown. The vaccine does promote a local inflammatory response that may be responsible for the antitumor effects.

In May of 2006, the FDA licensed a new vaccine to reduce older patients' risk of shingles. Shingles is a painful skin rash, often with blisters, that is also called herpes zoster. It is caused by the varicella zoster virus, the same virus that causes chickenpox. This vaccine (trade name, Zostavax), has been shown to prevent shingles in about 50% of patients who are age 60 or older, and can also reduce the pain associated with shingles.

A single dose of this vaccine is indicated for adults ages 60 or older. It is administered subcutaneously. No serious problems have been identified with the shingles vaccine.

✳ Apply Your Knowledge 11.4

The following questions focus on what you have just learned about immunizations for adults younger than age 65. *See Appendix E for the correct answers.*

MULTIPLE CHOICE

Select the correct answers from choices a–d.

1. Which of the following vaccines is not recommended for adults?

   a. Pertussis

   b. IgG

   c. Diphtheria

   d. Tetanus

2. The only routine immunization that is recommended for all normal adults between the ages of 18 and 65 years is a booster dose of:
   a. Adult varicella and rubella
   b. Adult varicella and pertussis
   c. Adult diphtheria and tetanus toxoid
   d. Adult typhoid and tetanus toxoid

3. Annual influenza immunization is recommended for all of the following, except:
   a. Those at high risk of influenza complications
   b. Those capable of nosocomial transmission of influenza to high-risk patients
   c. Those who are older than 65
   d. Healthy young adults between 20 and 35 years of age

4. The only disease for which an International Certificate of Vaccination may still be required is:
   a. Plague
   b. Pertussis
   c. Rubella
   d. Yellow fever

5. Which of the following vaccines is essential for health-care workers with exposure to human blood and tissues?
   a. Hepatitis A
   b. Hepatitis B
   c. HIV
   d. BCG

This vaccine has been tested in more than 38,000 adults 60 years of age or older. It has been found to be safe with no serious side effects. The duration of protection of this vaccine is unknown, but protection from herpes zoster has been demonstrated through four years of follow-up.

Standards of Immunization for Adults Older than Age 65

Evaluation of immune status and appropriate vaccination at age 65 is important to the quality of the later years of life. Every individual should continue to receive adult diphtheria and tetanus toxoid boosters every 10 years. If this has not been done, it is important to update these vaccinations at age 65. Unfortunately, many older Americans are susceptible to these diseases. Those at highest risk of fatal pneumococcal disease, such as individuals with **asplenia** (loss of the spleen), should receive a booster dose at 5 years after the initial dose of the pneumococcal vaccine (Pneumovax 23, Pnu-Immune 23) (see Table 11-4 ■).

Focus on Geriatrics

Influenza and Pneumonia Immunization

All individuals age 65 and older should receive annual influenza immunization and a single dose of pneumococcal vaccine. Those who received pneumococcal vaccine prior to age 65 should receive a booster dose if it has been 5 or more years since the first dose.

Table 11-4 ■ Adult Immunization Schedule

Recommended Adult Immunization Schedule
United States, October 2006–September 2007

Recommended adult immunization schedule, by vaccine and age group

Age group (yrs) ▶ Vaccine ▼	19–49 years	50–64 years	≥65 years
Tetanus, diphtheria, pertussis (Td/Tdap)[1]*	1-dose Td booster every 10 yrs Substitute 1 dose of Tdap for Td		
Human papillomavirus (HPV)[2]*	3 doses (females)		
Measles, mumps, rubella (MMR)[3]*	1 or 2 doses	1 dose	
Varicella[4]*	2 doses (0, 4–8 wks)	2 doses (0, 4–8 wks)	
Influenza[5]*	1 dose annually	1 dose annually	
Pneumococcal (polysaccharide)[6,7]	1–2 doses		1 dose
Hepatitis A[8]*	2 doses (0, 6–12 mos, or 0, 6–18 mos)		
Hepatitis B[9]*	3 doses (0, 1–2, 4–6 mos)		
Meningococcal[10]	1 or more doses		

Recommended adult immunization schedule, by vaccine and medical and other indications

Indication ▶ Vaccine ▼	Pregnancy	Congenital immunodeficiency; leukemia;[11] lymphoma; generalized malignancy; cerebrospinal fluid leaks; therapy with alkylating agents, antimetabolites, radiation, or high-dose, long-term corticosteroids	Diabetes, heart disease, chronic pulmonary disease, chronic alcoholism	Asplenia[11] (including elective splenectomy and terminal complement component deficiencies)	Chronic liver disease, recipients of clotting factor concentrates	Kidney failure, end-stage renal disease, recipients of hemodialysis	Human immunodeficiency virus (HIV) infection[3,11]	Health-care workers
Tetanus, diphtheria, pertussis (Td/Tdap)[1]*	1-dose Td booster every 10 yrs Substitute 1 dose of Tdap for Td							
Human papillomavirus (HPV)[2]*		3 doses for women through age 26 years (0, 2, 6 mos)						
Measles, mumps, rubella (MMR)[3]*	*(contraindicated)*	1 or 2 doses						
Varicella[4]*	*(contraindicated)*	2 doses (0, 4–8 wks)				*(contraindicated)*		2 doses
Influenza[5]*	1 dose annually		1 dose annually	1 dose annually				
Pneumococcal (polysaccharide)[6,7]	1–2 doses	1–2 doses						1–2 doses
Hepatitis A[8]*	2 doses (0, 6–12 mos, or 0, 6–18 mos)			2 doses (0, 6–12 mos, or 0, 6–18 mos)				
Hepatitis B[9]*	3 doses (0, 1–2, 4–6 mos)			3 doses (0, 1–2, 4–6 mos)				
Meningococcal[10]	1 dose		1 dose	1 dose				

* Covered by the Vaccine Injury Compensation Program

These recommendations must be read along with the footnotes, which can be found in Appendix D.

For all persons in this category who meet the age requirements and who lack evidence of immunity (e.g., lack documentation of vaccination or have no evidence of prior infection)	Recommended if some other risk factor is present (e.g., on the basis of medical, occupational, lifestyle, or other indications)	Contraindicated

Courtesy of Centers for Disease Control and Prevention, National Immunization Program http://www.cdc.gov/Nip/

Immunoglobulins

Globulins are proteins that contain antibodies and are present in blood. Immunoglobulins (Ig) are derived from human plasma containing antibodies that have been formed by the body to specific antigens. The antibody content is primarily IgG (90–98%) and their **isotypes** (atoms of a chemical element that have the same atomic number with nearly identical chemical properties, but different physical properties) such as IgG_1, IgG_2, IgG_3, and IgG_4. There are two types of immunoglobulins, one that should be administered intramuscularly and one that should be administered intravenously.

The immunoglobulin intramuscular (IGIM) products are aqueous solutions containing 15% protein, of which more than 90% is IgG. They are standardized for antibodies to measles, diphtheria, and poliovirus to ensure reasonable uniformity of product, but they contain antibodies specific for numerous bacteria, viruses, and fungi. Ig is given by injection into a muscle.

How do they work?
The immunoglobulins are given to provide passive immunity to one or more infectious diseases. Individuals receiving immunoglobulins receive antibodies only to the diseases to which the donor blood is immune. The onset of protection is rapid but of short duration (1 to 3 months).

How are they used?
The main indications of IGIM are for IgG-replacement therapy in disorders where there is a deficiency of IgG antibodies, and for the passive prevention or modification of hepatitis A and measles in susceptible persons, when given shortly after exposure. Passive immunization for measles is particularly important in children younger than 1 year of age because they are prone to measles complications and have not yet been vaccinated. IGIM is not standardized for hepatitis B, and the specific immunoglobulin should be used in this case. IGIM can be used for the prevention of varicella in immunocompromised patients if varicella-zoster immunoglobulin is not available. It has also been used to prevent fetal damage in women who are exposed to rubella during the first trimester of pregnancy. Immunoglobulins (IM or IV) are recommended to HIV-positive patients who are exposed to measles, regardless of their immunization status.

What are the adverse effects?
There are few adverse reactions associated with IGIM, except for local pain and tenderness at the injection site. As with all immunoglobulin products, serious anaphylactic reactions occur occasionally and are the most common selective immunoglobulin deficiency.

What are the contraindications and interactions?
IGIM must not be injected intravenously because it can cause serious anaphylactic reactions.

What are the important points patients should know?
Instruct patients to report signs and symptoms of hypersensitivity and infusion symptoms of nausea, chills, headache or chest tightness. Advise women to avoid breastfeeding without consulting a physician.

Focus Point

Site of Injection

The dosage and the site for the injection vary according to the amount of Ig required and the size of the person (typically, the site is in the buttocks for adults and the leg or arm for children).

✳ Apply Your Knowledge 11.5

The following questions focus on what you have just learned about immunoglobulins. *See Appendix E for the correct answers.*

MATCHING
Match the lettered term to the numbered description.

DESCRIPTION

1. _____ Proteins present in blood that contain antibodies
2. _____ May be administered intramuscularly or intravenously
3. _____ Immunoglobulin injection site for children
4. _____ Immunity provided by Ig
5. _____ Must not be injected intravenously

TERM

a. Leg or arm
b. Globulins
c. IGIM
d. Passive
e. Immunoglobulins

FILL IN THE BLANK
Select terms from your reading to fill in the blanks.

1. IGIM must not be injected intravenously because it can cause serious _____.
2. The onset of action of immunoglobulins is _____, but _____ in duration.
3. Immunoglobulin is given by _____ into _____.
4. Individuals with _____ are at highest risk of fatal pneumococcal disease.
5. Immunoglobulins are derived from human _____ containing antibodies that have been formed by the body to specific antigens.

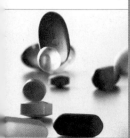

Chapter Capsule

This section repeats the objectives from the beginning of the chapter and then provides a summary of the most important concepts for that objective. Use this section as a quick review and to check your knowledge.

Objective 1: State the names and functions of blood cells involved in immunity.

■ White blood cells (lymphocytes)—manufacture antibodies to overcome infection and disease

■ T cells, B cells, and NK cells—attack viruses, fungi, bacteria, and other foreign cells that invade the body

Objective 2: List the major components of the lymphatic system.

■ Lymphatic vessels, lymph fluid, lymph nodes, the thymus gland, spleen, and tonsils

Objective 3: Discuss and contrast the various types of immunities.

■ Humoral immunity—B cells produce circulating antibodies to act against an antigen

- Cell-mediated immunity—T cells attack the antigens directly, rather than producing antibodies

Objective 4: Explain the differences between active and passive immunity.

- Active immunity—a form of acquired immunity that develops in response to an antigen either naturally acquired by exposure to an infectious disease or artificially acquired by receiving active immunizing agents (*vaccines*)
- Passive immunity—the transfer of immunoglobulins (antibodies) from an immune individual to another, occurring naturally in the active transport across the placental barrier of immunoglobulin G (IgG) antibodies from mother to fetus or by the transfer of IgA antibodies in the mother's milk

Objective 5: State the main action of immunizing agents.

- Prompt the body's immune system to become resistant to a specific disease or several diseases
- Sensitize immune cells for a possible subsequent reexposure to the organism, thus triggering an immune response

Objective 6: Contrast inactivated and attenuated vaccines.

- Inactivated vaccines—microorganisms in the vaccine are killed, prompting immunity in the injected individual; most bacterial vaccines are inactivated
- Attenuated (live) vaccines—these vaccines cause an infection within the patient to induce a protective immune response; they contain less immunogen than killed vaccines

Objective 7: List the most common adverse effects associated with vaccinations.

- Localized inflammation at the site of injection, mild fever, headache, malaise, nausea, and dizziness

Objective 8: Describe the most common childhood immunizations.

- *Hemophilus influenzae* type b (Hib) (meningitis, other bacterial diseases), *Salk* inactivated vaccine and the Sabin live vaccine (poliomyelitis), MMR (measles, mumps, rubella), diphtheria, tetanus, pertussis, hepatitis B, varicella-zoster (chickenpox)

Objective 9: List the most common adult immunizations.

- Influenza and pneumococcus vaccines annually; booster dose of adult diphtheria and tetanus toxoid every 10 years

Objective 10: Explain how immunoglobulins work to provide immunity.

- Immunoglobulins, derived from human plasma containing antibodies against specific antigens, provide passive immunity

Internet Sites of Interest

■ Immunization Action Coalition provides numerous articles offering vaccination information for health-care professionals: **www.immunize.org**

■ Safe injections are discussed on this World Health Organization Web site: **www.who.int/immunization_safety/safe_injections/en/**

■ The National Immunization Program of the Centers for Disease Control and Prevention (CDC) offers a quick reference chart, including frequently asked questions, a list of side effects, and current news related to various types of vaccines at: **www.cdc.gov/nip/vaccine/vac-chart-public.htm**

■ All that you need to know about getting vaccinated for travel to other countries can be found at: **www.cdc.gov/travel/vaccinat.htm**

■ The Johns Hopkins Bloomberg School of Public Health provides independent assessment of studies related to vaccine safety at: **www.vaccinesafety.edu**

■ More information from Facts & Comparison's ImmunoFacts Web site is available at: **www.immunofacts.com**. This Web site covers laws and regulations and government databases in addition to fact sheets, vaccine monographs, and bioterrorism information.

Chapter Objectives

After completing this chapter, you should be able to:

1. List the antipyretic properties of anti-inflammatory and analgesic drugs.

2. Describe the role of prostaglandins in inflammation.

3. Outline the dangers of aspirin use.

4. List the uses and side effects of anti-inflammatory drugs.

5. Identify the different types of analgesics.

6. Describe the function of naturally occurring opioids and their receptors.

7. Explain the rationale behind the use of narcotic analgesics.

8. Describe the problems associated with the use of narcotic analgesics.

Chapter 12

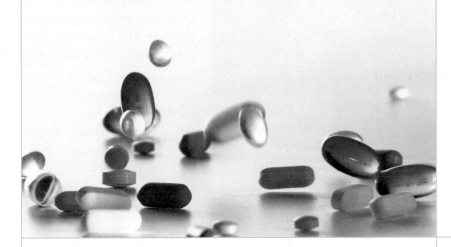

Analgesic, Antipyretic, and Anti-Inflammatory Drugs

Key Terms

Acute (page 246)

Analgesic (ah-nul-JEE-zik) (page 246)

Antipyretics (an-tih-pye-REH-tiks) (page 246)

Bradykinin (brah-dee-KYE-nin) (page 246)

Chronic (page 246)

Cyclooxygenase (sye-klo-OKS-ih-jeh-nase) (page 252)

Endogenous (en-DAH-jeh-nus) (page 255)

Endorphins (en-DOR-finz) (page 247)

Enkephalins (en-KEH-fuh-linz) (page 247)

Narcotic (page 255)

Neurotransmitters (noo-roh-TRANZ-mih-ters) (page 247)

Opiates (OH-pee-uts) (page 255)

Opioid (OH-pee-oyd) (page 255)

Prostaglandins (prah-stuh-GLAN-dinz) (page 246)

PRACTICAL SCENARIO

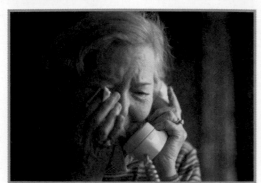

Janet is a 4-year-old girl who is found unconscious. Her grandmother calls the physician's office and speaks to the medical assistant. The grandmother states that she put her granddaughter down for a nap around 13:00 hours in the grandmother's bedroom. At about 15:30, she checked on Janet and found her on the floor of the bedroom, unconscious and unresponsive, with an open bottle of acetaminophen beside her. The grandmother says the bottle of 60 tablets was empty, and there were 7 to 10 tablets on the floor.

Critical Thinking Questions

1. What should the medical assistant tell the grandmother to do immediately?
2. In counseling the grandmother about this incident, what teaching information should the medical assistant present?
3. What are some of the complications of this child's overdose of acetaminophen?

Introduction

Analgesics are agents that relieve pain without significantly disturbing consciousness or altering the actions of the sensory nerves, which carry impulses to the brain. Therefore, many drugs that are used to relieve pain are not truly analgesics. For example, general anesthetics reduce pain but interfere with consciousness (see Chapter 16); local anesthetics reduce pain by blocking peripheral nerve fibers that carry other sensory input (see Chapter 16); antispasmodics indirectly relieve certain types of pain by relaxing smooth muscle (see Chapter 26); and steroids relieve pain associated with rheumatoid arthritis via their anti-inflammatory action (see Chapter 26).

Antipyretics are drugs that reduce elevated body temperature (fever) to normal levels. Certain analgesics and antipyretics also possess anti-inflammatory properties; such agents are used in the treatment of arthritis and other inflammatory conditions. The drugs considered in this chapter have demonstrated **analgesic**—or pain-relieving—action, with or without antipyretic or anti-inflammatory action.

What Is Pain?

Pain is considered to be the central nervous system's reaction to potentially harmful stimuli characterized by physical discomfort. It has been described by the *International Association for the Study of Pain* as an "unpleasant sensory and emotional experience associated with actual or potential tissue damage." **Acute** pain (severe pain with a sudden onset) serves as an early warning alert to seek medical help for preventing any further damage to our bodies. Although pain can play a beneficial role as a warning system and aid in diagnosis, some pain (such as that associated with the postoperative period or cancer patients) and types of **chronic** pain (lasting a long time or marked by frequent recurrence), have very few positive effects.

Pain stimuli may result from the process of inflammation that causes tissue injury, and the release of different substances such as histamine, **prostaglandins** (hormone-like substances that control blood pressure, contract smooth muscle, and modulate inflammation), serotonin, and **bradykinin** (a polypeptide that mediates inflammation, increases vasodilation, and contracts smooth muscle). Such chemical substances initiate an action potential along a sensory nerve fiber and/or sensitize pain receptors. These pain receptors, called *nociceptors,* are free nerve endings strategically located throughout the body. The pain enters from a pain receptor and sensory fibers, moving into the spinal cord and the brain. Once perceived, interpretation of the pain impulse occurs in the brain cortex, and appropriate autonomic and reflex responses occur to deal with the pain (see Figure 12-1 ■).

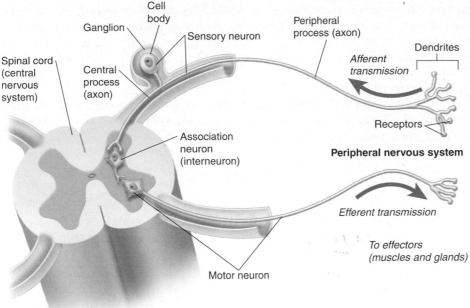

Figure 12-1 ■ Reflex responses to pain.

The transmission of pain impulses relates to the actions of certain chemical substances called **neurotransmitters** that are concentrated in various parts of the central nervous system (CNS) and allow communication from nerve cell to nerve cell. These neurotransmitters are known as **endorphins** and **enkephalins** and are capable of binding with opiate receptors in the CNS, and thereby inhibit the transmission of pain impulses, providing an analgesic effect. These analgesic compounds are released when painful stimuli affect the body (see Figure 12-2 ■).

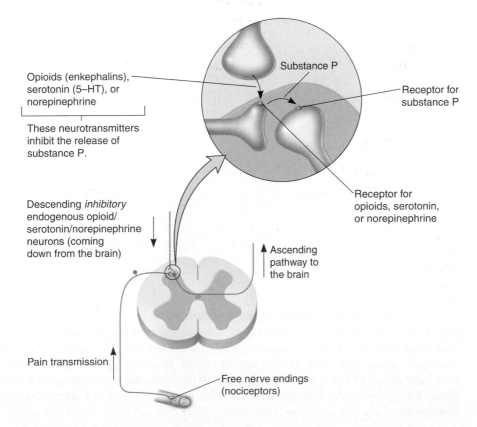

Figure 12-2 ■ Endogenous analgesic compounds released after pain stimuli.

Nonsteroidal Anti-Inflammatory Drugs

Nonsteroidal anti-inflammatory drugs (NSAIDs) are used to relieve some symptoms caused by arthritis, such as inflammation, swelling, stiffness, and joint pain. However, these medicines do not cure arthritis and help patients only as long as they continue to take them. Some of these drugs are also used to relieve other kinds of pain or to treat other painful conditions such as menstrual cramps, gout attacks, bursitis, tendonitis, sprains, and muscle strains.

The salicylate group of analgesics and antipyretics is a subset of NSAIDs and are commonly used. These agents are consumed at a rate in excess of 10,000 tons annually, primarily for antiplatelet effects.

ASPIRIN

Of all the salicylate drugs, aspirin, or acetylsalicylic acid (Bayer, Ecotrin, St. Joseph's), is the most commonly used. All commercially available salicylates have similar pharmacologic properties, so aspirin is discussed as the prototype for this group.

How does it work?

Aspirin's mechanism of action is unknown. It may produce analgesia and block pain impulses by inhibiting synthesis of prostaglandin in the CNS. It is thought to relieve fever by central action in the hypothalamic heat-regulating center. In low doses, aspirin also appears to impede clotting in the blood by blocking prostaglandin synthesis, which prevents formation of the platelet-aggregating substance, thus helping to prevent strokes and heart attacks.

How is it used?

Aspirin is employed as an antipyretic and analgesic in a variety of conditions. It is used for the relief of pain from simple headache, discomfort, and fever associated with the common cold, and minor muscular aches and pains. When aspirin is used for lowering a fever, it is one of the most effective and safest drugs.

What are the adverse effects?

Though uncommon, adverse effects of aspirin taken in usual doses may include dyspepsia, nausea, vomiting, and occult bleeding (blood in the stool). Prolonged administration of large doses (3.6 g/day or higher) results in occult bleeding and anemia. Massive GI hemorrhage can also occur, particularly in elderly clients.

What are the contraindications and interactions?

In general, salicylates are contraindicated in hypersensitive people and in patients who have GI disturbances, particularly hemorrhaging ulcers. Salicylates also should be used with caution in patients on anticoagulant therapy and avoided in patients who are taking *uricosurics*, agents that promote excretion of uric acid in the urine. Salicylates interact with a wide variety of agents, including antidiabetic drugs (causing increased hypoglycemia) and oral anticoagulants (causing increased anticoagulant effects).

What are the important points patients should know?

Any condition involving bleeding may be worsened by taking aspirin. Advise menstruating women, to avoid aspirin if menstrual bleeding is heavy or during the last 3 months of pregnancy or while breastfeeding. Instruct patient to discontinue aspirin use 1 week before or after surgery, including oral surgery. Advise patients not to use aspirin if symptoms of meningitis exist and to avoid alcohol when taking large doses of aspirin.

Focus on Pediatrics

Aspirin and Reye's Syndrome

The use of aspirin in the treatment of fever in children who have varicella (chickenpox), a common cold, or influenza virus infections may result in the development of Reye's syndrome. The current opinion is that aspirin should not be prescribed for children who have upper respiratory viral infections. If control of fever, aches, and pains is necessary, alternative measures should be employed.

Focus on Geriatrics

Salicylates and GI Bleeding

Administration of salicylates to elderly patients who are vulnerable to GI bleeding may cause this bleeding to become severe. Emergency help should be requested if any of these symptoms occurs: bloody urine, loss of hearing or vision, confusion, convulsions, diarrhea, difficulty swallowing, dizziness, severe drowsiness, severe excitement, abnormal respiration, change in skin color, hallucinations, sweating, increased thirst, nausea or vomiting, stomach pain, swelling, fever, or a flapping movement of the hands.

Nonsalicylate NSAIDs

Little distinguishes the clinical profile of this group of NSAIDs from the others. In this chapter, only two of these drugs will be discussed (ibuprofen and indomethacin) as examples of NSAIDs.

IBUPROFEN

Ibuprofen (Motrin, Advil) is an NSAID that possesses analgesic, anti-inflammatory, and antipyretic activities.

How does it work?

Ibuprofen, like other NSAIDs, has a mechanism of action that is likely related to its inhibition of prostaglandin synthesis.

How is it used?

Ibuprofen is used for rheumatoid arthritis, osteoarthritis, and arthritis. It is also indicated for mild to moderate pain, dysmenorrhea, and fever.

What are the adverse effects?

Ibuprofen may cause headache, dizziness, nervousness, peripheral edema, fluid retention, and tinnitus. Common adverse effects of ibuprofen include nausea, occult blood loss, peptic ulceration, diarrhea, constipation, abdominal pain, dyspepsia, flatulence, heartburn, and decreased appetite. Severe adverse effects from ibuprofen are azotemia (abnormally high nitrogen-type wastes in the bloodstream), cystitis, hematuria, aplastic anemia, hypoglycemia, and hyperkalemia.

What are the contraindications and interactions?

Ibuprofen is contraindicated in patients who are hypersensitive to the drug and in those with angioedema, nasal polyps, or bronchospastic reaction to aspirin or other NSAIDs. Pregnant women should avoid ibuprofen. Individuals with GI disorders, history of peptic ulcer, hepatic or renal disease, hypertension, and preexisting asthma should use ibuprofen cautiously. Ibuprofen may interact with antihypertensives, furosemide, and thiazide diuretics and may decrease the effectiveness of diuretics or antihypertensive drugs.

What are the important points patients should know?

Advise patients to notify their physician if blood appears in the stool, vomitus, or urine, or if there is onset of skin rash, pruritus, or jaundice. Driving a vehicle is not advised until individual patient response to ibuprofen has been assessed. Instruct patients to not take ibuprofen with aspirin, alcohol, or NSAIDs. Breastfeeding women should not take ibuprofen.

INDOMETHACIN

Indomethacin (Indocin) is a nonsteroidal drug with anti-inflammatory, antipyretic, and analgesic properties. It is not a simple analgesic, because of its potential serious adverse effects, and should not be used for minor pain.

How does it work?

Indomethacin produces anti-inflammatory, analgesic, and antipyretic effects by inhibiting prostaglandin synthesis.

How is it used?

Indomethacin is indicated for the treatment of rheumatoid arthritis, rheumatoid spondylitis, osteoarthritis, bursitis, tendonitis, gouty arthritis, and *patent ductus arteriosus* (abnormal fetal connection of the left pulmonary artery and the descending aorta) in premature neonates.

What are the adverse effects?

The most common adverse effects of indomethacin include GI ulcerations, hemorrhage, GI bleeding, increased pain in ulcerative colitis, gastritis, nausea, and vomiting. Indomethacin may also cause blurred vision, hepatic toxicity, aplastic anemia, hemolytic anemia, asthma, pruritus, urticaria, and skin rashes. Depression, mental confusion, coma, and convulsions are also reported.

What are the contraindications and interactions?

Indomethacin is contraindicated in patients hypersensitive to the drug and in those with a history of aspirin- or NSAID-induced asthma, rhinitis, or urticaria (hives). It must be avoided by pregnant or breastfeeding women and in neonates with untreated infection, active bleeding, and significant renal impairment. Indomethacin should be used cautiously in patients with epilepsy, parkinsonism, and hepatic or renal disease. Aminoglycosides, cyclosporine, and methotrexate may enhance the toxicity of indomethacin. Antihypertensives, furosemide, and thiazide diuretics may impair response to both drugs.

What are the important points patients should know?

Advise patients taking NSAIDs to notify their physician promptly if they develop signs of skin rash, breathing problems, or visual disturbances. These are signs of hypersensitivity to NSAIDs.

Focus Point

Allergy to Analgesics

If the patient is allergic to one analgesic, be cautious in giving another over-the-counter analgesics.

✳ Apply Your Knowledge 12.1 ━━━━━

The following questions focus on what you have just learned about pain and NSAIDs. *See Appendix E for the correct answers.*

FILL IN THE BLANK

Select terms from your reading to fill in the blanks.

1. The mechanism of action of aspirin may produce analgesia by inhibiting synthesis of _____ in the CNS.

2. Prolonged administration of large doses of aspirin results in _____, _____ _____, or _____.

3. Ibuprofen is an NSAID that possesses _____ and _____ activities.

4. Indomethacin should be used cautiously in patients with _____, _____, and _____ or _____ disease.

5. Reye's syndrome may develop in children when _____ is used to treat fever from _____ infections.

MULTIPLE CHOICE

Select the correct answers from choices a–d.

1. Which of the following chemical agents may be released in tissue injury during the process of inflammation?

   a. Heparin

   b. Renin

   c. Prostaglandin

   d. Secretin

2. Which of the following can prevent formation of the platelet-aggregating substance?

   a. Codeine

   b. Acetaminophen

   c. Naltrexone

   d. Aspirin

3. Which of the following agents is indicated for treatment of patients with ductus arteriosus?

   a. Indomethacin

   b. Ibuprofen

   c. Acetaminophen

   d. Celecoxib

4. Salicylates should be used with caution in patients on which of the following medications?

   a. Antianginal

   b. Anticoagulant

   c. Antibiotic

   d. Antidiarrheal

5. Ibuprofen may be given to patients in all of the following disorders or conditions, except:

   a. Dysmenorrhea

   b. Fever

   c. Peptic ulcer

   d. Rheumatoid arthritis

Selective COX-2 Inhibitors

NSAIDs play a major role in the management of inflammation and pain caused by arthritis. A new class of NSAIDs that selectively inhibits the **cyclooxygenase**-2 (COX-2) enzyme has been developed. Cyclooxygenase (COX) is the name for a group of enzymes required to produce prostaglandins from arachidonic acid. Two subtypes of cyclooxygenase have been identified: COX-1 and COX-2. COX-1 is available in all cells, especially in the platelets, GI tract, and kidneys, and helps maintain homeostasis in these cells. COX-2, on the other hand, appears to be made in macrophages in response to damage to local tissues. One of the first COX-2 inhibitors, celecoxib (Celebrex), is said to provide therapeutic benefit with less toxicity than traditional NSAIDs. Another COX-2 selective inhibitor, meloxicam (Mobic), has recently been introduced. COX-2 inhibitors and traditional NSAIDs do not appear to differ significantly in their effectiveness in alleviating pain or inflammation. They have similar GI side effects. However, short-term studies show fewer GI ulcers in patients treated with COX-2 inhibitors compared with traditional NSAIDs. On the other hand, at least one COX-2 inhibitor, rofecoxib (Vioxx), was voluntarily removed from the market by its manufacturer because of safety concerns: There was an increased risk of cardiovascular events (including heart attack and stroke).

How do they work?

The COX-2 inhibitors affect the synthesis of prostaglandins by selectively targeting only the COX-2 enzymes. These agents have similar anti-inflammatory activity without the adverse GI effects associated with COX-1 inhibition. COX-2 inhibitors exert anti-inflammatory and analgesic effects through the inhibition of prostaglandin synthesis, by blocking COX activity. The isoenzyme COX-2 is primarily associated with inflammation. Cytokines increase the expression of COX-2, mainly at inflammatory sites, producing prostaglandins that mediate inflammation, pain, and fever.

How are they used?

The FDA has labeled celecoxib (Celebrex) for the treatment of osteoarthritis and rheumatoid arthritis in adults. This agent is recommended in the lowest effective dosage for the shortest duration possible. Meloxicam (Mobic), the newest COX-2 inhibitor, has been labeled by the FDA for the treatment of osteoarthritis (see Table 12-1 ■).

What are the adverse effects?

Like traditional NSAIDs, the COX-2 inhibitors commonly cause abdominal pain, dyspepsia, and diarrhea. There is an increased risk of serious cardiovascular thrombotic events, even myocardial infarction and stroke, which can be fatal. This risk may increase with longer duration of use.

What are the contraindications and interactions?

Treatment with COX-2 inhibitors is contraindicated in patients who have hypersensitivity to these drugs, asthma, urticaria, or previous anaphylactic reactions after taking aspirin or NSAIDs. Because of potential aggravation of hypertension and lower extremity edema, caution should be exercised in prescribing COX-2 inhibitors to patients with congestive heart failure, fluid retention, or hypertension. COX-2 inhibitors are contraindicated in elderly patients, patients younger than 18 years, and in pregnant (third trimester) or lactating women. These agents should be avoided in patients with severe hepatic impairment or advanced renal disease. COX-2 inhibitors may diminish effectiveness of ACE inhibitors. Fluconazole (Diflucan), an antifungal, can increase celecoxib concentrations. COX-2 inhibitors may increase lithium (Eskalith) concentrations.

What are the important points patients should know?

Advise patients to tell their physician immediately if they experience unexplained weight gain, skin rash, nausea, fatigue, lethargy, jaundice, flu-like symptoms, black tarry stool, or upper GI distress; and to avoid alcohol, tobacco, and aspirin or other NSAIDs when taking meloxicam. Instruct women to avoid celecoxib during the third trimester of pregnancy. Neither celecoxib nor meloxicam should be used by women who are breastfeeding.

Table 12-1 ■ Selective COX-2 Inhibitors

GENERIC NAME	TRADE NAME	AVERAGE DOSAGE FOR ADULTS	ROUTE OF ADMINISTRATION
celecoxib	Celebrex	100–200 mg bid	PO
meloxicam	Movera	7.5 mg/d	PO

ACETAMINOPHEN

The analgesic efficacy of acetaminophen (Tylenol) is essentially equivalent to that of NSAIDs, but acetaminophen is not anti-inflammatory. Like aspirin, acetaminophen has analgesic and antipyretic actions.

How does it work?

The mechanism of action of acetaminophen is unknown. As with most nonopioid analgesics, the mechanism of action is thought to be inhibition of prostaglandin in the peripheral nervous system (PNS), making the sensory neurons less likely to receive pain signals. Acetaminophen blocks the peripheral pain impulses to a lesser degree than other NSAIDs. It lacks the anti-inflammatory action of the salicylates; hence, it is of only limited usefulness in inflammatory rheumatic disorders and is often not considered to be an NSAID agent.

How is it used?

Acetaminophen is effective in the treatment of a wide variety of arthritic and rheumatic conditions involving musculoskeletal pain as well as headache, dysmenorrhea, myalgias, and neuralgias. This agent also is useful in diseases accompanied by fever, discomfort, and pain, such as the common cold and other viral infections. Acetaminophen is particularly useful as an analgesic-antipyretic in patients who experience adverse reactions to aspirin.

What are the adverse effects?

The adverse effects of acetaminophen are rare in therapeutic doses, and the drug is usually well tolerated by aspirin-sensitive patients. Sensitivity reactions may occur—in this case, the drug should be stopped. Over long-term use, adverse effects include skin eruptions and urticaria, hypotension, and hepatotoxicity. Acetaminophen frequently is combined with other drugs, such as caffeine, aspirin, and opiates such as codeine and oxycodone. An overdose can cause hepatotoxicity, coma, and internal bleeding. If overdose occurs, the antidote for acetaminophen is acetylcysteine (Mucomyst).

What are the contraindications and interactions?

Acetaminophen is contraindicated in patients with a history of hypersensitivity to this drug. It must be used cautiously in children younger than age 3, unless directed by a physician. Repeated administration to patients with anemia or hepatic disease, or to children younger than 12 years who are affected by rheumatoid conditions, should be avoided. Acetaminophen should be avoided in patients with alcoholism, malnutrition, or thrombocytopenia (a platelet deficiency often caused by anticancer drugs). Safety during pregnancy or lactation is not established.

What are the important points patients should know?

Acetaminophen may cause acute liver damage or failure in patients who consume 3 or more alcoholic drinks per day, but a person does not have to be a chronic drinker to suffer damage. Taking acetaminophen after a weekend of drinking can prove fatal. Advise patients to avoid this combination of drugs if possible. The use of acetaminophen with barbiturates (Nembutal, Seconal), carbamazepine (Tegretol), phenytoin (Dilantin), and rifampin (Rifadin, Rimactane) may increase potential hepatotoxicity. With other drugs, such as cholestyramine (Questran), the absorption of acetaminophen is decreased.

Focus Point

Differences Among OTC Analgesics

Over-the-counter (OTC) analgesics include salicylates, acetaminophen, and NSAIDs. All are antipyretics, but acetaminophen does not have an anti-inflammatory effect. Salicylates are also used to prolong clotting time by preventing platelets from binding together.

✷ Apply Your Knowledge 12.2

The following questions focus on what you have just learned about selective COX-2 inhibitors and acetaminophen. *See Appendix E for the correct answers.*

MULTIPLE CHOICE
Select the correct answers from choices a–d.

1. The isoenzyme COX-2 is primarily associated with which of the following?
   a. Inflammation
   b. Hypertension
   c. Heart attack
   d. Hypercalcemia

2. Acetaminophen lacks which of the following actions?
   a. Analgesic
   b. Antipyretic
   c. Anti-inflammatory
   d. All of the above

3. Like traditional NSAIDs, the COX-2 inhibitors cause all of the following adverse effects, except:
   a. Diarrhea
   b. Dyspepsia
   c. Osteoarthritis
   d. Abdominal pain

4. The adverse effects of acetaminophen are:
   a. Rare
   b. Severe coughing
   c. Headache
   d. GI bleeding

5. The FDA has labeled celecoxib for the treatment of which of the following?
   a. Migraine
   b. Tension headache
   c. Abdominal pain
   d. Rheumatoid arthritis

MATCHING

Match the letter trade name to the numbered generic drug name.

GENERIC NAME	TRADE NAME
1. _____ acetaminophen	a. Celebrex
2. _____ meloxicam	b. Talwin
3. _____ celecoxib	c. Revex
4. _____ pentazocine/naloxone	d. Tylenol
5. _____ nalmefene HCl	e. Movera

Opiates

The analgesic properties of opium and its derivatives have been known for centuries. **Opiates** are drugs derived from opium poppies and include, for example, morphine and codeine. **Opioid** is a general term referring to natural, synthetic, or **endogenous** (related to internal structures of function) morphine-related substances. Narcotics are drugs of certain legal status and in general are considered Schedule II drugs. They are controlled substances (see Chapter 2) and are used to treat moderate to severe pain. Narcotics obtained from the raw opium plant include opium, morphine, and codeine.

Raw opium consists of the air-dried milky exudates obtained by incision of unripe capsules of *Papaver somniferum*, which contains approximately 9.5% morphine. Opium, as a medicinal drug, has been known for many centuries.

The principal opium-exporting countries traditionally have been Iran, Turkey, India, and Yugoslavi. Drugs derived from opium, called *opiates*, owe their activity to the opioid alkaloids. Opium's chief pharmacologic effects are due to its morphine content, and the presence of other alkaloids in amounts insufficient to significantly modify the morphine type of action. Thus, opium has many of the same uses as morphine, but morphine nearly always is preferred. Opiates have analgesic and other opioid effects.

MORPHINE

Morphine (Astramorph PF, Duramorph) can be treated chemically to produce semisynthetic narcotics, such as hydromorphone, oxycodone, oxymorphone, and heroin. These are classified as Schedule II drugs, except for heroin, a Schedule I drug, (see Chapter 2) which is an illegal **narcotic** (a medication that induces sleep or stupor and alters mood and behavior) in the United States and is not used in medicine. The properties and actions of synthetic opioids are similar to those of the natural opiates. Synthetic narcotic analgesics include meperidine (Demerol), methadone (Dolophine), remifentanil (Ultiva), and levorphanol (Levo-Dromoran). Natural, synthetic, and semisynthetic narcotics are listed in Table 12-2 ■.

How does it work?

Morphine produces its effects by binding to the opioid receptors. Opioid receptors are located presynaptically and postsynaptically along the pain transmission pathways. High densities of receptors are found in the dorsal horn of the spinal cord and higher CNS. Opioid receptors in the brainstem are responsible for the respiratory depressant effects produced by opioid analgesics. Opioid receptors in the higher CNS probably account for the effect of opioid analgesics on pain perception.

There are three major types of opioid receptors: the *mu, kappa,* and *delta* receptors. Most of the currently used opioid analgesics act primarily at mu receptors; some have varying degrees of activity at the other types of receptors.

How is it used?

Morphine is used in the management of almost all types of moderate to severe pain. Derivatives of morphine are also prescribed for cough inhibition, treatment of GI pain, and for relieving pain associated with myocardial infarction.

What are the adverse effects?

Morphine causes nausea, vomiting, constipation, dry mouth, biliary tract spasms, dizziness, sedation, and pruritus. The major adverse effect of opioid analgesics such as morphine is respiratory depression. Physical and psychological dependence can occur with opioid analgesics. For this reason, health-care providers often hesitate to administer the proper doses, fearing that the patient will become dependent or respiratory depression will occur. When used as directed, these drugs are safe and do not cause dependent or adverse effects. Patients should always be properly medicated for pain alleviation.

What are the contraindications and interactions?

Opioid analgesics are contraindicated in patients with known hypersensitivity. They are also contraindicated in patients who have asthma, emphysema, or head injury. Opioid analgesics must be avoided in patients with increased intracranial pressure, severe liver or kidney dysfunction, acute ulcerative colitis, or convulsive disorders. Opioid analgesics must be used cautiously in patients with prostatic hypertrophy because urine retention can occur.

Opioids or opiates can interact with alcohol, causing CNS depression with subsequent respiratory depression. Meperidine (Demerol) undergoes a potentially fatal reaction with monoamine oxidase (MAO) inhibitors (antidepressants). Morphine (Astramorph PF, Duramorph) and meperidine should not be mixed because they potentiate each other and are physically incompatible.

What are the important points patients should know?

Inform patients that the most serious adverse effect of narcotic analgesics is respiratory depression. Narcotic analgesics should not be taken if respirations are less than 12 per minute or systolic blood pressure is less than 110 mm Hg in adults. Narcotic analgesics may cause constipation, so advise patients to request symptomatic relief from their health-care provider.

Table 12-2 ■ Classifications of Opioid Analgesics

GENERIC NAME	TRADE NAME	ADULT COMMON DOSAGE RANGE	ROUTE OF ADMINISTRATION
Natural Opioid Analgesics			
codeine	Codeine	15–60 mg analgesic	PO, IM, subcutaneously
morphine	Duramorph, Avinza	10–30 mg q4h PRN or 15–30 mg sustained release of 8–12 h	PO
		2.5–15 mg q4h or 0.8–10 mg/h by continuous infusion	IV
		5–20 mg q4h	IM or subcutaneously
		10–20 mg q4h PRN	By rectum
opium tincture	Laudanum	0.6–1 mL qid (max: 6 mL/d)	PO

Table 12-2 ■ Classifications of Opioid Analgesics

GENERIC NAME	TRADE NAME	ADULT COMMON DOSAGE RANGE	ROUTE OF ADMINISTRATION
Semisynthetic Opioid Analgesics			
hydrocodone	Hycodan, Robindone_A	5–10 mg q4–6h PRN (max: 15 mg/dose)	PO
hydrocodone with acetaminophen	Lortab, Vicodin	500–1000 mg q4–6h PRN	PO
levorphanol	Levo-Dromoran	2–3 mg q6–8h PRN	PO
		1–2 mg q6–8h PRN	Subcutaneously, IM
		Up to 1 mg q3–6h PRN	IV
oxycodone	OxyContin, Percolone	5–10 mg q6h PRN (OxyContin can be dosed q8h)	PO
oxycodone acetaminophen	Endocet, Percocet	Comb. drug: 325–650 mg q4–6h PRN	PO
oxycodone–aspirin	Endodan, Percodan	Comb. drug: 325–650 mg q6h PRN	PO
Synthetic Opioid Antagonists			
naloxone	Narcan	0.1–2 mg q2–3 min up to 3 doses if necessary	IV
naltrexone	Trexan, ReVia	25 mg followed by another 25 mg in 1 h if no withdrawal response (max: 800 mg/d)	PO
Synthetic Opioid Agonist/Antagonists _—Antidote for codine_			
buprenorphine	Buprenex, Subutex	0.3 q6h up to 0.6 mg q4h or 25–50 mcg/h by IV infusion	IV, IM
butorphanol	Stadol, Stadol NS	1–4 mg q3–4h PRN (max: 4 mg/dose)	IM
		0.5–2 mg q3–4h PRN	IV
fentanyl	Duragesic, Sublimaze	50–100 mcg q1–2h PRN	IV
		25 mcg/h patch q3d	Transdermal
meperidine	Demerol	50–150 mg q3–4h PRN	PO, subcutaneously, IM, IV
methadone	Dolophine, Methadone	2.5–20 mg q3–8h PRN	PO, subcutaneously, IM
pentazocine	Talwin, Talwin NX	50–100 mg q3–4h (max: 600 mg/d)	PO
		30 mg q3–4h (max: 360 mg/d)	IM, IV, subcutaneously

Focus Point

Age Differences in Narcotic Metabolism

The metabolism of narcotics is slower in elderly patients. Therefore, opioid use may have undesirable effects, such as confusion and respiratory depression. In pediatric patients, dosing is difficult because elimination occurs at a different rate. Premature infants with chronic lung disease often have depressed hypoxic drive and require careful monitoring after administration of opioids.

CODEINE

Although some codeine is obtained from opium directly, the quantity is not sufficient to meet the extensive use of this alkaloid as a valuable medicinal agent. Much more codeine is used than morphine. This need is met by producing it via partial synthesis from morphine. Codeine does not produce proportionately greater analgesia as the dose is increased.

How does it work?

Codeine, like morphine and all other opiates, binds to opioid receptors in the brain and spinal cord, thereby relieving pain.

How is it used?

Codeine is useful for inducing sleep in the presence of mild pain. This drug, like morphine, is employed as an analgesic, sedative, hypnotic, antiperistaltic, and antitussive agent. It commonly is given in combination with aspirin, acetaminophen, or other agents. Administered alone, codeine is a Schedule II drug. In combination with aspirin-like drugs, it is classified as Schedule III (see Chapter 2).

What are the adverse effects?

Codeine is less apt than morphine to cause nausea, vomiting, constipation, and miosis (contraction of the pupils). Tolerance, dependence, and addiction can occur. Codeine, like morphine, produces cortical and respiratory depression, but serious degrees of either are practically unknown. Patients may also have postural hypotension.

What are the contraindications and interactions?

Codeine is contraindicated in advanced respiratory insufficiency, bronchial asthma, and in patients with raised intracranial pressure. Its effects are increased by use with other drugs that have centrally suppressing effects, including alcohol, or with cimetidine (Tagamet). Antidepressive agents and neuroleptics can completely halt the analgesic effects of codeine.

What are the important points patients should know?

Instruct patients to comply with the physician-ordered drug regimen because overuse may lead to dependence and to avoid alcohol and other CNS depressants. Advise patients to report urine retention or severe constipation and to rise slowly from a lying position to prevent postural hypotension.

✳ Apply Your Knowledge 12.3

The following questions focus on what you have just learned about opioid analgesics. *See Appendix E for the correct answers.*

MULTIPLE CHOICE

Select the correct answer from choices a–d.

1. Semisynthetic narcotics include which of the following?

   a. Meperidine

   b. Oxycodone

   c. Methadone

   d. Levorphanol

2. The adverse effects of morphine include all of the following except:

   a. Dry mouth

   b. Constipation

   c. Hypertension

   d. Biliary tract spasms

3. Opioids or opiates can interact with alcohol and cause:

   a. CNS stimulation

   b. Hypertensive crisis

   c. Increased appetite

   d. Respiratory depression

4. Hydrocodone is classified as:

   a. Schedule II

   b. Schedule IV

   c. Schedule I

   d. Schedule III

5. Oxycodone is classified as which of the following schedules?

   a. I

   b. II

   c. III

   d. IV

FILL IN THE BLANK

Select terms from your reading to fill in the blanks.

1. Opioids may be natural, synthetic, or _____ morphine-related substances.

2. The unripe capsules of *Papaver somniferum* contain approximately 9.5% _____.

3. Opium owes its activity to the _____.

4. Of these semisynthetic narcotics, hydromorphone, heroin, oxymorphone, and oxycodone, only _____ is an illegal narcotic in the United States and is not used in medicine.

5. The three major types of opioid receptors are called the _____, _____, and _____ receptors.

Semisynthetic Opioid Analgesics

Semisynthetic opioid analgesics are modifications of the natural alkaloids of opium. These agents have the same advantages of morphine or codeine, without their disadvantages. Examples of semisynthetic opioids include hydrocodone, oxycodone, and oxymorphone (see Table 12-2).

HYDROCODONE

Hydrocodone (Hycodan) is a morphine derivative similar to codeine, but more addicting, and with slightly greater antitussive activity and analgesic effects. This CNS depressant relieves moderate to severe pain. Hydrocodone is a Schedule III. Hydrocodone is combined with other drugs, such as aspirin-like analgesics, antihistamines, expectorants, and sympathomimetics (drugs that increase cardiac output, dilate bronchioles, and constrict blood vessels).

How does it work?

Hydrocodone suppresses the cough reflex by direct action on the cough center in the medulla of the brain. It also acts as a CNS depressant, which relieves moderate to severe pain.

How is it used?

Hydrocodone is used for relief of nonproductive cough and for moderate to severe pain.

What are the adverse effects?

The most common adverse effects include dry mouth, nausea, vomiting, constipation, sedation, dizziness, and drowsiness. Other adverse effects are euphoria, dysphoria, respiratory depression, pruritus, and skin rashes.

What are the contraindications and interactions?

Hydrocodone is contraindicated in patients with a history of hypersensitivity to this drug or in women who are lactating. It should be used cautiously in patients with asthma, emphysema, history of drug abuse, and respiratory depression. This drug can be prescribed with caution in children younger than 1 year and in pregnant women. Hydrocodone with alcohol and other CNS depressant compounds may interact and cause severe CNS depression.

What are the important points patients should know?

Instruct patients taking hydrocodone to avoid hazardous activities until response to the drug is determined. Advise patients to drink plenty of liquids to ensure adequate hydration. Because the abuse potential of hydrocodone is high, advise patients to take only the dose prescribed. Patients should never breast feed while taking this drug.

OXYCODONE

Although oxycodone (OxyContin) has less analgesic capability than morphine, it possesses comparable addiction potential and is a Schedule II drug. It frequently is used in combination with aspirin or acetaminophen.

How does it work?

The most prominent actions of oxycodone affect the CNS and organs composed of smooth muscle. Oxycodone binds with specific receptors in various sites of the CNS to alter both perception of pain and emotional response to pain, but its precise mechanism of action is not clear. Oxycodone is as potent as morphine and 10 to 12 times more potent than codeine.

How is it used?

This agent is used for relief of moderate to severe pain, such as the type that may occur with bursitis, dislocations, simple fractures, and other injuries. Oxycodone is also indicated to relieve postoperative and postpartum pain.

What are the adverse effects?

The adverse effects of oxycodone include euphoria, dysphoria, light-headedness, dizziness, sedation, anorexia, nausea, vomiting, constipation, jaundice, hepatotoxicity, and respiratory depression.

What are the contraindications and interactions?

Oxycodone is contraindicated in patients with hypersensitivity to this drug and during pregnancy or lactation. It is also contraindicated in children younger than 6 years of age. It must be used cautiously in people with alcoholism, renal or hepatic disease, and viral infections. Oxycodone is also prescribed with caution in patients with chronic ulcerative colitis, gallbladder disease, head injury, acute abdominal conditions, hypothyroidism, prostatic hypertrophy, and respiratory disease.

What are the important points patients should know?

Instruct patients to take oxycodone in the form prescribed without crushing, chewing, or breaking the medication—it is formulated to be released into the blood slowly. Advise patients to avoid driving, operating heavy machinery, or performing other hazardous activities because oxycodone causes drowsiness or dizziness. Alcohol must also be avoided. This drug may increase the effects of antidepressants, antihistamines, pain relievers, anxiety medications, seizure medications, and muscle relaxants. Instruct patients to take only the dose that was prescribed—taking too much of this drug could result in serious adverse effects and even death.

Synthetic Opioid Antagonists

The term *antagonist*, as used in this section, applies to naloxone and naltrexone, which are antagonists with little or no agonist actions. These competitive opioid antagonists are effective in the management of severe respiratory depression induced by opioid drugs, and of asphyxia neonatorum (respiratory distress in the newborn) caused by administration of these drugs to the expectant mother, and for the diagnosis or treatment of opioid addiction.

NALOXONE

Naloxone (Narcan) is a synthetic opioid antagonist essentially devoid of opioid-agonist properties. Hence, it does not possess morphine-like properties, such as respiratory depression, psychotomimetic effects, and pupillary constriction, which are characteristic of other opioid antagonists.

How does it work?
Available evidence suggests that naloxone antagonizes these opioid effects by competing for the same receptor sites.

How is it used?
Naloxone is prescribed for narcotic overdose and complete or partial reversal of narcotic depression, including respiratory depression induced by natural and synthetic narcotics. Naloxone is a drug of choice when the nature of a depressant drug is not known and for the diagnosis of suspected acute opioid overdose.

What are the adverse effects?
Naloxone may cause reversal of analgesia, tremors, slight drowsiness, hyperventilation, sweating, nausea, vomiting, hypertension, and tachycardia.

What are the contraindications and interactions?
Naloxone is contraindicated in patients who suffer from respiratory depression due to nonopioid drugs. Safety during pregnancy or lactation is not established. Naloxone must be used cautiously in neonates and children. It must be avoided in patients who are suspected to be dependent on narcotics and for those with cardiac irritability.

What are the important points patients should know?
Naloxone reverses the analgesic effects of narcotic agents and may cause withdrawal symptoms, or the patient may experience a return of the pain that the narcotic agents were originally prescribed to treat. Instruct patients to tell their physician about postoperative pain that emerges after naloxone is administered.

NALTREXONE

Naltrexone (Trexan, ReVia) generally has little or no agonist activity. Its opioid antagonist activity is reported to be 2 to 9 times that of naloxone.

How does it work?
The mechanism of action of naltrexone is not clearly known, but it appears that its competitive binding at opioid receptor sites reduces euphoria.

How is it used?
Naltrexone is used as an adjunct to the maintenance of an opioid-free state in detoxified addicts who are and desire to remain narcotic free. It is also used in the management of alcohol dependence as an adjunct to social and psychotherapeutic methods.

What are the adverse effects?

Naltrexone causes dry mouth, anorexia, nausea, vomiting, constipation, abdominal cramps, and hepatotoxicity. This agent may also cause muscle and joint pains, headache, nervousness, irritability, dizziness, and depression.

What are the contraindications and interactions?

Naltrexone is contraindicated in patients receiving opioid analgesics or in acute opioid withdrawal and opioid-dependent patients. It must be avoided in patients with acute hepatitis and liver failure. Naltrexone is also contraindicated in any individual who has a positive urine screen for opioids. Safety during pregnancy, lactation, or in children younger than age 18 is not established.

Phenothiazines (antipsychotics such as Thorazine and Mellaril) may interact with administration of naltrexone and cause increased somnolence and lethargy. Naltrexone reverses the analgesic effects of narcotic agonists and narcotic agonist–antagonists.

What are the important points patients should know?

Naltrexone may put patients in danger of fatally overdosing if they are using opiates. Advise patients to check with their physicians before taking OTC drugs with naltrexone because opioids are present in many OTC preparations, including cough medicines. Instruct patients to tell their physician or dentist that they are taking naltrexone before undergoing treatment and to wear medical alert jewelry indicating naltrexone use. Warn female patients to avoid breastfeeding while using naltrexone without first consulting their physicians. Patients taking methadone (Dolophine) for treatment of opioid dependency or addiction may be able to transfer from methadone to naltrexone after gradual withdrawal and final discontinuation of methadone.

✳ Apply Your Knowledge 12.4

The following questions focus on what you have just learned about synthetic and semisynthetic opioid antagonists. *See Appendix E for the correct answer.*

MATCHING
Match the lettered drug to its numbered description.

DESCRIPTION

1. _____ Drug of choice to treat overdose when the nature of a depressant drug is not known

2. _____ Used for relief of nonproductive cough

3. _____ Possesses no morphine-like properties such as pupillary constriction or respiratory depression

4. _____ Indicated to relieve postoperative and postpartum pain

DRUG

a. Oxycodone
b. Naltrexone
c. Naloxone
d. Hydrocodone

FILL IN THE BLANK
Select terms from your reading to fill in the blanks.

1. The safety of naloxone during pregnancy or lactation is _____.

2. Naloxone is ordered for _____.

3. _____ is contraindicated in patients receiving opioid analgesics or in acute opioid withdrawal.

4. Phenothiazines may interact with naltrexone and cause increased _____ and _____.

5. Naloxone and naltrexone are _____.

Synthetic Opioid Analgesics

Synthetic opioid analgesics have the properties of morphine as analgesics but have fewer undesirable effects and less addiction potential. Currently available synthetic agents have valuable analgesic and pharmacologic properties that are described in this section.

BUPRENORPHINE

Buprenorphine (Buprenex) is a centrally acting synthetic and narcotic analgesic. This opiate agonist–antagonist has agonist activity approximately 30 times that of morphine and antagonist activity equal to or up to 3 times greater than that of naloxone.

How does it work?

Dose-related analgesia results from a high affinity of buprenorphine for mu-opioid receptors and an antagonist at the kappa-opiate receptors in the CNS.

How is it used?

Buprenorphine is used principally for moderate to severe postoperative pain. It is also administered for pain associated with cancer, accidental trauma, urethral calculi, and myocardial infarction.

What are the adverse effects?

Buprenorphine may cause sedation, drowsiness, vertigo, dizziness, headache, amnesia, euphoria, and insomnia. This agent can also cause hypotension, miosis, nausea, vomiting, diarrhea, and constipation.

What are the contraindications and interactions?

Buprenorphine is contraindicated in known hypersensitivity to this agent or to naloxone. Safety during pregnancy, lactation, or in children younger than 13 years is not established. Buprenorphine may interact with alcohol and cause CNS depression. Diazepam (Valium) may cause respiratory or cardiovascular collapse.

What are the important points patients should know?

Instruct patients to avoid driving or engaging in hazardous activities until response to this drug is known and to avoid alcohol or other CNS depressants. Advise female patients to avoid breastfeeding while using this drug without consulting their physician.

FENTANYL

Fentanyl (Duragesic, Sublimaze) is a potent and synthetic narcotic agonist analgesic agent with pharmacologic actions similar to those of morphine and meperidine.

How does it work?

The principal mechanism of action of fentanyl is analgesia and sedation, but its action is more prompt and less prolonged than that of morphine or meperidine.

How is it used?

Fentanyl is a short-acting analgesic drug used during operative and perioperative periods. This agent is prescribed as a narcotic analgesic supplement in general and regional anesthesia with diazepam (Valium) or droperidol (Inapsine) to produce neuroleptanalgesia (a form of analgesia accompanied by general quieting of the patient and indifference to environmental stimuli, without loss of consciousness). Fentanyl is also given with oxygen and a skeletal muscle relaxant to select, high-risk patients, such as those undergoing open heart surgery.

What are the adverse effects?

The adverse effects of fentanyl include sedation, euphoria, dizziness, delirium (excitement and mental confusion with hallucinations), and convulsions with high doses.

This agent may also cause hypotension, bradycardia, cardiac arrest, and respiratory arrest. In some patients, blurred vision and miosis are reported. Other common adverse effects of fentanyl include nausea, vomiting, and constipation.

What are the contraindications and interactions?
Fentanyl is contraindicated in the management of acute or postoperative pain and in mild or intermittent pain that can be otherwise managed by less potent agents. It is also contraindicated at high doses at the initiation of opioid therapy and in patients with hypersensitivity to this agent. This agent may interact with alcohol and other CNS depressants, increasing their effects. Fentanyl may also interact with MAO inhibitors to cause hypertensive crisis.

What are the important points patients should know?
Instruct patients to report muscle rigidity or weakness; unusual postoperative muscle movement of the extremities, eyes, or neck; and any problems breathing after taking this drug.

MEPERIDINE
Meperidine (Demerol) is a synthetic opioid analgesic with multiple actions qualitatively similar to those of morphine.

How does it work?
The most prominent of drug actions are on the CNS and on organs composed of smooth muscle. It acts principally to induce analgesia and sedation.

How is it used?
Meperidine is indicated for preoperative use, relief of moderate to severe pain, supportive anesthesia, and obstetric analgesia.

What are the adverse effects?
Major adverse effects include respiratory depression or arrest, circulatory depression, shock, and cardiac arrest. The most common untoward effects include dizziness, sedation, nausea, vomiting, and sweating. Other adverse effects include euphoria, headache, weakness, agitation, tremor, seizures, disorientation, and hallucinations.

What are the contraindications and interactions?
Meperidine is contraindicated in patients taking MAO inhibitors; it inconsistently has precipitated severe and occasionally fatal reactions within 14 days. The drug should be used with caution and in reduced dosage in patients taking other opioid analgesics, general anesthetics, phenothiazines, sedatives, tricyclic antidepressants, and other CNS depressants.

What are the important points patients should know?
Advise patients to ambulate carefully and to avoid smoking. Instruct patients to avoid driving or engaging in hazardous activities until drowsiness and dizziness have passed. CNS depressants and alcohol should be avoided. Female patients should not breastfeed while using this drug.

Focus on Geriatrics

Oversedation in Elderly Patients
Sedatives and narcotics must be given with extreme caution to elderly people who may easily become oversedated.

METHADONE

Methadone (Dolophine) is a synthetic opioid analgesic with multiple actions quantitatively similar to morphine.

How does it work?

Methadone binds with opiate receptors in the CNS, altering both perception of and emotional response to pain.

How is it used?

Methadone is indicated for the relief of moderate to severe chronic pain. It is also used for detoxification of opioid addiction and for temporary or sometimes long-term maintenance treatment of opioid addiction.

What are the adverse effects?

The adverse effects of methadone are similar to those for other opioid analgesics, especially meperidine (Demerol).

What are the contraindications and interactions?

Methadone is contraindicated in patients with known hypersensitivity. The drug should be used with caution, and in reduced dosage in patients taking other opioid analgesics, general anesthetics, phenothiazines and other tranquilizers, sedative-hypnotics, tricyclic antidepressants, MAO inhibitors, and other CNS depressants. The safe use of methadone in pregnancy has not been established. It is not recommended for obstetric analgesia because its long duration may induce respiratory depression in the newborn.

What are the important points patients should know?

Instruct patients to make position changes slowly, especially from supine to upright position, and to sit or lie down if they feel dizzy or faint. Advise patients to avoid driving or engaging in potentially hazardous activities until response to this drug is known. Female patients should not breastfeed while taking this drug without consulting their physician.

PENTAZOCINE

Pentazocine (Talwin) is a synthetic narcotic agonist–antagonist analgesic that is classified as a controlled substance (Schedule IV).

How does it work?

Pentazocine has a similar mechanism of action to that of morphine, but with only one third the strength. Large doses of pentazocine may increase blood pressure and heart rate. When given in usual parenteral doses, it is as effective in relieving moderate to severe pain as the usual parenteral doses of morphine, meperidine, butorphanol, or nalbuphine.

How is it used?

Pentazocine is indicated for the control of moderate to severe pain. It is also used for preoperative analgesia or sedation and as a supplement to surgical anesthesia.

What are the adverse effects?

Pentazocine causes nausea, vomiting, diarrhea, constipation, dry mouth, and alterations of taste. This agent may also cause dizziness, light-headedness, sedation, euphoria, headache, disturbed dreams, insomnia, syncope (fainting), and visual blurring. Hypotension, tachycardia, and respiratory depression have also been included among its adverse effects.

What are the contraindications and interactions?

Pentazocine is contraindicated in patients with a history of hypersensitivity. This agent must be avoided in patients with head injuries or increased intracranial pressure, in emotionally unstable patients, or in those with a history of drug abuse. Safety during pregnancy or lactation or in children younger than age 12 is not established. Pentazocine must be used cautiously in patients with impaired kidney or liver function, respiratory depression, biliary surgery, and myocardial infarction with nausea and vomiting. Alcohol and other CNS depressants add to CNS depression with the use of pentazocine.

What are the important points patients should know?

Instruct patients to avoid driving and other hazardous activities until response to this drug is known. Pentazocine should not be discontinued abruptly after extended use, and female patients should not breastfeed while taking this drug.

✳ Apply Your Knowledge 12.5

The following questions focus on what you have just learned about hydrocodone, oxycodone, and synthetic opioid analgesics. See *Appendix E for the correct answer.*

MATCHING

Match the lettered description to the numbered drug.

DESCRIPTION

1. _____ Often used with aspirin or acetaminophen

2. _____ Often used during open-heart surgery

3. _____ Used for detoxification of opioid addiction

4. _____ Fewer undesirable effects than morphine

5. _____ More addicting than codeine

6. _____ Has caused fatal reactions within 14 days

DRUG

a. Hydrocodone

b. Oxycodone

c. Synthetic opioid analgesics

d. Fentanyl

e. Meperidine

f. Methadone

FILL IN THE BLANK

Select terms from your reading to fill in the blanks.

1. The principal mechanisms of action for fentanyl are _____ and _____, but its action is more prompt and less prolonged than morphine.

2. Pentazocine is contraindicated in patients with _____, _____, or a history of _____.

3. Buprenorphine is an opiate agonist–antagonist with agonist activity about _____ times that of morphine and antagonist activity equal to _____ times greater than that of naloxone.

4. Methadone is a _____ opioid analgesic with multiple actions similar to morphine.

5. The adverse effects of buprenorphine on the CNS include _____, _____, _____, _____, _____, _____, _____, and _____.

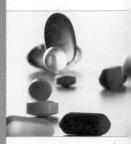

Chapter Capsule

This section repeats the objectives from the beginning of the chapter and then provides a summary of the most important concepts for that objective. Use this section as a quick review and to check your knowledge.

Objective 1: List the antipyretic properties of anti-inflammatory and analgesic drugs.

- Inhibition of prostaglandin synthesis in the CNS
- Central action in the hypothalamic heat-regulating center

Objective 2: Describe the role of prostaglandins in inflammation.

- Postglandins—hormone-like substances that modulate inflammation. Initiate an action potential along a sensory nerve fiber or sensitize pain receptors

Objective 3: Outline the dangers of aspirin use.

- Possible massive GI hemorrhage, dyspepsia, nausea and vomiting, occult bleeding

Objective 4: List the uses and side effects of anti-inflammatory drugs.

- Used for rheumatoid arthritis, osteoarthritis, arthritis, moderate pain, and fever
- Side effects—dizziness, nervousness, occult blood loss, peptic ulceration, GI bleeding, and others

Objective 5: Identify the different types of analgesics.

- Nonopioid analgesics
- Opioid analgesics

Objective 6: Describe the function of naturally occurring opioids and their receptors.

- Naturally occurring opioids bind to opioid receptors to block pain transmission

Objective 7: Explain the rationale behind the use of narcotic analgesics.

- Effective for almost all types of moderate and severe pain and for cough inhibition
- Mimic endogenous opioids to block pain transmission

Objective 8: Describe the problems associated with the use of narcotic analgesics.

- Can cause respiratory depression
- Can produce physical and psychological dependence

Internet Sites of Interest

- The International Association for the Study of Pain (IASP) offers a discussion about tolerance to opioids at: **www.iasp-pain.org/PCUO1-5.html**
- *Pain Management: The Online Series* is a continuing education program on pain offered by the American Medical Association at: **www.ama-cmeonline.com**

■ The National Institutes of Health (NIH) offer information on drugs and other medical conditions at its MedLine Web site at: **www.nlm.nih.gov/medlineplus**. Search for NSAIDs.

■ An explanation of antipyretics can be found on Wikipedia at: **http://en.wikipedia.org/wiki/Antipyretic**. However, always be aware that Wikipedia sites are written by numerous people, not all of whom may be experts in the topic. Therefore, double-check information you find there with other reputable sources.

■ The World Health Organization (WHO) has developed a widely recognized protocol for use of pain medications, called the WHO Pain Ladder. An example can be found at: **http://www.who.int/cancer/palliative/painladder/en/**

Chapter Objectives

After completing this chapter, you should be able to:

1. List the seven warning signs of cancer.

2. Summarize the basic cell cycle and its importance in the use of antineoplastic agents.

3. List commonly used antineoplastic agents in each class.

4. Explain the mechanism of action of each class of antineoplastic agents.

5. Discuss how steroids, estrogens, progestins, antiestrogens, and antiandrogens work in the treatment of cancer.

6. Explain how biologic response modifiers are created and how they work.

7. Describe the advantages of using monoclonal antibodies in the treatment of cancer.

8. Identify common side effects of chemotherapy treatment.

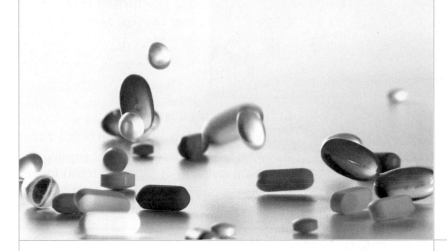

Chapter 13

Antineoplastic Agents

Key Terms

PRACTICAL SCENARIO

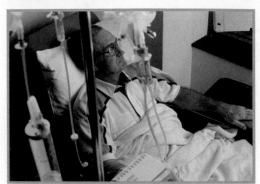

A 68-year-old man has undergone adjuvant chemotherapy for completely resected colon cancer that involved several pericolonic lymph nodes at the time of his surgical resection. After a few days of experiencing diarrhea, he calls his physician. He tells his physician that he has experienced approximately five to six loose, watery stools per day over the past few days. He is mildly light-headed when walking around.

Critical Thinking Questions

1. What is the most likely cause of this patient's ongoing diarrhea?
2. What are the consequences of ongoing diarrhea, and why do you think the physician might instruct this patient to report to the clinic or emergency room immediately?
3. What advice on diet might you offer this patient after he has been seen by his physician?

Introduction

Cancer is the second most common cause of death in the United States after cardiovascular disease, causing more than 500,000 fatalities annually. The most common cancers are breast, prostate, lung, and colorectal. The leading cause of cancer death is lung cancer. Cancer is a group of more than 100 different diseases, characterized by uncontrolled cellular division and **hyperplasia** (abnormal cell growth), local tissue *invasion* (breaking through boundaries that separate cell types within some organs), and **metastasis** (spreading of cancer cells from the primary site to secondary sites). Cancer cells are also referred to as *tumors,* or *neoplasms.* Tumors can be benign or malignant. **Benign** tumors are generally slow growing and resemble normal cells. They are localized and not harmful. **Malignant** tumors often proliferate more rapidly and have an atypical appearance. This atypical appearance is because cancer cells, unlike normal cells, do not continue to mature. Instead, their rapid multiplication causes them to become more and more atypical, a process often called *differentiation.* They invade and destroy surrounding tissues, and they induce the formation of new blood vessels (*angiogenesis)* that act as the tumor's own blood supply to help spread malignant cells to other tissues.

Chemotherapy uses chemical agents to interact with cancer cells to stop or control the growth of the cancer. For example, during World War II, soldiers exposed to nitrogen mustard suffered from low white blood cell (WBC) counts. Today, nitrogen mustard is used to treat patients with lymphoid leukemia and lymphomas. However, because chemotherapeutic drugs cannot distinguish between normal cells and cancer cells, both types of cells are affected by chemotherapy. But the killing effect of chemotherapeutic agents has selectivity for cancer cells over normal host cells, and, thus, normal host cells are able to repair themselves and continue to grow.

Chemotherapy, as used for the treatment of cancer, may be termed *primary, palliative, adjuvant,* or *neoadjuvant* agent. For some cancers, chemotherapy alone can destroy all the cancer cells and cure the cancer, which is *primary* treatment. As an **adjuvant** treatment (one that aids or contributes), chemotherapy is given prior to or after other methods of treatment such as surgery and radiation to reduce the risk of recurrence or to prolong survival. **Palliative** treatment, which eases a disease's effects but does not cure, may be used if a cure is not possible, to minimize the discomfort caused by cancer or to slow the progression of the disease and prolong the patient's life.

Chemotherapy may also be given in the *neoadjuvant,* or preoperative setting. The goal in this setting is to make other treatments more effective by reducing tissue damage, decreasing tumor size, or destroying micrometastases.

Neoplasms

Tumors arise from any of the four basic tissue types: epithelial tissue, connective tissue (blood, bone, and cartilage), muscle tissue, and nerve tissue. Benign tumors are named by adding the suffix *-oma* to the name of the cell type. For example, *adenomas* are benign growths of glandular origin. On the other hand, *carcinomas* are malignant growths arising from epithelial cells. An **adenocarcinoma** is a malignant tumor arising from glandular origin. Malignant growths of muscle or connective tissue are called **sarcomas**. Another term used frequently in the description of malignancy is *carcinoma in situ*. In this instance, the cancer is limited to the epithelial cells where it began. Because cancers are most curable with surgery or radiation before they have metastasized, early detection and treatment is very important. In addition, small tumors are more responsive to chemotherapy than are large tumors. Early diagnosis is difficult for many cancers because they do not produce clinical signs or symptoms until they have become large or have metastasized.

Tumors are constantly shedding neoplastic cells into the systemic circulation or surrounding lymphatic nodules. Cells of benign tumors resemble the cells from which they developed. These masses seldom metastasize, and once removed, they rarely recur. In contrast, malignant tumors invade and destroy the surrounding tissues. Malignant tumors tend to metastasize and, therefore, recurrences are common after removal or destruction of the primary tumor.

ONCOGENES

Recent explorations into the causes of cancer have centered on the role of genes that cause cancer. There are two major classes of genes involved in carcinogenesis: *oncogenes* and *tumor suppressor genes*. **Oncogenes** develop from normal genes, termed *protooncogenes*. Protooncogenes are present in all cells and are essential regulators of normal cellular functions, including the cell cycle. Genetic alteration of the protooncogenes may activate the oncogenes. These genetic alterations may be caused by **carcinogenic** (cancer-causing) agents such as radiation, chemicals, or viruses. **Tumor suppressor genes** are another category of genes involved in carcinogenesis. The normal function of these genes is to regulate and inhibit inappropriate cellular growth and proliferation. Gene loss or mutation can result in loss of control over normal cell growth.

THE CELL CYCLE AND MOLECULAR BIOLOGY

The ability of chemotherapy to kill cancer cells depends on its ability to stop cell division. Usually, cancer drugs work by damaging the ribonucleic acid (RNA) or deoxyribonucleic acid (DNA) that tells the cell how to copy itself for division. If the cancer cells are unable to divide, they die. The faster that cancer cells divide, the more likely it is that chemotherapy will kill the cells, causing the tumor to shrink. Both cancer cells and normal cells reproduce themselves in a series of steps known as the *cell cycle*. There are usually four steps after the resting (G_0) stage, as follows:

G_0: The resting or dormant stage when cells have not started to divide. Cells spend much of their lives in this phase. Depending on their type, different cells can last just a few hours or a few years. When cells receive a signal to reproduce, they move into the G_1 phase (Figure 13-1 ■).

G_1: The first gap phase. The cell starts making proteins to prepare for division. This phase lasts about 18 to 30 hours.

S: DNA synthesis occurs. The chromosomes containing the genetic code are copied so that both of the new cells formed have the right amount of DNA. This phase lasts about 18 to 20 hours.

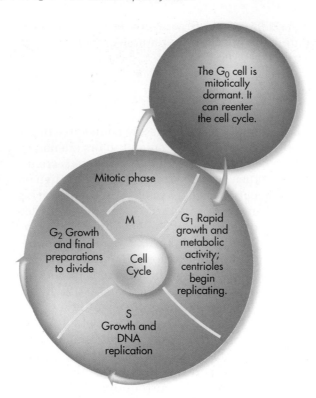

Figure 13-1 ■ The four steps of the cell cycle.

G_2: The second gap phase. This occurs just before the cell starts splitting into two cells. It lasts from 2 to 10 hours.

M: **Mitosis** (when one cell splits into two new cells) occurs. This lasts only 30 to 60 minutes.

Most human cells exist in the G_0 phase, and most cancer cells in the G_0 stage are not sensitive to the effects of chemotherapy. Not all cancer cells proliferate faster than normal cells. Many anticancer drugs target rapidly proliferating cells, and these agents may act at selective or multiple sites of the cell cycle. Agents with major activity in a particular phase of the cell cycle are known as *cell cycle phase–specific agents.* Many antineoplastic agents interfere with the cellular synthesis of DNA, RNA, and proteins. The genetic information is encoded in DNA by precise sequencing of basic structural subunits of DNA, known as **nucleotides**. The goal of chemotherapy is to selectively destroy tumor cells, which can be achieved by targeting specific growth characteristics of most tumors. Agents used in cancer chemotherapy are commonly categorized by their mechanism of action or by their origin.

Focus Point

The Seven Warning Signs of Cancer

1. Change in bowel or bladder habits
2. A sore that does not heal
3. Unusual bleeding or discharge
4. Thickening or lump in breast or elsewhere
5. Indigestion or difficulty swallowing
6. Obvious change in a wart or mole
7. Nagging cough or hoarseness

Focus on Pediatrics

Warning Signs of Cancer in Children

1. Unexplained or persistent lump
2. Unexplained or persistent limping
3. Unexplained normocytic anemia
4. Unexplained thrombocytopenic bruising
5. Unexplained weight loss
6. Abdominal mass
7. Unexplained persistent headache and/or vomiting on awakening

✳ Apply Your Knowledge 13.1

The following questions focus on what you have just learned about various cancer cells and molecular biology. *See Appendix E for the correct answers.*

FILL IN THE BLANK

Select terms from your reading to fill in the blanks.

1. Benign tumors are named by adding the suffix _____ to the name of the cell type.

2. Cancer is the second most common cause of death in the _____, causing more than _____ fatalities _____.

3. Cancers are most curable with _____ or _____ before they have metastasized.

4. There are two major classes of genes involved in carcinogenesis: oncogenes and _____.

5. G_0 in the cell cycle is the resting or dormant stage, during which cells have not started to divide. When the cell is signaled to reproduce, it moves into the _____ stage.

6. The M-phase of the cell cycle is when mitosis occurs. This is when the cell actually _____.

7. Agents used in cancer chemotherapy are commonly categorized by the _____, or by their origin.

8. Tumors may be either _____ or _____.

MATCHING

Match the lettered term to the numbered description.

DESCRIPTION

1. _____ The process by which cancer cells become more and more atypical
2. _____ Uncontrolled cell division
3. _____ Break through boundaries that separate cell types within some organs
4. _____ Spreading of primary cancer cells to other tissues
5. _____ Formation of blood vessels

TERM

a. Hyperplasia
b. Invasiveness
c. Metastasis
d. Angiogenesis
e. Differentiation

Cancer Therapy

Five primary methods are employed in the approach to cancer treatment: surgery, radiation therapy, chemotherapy, immunotherapy, and hormonal therapy. Surgery remains the treatment of choice for many solid tumors. Radiation treatment was first used for cancer treatment in the late 1800s. Though very effective for treating many types of cancer, surgery and radiation are local treatments. Systemic diseases such as leukemia cannot be treated this way. Chemotherapy and hormonal therapy access the systemic circulation. Immunotherapy uses the stimulation of the host's immune system to fight against the cancer. The response to chemotherapy may be described as *cure*, *complete response*, **partial response**, **stable disease**, or *progression of disease*. A *cure* implies that the patient is entirely free of disease and has the same life expectancy as a cancer-free individual. *Complete response* means complete disappearance of all cancer, and no evidence of new disease for at least 1 month after treatment. A *partial response* is defined as a 50% or greater decrease in the tumor size, or other objective disease markers, and no evidence of any new disease for at least 1 month. A patient whose tumor size neither grows nor shrinks significantly has stable disease.

Depending on the type of cancer, and the drug used, chemotherapy agents may be administered orally, intramuscularly (IM), subcutaneously, or intravenously (IV). IV administration is the most common method of administration. Oral chemotherapy is becoming more popular than ever because of its ease of use. The most common antineoplastic agents are listed in Table 13-1 ■.

Table 13-1 ■ Common Agents Used in the Treatment of Cancer

GENERIC NAME	TRADE NAME	COMMON DOSAGE RANGE	ROUTE OF ADMINISTRATION
Alkylating Agents			
chlorambucil (nitrogen mustard)	Leukeran	0.1–0.2 mg/kg/d	PO
cyclophosphamide	Cytoxan	1–5 mg/kg/d	PO
		10–15 mg/kg q7–10d or 3–5 mg/kg twice weekly	IV
ifosfamide	Ifex	1.2 g/m^2/d for 5 d	IV
mechlorethamine (nitrogen mustard)	Mustargen	0.4 mg/kg in 1–4 divided doses	IV, intracavity
melphalan	Alkeran	2–10 mg/d (0.15 mg/kg/d) for 7 d	PO
Ethyleneimines			
altretamine	Hexalen	260 mg/m^2/d for 14 or 21 d in a 28-d cycle	PO
thiotepa	Immunex	0.3–0.4 mg/kg	IV
		0.6–0.8 mg/kg	Intravesicular directly into the bladder
Alkyl Sulfonate			
busulfan	Busulfex	4–8 mg/d	PO
		0.8 mg/kg q6h for 4 d	IV

Table 13-1 ■ Common Agents Used in the Treatment of Cancer

GENERIC NAME	TRADE NAME	COMMON DOSAGE RANGE	ROUTE OF ADMINISTRATION
Miscellaneous			
carboplatin	Paraplatin	On Day 1 every 4 weeks	IV infusion
cisplatin	Platinol-AQ	20–100 mg/m^2/d (schedule depends on type of cancer; up to 360 mg/m^2)	IV
procarbazine	Matulane	2–4 mg/kg/d for 1 wk; then 4–6 mg/kg/d until WBCs are less than 4,000/mm^3	PO
Antimetabolites			
capecitabine	Xeloda	2,500 mg/m^2/d in 2 divided doses for 2 wk	PO
fluorouracil	5-FU, Efudex, Adrucil	6–12 mg/kg/d	IV
mercaptopurine	6-MP, Purinethol	1.5–2.5 mg/kg/d	PO
methotrexate	Rheumatrex, Folex, Trexall	10–30 mg/d for 4–8 d with 7–10-d rest interval	PO
		10–30 mg	IM
		20–500 mg/m^2	IV
Mitotic Inhibitors (Plant Alkaloids)			
etoposide	VePesid, Toposar, VP-16	35–100 mg/m^2/d	PO, IV
teniposide	Vumon	165 mg/m^2 in combination twice weekly for 4.5 wk	IV
vinblastine	Velban	3.7–11.1 mg/m^2	IV
vincristine	Oncovin, Vincasar PFS	1.4 mg/m^2	IV
vinorelbine	Navelbine	15–30 mg/m^2	IV
Antitumor Antibiotics			
bleomycin	Blenoxane	0.25–0.50 units/kg/d	IM, IV, subcutaneously
daunorubicin	Cerubidine	30–60 mg/m^2/d	IV
doxorubicin	Adriamycin	20–75 mg/m^2	IV
epirubicin	Ellence	100–120 mg/m^2 infused over 3–5 min on Day 1 of a 3–4 wk cycle, or 50–60 mg/m^2 on Day 1 and Day 8 of a 3–4 wk cycle	IV
idarubicin	Idamycin	12 mg/m^2/d for 3 d	IV
mitomycin C	Mutamycin	10–20 mg/m^2	IV
plicamycin	Mithracin	20 30 mcg/kg/day for 8–10 d	IV
valrubicin	Valstar	800 mg in 75 mL of solution once a week for 6 wk	Instilled into the urinary bladder

(continued)

Table 13-1 ■ Common Agents Used in the Treatment of Cancer (*continued*)

GENERIC NAME	TRADE NAME	COMMON DOSAGE RANGE	ROUTE OF ADMINISTRATION
Hormonal Therapy			
Corticosteroids			
dexamethasone	Provera	0.25–4 mg bid to qid	PO
	Depo-Provera	8–6 mg every 1–3 wk	IM
prednisone	Deltasone	5–60 mg/d in single or divided doses	PO
Estrogens			
estramustine	Emcyt	10–16 mg/kg/d in 3–4 divided doses for up to 3 y	PO
tamoxifen	Nolvadex	10–20 mg 1–2 times/d	PO
Progestins			
megestrol	Megace	40–320 mg/d in divided doses	PO
Gonadotropins			
goserelin	Zoladex	3.6 mg once every 4 wk, or 10.8 mg depot every 3 mo	Subcutaneous implants
leuprolide	Lupron,	1 mg/d	Subcutaneous
	Eligard	7.5 mg monthly as depot injection	IM
Antiandrogens			
bicalutamide	Casodex	50 mg/d	PO
flutamide	Eulexin	250 mg 3 times/d at 8-h intervals	PO
nilutamide	Nilandron	300 mg/d for 3 d	PO

Focus Point

Bone-Marrow Depression

Depression of bone marrow is usually the most serious limiting toxicity of cancer chemotherapy.

Alkylating Agents

Alkylating agents cause replacement of hydrogen by an alkyl group, specifically one that inhibits cell division and growth. There are five major types of alkylating agents:

1. Nitrogen mustards
2. Ethyleneimines
3. Alkyl sulfonates
4. Nitrosoureas
5. Temozolomide

Acquired resistance to alkylating agents is a common event, but resistance of a cancer to one alkylating agent does not always imply cross-resistance to others.

How do they work?

Alkylating agents act directly on DNA, causing cross-linking of DNA strands, abnormal base pairing, or DNA strand breaks, thus preventing the cells from dividing. They are cell cycle phase–nonspecific, but are most active in the resting phase.

How are they used?

Alkylating agents are generally of greatest value in treating slow-growing cancers. They are not as effective on rapidly growing cells.

What are the adverse effects?

This class has a dose-limiting toxicity to bone marrow and intestinal mucosa. Alkylating agents cause oral mucosa ulceration and intestinal denudations. All alkylating agents can cause instances of pulmonary fibrosis and venoocclusive disease in the liver; renal failure; or central neurotoxicity with seizures, coma, and at times, death. Most alkylating agents cause **alopecia** (hair loss). Central nervous system (CNS) toxicity is indicated by nausea and vomiting. Ifosfamide (Ifex) is the most neurotoxic of this class, producing altered mental status, coma, generalized seizures, and paralysis. All alkylating agents have toxic effects on the reproductive system.

What are the contraindications and interactions?

Alkylating agents are contraindicated during pregnancy, especially during the first trimester, because they are **teratogenic** (able to cause birth defects in the fetus). Alkylating agents may interact with antidepressants, other anticancer medications, warfarin (Coumadin), and both prescription and nonprescription medications such as certain vaccines, aspirin, and vitamins.

What are the most important points patients should know?

Teach patients about the manifestation of bone-marrow depression. Advise patients to avoid contact with people who are suffering from colds or other infections during susceptible times (for example, following a course of therapy). Warn patients that hair loss may occur from the head, eyelashes, nose, and pubic area, but reassure them that hair will grow back once the course of therapy is complete.

Focus Point

Tyramine and Procarbazine

Procarbazine (Matulane) is available as a 50-mg capsule. It can cause acute disulfiram-like reaction (flushing, headache, acute vomiting, and chest or abdominal pain) with alcohol. Avoid tyramine-containing foods (aged cheese, chocolate, pickles, aged meat, wine, etc.), which can cause a life-threatening elevation in blood pressure.

Antimetabolites

Antimetabolites prevent cancer cell growth by affecting DNA production. They are only effective against cells that are actively participating in cell metabolism. The classes of antimetabolites include the following:

1. Purine antagonists: mercaptopurine

2. Adenosine antagonists: fludarabine

3. Pyrimidine antagonists: fluorouracil

4. Folic-acid antagonists: methotrexate

How do they work?

Antimetabolites replace natural substances as building blocks in DNA molecules, altering the function of enzymes required for cell metabolism and protein synthesis. They are cell cycle phase–specific and are most effective during the S-phase of cell division.

How are they used?

Mercaptopurine (Purinethol) is useful in maintenance therapy of children with acute and chronic myelocytic leukemia. Fludarabine (Fludara) is used in the treatment of chronic lymphocytic leukemia and non-Hodgkin's lymphoma. Capecitabine (Xeloda) is used for metastatic breast and colorectal cancers. It is a *prodrug* (a modified, pharmacologically inactive form of a pharmacologic agent) of fluorouracil (Adrucil) and undergoes hydrolysis in the liver to form the active drug. Fluorouracil is prescribed for treatment of *keratoses* (overgrowths of horny skin tissue) and basal cell carcinomas (skin cancer). Methotrexate (Trexall) is used for acute lymphoblastic leukemia, meningeal leukemia, and head and neck cancers (and for noncancerous disorders such as rheumatoid arthritis and psoriasis).

What are the adverse effects?

The adverse effects of mercaptopurine include anorexia, nausea, vomiting, hepatotoxicity, bone-marrow depression, and hyperuricemia. Fludarabine may cause headache, hearing loss, sleep disorders, and depression. It may also cause bone-marrow toxicity, pneumonia, dyspnea (difficulty breathing), epistaxis (nosebleed), and edema. Fluorouracil causes marked myelosuppression. It can also result in gastrointestinal (GI) disturbances, alopecia, dermatitis, and nail changes.

Methotrexate commonly causes skin rashes, hyperpigmentation, photosensitivity, hyperuricemia, inflammation of the tongue, and alopecia. Serious adverse effects include severe leukopenia, bone-marrow aplasia, and thrombocytopenia.

What are the contraindications and interactions?

Mercaptopurine is contraindicated in patients with a history of resistance to this agent. It must be avoided in the first trimester of pregnancy, in women who are lactating, and in those patients who have acute infectious diseases. Fluorouracil, mercaptopurine, and methotrexate are contraindicated in patients with severe bone-marrow depression and renal dysfunction. Mercaptopurine may interact with allopurinol (Zyloprim), warfarin (Coumadin), and certain drugs used to treat ulcerative colitis, such as mesalamine (Asacol), olsalazine (Dipentum), and sulfasalazine (Azulfidine). Patients should be instructed not to start or stop any prescription or nonprescription medications while taking this drug, and to tell their health-care provider about all medications they are currently taking before taking mercaptopurine.

What are the most important points patients should know?

Advise patients that antimetabolites may cause bone-marrow suppression and damage to the GI lining, such as stomatitis (a group of diseases affecting the mucous membranes of the mouth) and ulceration.

Focus on Natural Products

Green Tea as an Antioxidant

Green tea has a reputation as a healthful drink, with studies suggesting that it may reduce the incidence of a variety of cancers, including cancers of the colon, pancreas, and stomach. Green tea contains high levels of polyphenols, which exhibit antioxidant and chemopreventive properties. However, green tea is not a proven cure for cancer. As often happens with natural supplements that are supported primarily by observational trials, results of these studies are inconsistent. Also, green tea should not be given to infants or young children.

Mitotic Inhibitors (Plant Alkaloids)

Plant alkaloids are typically physiologically active organic bases containing nitrogen (and usually, oxygen) that occur in seed plants. They are called *mitotic inhibitors* because they prevent cell division (or *meiosis*). The primary plant alkaloids are vincristine (Oncovin) and vinblastine (Velban). Examples of plant alkaloids are listed in Table 13-1.

How do they work?

Mitotic inhibitors act throughout the cell cycle, and some of these agents are more effective during the S- and M-phases of the cell cycle. They inhibit DNA and RNA synthesis.

How are they used?

Mitotic inhibitors are used to treat cancer of the breast, bladder, ovaries, and lungs, as well as leukemias, lymphomas, and testicular cancer.

What are the adverse effects?

These agents may cause nausea, vomiting, diarrhea, alopecia, dizziness, weakness, headache, depression, and stomatitis. The adverse effects of mitotic inhibitors also may cause anemia and hyperpigmentation of the nails, tongue, or oral mucosa.

What are the contraindications and interactions?

Mitotic inhibitors are contraindicated in severe cardiac disease, hypocalcemia, bleeding disorders, myelosuppression, and pregnancy. Some of these drugs, such as plicamycin (Mithracin), must be used cautiously in patients with hepatic or renal impairment. Mitomycin (Mutamycin) may cause acute shortness of breath and severe bronchospasm if it is used with mitotic inhibitors. These agents may decrease phenytoin (Dilantin) levels. Erythromycin (Eryc) and itraconazole (Sporanox) may increase vinblastine toxicity.

What are the important points patients should know?

Be sure patients are aware that mitotic inhibitors may produce serious toxicity with bone-marrow depression and GI damage. Advise them that, if they have diarrhea, to avoid foods that are likely to cause GI irritation, such as coffee, spicy foods, fruits, and raw vegetables.

Focus on Geriatrics

Toxicity of Antineoplastic Drugs in Elderly Patients

Older adults—many of whom may have chronic diseases such as cardiovascular disease or kidney impairment—are at higher risk for adverse effects when they are being treated with antineoplastic drugs. As a result, lower dosages of antineoplastics should be administered to these patients. Creatinine clearance is used to monitor renal function in elderly patients.

Hormonal Therapy

Hormonal agents are frequently prescribed in antineoplastic therapy. These agents may selectively suppress the growth of certain tissues of the body without causing a cytotoxic action. The sex hormones, such as estrogens, progestins, and androgens, are generally employed to change the hormonal environment of tissues dependent on these agents for their growth. For example, the administration of antiandrogens or estrogens is beneficial in the treatment of prostatic cancer. On the other hand, these hormones can be useful in treating breast or endometrial cancers.

How do they work?

Hormonal agents are a class of heterogeneous compounds that have various effects on cells. These agents block either hormone production or hormone action. Their action on malignant cells is highly selective. Steroids inhibit migration of white blood cells (WBCs) and inhibit production of products of the arachidonic acid cascade. Estrogen works by promoting the release of calcitonin and by enhancing the availability of vitamin D_3 to increase bone formation in postmenopausal patients with breast cancer.

Progestins inhibit secretion of pituitary gonadotropins by positive feedback. Antiestrogens bind to estrogen receptors, which prevents estrogen from binding to these receptors. Antiandrogens act by blocking the synthesis of endogenous testosterone.

How are they used?

Hormones and their antagonists have various uses in the treatment of malignant tumors. Steroids are especially useful in treating acute lymphocytic leukemia. They are also used in conjunction with radiation therapy to reduce radiation edema. Sex hormones are used in carcinomas of the reproductive tract; for example, estrogen may be given to a patient with testicular cancer or to patients with certain carcinomas of the breast.

What are the adverse effects?

GI disturbances are common adverse effects associated with these drugs. Impaired fertility may result from treatment with sex hormone antagonists. In women, menstrual irregularities may develop, depending on premenopausal or menopausal stages of life.

What are the contraindications and interactions?

Most hormones are contraindicated during pregnancy because they are harmful to the fetus. These drugs should be used during pregnancy only in circumstances in which the benefits of treatment far outweigh the risk of harm to the fetus. Interactions with hormonal therapies occur with tamoxifen (Nolvadex), alcohol, St. John's wort, zinc, magnesium, vitamin B, and thyroid supplements.

What are the important points patients should know?

Warn patients that hormonal agents are contraindicated during pregnancy and that menstrual irregularities are common. If appropriate, advise female patients to use strict contraception and avoid pregnancy for 3 to 4 months after completing the course. Some sources advise that both men and women should avoid conceiving a child for about 2 years after treatment.

Focus Point

Possibility of Infertility

It is important to instruct patients that infertility, which may occur with antineoplastic agents, may not be reversible.

Antitumor Antibiotics

Antitumor antibiotics are made from natural products produced by species of the soil fungus *Streptomyces*. They are very effective in the treatment of certain tumors. The classifications of these agents are listed in Table 13-1.

How do they work?

The majority of antitumor antibiotics inhibit DNA and RNA synthesis, causing cell death.

How are they used?

Antitumor antibiotics are used only to treat cancer and are not used to treat infections. The effects of each of the antitumor antibiotics are as follows:

✳ Doxorubicin (Adriamycin) is used in the treatment of breast, ovarian, and bone cancers. It is also used for therapy of acute lymphoblastic and myeloblastic leukemias. Doxorubicin is generally used in combination with surgery, radiation, and immunotherapy.

✳ Daunorubicin (Cerubidine) is the first-line treatment for advanced HIV-associated Kaposi's sarcoma. It is also used for testicular cancer, Wilms' tumor, and chorio-carcinoma.

✳ Idarubicin (Idamycin) can be used for treating acute monocytic leukemia and solid tumors.

✳ Plicamycin (Mithracin) is used to treat hypercalcemia associated with advanced neoplasms and testicular cancer.

✳ Bleomycin (Blenoxane) is used in squamous cell carcinomas (skin cancer) of the head, neck, penis, and cervix. It is also used for the treatment of lymphomas and testicular carcinoma.

✳ Mitomycin (Mutamycin) is used in combination with other chemotherapeutic agents in palliative and adjunctive treatment of breast, stomach, and pancreatic cancers.

What are the adverse effects?

Bone-marrow suppression is a major adverse effect of antitumor antibiotics. Stomatitis, GI upset, and alopecia can occur during treatment but cease when treatment is discontinued. Bleomycin is less toxic to bone marrow but tends to cause hyperpigmentation, redness, and sometimes ulceration of the skin. Pulmonary fibrosis can occur during therapy. Mitomycin may induce serious renal impairment.

What are the contraindications and interactions?

Antitumor antibiotics are contraindicated in patients with known hypersensitivity to these agents. Some antitumor antibiotics have toxic effects on the heart, kidneys, and liver. Therefore, they are contraindicated in patients with diseases of these organs. Plasma digoxin (Lanoxin) levels may decrease when administered with bleomycin. When bleomycin is used with cisplatin (Platinol), there is an increased risk of bleomycin toxicity. Mitomycin and plicamycin may have an additive bone-marrow depressant effect when used with other antineoplastic agents. There is an increased risk of bleeding when plicamycin is administered with aspirin, heparin (Hep-Lock), warfarin (Coumadin), or nonsteroidal anti-inflammatory drugs (NSAIDs).

What are the important points patients should know?

Advise patients that bone-marrow suppression is a major adverse effect of these drugs. Because cardiac toxicity is observed with antitumor antibiotics, instruct patients to report to their physician if they experience cardiac problems.

✳ Apply Your Knowledge 13.2 ▬▬▬▬

The following questions focus on what you have just learned about various cancer therapies. *See Appendix E for the correct answers.*

MATCHING

Match the lettered generic drug name to its numbered classification.

DRUG CLASSIFICATION

1. _____ Alkylating agent
2. _____ Antimetabolite
3. _____ Antitumor antibiotic
4. _____ Hormonal therapy
5. _____ Mitotic inhibitor

GENERIC DRUG

a. Vinblastine
b. Plicamycin
c. Prednisone
d. Mercaptopurine
e. Melphalan

FILL IN THE BLANK

Select terms from your reading to fill in the blanks.

1. All alkylating agents have caused instances of pulmonary fibrosis and _____.
2. Mercaptopurine is useful in maintenance therapy of children with _____.
3. Mitotic inhibitors are contraindicated in _____.
4. Alkylating agents are generally effective on _____.
5. Mitotic inhibitors are used to treat cancer of _____.

MULTIPLE CHOICE

1. Which of the following is the mechanism of action of antitumor antibiotics?
   a. Inhibition of cancer cell membranes
   b. Inhibition of DNA and RNA synthesis
   c. Prevention of DNA synthesis only
   d. Prevention of RNA synthesis only

2. Which of the following is the first-line treatment for advanced HIV-associated Kaposi's sarcoma?
   a. Daunorubicin (antitumor antibiotic)
   b. Progestin (hormonal agent)
   c. Nitrogen mustards (alkylating agents)
   d. Mercaptopurine (antimetabolite agent)

3. All of the following agents are antitumor antibiotics, except:
   a. Plicamycin
   b. Bleomycin
   c. Melphalan
   d. Mitomycin

4. Sex hormones are used to treat carcinomas of which of the following body systems?
   a. Respiratory
   b. Urinary
   c. Nervous
   d. Reproductive

5. Which of the following agents are especially useful in treating acute lymphocytic leukemia?

    a. Radiation

    b. Estrogen

    c. Calcitonin

    d. Steroids

Biologic Response Modifiers

Biologic response modifiers include agents that affect the patient's biologic response to a neoplasm in a beneficial way. Included in this class are agents that act indirectly to mediate antitumor effects or directly on the tumor cells. Recombinant DNA technology has greatly facilitated the identification and production of a number of human proteins, with potent effects on the function and growth of both normal and neoplastic cells. Interferons, interleukin-2, tumor necrosis factor (TNF), and monoclonal antibodies are types of human proteins. An example of how the biologic response modifiers are produced is that of **monoclonal antibodies**. These are produced by fusing a single immune cell to tumor cells that are grown in cultures, known as **hybridomas**. Large quantities of these identical antibody cells are produced (rather like clones), all with the same specific antigen as their target. The advantage of monoclonal antibodies is that they can be used to target and then purify the *specific* protein that induced their formation. Interferons are another type of biologic response modifiers that are discussed in detail in this chapter.

INTERFERONS

Interferons are a group of blood proteins that have antiviral effects. The genes that produce some of the interferons have been isolated, and those interferons are now commercially produced by means of genetic engineering. Interferons are naturally produced in response to viral infections, or other biological inducers, such as some tumors.

There are three types of interferons: alpha (2a and 2b), beta, and gamma.

✳ Alfa (called *alfa* when referring to drugs)—produced by white blood cells (WBCs)

✳ Beta—produced by connective tissue cells

✳ Gamma—produced by T lymphocytes

Only interferon alfa-2b (Intron A) is effectively used for some cancers. Thus, only alfa-2b will be discussed here.

How does it work?

Interferon alfa-2b (Intron A) is a natural product induced virally in peripheral WBCs. Interferon alfa-2b is obtained by recombinant DNA technology of *Escherichia coli* bearing an interferon alfa-2b gene from human leukocytes.

How is it used?

Interferon alfa-2b is a chemotherapy agent that has been used for years to treat kidney cancers, lymphoma, and melanoma. It is given IV or IM, with the method and schedule of administration determined by the actual cancer type and the extent of its growth. It is usually administered daily for a specific period of days.

What are the adverse effects?

Patients receiving high IV doses of this agent are closely monitored in a hospital for adverse effects, which may include nausea, vomiting, weight gain, fluid retention, and damage to the liver, lungs, nerves, or kidneys.

What are the contraindications and interactions?

Contraindications include hypersensitivity to interferon alfa-2b or to any components of this product. Safe use during pregnancy, lactation, or in children younger than 18 years is not established.

Interferon alfa-2b should be used cautiously in severe, preexisting cardiac, renal, or hepatic disease; pulmonary disease; diabetes mellitus; or in those prone to ketoacidosis. This agent may increase theophylline (Elixophyllin) levels, and zidovudine (Retrovir) may increase hematologic toxicity.

What are the important points patients should know?

Teach patients techniques for reconstituting and administrating these drugs. Warn them not to change brands of interferon without first consulting their physician. Advise patients about adverse effects and when to notify their physician about those that cause significant discomfort. Advise women not to breast feed while taking these drugs without consulting their physician.

Focus Point

Interferon Administration Changes

All changes in interferon administration must be directed by a physician. Patients should never change the times or doses specified for taking interferons.

✳ Apply Your Knowledge 13.3

The following questions focus on what you have just learned about biologic response modifiers. *See Appendix E for the correct answers.*

FILL IN THE BLANK

Select terms from your reading to fill in the blanks.

1. Interferon beta is produced by _____.

2. Interferon alfa-2b has been used for years to treat _____ cancers, lymphoma, and _____.

3. Interferon alfa-2b is a natural product induced virally in peripheral _____.

4. Recombinant DNA technology has greatly facilitated the identification and production of a number of human _____.

5. Interferons, interleukin-2, tumor necrosis factor, and _____ are some examples of human proteins.

6. Adverse effects of interferon alfa-2b include nausea, vomiting, weight gain, fluid retention, and damage to the nerves, _____, _____, and _____.

7. Only a _____ can change the type or administration of interferon alfa-2b.

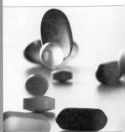

Chapter Capsule

This section repeats the objectives from the beginning of the chapter and then provides a summary of the most important concepts for the objective. Use this section as a quick review and to check your knowledge.

Objective 1: List the seven warning signs of cancer.

- Changes in bowel or bladder habits
- A sore that does not heal
- Unusual bleeding or discharge
- Thickening or lump in breast or elsewhere
- Indigestion or difficulty swallowing
- Obvious change in a wart or mole
- Nagging cough or hoarseness

Objective 2: Summarize the basic cell cycle and its importance in the use of antineoplastic agents.

- The basic cell cycle—G_0 (resting or dormant stage); G_1 (the first gap phase); S (DNA synthesis occurs); G_2 (the second gap phase); and M (mitosis occurs)
- Some antineoplastic agents target cancer cells in various stages of the cell cycle, which, in part, determines how and when they are used

Objective 3: List commonly used antineoplastic agents in each class.

- Alkylating agents—nitrogen mustards, ethyleneimines, alkyl sulfonates, nitrosoureas, and triazenes
- Antimetabolites—purine antagonists, adenosine antagonists, pyrimidine antagonists, and folic-acid antagonists
- Mitotic inhibitors (plant alkaloids)—vincristine and vinblastine
- Hormonal therapy—estrogens, progestins, and androgens
- Antitumor antibiotics—doxorubicin, daunorubicin, idarubicin, plicamycin, bleomycin, and mitomycin
- Biologic response modifiers—interferons, interleukin-2, TNF, and monoclonal antibodies

Objective 4: Explain the mechanism of action of each class of antineoplastic agents.

- Alkylating agents—cell cycle phase–nonspecific; most active in resting phase; act directly on DNA, causing cross-linking of DNA strands, abnormal base pairing, or DNA strand breaks, thus preventing the cell from dividing
- Antimetabolites—cell cycle phase–specific; most effective during S-phase; replace natural substances as building blocks in DNA molecules, altering the function of enzymes required for cell metabolism and protein synthesis
- Mitotic inhibitors—act throughout cell cycle; some are most effective during S- and M-phases; inhibit DNA and RNA synthesis
- Hormonal agents—highly selective; either block hormone production or block hormone action
- Antitumor antibiotics—most inhibit DNA and RNA synthesis, causing cell death
- Biologic response modifiers—affect biologic responses to a neoplasm in beneficial ways, sometimes acting indirectly to mediate antitumor effects or directly on the tumor cells

Objective 5: Discuss how steroids, estrogen, progestins, antiestrogens, and antiandrogens work in the treatment of cancer.

■ Steroids—inhibit migration of WBCs and inhibit production of products of the arachidonic acid cascade

■ Estrogens—promote the release of calcitonin and enhance the availability of vitamin D3 to increase bone formation in postmenopausal patients with breast cancer

■ Progestins—inhibit secretion of pituitary gonadotropins by positive feedback

■ Antiestrogens—bind to estrogen receptors, preventing estrogen from binding to these receptors

■ Antiandrogens—block the synthesis of endogenous testosterone

Objective 6: Explain how biologic response modifiers are created and how they work.

■ Human proteins modified by recombinant DNA technology to produce agents with potent effects on the function and growth of both normal and neoplastic cells

■ Examples—interferon, interleukin-2, tumor necrosis factor, and monoclonal antibodies

Objective 7: Describe the advantages of using monoclonal antibodies in the treatment of cancer.

■ Monoclonal antibodies—can be used to specifically track down and purify the specific protein that induced their formation

Objective 8: Identify common side effects of chemotherapy treatment.

■ Alkylating agents—oral mucosal ulceration and intestinal denudations, pulmonary fibrosis and venoocclusive disease in the liver, renal failure, or central neurotoxicity with seizures, coma, and at times, death; most of these agents cause hair loss; some cause nausea and vomiting; ifosfamide is the most neurotoxic of this class, producing altered mental status, coma, generalized seizures, and paralysis. All of these agents have toxic effects on the reproductive system.

■ Antimetabolites—nausea, vomiting, hepatotoxicity, bone-marrow depression, headache, hearing loss, sleep disorders, depression, myelosuppression, GI disturbances, hair loss, dermatitis, nail changes, skin rashes, hyperpigmentation, photosensitivity, hyperuricemia, inflammation of the tongue. Methotrexate may cause serious adverse effects, including severe leukopenia, bone-marrow aplasia, and thrombocytopenia.

■ Mitotic inhibitors (plant alkaloids)—nausea, vomiting, diarrhea, hair loss, dizziness, weakness, headache, depression, stomatitis, anemia, and hyperpigmentation of the nails, tongue, and oral mucosa

■ Hormonal therapy—GI disturbances, possible impaired fertility, menstrual irregularities

■ Antitumor antibiotics—bone-marrow suppression, stomatitis, GI upset, hair loss, hyperpigmentation, skin ulceration, pulmonary fibrosis, serious renal impairment

■ Biologic response modifiers—nausea, vomiting, weight gain, fluid retention, and damage to the liver, lungs, nerves, or kidneys

Internet Sites of Interest

- Health-care workers who are exposed to antineoplastic agents when working with patients are at risk for toxicity. See the Centers for Disease Control and Prevention (CDC) publication about occupational hazards at: **www.cdc.gov/niosh/docs/2004-102**

- The Virtual Library of Biochemistry, Molecular Biology, and Cell Biology provides information on the cell cycle. Click on the Cell Cycle link at: **www.biochemweb.org/**. Many other resources are available from this Web site.

- Hormone therapy for treatment of reproductive cancers is discussed on the Mayo Clinic Web site at: **www.mayoclinic.com**. Search "reproductive cancer."

- The American Cancer Society (ACS) has a wealth of information for patients and health-care providers on its Web site at: **http://www.cancer.org/**

Checkpoint Review 3

Select the best answer for the following questions.

1. Vitamin requirements are measured by which of the following units?

   a. Milligrams
   b. Centigrams
   c. Micrograms
   d. a and c

2. Vitamin B_1 is also called:

   a. Riboflavin
   b. Cobalamin
   c. Thiamine
   d. Retinol

3. Which of the following is the newest COX-2 inhibitor for the treatment of osteoarthritis?

   a. Celecoxib (Celebrex)
   b. Meloxicam (Mobic)
   c. Oxycodone (Percolone)
   d. Fentanyl (Duragesic)

4. Which of the following vaccines is used for the prevention of viral infections?

   a. Q fever
   b. Pertussis
   c. Yellow fever
   d. Plague

5. Which of the following minerals acts in bone formation, impulse conduction, myocardial contractions, and the blood-clotting process?

   a. Sodium
   b. Phosphorus
   c. Iodine
   d. Calcium

6. Which of the following is the trade name of naloxone?

   a. Demerol
   b. Talwin
   c. Narcan
   d. Stadol

7. Zinc is a very important trace element for which of the following conditions?

   a. During hemoglobin synthesis and energy production
   b. During periods of rapid tissue growth
   c. Gaining too much weight
   d. Kidney failure

8. Which of the following vitamins is an antioxidant?

   a. Tocopherol (vitamin E)
   b. Cholecalciferol (vitamin D)
   c. Phylloquinone (vitamin K)
   d. Cobalamin (vitamin B_{12})

9. Patients should be instructed to drink several full glasses of water when taking which of the following antimicrobial drugs?

   a. Penicillins
   b. Sulfonamides
   c. Fluoroquinolones
   d. Aminoglycosides

10. Acetaminophen should be avoided in which of the following patients?

    a. Those taking antacids
    b. Those drinking milk
    c. Those drinking alcohol
    d. Those taking antibiotics

11. The sulfonamides block the biosynthetic pathway of which of the following?

    a. Folic acid
    b. Bacterial proteins
    c. Bacterial nucleic acid
    d. Bacterial lipids

12. The presence of food in the GI tract reduces is the absorption of many anti-infective agents, except:

    a. Penicillin V
    b. Doxycycline
    c. Minocycline
    d. All of the above

13. Which of the following foods contains very high amounts of tyramine, that may interact with MAO inhibitors and cause hypertensive crises?

    a. Bananas
    b. Cottage cheese
    c. Red meat
    d. Red apples

14. Ethanol impairs absorption of which of the following vitamins?

    a. Thiamine (vitamin B_1)
    b. Cobalamin (vitamin B_{12})
    c. Ascorbic acid (vitamin C)
    d. Tocopherol (vitamin E)

15. Black "hairy" tongue (temporary overgrowth of harmless bacteria or yeast in the mouth) is a side effect of oral administration of which of the following antibacterials?

 a. Tetracycline
 b. Erythromycin
 c. Penicillin
 d. Streptomycin

16. Opioid receptors in the brainstem are responsible for the respiratory depressant effects produced by which of the following?

 a. Nonopioid analgesics
 b. Nonopioid antagonists
 c. Opioid antagonists
 d. Opioid analgesics

17. Fluoride's main function in human nutrition is to prevent:

 a. Retarded physical growth
 b. Formation of kidney stones
 c. Dental caries
 d. Wilson's disease

18. Which of the following is the major adverse effect of aminoglycosides?

 a. Hepatotoxicity
 b. Nephrotoxicity
 c. Neurotoxicity
 d. GI toxicity

19. Most of the currently used opioid analgesics act primarily at which of the following receptors?

 a. Mu
 b. Delta
 c. Kappa
 d. Gamma

20. Which of the following is the major adverse effect of meperidine?

 a. Hypertensive crisis
 b. Agitation
 c. Hallucinations
 d. Respiratory depression

21. Essential fatty acids are required for the formation of:

 a. Prostaglandins
 b. Insulin
 c. Vitamin K
 d. Enzymes

22. Aspirin appears to impede clotting by blocking which of the following?

 a. Opioid receptors
 b. Calcium channels
 c. Prostaglandin formation
 d. All of the above

23. Which of the following antibiotics may impair bone growth and discolor the teeth in children?

 a. Macrolides
 b. Aminoglycosides
 c. Sulfonamides
 d. Tetracyclines

24. Talwin is the trade name of:

 a. Meperidine
 b. Pentazocine
 c. Fentanyl
 d. Naloxone

25. Patients should notify their physician if blood appears in their stools, vomitus, or urine if they are taking:

 a. Indomethacin
 b. Antacids
 c. Acetaminophen
 d. Benzodiazepines

26. All of the following infections may be transmitted by mosquitoes, except:

 a. West Nile virus
 b. Malaria
 c. Rabies
 d. Encephalitis

27. Which of the following antibiotics is in the class of macrolides?

 a. Erythromycin
 b. Ciprofloxacin
 c. Doxycline
 d. Rifampin

28. Which of the following is the most common adverse effect of vaccinations?

 a. Convulsions
 b. Liver impairment
 c. Malaise
 d. Allergic reaction

29. A booster dose of adult diphtheria and tetanus toxoid is recommended every:

 a. 2 years
 b. 5 years
 c. 10 years
 d. Not required

30. Ganciclovir is used for prophylaxis and systemic treatment of which of the following infections?

 a. Respiratory syncytial virus
 b. Hepatitis C virus
 c. Advanced HIV
 d. Cytomegalovirus

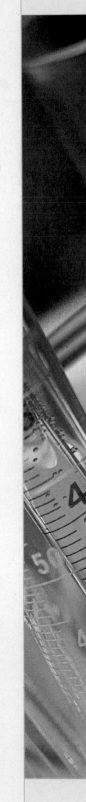

31. Which of the following was the leading cause of invasive bacterial disease (meningitis) among children until pediatric immunization was introduced in 1988?

    a. Measles
    b. Polio
    c. *Haemophilus influenzae* type b
    d. Varicella

32. Which of the following is the trade name for doxyccyline?

    a. Minocin
    b. Vibramycin
    c. Terramycin
    d. Aureomycin

33. Which of the following vaccines may be given at birth?

    a. Varicella (chickenpox)
    b. Rubella (German measles)
    c. Hepatitis B
    d. Influenza

34. Which of the following agents may cause a reddish-orange discoloration of body fluids including tears, urine, and saliva?

    a. Isoniazid
    b. Chloramphenicol
    c. Spectinomycin
    d. Rifampin

35. Amantadine is used to prevent or treat symptoms of:

    a. Mumps
    b. Influenza A
    c. Hepatitis A
    d. Hepatitis C

36. Which of the following vaccines is recommended every year for those at high-risk for complications?

    a. Influenza
    b. Meningococcal
    c. Typhoid
    d. Cholera

37. Meningococcal polysaccharide vaccine must be administered via which of the following routes?

    a. Subcutaneously
    b. Intramuscularly
    c. Intravenously
    d. Inhalation

38. The second most common cause of death in the United States is:

    a. Cardiovascular disease
    b. Car accidents
    c. Cancer
    d. Infectious diseases

39. The ability of chemotherapy to kill cancer cells depends on which of the following factors?

    a. Its ability to destroy specific tissues
    b. Its ability to stop cell division
    c. Its ability to cause necrosis of tissues
    d. All of the above

40. Which of the following vaccines is recommended only in extremely high-risk individuals in whom other controls are impractical?

    a. Q fever
    b. Rabies
    c. Tuberculosis
    d. Typhoid

41. DNA synthesis occurs in which of the following phases of the cell cycle?

    a. G_0
    b. G_1
    c. S
    d. M

42. Chemotherapy agents may be administered by which of the following routes?

    a. Intramuscularly
    b. Orally
    c. Subcutaneously
    d. All of the above

43. Which of the following vaccines is recommended between 12 and 15 months of age?

    a. Hepatitis B
    b. *Hemophilus influenzae* b
    c. Diphtheria, tetanus, pertussis
    d. Measles, mumps, rubella

44. Which of the following is an example of antimetabolites?

    a. Nitrogen mustards
    b. Ethyleneimines
    c. Adriamycin
    d. Fluorouracil

45. Which of the following antitumor antibiotics is the first-line treatment for advanced HIV-associated Kaposi's sarcoma?

    a. Doxorubicin (Adriamycin)
    b. Daunorubicin (Cerubidine)
    c. Idarubicin (Idamycin)
    d. Plicamycin (Mithracin)

46. Interferons are a group of blood proteins that have which of the following effects?

    a. Antiviral
    b. Antiprotozoal
    c. Antibiotic
    d. None of the above

47. Acyclovir is used to treat all of the following, except:
    a. Chickenpox
    b. Hepatitis B
    c. Herpes zoster (shingles)
    d. Herpes simplex encephalitis

48. Which of the following is the major adverse effect of didanosine (antiviral drug)?
    a. Hepatitis and heart failure
    b. Peripheral neuropathies and pancreatitis
    c. Nephritis and pulmonary edema
    d. Ototoxicity and glaucoma

For questions 49–53, match lettered drug to the numbered description.

DESCRIPTION

_____ 49. Used for the relief of nonproductive cough and for moderate to severe pain

_____ 50. Related to its inhibition of prostaglandin

_____ 51. Used for the treatment of osteoarthritis and rheumatoid arthritis in adults

_____ 52. Has caused liver damage in patients who consume three or more alcoholic drinks per day

_____ 53. Used for narcotic overdose

TERM

a. celecoxib
b. naloxone
c. acetaminophen
d. ibuprofen
e. hydrocodone

For questions 54–58, match lettered term to the numbered description.

DESCRIPTION

_____ 54. A fungal is also called this

_____ 55. A common opportunistic infection (candidiasis) is also known as this

_____ 56. Caused by _Plasmodium vivax_

_____ 57. Responsible for causing dysentery

_____ 58. Caused by the flagellated protozoan lamblia

TERM

a. _Entamoeba histolytica_
b. Giardiasis
c. Moniliasis
d. Malaria
e. Mycosis

Select terms from your reading to fill in the blanks.

59. _____ is prescribed for asymptomatic and symptomatic trichomoniasis in females and males.

60. Iodoquinol is an anti-infective, antiamebicide, and _____ agent.

61. Substances produced by microorganisms that, in low concentrations, are able to inhibit or kill other microorganisms are called _____.

62. The most common sources of natural antibiotics are molds and _____.

63. Systemic antibacterial agents that are able to kill microbes are called _____.

64. Today, sulfamethoxazole is the most commonly used sulfonamide and is usually combined with trimethoprim, and abbreviated _____.

65. The cephalosporins are a group of antibiotics closely related to the _____.

66. First-generation cephalosporins have their highest activity against _____ bacteria.

67. The serious adverse effects of aminoglycosides include ototoxicity and _____.

68. Macronutrients are needed by the body in relatively _____ _____ and constitute the bulk of the diet.

69. The daily requirement for carbohydrates is _____% to _____% of total caloric intake.

70. Deficiency of thiamine (vitamin B_1) leads to the disease called _____.

71. Pyridoxine (vitamin B_6) is prescribed to treat _____ during pregnancy.

72. _____ is the ability to resist infection and disease through the activation of specific defenses.

73. Active immunity is a form of acquired immunity that develops in an individual in response to an _____.

74. Immune globulin is produced by _____.

75. The treatment of patients with diphtheria requires a specific _____.

Unit 4

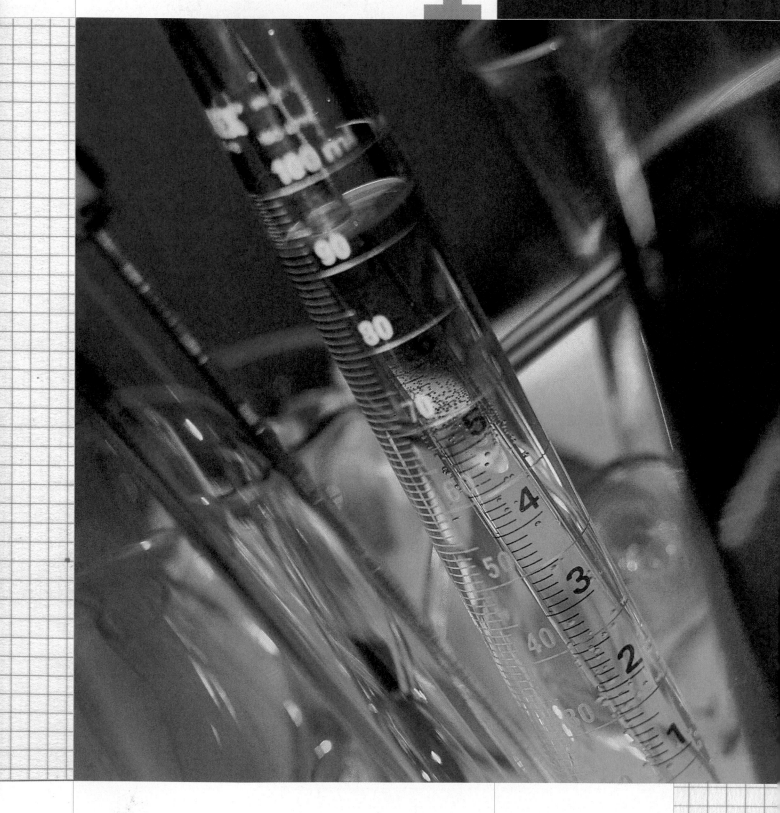

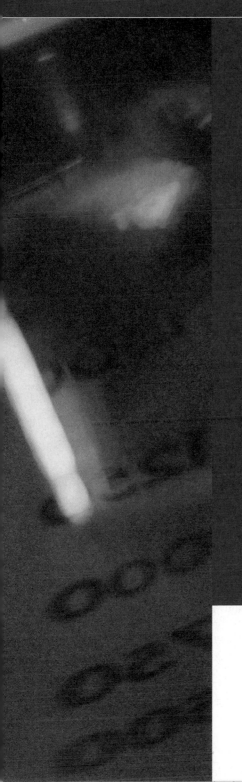

EFFECTS OF DRUGS ON SPECIFIC SYSTEMS

" Both the nervous and endocrine systems involve high-level integration in the brain and have the ability to influence processes in distant regions of the body and to extensively use negative feedback. "

Chapter 14

Chapter

Effects of Drugs on the Central Nervous System

Key Terms

PRACTICAL SCENARIO

The father of an 18-year-old teenager calls the physician's office, stating that his son, who has schizophrenia, has become increasingly withdrawn and does not seem interested in doing anything at all. He says his son is taking the antipsychotic clozapine (Clozaril), and therefore, he should be better. His father states that he is worried because his son also seems to have strange movements—he seems to move very slowly.

Critical Thinking Questions

1. As the medical assistant who takes the phone call, what might you say to alleviate some of the father's anxiety as you take down the details to relay to the physician?

2. What questions would you ask the father about his son's personality, mood, and physical changes?

3. What teaching points might you offer the father during the phone call?

Introduction

Thinking, remembering, feeling, moving, and being aware of the world require activity from the nervous system. The human brain has about 100 billion **neurons** (or nerve cells) that help to coordinate all other body functions to maintain homeostasis and to enable the body to respond to changing conditions. The neurons release chemical substances called neurotransmitters that allow communication from one nerve cell to another. The most common neurotransmitters are acetylcholine, norepinephrine, dopamine, serotonin, gamma-aminobutyric acid (GABA), and glutamate. Some mental disorders or conditions are associated with abnormal changes in the activity or amount of a specific neurotransmitter.

The Nervous System

The organs of the nervous system can be divided into two groups. One group, consisting of the brain and spinal cord, forms the **central nervous system** (CNS). The other group, composed of the nerves (peripheral nerves) that connect the central nervous system to other body parts, is called the **peripheral nervous system** (PNS). Together, these systems provide three general functions: sensory, integrative, and motor (see Figure 14-1 ■).

The brain can be divided into four major portions—the cerebrum, the diencephalon, the brainstem, and the cerebellum. The **cerebrum** (the largest part of the brain) includes nerve centers associated with sensory and motor functions and provides higher mental functions, including memory and reasoning. The cerebrum is composed of an outer cerebral cortex and inner cerebral medulla. In the medulla, there is a group of cell bodies (gray matter) known as the **basal ganglia**. The basal ganglia are involved in the regulation of motor activity. Degeneration of certain neurons within the basal ganglia is responsible for Parkinson's disease. The *diencephalon* also processes sensory information. Nerve pathways in the brainstem connect various parts of the nervous system and regulate certain visceral activities. The cerebellum includes centers that coordinate voluntary muscular movements.

The spinal cord is a slender nerve column that passes downward from the brain into the vertebral canal, continuing on to the peripheral organs and skeletal muscle,

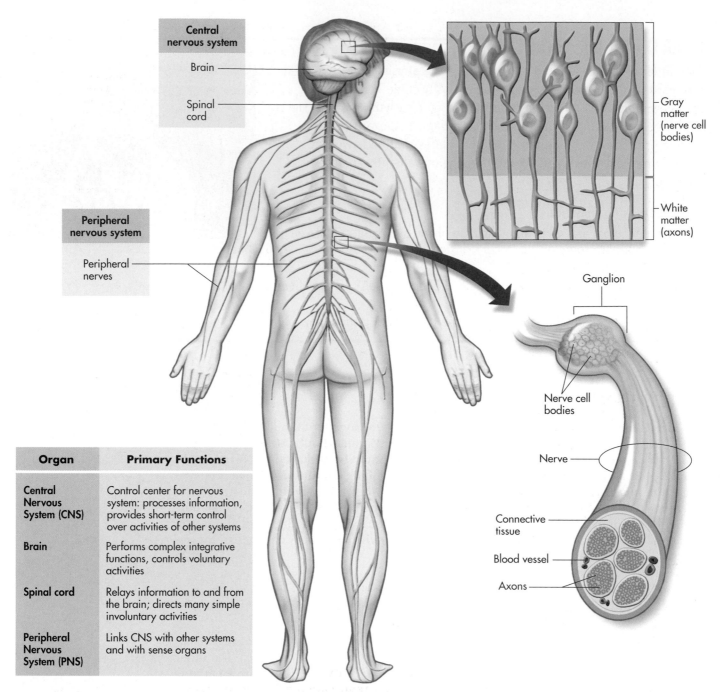

Figure 14-1 ■ The central nervous system (CNS) includes the brain and spinal cord. The peripheral nervous system includes the nerves throughout the body that exit from the spinal cord.

carrying motor impulses. Nerve axons travel from the peripheral parts of the body, such as the skin, muscles, and visceral organs to the brain, carrying sensory information (see Figure 14-2 ■).

CNS Stimulants

The CNS stimulants are a diverse group of pharmacologic agents. Many are used therapeutically and are prescription drugs—for example, the psychostimulant amphetamines.

How do they work?
The exact mechanism of action of CNS stimulants is not clear, but they stimulate the cerebral cortex and increase the activity of norepinephrine, dopamine, and other cate-

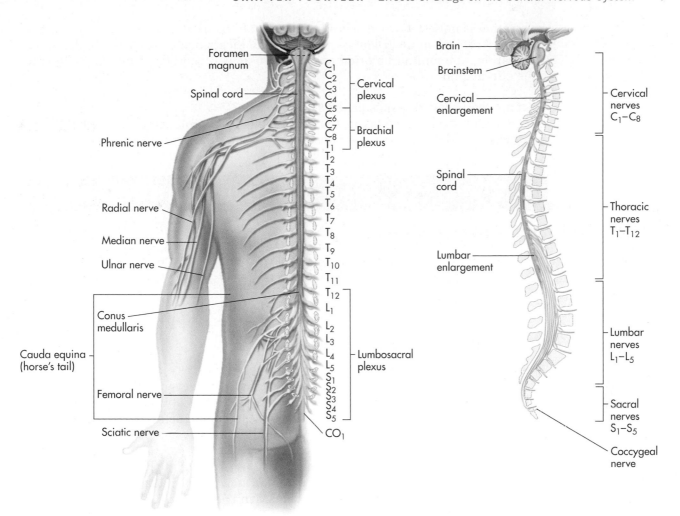

Figure 14-2 ■ The spinal cord.

cholamines at CNS **synapses** (the point of contact between nerve cells with each other or other types of cells). This increased activity can lead to many effects, which include euphoria, reduced appetite, insomnia, and wakefulness.

How are they used?

The indirect-acting sympathomimetics (for example, methylphenidate [Ritalin] and the amphetamines) are more potent CNS stimulants than caffeine but have limited therapeutic use. They are used in the treatment of attention deficit–hyperactivity disorder (ADHD), narcolepsy, and obesity. However, because these CNS stimulants convey a sense of self-confidence, well-being, and euphoria, they are highly addictive. Some of these agents are widely abused (such as amphetamines, and especially methamphetamine).

What are the adverse effects?

The most common adverse effects include headache, palpitations, cardiac dysrhythmias, hypertension, nervousness, and nausea.

What are the contraindications and interactions?

CNS stimulants are contraindicated in persons who are hypersensitive to sympathomimetic amines; have a history of drug abuse; are severely agitated; have hyperthyroidism, diabetes mellitus, moderate to severe hypertension, advanced arteriosclerosis, angina pectoris, or other cardiovascular disorders, or glaucoma. Safety during pregnancy or lactation is not established. These agents should be used cautiously in mild hypertension. Acetazolamide (Diamox) and sodium bicarbonate decrease amphetamine elimination; ammonium chloride and ascorbic acid (Ascorbicap) increase amphetamine elimination.

What are the important points patients should know?

Advise patients that when taking CNS stimulants for a prolonged period, withdrawal symptoms could occur. A gradual decrease is essential to prevent withdrawal effects.

Focus on Pediatrics

The Need for Counseling in ADHD

Families of children with attention deficit–hyperactivity disorder (ADHD) should be encouraged to seek counseling for support and reassurance. Drug treatment alone is an insufficient form of therapy.

Anxiety and Insomnia

Anxiety is a very common disorder. In many cases, anxiety is self-limiting and recourse to medications is not necessary. Occasionally, however, anxiety is so stressful and mentally painful that drug therapy is required. Anxiety and stress are part of everyday life, and it is important that education programs include life skills that help people develop coping mechanisms. Furthermore, anxiety may be accompanied by mild reactive or even endogenous depression.

Sleep, and its importance for normal living, is a process that is still little understood. Sleep disturbances are extremely common and, if continuous, have the potential to seriously disrupt normal day-to-day living. Many people with a sleep disorder want to turn to drugs to solve their problem.

Sedatives and Hypnotics

A sedative diminishes the activity of the CNS. This effect on the CNS can, in many circumstances, relieve anxiety, which is why sedatives are often referred to as *anxiolytics*. *Hypnotic* is the term used to describe a substance that induces sleep. Many of the drugs in these categories are addictive if taken regularly for even short periods. In some cases, addiction has been known to occur in about 10 days. Thus, the use of these drugs is controversial. If prescribed, they should be taken for only limited periods (no more than 7 days, under normal circumstances).

The use of hypnotics in the treatment of short-term insomnia is often beneficial in cases in which the insomnia can be predicted. There are least two stages of sleep: one called *rapid eye movement (REM)*, which is the dreaming stage, and the other, *non-REM* stage. It seems that many hypnotics upset the REM stage of sleep.

Focus Point

Sleep with Hypnotics

It is important to remember that no currently available hypnotics induce what could be termed "natural sleep."

The difference between most hypnotics and anxiolytics is the dosage, not the drug. Therefore, the drugs will be dealt with according to their chemical classification and not their therapeutic classification, except when there is no overlap.

Table 14-1 ■ Commonly Used Benzodiazepines

GENERIC NAME	TRADE NAME	AVERAGE ADULT DOSAGE	ROUTE OF ADMINISTRATION
alprazolam	Xanax	0.25–0.5 mg tid up to 4 mg/d in divided doses	PO
chlordiazepoxide	Librium	5–25 mg tid–qid	PO
		25–100 mg; then 25–50 mg tid–qid PRN	IM/IV
clorazepate	Tranxene	7.5–60 mg in divided doses tid	PO
diazepam	Valium	2–10 mg bid–qid	PO
		2–20 mg; may be repeated in 1–4 h PRN	IM, IV
		0.2 mg/kg only once q5d	Rectal
estazolam	ProSom	1–2 mg at bedtime	PO
flurazepam	Dalmane	30 mg at bedtime; 15 mg may suffice	PO
halazepam	Paxipam	20–40 mg tid–qid	PO
lorazepam	Ativan	1–10 mg/d in divided doses with largest dose at bedtime	PO
		0.05–4 mg/kg	IM
		0.044 mg/kg, but no greater than 2 mg/kg total	IV
midazolam	Versed	0.07–0.08 mg/kg 30–60 min before procedure	IM
		1–1.5 mg; may repeat in 2 min PRN	IV
oxazepam	Serax	10–30 mg tid–qid	PO
quazepam	Doral	7.5–15 mg until desired response is seen	PO
temazepam	Restoril	15–30 mg at bedtime	PO
triazolam	Halcion	0.125–0.5 mg at bedtime	PO

BENZODIAZEPINES

Benzodiazepines may be used as sedatives or hypnotics. However, it is wise to attempt treatment options with less addictive potential prior to using a benzodiazepine for this purpose. Table 14-1 ■ shows some of the most commonly prescribed benzodiazepines.

How do they work?

The mechanism of action of benzodiazepines on the CNS appears to be closely related to their ability to increase the action of the neurotransmitter GABA.

How are they used?

Indications for the use of benzodiazepines include generalized anxiety disorders, panic disorders, insomnia, myoclonic and **absence seizures** (brief seizures characterized by arrest of activity and occasional muscle contractions and relaxations), status epilepticus, and muscle relaxation. In **seizures** (abnormal electrical activity in the brain), injectable forms of diazepam (Valium) and lorazepam (Ativan) are commonly used initially to stop the repetitive seizure activity, and then, long-acting drugs such as phenytoin (Dilantin) are given to prevent the recurrence of seizures.

What are the adverse effects?

The adverse effects of benzodiazepines include drowsiness, **ataxia** (an inability to coordinate muscle activity), impaired judgment, rebound insomnia, and the development of tolerance. Overdosage may result in CNS and respiratory depression, as well as hypotension and coma. Gradual withdrawal of these drugs is recommended.

What are the contraindications and interactions?

The benzodiazepines, if taken during pregnancy, are likely to cause fetal abnormalities, and flurazepam (Dalmane) is entirely contraindicated during pregnancy. Benzodiazepines are also contraindicated in severe liver or kidney disorders and in children who are hyperactive.

Benzodiazepines increase CNS depression with alcohol and omeprazole (Prilosec). They also increase pharmacologic effects if combined with cimetidine (Tagamet), disulfiram (Antabuse), or hormonal contraceptives. The effects of benzodiazepines decrease with theophylline (Bronkodyl) and ranitidine (Zantac).

What are the important points patients should know?

Instruct patients about methods such as relaxation, they can use to decrease anxiety. Advise patients not to stop the medication abruptly after prolonged use because withdrawal symptoms may occur. Warn patients not to drink alcohol or take other CNS depressants while taking hypnotics or anxiolytics.

Instruct patients about methods to assist with sleep, such as avoiding coffee, heavy meals, and excessive stimuli close to bedtime. Caution them against driving or operating machinery, because dizziness or drowsiness might occur.

Focus Point

Oral Contraceptives and Benzodiazepines

Women who are taking benzodiazepines should not use oral contraceptives because the drug combination may cause increased sedative effects, and high levels of the benzodiazepine may accumulate in the blood plasma.

Focus on Geriatrics

Diazepam

Elderly patients usually require lower dosages of diazepam to decrease ataxia and avoid oversedation. Apnea and cardiac arrest may occur when diazepam is given to elderly patients, very ill people, and individuals with limited pulmonary reserve.

BARBITURATES

Barbiturates are classified as CNS agents, anticonvulsants, and sedative–hypnotic drugs.

How do they work?

The sedative and hypnotic effects of barbiturates such as phenobarbital (Luminal) appear to be due primarily to interference with impulse transmission of the cerebral cortex by inhibition of the reticular activating system (a part of the brain that appears to control sleep and wakefulness). CNS depression may range from mild sedation to coma, depending on dosage, route of administration, degree of nervous system excitability, and drug tolerance. Initially, barbiturates suppress REM sleep, but with chronic therapy, REM sleep returns to normal. In seizure disorders, phenobarbital limits the spread of seizure activity by increasing the threshold for motor cortex stimuli. Barbiturates are habit forming.

How are they used?

Barbiturates are primarily used to treat insomnia, although they are also used for partial **epilepsy** (brain dysfunction that is caused by excessive discharge of neurons) and tonic-clonic seizures.

What are the adverse effects?

The most common adverse effect associated with barbiturates is sedation, which can range from mild sleepiness or drowsiness, to somnolence. The barbiturate phenobarbital may also cause nausea, vomiting, constipation or diarrhea, bradycardia, skin rash, fever, and headache. The toxic effects of barbiturates include respiratory depression, circulatory shock, and renal or hepatic damage.

What are the contraindications and interactions?

Barbiturates such as phenobarbital are contraindicated in anyone with a familial history of **porphyria** (a genetic disorder caused by deficiency of enzymes of the heme biosynthetic pathway) and in cases of severe respiratory or kidney disease. They should be avoided in patients with a history of previous addiction to sedative-hypnotics or uncontrolled pain, and in women who are pregnant or lactating. Alcohol may interact with barbiturates because of these agents' similar CNS depressant qualities. The barbiturate phenobarbital may decrease absorption and increase metabolism of oral anticoagulants and may also increase metabolism of corticosteroids and oral contraceptives.

What are the important points patients should know?

Instruct patients about methods such as relaxation, they can use to decrease anxiety. Advise patients not to stop the medication abruptly after prolonged use because withdrawal symptoms may occur. Warn patients not to drink alcohol or take other CNS depressants while taking hypnotics or anxiolytics.

Instruct patients about methods to assist with sleep, such as avoiding coffee, heavy meals, and excessive stimuli close to bedtime. Caution them against driving or operating machinery, because dizziness or drowsiness that might occur.

✱ Apply Your Knowledge 14.1

The following questions focus on what you have just learned about the nervous system, CNS stimulants, and sedatives and hypnotics. *See Appendix E for the correct answers.*

FILL IN THE BLANK

Select terms from your reading to fill in the blanks.

1. Name 5 common neurotransmitters:_____, _____, _____, _____, and _____.

2. When a patient is taking CNS stimulants for a prolonged period, _____ symptoms can occur.

3. List three general functions of the nervous system: _____, _____, and _____.

4. Injury to certain neurons within the basal ganglia may cause _____.

5. Amphetamines (CNS stimulants) are used in the treatment of _____, _____, and _____.

MATCHING

Match the lettered term to the numbered description.

DESCRIPTION	TERM
1. _____ A slender nerve column in which nerve axons travel from the peripheral parts of the body	a. Brainstem
2. _____ Provides higher mental functions such as reasoning	b. Cerebrum
3. _____ Processes sensory information	c. Diencephalon
4. _____ Regulates certain visceral activities	d. Cerebellum
5. _____ Coordinates voluntary muscular movements	e. Spinal cord

(continued)

Apply Your Knowledge 14.1 (continued)

MULTIPLE CHOICE

Choose the correct answers from choices a–d.

1. Phenobarbital is contraindicated in which of the following disorders or conditions?

   a. Insomnia

   b. Porphyria

   c. Partial seizure

   d. Tonic-clonic seizure

2. When elderly patients are given diazepam, which of the following complications may occur?

   a. Epilepsy

   b. Heart attack

   c. Hypertension

   d. Cardiac arrest

3. Overdosage of benzodiazepines may result in which of the following?

   a. Epilepsy

   b. Heart attack

   c. Hypertension

   d. Cardiac arrest

4. Which of the following explains the mechanism of action of barbiturates?

   a. Interference with impulse transmission of the cerebral cortex

   b. Interference with impulse transmission of the diencephalon

   c. Inhibition of releasing hormone from the hypothalamus

   d. The mechanism of action is not clear

5. Which of the following drugs may increase CNS depression when it is used with benzodiazepines?

   a. Niacin

   b. Neomycin

   c. Alcohol

   d. Amantadine

Epilepsy

The terms **convulsion** (violent spasms) and *seizure* are often used interchangeably and basically have the same meaning. A seizure is a periodic attack of disturbed cerebral function. A seizure may also be defined as an abnormal disturbance in the electrical activity in one or more areas of the brain.

Seizures may be classified as follows: generalized **tonic–clonic** (contraction–relaxation) seizures (previously termed *grand mal*), generalized absence seizures (previously called *petit mal*), generalized myoclonic seizures, and partial seizures. Status epilepticus is an emergency condition that may result in brain injury or death if not treated immediately.

Epilepsy is a permanent, recurrent seizure disorder. Examples of the known causes of epilepsy include brain injury at birth, head injuries, and inborn errors of metabolism. In some patients, the cause of epilepsy is never determined.

Antiseizure Drugs (Anticonvulsants)

The categorizations of antiseizure drugs that follow are based on chemical structure and mechanism of action. Chemical groupings include the hydantoins, succinimides, benzodiazepines, and barbiturates.

In addition, several miscellaneous drugs are used as anticonvulsants, such as carbamazepine (Tegretol), valproic acid or valproate (Depakote), primidone (Mysoline), gabapentin (Neurontin), and lamotrigine (Lamictal). All can depress abnormal neural discharges in the CNS, resulting in an inhibition of seizure activity. Drugs that control generalized tonic–clonic seizures are not effective for absence seizures. If both conditions are present, then combined drug therapy is required. Table 14-2 ■ lists the most commonly used antiseizure medications.

Table 14-2 ■ **Most Commonly Prescribed Antiseizure Drugs**

GENERIC NAME	TRADE NAME	AVERAGE ADULT DOSAGE	ROUTE OF ADMINISTRATION
Hydantoins			
fosphenytoin	Cerebyx	Individualized	IM, IV
phenytoin	Dilantin	50–200 mg bid–tid	PO
Succinimides			
ethosuximide	Zarontin	500 mg/d	PO
methsuximide	Celontin	300–1,200 mg/d	PO
phensuximide	Milontin	1–3 g/d in divided doses	PO
Benzodiazepines			
diazepam	Valium	5–10 mg, repeat if needed at 10- to 15-min intervals to 30 mg; then repeat if needed q2–4h	IM, IV
lorazepam	Ativan	4 mg injected slowly at 2 mg/min; may repeat once after 10 min	IV
Barbiturates			
mephobarbital	Mebaral	400–600 mg/d in divided doses	PO
		Anticonvulsant: 100–300 mg/d	PO
phenobarbital	Barbital	Anticonvulsant: 200–600 mg up to 20 mg/kg	IM, IV
		Status epilepticus: 15–18 mg/kg in single or divided doses (max: 20 mg/kg)	IV
Miscellaneous Antiseizure Drugs			
carbamazepine	Tegretol	100–400 mg tid	PO
gabapentin	Neurontin	100–800 mg tid–qid	PO
lamotrigine	Lamictal	500 mg bid (maintenance) Starting dosage depends on patient weight and other variables	PO
primidone	Mysoline	250 mg–2 g in divided doses	PO
valproate	Depakote	125–250 mg tid–qid	PO
valproic acid	Depakene	100–200 mg bid–tid	PO

Focus on Natural Products

Drug Interactions with Kava

The dried crushed roots and rhizome of the kava plant, an Australasian shrubby pepper found in abundance on the islands of the South Pacific, are often used as an antiepileptic and dietary supplement to reduce stress and anxiety. Kava is available in many different oral forms, such as teas, cold drink powders, and paste. It should not be used in patients who have Parkinson's disease, and concurrent use with carbidopa and levodopa is contraindicated. Antipsychotics taken with kava may result in neuroleptic movement disorders. Barbiturates, benzodiazepines, and CNS depressants in general may cause increased sedation when taken with kava.

PHENYTOIN

The most commonly used and recognizable drug in this group is phenytoin (Dilantin), which was first synthesized in 1908. It is the sole clinical representative of the hydantoins in use as an antiseizure drug.

How does it work?

Phenytoin is a hydantoin derivative chemically related to phenobarbital (Luminal). The precise mechanism of anticonvulsant action is not known, but use of this drug is accompanied by reduced voltage, frequency, and spread of electrical discharges within the motor cortex.

How is it used?

Phenytoin is approved by the FDA for partial seizures with complex symptomatology, and tonic–clonic seizures, psychomotor, and nonepileptic seizures, such as those caused by head trauma. It is also used to prevent or treat seizures occurring during or after neurosurgery. Phenytoin is prescribed as an antiarrhythmic agent, especially in the treatment of digitalis-induced arrhythmias.

What are the adverse effects?

Phenytoin may cause blurred vision, dizziness, drowsiness, fatigue, thrombocytopenia, and aplastic anemias. Patients should be advised to use caution when driving or operating machinery, or performing tasks that require mental alertness. Serum levels above the optimal range may produce confusion, delirium, or psychosis. Dose adjustments may be necessary in patients with renal disease. Chronic use may cause gingival hyperplasia.

What are the contraindications and interactions?

Phenytoin is contraindicated in patients who are hypersensitive to the drug. It must be avoided in patients with seizures caused by hypoglycemia, sinus bradycardia, and complete or incomplete heart block, or in pregnant or lactating patients.

There are numerous drug–drug interactions with phenytoin including antacids, antidiabetic agents, **antipsychotics** (*neuroleptic* drugs that can improve thought disorders), anxiolytics, barbiturates, calcium channel blockers, cardiac glycosides, corticosteroids, estrogens, neuromuscular-blocking agents, opiate agonists, oral contraceptives, progestins, salicylates, sulfonamides, thyroid hormones, tricyclic antidepressants (TCAs), vinca alkaloids, and vitamin D analogues. Phenytoin should be used cautiously in patients with impaired liver or kidney function, alcoholism, blood disorders, and hypotension.

What are the important points patients should know?

Advise patients taking phenytoin that their urine might become discolored to a pink or red-brown color. This discoloration is harmless. For the patient with diabetes who is taking phenytoin, advise him or her that the blood glucose level should be checked more closely because phenytoin can inhibit insulin release. Also advise patients about the importance of oral hygiene and regular dental checkups to prevent gingivitis and gingival hyperplasia.

Focus on Geriatrics

Phenytoin

Phenytoin should be used cautiously, and at lower doses, in elderly patients to avoid toxicity.

VALPROIC ACID

Valproic acid (Depakote) is used to treat simple and complex absence seizures. It has been used for other generalized seizures, including primary generalized tonic–clonic, atypical absence, myoclonic, or atonic seizures.

How does it work?

The mechanism of action of valproic acid is unknown. It may be related to the increased bioavailability of the inhibitor neurotransmitter GABA to brain neurons.

How is it used?

Valproic acid is used alone or with other anticonvulsants in the management of absence and mixed seizures, mania, and in migraine headache prophylaxis. It is the drug of choice for symptomatic and idiopathic generalized seizures, juvenile myoclonic epilepsy, and childhood absence seizures.

What are the adverse effects?

Adverse effects of valproic acid include nausea, vomiting, hypersalivation, abdominal cramps, liver failure, and cases of life-threatening pancreatitis. Sedation and drowsiness are the most frequently reported. There are considerable hematologic effects, and because it inhibits the secondary phase of platelet aggregation, it may prolong bleeding time.

What are the contraindications and interactions?

Safe use of valproic acid during pregnancy has not been established. Patients taking valproic acid may develop clotting abnormalities. Additive CNS depression may occur when valproic acid is administered with other CNS depressants. Valproic acid may potentiate the effects of monoamine oxidase inhibitors (MAOIs) and other antidepressant drugs. This drug may alter some laboratory tests such as thyroid function and urinary ketones. Alcohol and other CNS depressants potentiate its depressant effects. Haloperidol (Haldol), loxapine (Loxitane), maprotiline (Maprotiline HCl), phenothiazines, and TCAs can increase CNS depression or lower seizure thresholds. Aspirin and warfarin (Coumadin) increase the risk of spontaneous bleeding and decrease clotting. Cimetidine (Tagamet) may increase valproic acid levels and toxicity.

What are the important points patients should know?

Valproic acid may irritate the mouth, throat, and stomach, so if patients are taking the capsule form, instruct them to swallow the capsules whole and not chew, crush, or break them. The syrup form of valproic acid may be added to foods or liquids for a better taste. It is advisable to take valproic acid with meals or snacks to reduce stomach upset.

ETHOSUXIMIDE

Succinimides are anticonvulsant agents. There is only one member of this group still used in clinical practice—ethosuximide (Zarontin). Ethosuximide is the drug of choice for control of uncomplicated absence seizures. It is generally considered to be the safest of the succinimide drugs. The FDA approved ethosuximide in 1960 as a succinimide-derived anticonvulsant.

How does it work?

Ethosuximide acts to stabilize neuronal excitability, thereby raising the threshold of uncontrolled cerebral discharges (especially within the motor cortex). It does this by delaying the entry of calcium into neuron cells by blocking calcium channels. It suppresses the electroencephalogram (EEG) pattern associated with lapses of consciousness in absence seizures. Its actual mechanism of action is not understood, but it may act to inhibit neuronal systems.

How is it used?

Ethosuximide is used to manage absence seizures in adults and children older than 6 years, myoclonic seizures, and akinetic epilepsy. This agent may be administered with other anticonvulsants when other forms of epilepsy coexist with absence seizures. It is the drug of choice for absence seizures during pregnancy because it is much less teratogenic than other drugs in this category.

What are the adverse effects?

Common adverse effects of ethosuximide include drowsiness, hiccups, ataxia, dizziness, headache, euphoria, restlessness, anxiety, blurred vision, and aggressiveness. Pancytopenia (abnormal reduction in red and white blood cells and platelets), nausea, vomiting, anorexia, abdominal pain, weight loss, diarrhea, and gingival hyperplasia are also seen. Vaginal bleeding, agranulocytosis (depression of granulocyte-producing bone marrow), aplastic anemia, alopecia (hair loss), and muscle weakness have been associated with ethosuximide therapy. Abnormal liver and kidney function test results are sometimes seen.

What are the contraindications and interactions?

Contraindications include hypersensitivity to succinimides and severe liver or kidney disease. Safety during pregnancy, lactation, or in children younger than 3 years is not established. Ethosuximide decreases serum levels of primidone (Mysoline). Carbamazepine (Tegretol) decreases ethosuximide levels, and isoniazid (Nydrazid, Laniazid) significantly increases ethosuximide levels.

What are the important points patients should know?

Advise patients about the possibility of blood disorders and instruct them to report any signs of a sore throat, fever, or bruising of unknown cause to their physician. Warn them against driving or working with heavy machinery because of the adverse effects of succinimides.

CARBAMAZEPINE

Carbamazepine (Tegretol) is an oral anticonvulsant drug similar to TCAs. It is used to treat partial seizures, both simple and complex, and for tonic–clonic seizures. It is the drug of choice in symptomatic partial seizures. This drug is preferred over phenobarbital because it has fewer adverse effects on behavior and alertness. Carbamazepine is also the drug of choice in treatment of neuralgias, particularly trigeminal neuralgia (intense pain in the lips, eyes, nose, scalp, forehead, and upper or lower jaw).

How does it work?

Carbamazepine promotes sodium **efflux** (the process of flowing out) across the nerve membranes. As a consequence, carbamazepine reduces neuronal excitability, especially repeated firing of the same neuron. Unlike phenytoin, carbamazepine leaves the motor cortex relatively unaffected.

How is it used?

FDA-approved uses are for partial seizures, tonic–clonic seizures, and trigeminal neuralgia. However, this drug is often used to treat many other disorders, such as depression and bipolar disorder.

What are the adverse effects?

Severe cardiovascular disturbances, blood disorders, altered urination, and liver or kidney dysfunctions are adverse effects of carbamazepine, in addition to those generally associated with antiseizure drugs. Elderly patients may be more susceptible to confusion or agitation. Carbamazepine commonly causes blurred vision, dizziness, drowsiness, and fatigue.

What are the contraindications and interactions?

Absolute contraindications for use of carbamazepine are hypersensitivity and cardiac or liver impairment. It should be used with extreme caution in pregnant women because it crosses the placenta and has been implicated in a number of fetal abnormalities.

Drug interactions occur with antineoplastic agents, antiretroviral protease inhibitors, barbiturates, calcium channel blockers, corticosteroids, MAOIs, neuromuscular blockers, opiate agonists, oral contraceptives, progestins, estrogens, halogenated anesthetics, thyroid hormones, and TCAs.

What are the important points patients should know?

Inform patients about the possibility of blood disorders. Advise them to report any signs of a sore throat, mucosal ulceration, petechiae (minute hemorrhagic spots in the skin), or bruising of unknown cause.

✳ Apply Your Knowledge 14.2 ▬

The following questions focus on what you have just learned about the antiseizure medications. *See Appendix E for the correct answers.*

MULTIPLE CHOICE
Choose the correct answers from choices a–d.

1. The only clinical representative of hydantoins in use as an antiseizure drug is:
   a. Valproic acid
   b. Phenobarbital
   c. Carbamazepine
   d. Phenytoin

2. The formerly used name for tonic–clonic seizures was which of the following?
   a. Grand mal
   b. Petit mal
   c. Psychomotor
   d. Nonepileptic

3. Dose adjustments for patients who use phenytoin may be necessary in patients with which of the following disorders?
   a. Seizures
   b. Fever
   c. Renal disease
   d. Lyme disease

(continued)

Apply Your Knowledge 14.2 (continued)

4. Valproic acid is used to treat simple and complex absence seizures. These types of seizures were formerly termed:

   a. Grand mal

   b. Petit mal

   c. Neuroclonic

   d. Atomic

5. The most frequently reported adverse nervous system effects of valproic acid are:

   a. Hyperactivity and hunger

   b. Thirst and chest pains

   c. Headache and palpitations

   d. Sedation and drowsiness

6. Which of the following is the drug of first choice in the treatment of absence seizures during pregnancy?

   a. Primidone

   b. Valproic acid

   c. Ethosuximide

   d. Phenytoin

MATCHING
Match the lettered drug trade name to the numbered generic drug name.

GENERIC NAME	TRADE NAME
1. _____ methsuximide	a. Dilantin
2. _____ lorazepam	b. Mebaral
3. _____ fosphenytoin	c. Valium
4. _____ ethosuximide	d. Celontin
5. _____ mephobarbital	e. Milontin
6. _____ phensuximide	f. Cerebyx
7. _____ phenytoin	g. Ativan
8. _____ diazepam	h. Zarontin

Parkinson's Disease

Parkinson's disease was first described by the English physician James Parkinson in 1817. It is a disease that principally occurs in elderly individuals, but can develop in middle-aged people as well. Parkinson's disease is a nervous system disorder characterized by movement abnormalities such as tremor of the extremities and head, and great difficulty in coordination of fine muscle movement. The other salient feature is *hypokinesia,* an inability or slowness in initiating movements. Other signs and symptoms include a shuffling gait and skeletal muscle rigidity. Often, the affected person breaks into a run to stop from falling.

The incidence of Parkinson's disease is about 1% in people older than 60 years, so it is not an uncommon disease. Its cause is unknown, but a considerable amount is known about the CNS defect that leads to the illness.

This defect is in the basal ganglia portion of the midbrain known as the **substantia nigra** (a large cell mass involved in metabolic disturbances associated with Parkinson's disease). This part of the brain is important in the initiation and control of muscular movement. Skeletal muscle movements are initiated in the motor cortex of the brain, and pass through the basal ganglia and thalamus to the spinal cord along the corticospinal tract.

In the pathways of the substantia nigra, there is a balance between dopamine and acetylcholine in normal individuals. In patients with Parkinson's disease, a lack of dopaminergic activity leads to an imbalance between these neurotransmitters (Figure 14-3 ■).

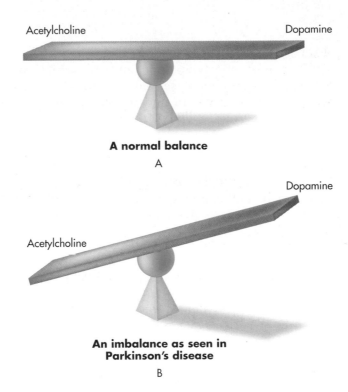

A normal balance

A

An imbalance as seen in Parkinson's disease

B

Figure 14-3 ■ (A) Normal and (B) abnormal balance between dopamine and acetylcholine.

Parkinsonism is a term that refers to the symptoms produced by certain drugs, poisons, and traumatic lesions in the basal ganglia. When the cause is known, the disease is termed *secondary parkinsonism*, as opposed to *primary parkinsonism*. Secondary parkinsonism is sometimes only temporary if the symptoms are caused by drugs. Secondary parkinsonism is not the same as Parkinson's disease.

There is no cure for Parkinson's disease. Drugs have been developed that can help patients manage many of the symptoms, but they do not stop the progression of the disease. However, patients who suffer from Parkinson's disease frequently experience dramatic swings in mobility and mood (known as being "on" or "off"), which may depend on the severity of the disease, or the timing of the medication doses.

Because surgical treatment is still experimental, the usual way to treat this condition is to try to rebalance dopamine and acetylcholine by using drugs. Two methods are used to correct the condition: decrease the muscarinic activity (by using antimuscarinic drugs) or increase the dopaminergic activity (by increasing dopamine levels, blocking its breakdown, or mimicking its action).

Anticholinergic Drugs (Muscarinic Antagonists)

The most commonly used agents in this class are benztropine (Cogentin) and trihexyphenidyl (Trihexy). Amantadine (Symmetrel) is sometimes useful for tremor or for making levodopa work better, but exactly how it works is not clear. It may also dramatically reduce dyskinesia (difficulty in making voluntary movements) in some patients.

How do they work?

Anticholinergic agents work by inhibiting the muscarine receptors in the basal ganglia, lessening the imbalance between the extrapyramidal and pyramidal pathways by blocking the effect of acetylcholine. Table 14-3 ■ lists anticholinergic drugs used for Parkinson's disease.

How are they used?

Only centrally acting anticholinergic drugs are effective for Parkinson's disease. These medications can also be prescribed in combination with other antiparkinsonian drugs.

What are the adverse effects?

CNS adverse effects include anxiety, which is experienced by 30 to 50% of all patients, and more seriously, agitation or confusion. The anticholinergic effects include dry mouth and decreased sweating and heat release. Other serious adverse reactions include urticaria, urine retention, paresthesias, and sinus tachycardia.

What are the contraindications and interactions?

Safe use of anticholinergic agents in pregnant patients has not been established. They should not be given with other antimuscarinics because additive effects may occur.

What are the important points patients should know?

Instruct patients to avoid alcohol consumption because this combination may intensify the CNS depressant effects. Advise patients that constipation can occur and urge them to consume a high-fiber diet. Because drowsiness is a common effect of these drugs, advise patients to avoid driving a car or operating heavy machinery.

Table 14-3 ■ Anticholinergic Drugs Used for Parkinson's Disease

GENERIC NAME	TRADE NAME	AVERAGE ADULT DOSAGE	ROUTE OF ADMINISTRATION
benztropine	Cogentin	0.5–1 mg/d; gradually increase as needed up to 6 mg/d	PO
biperiden	Akineton	2 mg 1–4 times/d	PO
diphenhydramine	Benadryl	25–50 mg tid–qid	PO
procyclidine	Kemadrin	2.5–5 mg tid	PO
trihexyphenidyl	Artane	1 mg for Day 1; 2 mg on Day 2; then increase by 2 mg every 3–5 d up to 6–10 mg/d	PO

Dopaminergic Drugs

The first drug approved specifically for Parkinson's disease (in 1970)—and still the most commonly administered therapy—is levodopa (Larodopa). In most patients, it significantly improves mobility and allows them to function relatively normally.

A number of chemicals, such as carbidopa (a drug that prevents peripheral metabolism of levodopa and is marketed as Lodosyn), are able to prolong the effects of levodopa and help reduce its effects. The combination drug carbidopa–levodopa is marketed in the United States as Sinemet. Dopaminergic agents used for Parkinson's disease are listed in Table 14-4 ■.

How do they work?

Dopaminergic agents such as levodopa are metabolic precursors of dopamine, a catecholamine neurotransmitter. Unlike dopamine, levodopa readily crosses the blood–brain barrier. Its precise mechanism of action is unknown.

How are they used?

The dopaminergic agent levodopa is used in idiopathic Parkinson's disease, postencephalitic and arteriosclerotic parkinsonism, and in parkinsonism symptoms associated with manganese and carbon monoxide poisoning.

What are the adverse effects?

The debilitating side effects of dopaminergic agents include dyskinesia, hallucinations, and mental confusion. A major long-term complication is loss of efficacy after about 5 years of therapy. Abrupt discontinuation should be avoided because some patients experience a complex called *neuroleptic malignant syndrome (NMS)*, especially if they are also taking **neuroleptic** agents (psychotropic drugs used to treat psychosis). Manifestations of NMS include tachycardia, muscular rigidity, fever, mental status changes, diaphoresis, tachypnea, and increases in serum creatinine levels.

What are the contraindications and interactions?

Dopaminergic agents should be administered with extreme caution to patients who have cardiac disease. Other drugs work differently. So-called *dopamine agonists,* such as bromocriptine (Parlodel), ropinirole (Requip), pergolide (Permax), and pramipexole dihydrochloride (Mirapex), work directly on the target cells of the substantia nigra in a way that imitates dopamine. Dopamine agonists are often used in combination with levodopa.

Unfortunately, all drugs used to treat Parkinson's disease may have side effects. Although some people never experience such side effects, others are very sensitive to the medications and may be unable to tolerate them. Most commonly, the side effects of antiparkinsonian drugs are mental confusion, hallucinations, and dyskinesia. Because effective treatment of Parkinson's disease is often a matter of balancing beneficial effects of drugs against their side effects, many people prefer to see experienced specialists.

What are the important points patients should know?

Instruct patients to take dopaminergic agents such as levodopa with food to avoid gastrointestinal (GI) irritation. Levodopa may discolor urine and perspiration. Advise patients to avoid foods rich in vitamin B_6 (such as beans and cereals) and alcohol. Bromocriptine can cause postural hypotension; so advise patients to rise slowly from a lying position. Also instruct patients to regularly visit their dentist to prevent dental problems caused by the inhibition of salivation. Dopaminergic agents should never be stopped abruptly because of possible rebound of parkinsonism.

Table 14-4 ▪ Dopaminergic Drugs Used for Parkinson's Disease

GENERIC NAME	TRADE NAME	AVERAGE ADULT DOSAGE	ROUTE OF ADMINISTRATION
amantadine	Symmetrel	100 mg bid	PO
bromocriptine	Parlodel	1.25–2.5 mg/d up to 100 mg/d in divided doses	PO
carbidopa–levodopa	Sinemet	1 tablet containing 10 mg carbidopa/100 mg levodopa or 25 mg carbidopa/100 mg levodopa tid; increased by 1 tablet every day or every other day up to 6 tablets/d	PO
levodopa	L-Dopa, Larodopa	500 mg–1 g/d	PO
pergolide	Permax	Start with 0.05 mg/d for 2 d; then increase by 0.1 or 0.15 mg/d q3d for 12 d; and then increase by 0.25 mg every 3rd day until reaching the desired effect	PO
pramipexole	Mirapex	Start with 0.125 mg tid for 1 wk; double this dose for the next week; continue to increase by 0.25 mg/dose tid q1wk to the desired dose of 1.5 mg tid	PO
ropinirole	Requip	Start with 0.25 mg tid; increase q1wk by 0.25 mg/dose to the target dose of 1 mg tid	PO
tolcapone	Tasmar	100 mg tid (max: 600 mg/d)	PO

✳ Apply Your Knowledge 14.3

The following questions focus on what you have just learned about Parkinson's disease and antiparkinsonian drugs. *See Appendix E for the correct answers.*

FILL IN THE BLANK
Select terms from your reading to fill in the blanks.

1. Parkinsonism refers to the symptoms that are caused by traumatic lesions or certain drugs in the _____.
2. The first drug approved specifically for Parkinson's disease (in 1970) was _____.
3. Dopaminergic drugs are metabolic precursors of _____.
4. The incidence of Parkinson's disease is about _____ in people older than age _____.
5. In the pathways of the substantia nigra, there is a balance between dopamine and _____ in normal individuals.
6. Difficulty in making voluntary movements in some patients is called _____.
7. Since surgical treatment for Parkinson's disease is still experimental, the usual way to treat this condition is to try to rebalance _____ and _____ through drug therapy.
8. Anticholinergic agents work by inhibiting the _____ receptors in the basal ganglia.

MATCHING
Match the lettered drug trade name to the numbered generic name.

GENERIC NAME	TRADE NAME
1. _____ pergolide	a. Mirapex
2. _____ tolcapone	b. Tasmar
3. _____ amantadine	c. Parlodel
4. _____ bromocriptine	d. Symmetrel
5. _____ pramipexole	e. Permax

Schizophrenia

Schizophrenia is one of the most common psychotic disorders. Almost 1.6% of the population (about 2 million people in the United States), across all cultural groups, are affected by this disorder during their lifetimes. It occurs more commonly in urban populations and in lower socioeconomic groups. The cause of schizophrenia is unknown.

Manifestations of schizophrenia include either positive or negative symptoms. Positive symptoms tend to be exaggerations of normal functioning. For example, a distortion of perceptions may manifest as hallucinations (hearing or seeing things that are not real) and as distortions of thought processes, which may manifest as delusions. Negative symptoms include terseness in speech, social withdrawal, anhedonia (the inability to experience pleasure), and apathy. Symptoms usually manifest during the early years of adulthood. The illness is chronic, and less than 20% of patients recover fully from a single episode of psychosis.

PSYCHOACTIVE DRUGS

The past three decades of research in the neurosciences have dramatically increased our understanding of the neurobehavioral aspects of mental illness. The 1990s were referred to as the *decade of the brain*, and the more recent discovery of the human genome was accomplished in 2000. Historically, the advent of the first psychotropic medications in the 1950s significantly changed the treatment of the mentally ill.

More than 1,500 compounds, classified as *psychoactive* or *psychotropic* drugs, have been described. Approximately 20% of all prescriptions written in the United States are for medications intended to alter mental processes and behavior. Those agents used in the treatment of psychotic illnesses and depressant disorders are the focus of this chapter. One of the major uses of the antipsychotic drugs is the treatment of schizophrenia.

Antipsychotic Drugs

The terms *antipsychotic* and *neuroleptic* are used interchangeably to denote a group of drugs that have been used mainly for treating schizophrenia but are also effective in some other psychoses and agitated states. A new type of antipsychotic medication became available with the introduction of clozapine (Clozaril) in 1990. After its success, other medications with similar clinical profiles were developed. These *atypical* antipsychotic agents are effective against both the positive and the negative symptoms of schizophrenia. Although the atypical agents are more expensive than the typical drugs, recent evaluations of the total costs of treatment show that the atypical drugs are economically superior. This is because the increased efficacy and higher rate of compliance result in fewer hospital admissions and other emergency interventions.

Typical antipsychotics are available in several different groups. Structurally, they can be divided into phenothiazines, thioxanthenes, butyrophenones, dihydroindolone derivatives, and dibenzodiazepines. Common typical and atypical antipsychotic drugs are listed in Table 14-5 ■.

How do they work?

The mechanism of action of the antipsychotic agents is complex, and many details remain to be established. However, evaluation of properties shared by effective antipsychotic agents provides clues to their mechanism of action. All of the typical antipsychotic agents block postsynaptic dopaminergic receptors and act as competitive antagonists of dopamine centrally and peripherally.

How are they used?

Antipsychotic drugs are effective mainly against the positive symptoms of schizophrenia. In addition to their use in treating schizophrenia, several of these drugs are also effective antiemetic and antinausea agents.

What are the adverse effects?

The main adverse effects of antipsychotic drugs include sedation, dry mouth, sexual dysfunction, **akathisia** (difficulty in initiating muscle movement), **bradykinesia** (extremely slow movement), rigidity, and sometimes, **tardive dyskinesia** (slowed ability to make voluntary movements).

What are the contraindications and interactions?

Many of the contraindications to the use of these drugs are similar. They are contraindicated in comatose patients who have received large amounts of CNS depressant drugs (such as alcohol and barbiturates).

What are the important points patients should know?

Advise family members of psychiatric outpatients about the adverse effects of drug therapy and any adverse reactions that may occur because they will be responsible for administering antipsychotic drugs to the patient. They should suggest that the patient use hard candy or ice chips for a dry mouth. Inform the patient not to drive a car or operate machinery until a maintenance dose has been established. Instruct patients who are taking phenothiazines such as chlorpromazine (Thorazine) that their urine may turn pink or red-brown and that this discoloration is not harmful.

Table 14-5 ■ Common Typical and Atypical Antipsychotic Drugs

GENERIC NAME	TRADE NAME	AVERAGE ADULT DOSAGE	ROUTE OF ADMINISTRATION
Typical			
chlorpromazine	Thorazine	25–100 mg tid–qid up to 1,000 mg/d	PO
		25–50 mg up to 600 mg q4–6h. Switch to oral dosage as soon as possible.	IM
fluphenazine	Permitil, Prolixin	0.5–10 mg/d in divided doses q6–8h; usual daily dose is less than 3 mg	PO
		2.5–10 mg/d (range: 2.5–10 mg) q6–8h	IM
haloperidol	Haldol	Initial dosage range: 0.5–5 mg bid–tid	PO
		2–5 mg (up to 10–30 mg) q60 min or q4–8h PRN. Switch to oral dose as soon as possible.	IM
lithium	Eskalith, Lithobid	600 mg tid or 900 mg slow-release form bid to produce effective serum levels of 1–1.5 mEq/L	PO
loxapine	Loxitane	Initially, 10 mg bid, rapidly increased to 60–100 mg/d in 2–4 divided doses	IM
		12.5–50 mg q4–6h; once controlled, change to oral dose	IM
mesoridazine	Serentil	Initially, 50 mg tid up to 400 mg/d	PO
		25 mg; may repeat in 30–60 min	IM
molindone	Moban	50–75 mg/d in 3–4 divided doses; may be increased to 100 mg/d in 3–4 d	PO

Table 14-5 ■ Common Typical and Atypical Antipsychotic Drugs

GENERIC NAME	TRADE NAME	AVERAGE ADULT DOSAGE	ROUTE OF ADMINISTRATION
perphenazine	Trilafon	4–16 mg bid–qid; reduce as soon as possible; avoid dosages greater than 64 mg/d	PO
		Initially 5–10 mg q6h not exceeding 30 mg/d	IM
		Dilute to 0.5 mg per mL; give no more than 1 mg per injection at no less than 1- to 2-min intervals; do not exceed 5-mg total dose	IV
prochlorperazine	Compazine	Initially 5–10 mg tid–qid; gradually increase q2–3 d up to 50–150 mg/d	PO
		10–20 mg q2–4h; switch to oral therapy as soon as possible	IM
		2.5–10 mg q6–8h (max: 40 mg/d)	IV
		25 mg bid up to 40 mg/d	Rectal
promazine	Sparine	10–200 mg q4–6h up to 1,000 mg/d	PO/IM
thioridazine	Mellaril	50–100 mg tid; may increase up to 800 mg/d	PO
trifluoperazine	Stelazine	1–2 mg bid; may increase up to 20 mg/d in hospitalized patients	PO
		1–2 mg q4–6h (max: 10 mg/d)	IM
Atypical			
aripiprazole	Abilify	10–15 mg/d	PO
clozapine	Clozaril	25 mg/d in 1–2 doses; gradually increase by 25–50 mg/d up to 300–450 mg/d by end of Week 2	PO
olanzapine	Zyprexa	5–10 mg/d; increase by 5 mg/d at 1 wk intervals	PO
quetiapine	Seroquel	25 mg bid; increase by 25–50 mg bid up to 800 mg/d	PO
risperidone	Risperdal	1 mg bid; increase by 1 mg bid up to 3 mg bid	PO
risperidone	Risperdal	20 mg bid with food up to 80 mg bid	PO
ziprasidone	Geodon	40 mg/d	IM, PO

LITHIUM CARBONATE

Lithium carbonate (Eskalith) can control symptoms in both the manic and the depressive phases of psychotic disorders and is also used to treat bipolar disorder.

How does it work?

Lithium's exact mechanism of action is unclear. Therefore, therapeutic levels of lithium must be considered individually. Therapeutic effects usually take 1 to 2 weeks to be observed.

How is it used?

Lithium is used in the control and the prophylaxis of acute mania and the acute manic phase of mixed bipolar disorder.

What are the adverse effects?

Common adverse effects of lithium include nausea and tremors, which subside with continued treatment. Overdose may cause vomiting, diarrhea, dizziness, headache, drowsiness, tinnitus, loss of equilibrium, disorientation, and short-term memory loss. Toxic levels may cause kidney and heart damage. Therefore, serum concentration levels should be monitored on a regular basis.

What are the contraindications and interactions?

Lithium should be avoided in pregnant women or patients with thyroid disorders. Carbamazepine (Tegretol), haloperidol (Haldol), and phenothiazines increase the risk of neurotoxicity when they are used with lithium.

What are the important points patients should know?

Advise patients to drink plenty of fluids, at least 2 to 3 liters per day, during the stabilization period and at least 1–1-1/2 liters per day during ongoing therapy. Alert them that urine output will be increased and diluted, and that they may have persistent thirst. Dose reduction may be indicated. Instruct patients to contact their physician if diarrhea or fever develops. Warn patients to avoid hot environments and excessive use of caffeinated beverages. Warn patients against driving or engaging in other potentially hazardous activities until response to the drug is known.

Focus Point

Lithium, Contraception, and Pregnancy

Women who are taking lithium should use effective contraceptive measures. If therapy must be continued during pregnancy, serum lithium levels should be closely monitored to prevent toxicity.

✳ Apply Your Knowledge 14.4

The following questions focus on what you have just learned about psychoactive drugs. *See Appendix E for the correct answers.*

MATCHING

Match the lettered drug trade name to the numbered generic name.

GENERIC NAME	TRADE NAME
1. _____ lithium	a. Loxitane
2. _____ prochlorperazine	b. Haldol
3. _____ chlorpromazine	c. Mellaril
4. _____ haloperidol	d. Compazine
5. _____ clozapine	e. Stelazine
6. _____ trifluoperazine	f. Thorazine
7. _____ thioridazine	g. Eskalith
8. _____ loxapine	h. Clozaril

FILL IN THE BLANK

Select terms from your reading to fill in the blanks.

1. Atypical antipsychotic agents are effective against _____.

2. Therapeutic effects of lithium usually take a period of _____.

3. Patients who are taking _____ such as chlorpromazine (Thorazine) may notice that their urine turns pink or red-brown.

4. The increased efficacy and higher rate of compliance among patients taking _____ antipsychotics results in fewer hospital admissions and other emergency interventions than among those taking _____ antipsychotics.

5. A patient who uses lithium should drink plenty of liquids, at least _____ per day, during stabilization.

Depression

Major depression is one of the most common psychiatric disorders in the United States. About 5 to 6% of the population is depressed. Depression may be "reactive" (in response to a stimulus such as the loss of a loved one) or "endogenous" (a chemical disorder in the brain). The majority of antidepressant medications are used chiefly in the management of endogenous depression. Symptoms of depression include feelings of doom, lack of self-worth, the inability to sense pleasure, loss of energy, inability to concentrate, changes in sleep habits, and thoughts of suicide.

[handwritten margin notes: loss of hope / loss of appetite / suicide attempt / neglect physical appearance / isolation]

ANTIDEPRESSANTS

Antidepressants are classified into several groups on the basis of their chemical structures and antidepressant action in the brain. The most commonly used drugs are listed in Table 14-6 ■, and include TCAs, MAOIs, and selective serotonin reuptake inhibitors (SSRIs).

Table 14-6 ■ Classifications of Antidepressants

GENERIC NAME	TRADE NAME	AVERAGE ADULT DOSAGE	ROUTE OF ADMINISTRATION
Tricyclic Antidepressants			
amitriptyline	Elavil	Up to 300 mg/d in divided doses	PO
amoxapine	Asendin	Start at 50 mg bid–tid; may increase on Day 3 to 100 mg tid	PO
clomipramine	Anafranil	50–150 mg/d in single or divided doses	PO
desipramine	Norpramin	100–300 mg/d	PO
doxepin	Sinequan	25–30 mg/d in divided doses	PO
imipramine	Tofranil	75–300 mg/d in divided doses	PO
nortriptyline	Aventyl, Pamelor	25 mg tid–qid	PO
protriptyline	Vivactil	15–40 mg/d in 3–4 divided doses (max: 60 mg/d)	PO
trimipramine	Surmontil	100–300 mg/d in divided doses	PO
Monoamine Oxidase Inhibitors			
phenelzine	Nardil	15 mg tid rapidly increased to at least 60 mg/d; may need up to 90 mg/d	PO
tranylcypromine	Parnate	30–60 mg/d in divided doses at 3-wk interval	PO
Selective Serotonin Reuptake Inhibitors			
citalopram	Celexa	20–40 mg/d	PO
fluoxetine	Prozac, Prozac weekly, Sarafem	20 mg/d in morning; may increase by 40–80 mg/d in divided doses; weekly dose: 1 capsule/wk	PO
fluvoxamine	Luvox	50–300 mg/d in divided doses	PO
paroxetine	Paxil	20–50 mg/d	PO
sertraline	Zoloft	50–200 mg/d	PO

Tricyclic Antidepressants (TCAs)

Historically, drugs from this group have been the first choice in the treatment of depression and include imipramine (Tofranil), amitriptyline (Elavil), doxepin (Sinequan), and related drugs.

How do they work?
The TCAs increase the effect of both norepinephrine and serotonin in the CNS by blocking their reuptake by the neurons.

How are they used?
The TCAs are used for endogenous depression and occasionally for reactive depression.

What are the adverse effects?
Adverse effects derive from the fact that the TCAs have secondary actions, including antimuscarinic, antihistamine, and antiadrenergic activity. The first action accounts for dry mouth, blurred vision, constipation, urine retention, and tachycardia. Mental confusion and sedation arise from a central antihistamine action, and postural hypotension can occur as a result of an antiadrenergic effect. When used together with antihypertensive agents, orthostatic hypotension may increase. Norepinephrine and other sympathomimetics may increase cardiac toxicity when they are used with TCAs.

What are the contraindications and interactions?
TCAs are contraindicated in patients who are hypersensitive to these drugs. They must be avoided in patients during the acute recovery period after a heart attack, or in patients with severe renal or hepatic impairment. MAOIs may precipitate hyperpyrexic crisis, tachycardia, or seizures as a result of drug interaction with TCAs.

What are the important points patients should know?
Warn patients against stopping TCAs abruptly. Advise patients to take these drugs at bedtime to promote a normal sleep pattern. Instruct the patient to report having severe postural hypotension to their physician, and explain that the drug's effectiveness begins after about 2 weeks of use. Antidepressant treatment needs to continue even after recovery because of the potential for a relapse.

Focus on Geriatrics

Effect of TCAs on Prostate Gland

Elderly men with enlarged prostate glands are at higher risk for urine retention when taking TCAs.

Focus Point

TCAs and Other Medications

Patients taking TCAs should not take any medications, including over-the-counter (OTC) medications, without notifying their physician.

Focus on Natural Products

Drug Interactions with St. John's Wort

St. John's wort is a flower grown throughout the world and is used to treat mild to moderate depression and anxiety. It is administered orally for this purpose. St. John's wort should not be used during pregnancy and lactation. Interactions with St. John's wort occur with TCAs, MAOIs, selective serotonin reuptake inhibitors (SSRIs), alcohol, and foods high in tyramine or catecholamines. The major problem in using St. John's wort for depression and anxiety is that this herbal supplement may take 4–6 weeks to become effective. It may also cause increased photosensitivity.

Selective Serotonin Reuptake Inhibitors (SSRIs)

SSRIs are relatively newer antidepressants that have had a tremendous impact on prescribing patterns. They are now considered the first-line drugs in the treatment of major depression.

How do they work?

SSRIs primarily block the effect of serotonin reuptake. Clinical studies have found that generally, the SSRIs have comparable efficacy to the TCAs. However, the TCAs have been found to be more effective in the treatment of severe depression.

How are they used?

SSRIs are commonly used for depression, geriatric depression, obsessive–compulsive disorder, bulimia nervosa, and premenstrual dysphoric disorder.

What are the adverse effects?

In general, the adverse effects of SSRIs are relatively mild, of shorter duration than those of TCAs, and diminish as treatment continues. Cardiac toxicity and the risk of death after overdose are less likely than with the TCAs. Common adverse effects include headache, nausea, vomiting, tremor, insomnia, dizziness, and diarrhea.

What are the contraindications and interactions?

SSRI drugs must be avoided in patients who are hypersensitive to them. SSRI agents should not be used concurrently with MAOIs or thioridazine (Mellaril). These drugs should not be used during pregnancy or in children younger than 7 years. SSRI agents should be used with caution in patients with hepatic or renal impairment, renal failure, lactation, cardiac disease, or diabetes mellitus.

What are the important points patients should know?

Advise patients to report withdrawal symptoms, including abdominal pain, diarrhea, nausea, headache, sweating, and insomnia. Tell patients to take great care when driving or operating machinery while on antidepressant therapy, especially during the initial stages of treatment. Instruct patients to take SSRIs in the morning to minimize the incidence of insomnia and to avoid alcohol because of the additive CNS depressant effects.

Focus on Geriatrics

Taking SSRIs

All SSRIs should be administered with food. Patients—particularly older adults or nutritionally compromised patients—should be weighed weekly to monitor weight loss.

Monoamine Oxidase Inhibitors (MAOIs)

The therapeutic response rate with all antidepressants is similar, and the selection of the proper agent is dependent on the side effects that the patient experiences from the drugs. MAOIs are second- or third-line antidepressants because of the numerous interactions with prescription and OTC medications, as well as with certain foods and beverages.

How do they work?

MAOIs are thought to act by preventing the natural breakdown of neurotransmitters, but their precise mode of action is not known. It is also thought that MAOIs are able to inhibit hepatic microsomal drug-metabolizing enzymes; thus, they may intensify and prolong the effects of many drugs.

How are they used?

Until the availability of the SSRIs, the MAOIs were the most effective antidepressants available. These agents are used to manage endogenous depression, the depressive phase of manic–depressive (bipolar) psychosis, and severe exogenous (reactive) depression that is not responsive to more commonly used therapies.

What are the adverse effects?

Common adverse reactions of the MAOIs are less serious than those observed during TCA therapy, but consist of antimuscarinic and antiadrenergic effects. Orthostatic hypotension is a common adverse effect of MAOIs. Nausea, constipation, dry mouth, diarrhea, dizziness, vertigo, and headache are also seen. A serious hypertensive crisis may occur if a patient taking MAOIs eats a food containing tyramine (an amino acid present in some foods).

What are the contraindications and interactions?

The MAOIs are contraindicated in epilepsy, liver disease, and serious cardiovascular disease. These drugs are also contraindicated in patients with known hypersensitivity to them.

What are the most important points patients should know?

Instruct patients to avoid foods that contain tyramine and provide a list of these foods, which includes cheese, sour cream, yogurt, chicken liver, beef, coffee, tea, caffeinated sodas, chocolate, pickled herring, soy sauce, yeast extracts, fruits and vegetables (dried beans, fava beans, figs, raisins, avocados, bananas, and raspberries). Inform patients that the drug's effectiveness occurs after about 2 weeks of therapy.

Focus Point

Diet and MAOIs

Patients taking MAOIs must avoid foods containing tyramine to avoid severe hypertension, heart attack, adverse reactions, or death.

✳ Apply Your Knowledge 14.5

The following questions focus on what you have just learned about TCAs, SSRIs, and MAOIs. *See Appendix E for the correct answers.*

MULTIPLE CHOICE

Choose the correct answer from choices a–d.

1. TCAs increase the effect of which of the following substances?
   a. Epinephrine and acetylcholine
   b. Dopamine and carbidopa
   c. Norepinephrine and serotonin
   d. Norepinephrine and acetylcholine

2. SSRIs are commonly used for all of the following conditions, except:

   a. Obsessive–compulsive disorder
   b. Geriatric depression
   c. Parkinson's disease
   d. Bulimia nervosa

3. Which of the following medications is contraindicated in elderly men with enlargement of the prostate?

   a. TCAs
   b. SSRIs
   c. MAOIs
   d. Lithium

4. Which of the following are considered first-line drugs in the treatment of major depression?

   a. Benzodiazepines
   b. MAOIs
   c. TCAs
   d. SSRIs

5. Which of the following agents may precipitate hyperthermia crisis, tachycardia, or seizures?

   a. MAOIs
   b. SSRIs
   c. TCAs
   d. Valproic acid

FILL IN THE BLANK

Select terms from your reading to fill in the blanks.

1. The TCAs are used for endogenous depression and occasionally for _____ depression.

2. _____ activity of the TCAs accounts for dry mouth, blurred vision, constipation, urine retention, and tachycardia.

3. SSRIs primarily block the effect of _____ reuptake.

4. _____ should not be used by pregnant women or children younger than 7 years.

5. _____ is a common adverse effect of MAOIs.

6. Foods that contain tyramine should be avoided by patients taking _____.

Chapter Capsule

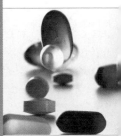

This section repeats the objectives from the beginning of the chapter and then provides a summary of the most important concepts for that objective. Use this section as a quick review and to check your knowledge.

Objective 1: Describe the four major parts of the brain.

- Cerebrum—the largest part, which includes nerve centers associated with sensory and motor functions, and provides higher mental functions, including memory and reasoning; composed of an outer cerebral cortex and inner cerebral medulla

- Diencephalon—also processes sensory information

- Brainstem—contains nerve pathways that connect various parts of the nervous system and regulate certain visceral activities

- Cerebellum—includes centers that coordinate voluntary muscular movements

Objective 2: Name three benzodiazepine hypnotic drugs and explain the mechanism by which they produce hypnotic effects.

- Diazepam—appears to act at the limbic and subcortical levels of the CNS
- Lorazepam—effects are mediated by GABA; it acts on the thalamic, hypothalamic, and limbic levels of the CNS
- Phenytoin—precise mechanism is not known, but it appears to reduce the voltage, frequency, and spread of electrical discharges within the motor cortex

Objective 3: List three different types of epilepsy.

- Generalized tonic–clonic seizures
- Generalized absence seizures
- Partial seizures

Objective 4: Name two drugs used specifically to treat each type of epilepsy.

- Phenytoin, carbamazepine—generalized tonic–clonic seizures
- Valproic acid, ethosuximide—generalized absence seizures
- Phenytoin, carbamazepine—partial seizures

Objective 5: Describe the mechanisms of action of drugs that increase dopamine or decrease acetylcholine levels in the basal ganglia.

- Anticholinergic agents—work by inhibiting the muscarine receptors in the basal ganglia, lessening the imbalance between the extrapyramidal and pyramidal pathways by blocking the effect of acetylcholine
- Dopaminergic drugs (such as levodopa)—exact mechanism of action is unknown

Objective 6: Describe five adverse effects associated with antianxiety drugs.

- Drowsiness
- Nausea
- Bradycardia
- Skin rash
- Fever

Note: There are more adverse effects, but these five are the most common.

Objective 7: Describe the common adverse effects and the specific neurologic conditions caused by antipsychotic drugs.

- Common adverse effects—nausea, vomiting, diarrhea, dizziness, headache, drowsiness, tinnitus, disorientation, short-term memory loss
- Neurological conditions—tremors, loss of equilibrium, neurotoxicity (when combined with carbamazepine, haloperidol, and phenothiazines)

Objective 8: Explain the use of lithium in mania and the adverse effects associated with its use.

- Lithium—controls symptoms in both the manic and depressive phases of psychotic disorders; used for the control and prophylaxis of acute mania and the acute manic phase of mixed bipolar disorder
- Adverse effects—nausea, tremors (which subside with continued treatment), vomiting, diarrhea, dizziness, headache, drowsiness, tinnitus, loss of equilibrium, short-term memory loss, and, at toxic levels, kidney and heart damage

Objective 9: Describe the main adverse effects of antipsychotic drugs.

- Sedation, dry mouth, sexual dysfunction, akathisia, bradykinesia, rigidity, and sometimes, tardive dyskinesia

Internet Sites of Interest

■ Find a concise description of sedative–hypnotic agents on the Psychology Today Web site at: **http://www.psychologytoday.com**. Search "Sedative."

■ The National Institute of Neurological Disorders and Stroke contains a comprehensive site for information on epilepsy, including support organizations and fact sheets for patients and caregivers at: **www.ninds.nih.gov/disorders/epilepsy/**

■ For an overview of anticonvulsant medications, click on "Neuro Med" and then look for "anticonvulsant" on Neuroland's site at: **http://neuroland.com/**

■ In-depth information on a variety of topics related to schizophrenia, including symptoms and diagnosis, drug therapy, support groups, and frequently asked questions can be found at: **www.schizophrenia.com**

■ Information about bipolar disorder and medications used to treat it can be found at: **www.pendulum.org**

■ The National Institute of Mental Health discusses the latest treatments for schizophrenia, depression, and other psychiatric disorders at: **http://www.nimh.nih.gov/**

Chapter Objectives

After completing this chapter, you should be able to:

1. List the two divisions of the nervous system and their subdivisions.
2. Explain the basic functional unit cell of the nervous system.
3. Define the terms *cholinergic* and *adrenergic*.
4. Describe the fight-or-flight response.
5. List the two main adrenergic receptors and what they respond to.
6. Explain the actions of adrenergic agonists.
7. Explain the actions of receptor agonists.
8. Define adrenergic antagonists.
9. List the two types of cholinergic receptors.
10. Discuss the source of atropine and how it works.

Chapter 15

Effects of Drugs on the Autonomic Nervous System

Key Terms

Adrenergic (add-ruh-NUR-jik) (page 328)

Alpha-adrenergic receptors (AL-fuh add-ruh-NUR-jik ree-SEP-ters) (page 332)

Anticholinergics (an-tee-kol-in-UR-jiks) (page 342)

Beta-adrenergic receptors (BAY-tuh add-ruh-NUR-jik) (page 332)

Catecholamines (kah-teh-KOH-luh-meenz) (page 331)

Cholinergic (kol-in-UR-jik) (page 328)

Cholinergic blockers (page 342)

Fight-or-flight response (page 330)

Muscarinic receptors (MUS-kah-RIN-ik) (page 340)

Nicotinic receptors (NIK-oh-TIN-ik) (page 340)

Parasympathetic nervous system (pair-ah-SIM-pah-THET-ik) (page 325)

Parasympatholytics (pair-ah-SIM-pa-tho-LIH-tiks) (page 342)

Peripheral nervous system (per-IF-urr-ul) (page 325)

Sympathetic nervous system (SIM-pah-THET-ik) (page 325)

Sympathomimetics (sim-pah-tho-MI-met-iks) (page 333)

PRACTICAL SCENARIO

The emergency medical services (EMS) team have brought a 54-year-old female patient to the emergency department (ED) where you are working. The EMS personnel state that the patient was found wandering in a nearby park by a jogger who called 911 from her cell phone after the woman screamed obscenities at her and then fell, seriously scraping her arm and face. The woman is bleeding, disoriented, combative, and accusing the EMS team of stealing her purse. Her hands are shaking severely, and she is shouting at the doctors and nurses that she needs a bottle. The woman's clothing is dirty, and you can smell stale body odor and urine.

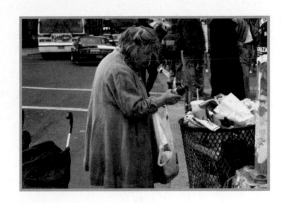

Critical Thinking Questions

1. Based on your first impressions of this patient's actions and appearance, what do you suspect she is suffering from? (*Hint*: Think about what you learned in Chapters 8 and Chapter 1.)
2. What short- and long-term health risks would you suspect this patient faces?
3. Why do you think the patient's hands are shaking, and what do you think causes her confusion and combativeness?
4. What assessments do you think are needed for this patient?

Introduction

The two major systems controlling bodily functions are the nervous system and the endocrine system. Both of these systems involve high-level integration in the brain and have the ability to influence processes in distant regions of the body as well as to extensively use negative feedback. Both use chemicals to transmit information. In the endocrine system, these chemicals (hormones) are released into the blood circulation and travel to interact with receptors in target tissue. In the nervous system, these chemicals (transmitters) are released from nerve terminals in the synaptic cleft (axons) and interact with receptors on neurons or effectors.

These two systems work closely with each other to control all of the body's functions. They are the most complicated and difficult parts of the anatomy and physiology of the body. For this reason, neuropharmacology is a challenging subject for allied health-care students.

Anatomy of the Autonomic Nervous System

The nervous system is divided into two main parts: the central nervous system (CNS), which comprises the brain and spinal cord, and the **peripheral nervous system**, that part of the nervous system that is outside the brain and spinal cord (Figure 15-1 ■). The autonomic nervous system is a division of the peripheral nervous system, which can itself be divided into two sections: motor and sensory neurons. In turn, motor neurons can be divided into two divisions that generally possess opposing functions: the **sympathetic nervous system** (which accelerates heart rate, constricts blood vessels, and raises blood pressure) and the **parasympathetic nervous system** (which slows the heart rate, increases intestinal and glandular activity, and relaxes muscles). This division is an anatomical division, rather than a strict neurotransmitter division. Each division uses two efferent neurons to carry neural signals to effector tissues with the specific receptors.

The neuron—is the basic functional unit cell of the nervous system. Therefore, these cells must communicate with each other and the other tissues of the body. The

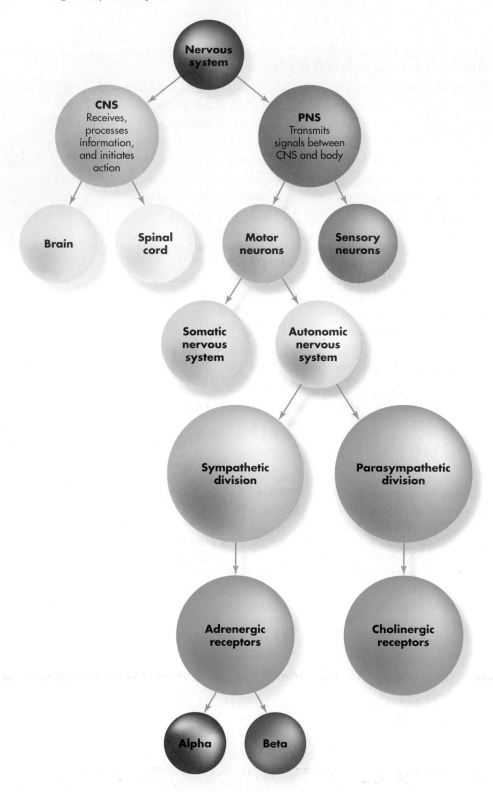

Figure 15-1 ■ Divisions of the nervous system.

communication sites of neurons are called synapses, which are actually junctions that nerve impulses pass across. The nerve starting the original impulse is known as the *presynaptic nerve*. The nerve that originates after the synapse is called *postsynaptic nerve*.

The space between each synapse (called the *synaptic* cleft) is bridged by chemicals called *neurotransmitters*. The two primary neurotransmitters in the autonomic

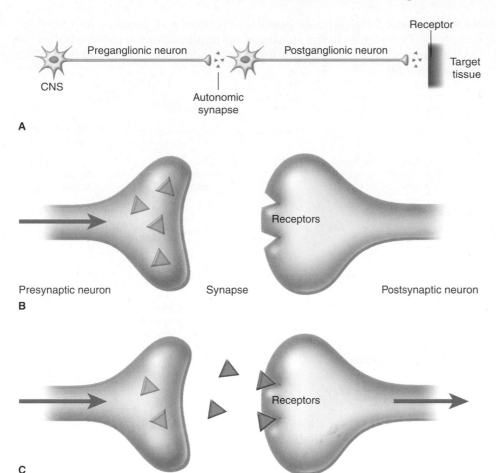

Figure 15-2 ■ (A) In the autonomic pathway, (B) nerve impulses (shown as arrows) travel along a presynaptic neuron to reach the junction between two neurons called the *synapses.* Chemicals called *neurotransmitters* (shown as triangles) must cross the synapses to carry the nerve impulse to the postsynaptic neuron. (C) When the neurotransmitters cross the synapses, they reach a receptor. Many drugs act as neurotransmitters, or they act by blocking the neurotransmitters from reaching a receptor or enhancing the activity of neurotransmitters so that more of them reach the receptor.

nervous system are *acetylcholine (ACh)* and *norepinephrine (NE),* although many different types of neurotransmitters exist throughout the nervous system. Many drugs act as neurotransmitters. Drugs can also be used to block or enhance the activity of these neurotransmitters (Figure 15-2 ■).

Sympathetic Nervous System

A *ganglion* is an aggregation of nerve cell fibers. Sympathetic preganglionic fibers exit the CNS through the thoracic and lumbar spinal nerves. Sympathetic preganglionic fibers terminate in ganglia located in the two paravertebral chains that lie on either side of the spinal cord. Thus, sympathetic preganglionic fibers are short and can activate diffuse numbers of postganglionic neurons. Acetylcholine is the neurotransmitter released by the preganglionic sympathetic neuron. Postganglionic sympathetic neurons project long fibers to innervate the sympathetic target tissue. The major neurotransmitter released by the postganglionic neuron is norepinephrine. However, in sweat glands, the postganglionic neuron releases acetylcholine. Dopamine serves as the postganglionic neurotransmitter in renal smooth muscle. The adrenal medulla also

[handwritten margin note: Chem. Transmitter / Epimephrine / Norepinephrine / Dobutamine]

receives sympathetic preganglionic fibers that release acetylcholine and bind to nicotinic receptors. This results in the release of epinephrine and norepinephrine into the blood circulation, where they act as hormones at adrenergic receptors throughout the body (Figure 15-3 ■).

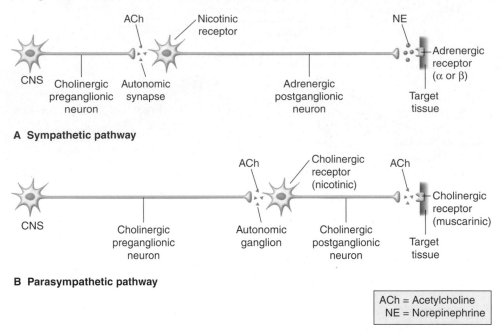

A Sympathetic pathway

B Parasympathetic pathway

ACh = Acetylcholine
NE = Norepinephrine

Figure 15-3 ■ Receptors in the autonomic nervous system: (A) sympathetic pathways (acetylcholine [ACh] and norepinephrine [NE]); (B) parasympathetic pathway (acetylcholine [ACh]).

Parasympathetic Nervous System

Parasympathetic preganglionic fibers exit the CNS through the cranial nerves and the sacral spinal roots and then travel to innervated tissues. Most preganglionic parasympathetic fibers terminate on ganglion cells. Innervation (neural or electrical arousal) of the target tissue is far less divergent than in the sympathetic nervous system. Just as in the sympathetic division, parasympathetic preganglionic neurons release acetylcholine at the ganglia. The parasympathetic postganglionic neurons also release acetylcholine, which binds to the target tissue.

Neurotransmitters of the Autonomic Nervous System

Neurons in the autonomic nervous system can be classified into two groups based on the neurotransmitter they release. Neurons that release acetylcholine are termed **cholinergic**. Cholinergic neurons include:

* Preganglionic neurons in both the sympathetic and parasympathetic nervous systems
* Parasympathetic postganglionic neurons
* Somatic transmission at the neuromuscular junction
* Sympathetic postganglionic fibers that innervate sweat glands

Accordingly, receptors to which acetylcholine binds are also termed *cholinergic*. There are more specific designations for cholinergic receptor–based selectivity for agonist/antagonist binding and anatomical location. Neurons that release norepinephrine, epinephrine, or dopamine are termed **adrenergic**. Similarly, receptors to which these adrenergic agonists bind are also termed *adrenergic*. Besides acting as direct agonists or antagonists at cholinergic and adrenergic receptors, drugs can affect the synthesis, storage, release, and termination of neurotransmitters in the autonomic nervous system.

✳ Apply Your Knowledge 15.1 ▬▬▬▬▬▬

The following questions focus on what you have just learned about the anatomy of the ANS. *See Appendix E for the correct answers.*

FILL IN THE BLANK

Select terms from your reading to fill in the blanks.

1. The nervous system is mainly divided into the _____ and _____ nervous systems.

2. The _____ nervous system accelerates heart rate, constricts blood vessels, and raises blood pressure.

3. The _____ nervous system slows heart rate, increases intestinal and glandular activity, and relaxes muscles.

4. A nerve cell that sends and receives electrical signals throughout the body is known as a _____.

5. A junction across which a nerve impulse passes is known as a _____.

6. In the sympathetic nervous system, the major neurotransmitter released by the postganglionic neuron is _____.

7. Neurons that release acetylcholine are termed _____.

8. Receptors to which adrenergic agonists bind are termed _____, which means "related to nerves that release _____ and _____."

MULTIPLE CHOICE

Choose the correct answers from choices a–d.

1. The major neurotransmitter released by the postganglionic sympathetic neuron is:

   a. Dopamine

   b. Norepinephrine

   c. Acetylcholine

   d. Epinephrine

2. Parasympathetic preganglionic neurons release which of the following neurotransmitters?

   a. Dopamine

   b. Epinephrine

   c. Norepinephrine

   d. Acetylcholine

3. Which of the following neurotransmitters is released from the parasympathetic postganglionic neurons?

   a. Norepinephrine

   b. Epinephrine

   c. Acetylcholine

   d. Dopamine

4. Which of the following is the effect of the sympathetic nervous system on the heart?

   a. Decreases heart rate

   b. Decreases occurrence of arrhythmias

   c. Increases heart rate

   d. No effect

Functions of the Autonomic Nervous System

The parasympathetic nervous system is required for life; it maintains essential body functions such as digestion and excretion. Its actions generally oppose those of the sympathetic system. At times of "rest and digest," the parasympathetic nervous system dominates the sympathetic nervous system. Rather than discharging as a complete system, the parasympathetic nervous system operates in discrete units based on the specific needs of the body. Discharging as a complete system would produce massive, undesirable symptoms (such as in organophosphate poisoning).

The sympathetic nervous system adjusts body function in response to stress such as trauma, fear, hypoglycemia, cold, or exercise. The **fight-or-flight** response (reaction in the body when faced by a sudden threat or source of stress) has been used to describe activation of the sympathetic nervous system during emergencies (Figure 15-4 ■).

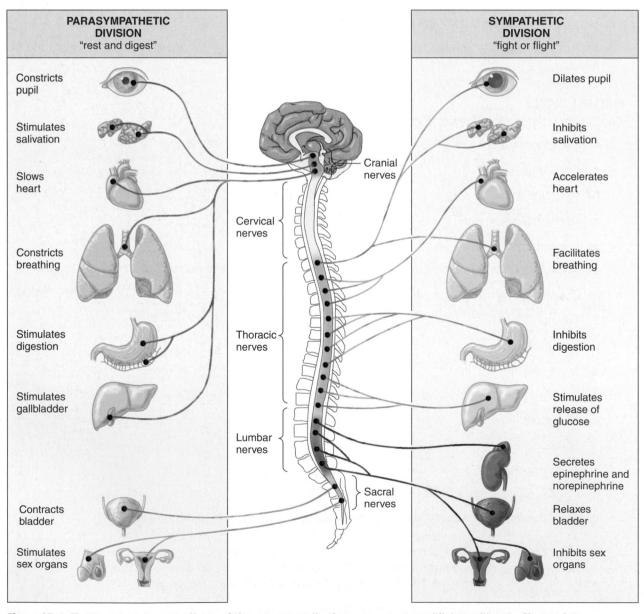

Figure 15-4 ■ "Rest and digest" effects of the parasympathetic nervous system; "fight-or-flight" effects of the sympathetic nervous system.

Remember that because of the sympathetic nervous system's anatomic wiring and release of epinephrine from the adrenal medulla, all of the sympathetic effector organs and tissues are activated. Heart rate, cardiac output, and blood pressure are increased; blood flow is diverted from the skin and internal organs to skeletal muscle; energy stores are mobilized; and pupils and bronchioles dilate. Autonomic regulation of target organs and tissues is listed in Table 15-1 ■.

Table 15-1 ■ Autonomic Regulation of Target Organs and Tissues

ORGANS OR TISSUES	SYMPATHETIC	PARASYMPATHETIC
Eyes		
Pupillary response	Causes dilation (mydriasis)	Causes constriction (miosis)
Heart		
	Increases heart rate	Decreases heart rate
	Increases arrhythmias	No effect
Blood vessels		
Skin	Causes vasoconstriction	No effect
Skeletal muscle vessels	Relaxes; causes vasodilation	No effect
Bronchial smooth muscle		
	Causes bronchodilation	Causes bronchoconstriction
Gastrointestinal tract		
Smooth muscle walls	Relaxes: decreases motility and tone	Contracts: increases motility and tone
Smooth muscle sphincter	Contracts	Relaxes
Secretion	No effect	Increases
Genitourinary smooth muscle		
Bladder wall	Relaxes: decreases pressure	Contracts: increases pressure
Sphincter	Contracts	Relaxes
Uterus (pregnant)	Relaxes/contracts	No effect
Penis	Causes ejaculation	Causes erection
Skin		
Sweat glands	Increases	No effect

ADRENERGIC RECEPTORS

The effects of stimulation of the sympathetic nervous system are mediated by the release of norepinephrine from postganglionic nerve terminals and epinephrine from the adrenal medulla. Norepinephrine and epinephrine are two types of endogenous **catecholamines** (chemical compounds containing nitrogen that is derived from the amino acid *tyrosine*) that bind to adrenergic receptors and produce sympathetic effects.

The two main adrenergic receptors are alpha and beta. Alpha-adrenergic receptors are divided into α_1 and α_2, whereas beta-adrenergic receptors are divided into β_1 and β_2.

Alpha-adrenergic receptors (parts of cells that respond to adrenaline) are found in vascular smooth muscle and, when stimulated by norepinephrine or epinephrine, cause vasoconstriction.

Beta-adrenergic receptors (receptors that respond to norepinephrine or epinephrine) are found on both smooth and cardiac muscle membranes. In the heart, the predominant beta-adrenergic receptors are β_1 receptors, which, when stimulated by norepinephrine and epinephrine, increase heart rate and force of contraction. In smooth muscle, the predominant beta-adrenergic receptors are β_2 receptors. When stimulated by epinephrine, β_2 receptors produce vasodilation, particularly in the coronary arteries and skeletal muscle blood vessels. β_2 receptors can produce relaxation of bronchiolar smooth muscle. Norepinephrine does not affect β_2 receptors.

CHOLINERGIC RECEPTORS

The parasympathetic nervous system, also known as the *cholinergic nervous system*, releases the neurotransmitter acetylcholine. Receptors that respond to cholinergic stimulation are called *cholinergic receptors*. Drugs that bind to cholinergic receptors are referred to as *cholinergic drugs* and exhibit effects similar to those of acetylcholine. Agents that bind to cholinergic receptors and prevent acetylcholine from acting on its receptors (antagonism) are called *cholinergic-blocking drugs* (see Figure 15-3).

✳ Apply Your Knowledge 15.2

The following questions focus on what you have just learned about the functions of the ANS. *See Appendix E for the correct answers.*

FILL IN THE BLANK
Select terms from your reading to fill in the blanks.

1. Catecholamine is a chemical compound derived from the amino acid called _____.

2. _____ is released from the adrenal medulla.

3. The "fight-or-flight" response has been used to describe activation of the _____ nervous system during emergencies.

4. Alpha-adrenergic receptors are found in vascular smooth muscle and cause _____.

5. Agents that bind to cholinergic receptors and do not cause any effect are known as _____.

6. Beta$_2$ receptors can produce _____ of bronchiolar smooth muscle.

MATCHING
Match the letter action to the numbered agonist that produces the action. type that produces the lettered action. Some agonists may have more than one action.

AGONIST	ACTION
1. _____ β_1	a. Vasodilation
2. _____ β_2	b. Increase in heart rate and force of contraction
3. _____ α_1	c. Relaxation of bronchiolar smooth muscle
4. _____ α_2	d. Pupil dilation
	e. Stimulation of sweat glands
	f. Decrease in systolic blood pressure

Focus on Geriatrics

Effects of Stress in Elderly Patients

Elderly people experience many losses and changes in their lives. These changes may be incremental and, over time, become stressful, and possibly overwhelming. Stress can have physical, emotional, intellectual, social, and spiritual consequences. Usually, the effects are mixed because stress affects every person uniquely.

Drug Effects on the Autonomic Nervous System

Autonomic drugs are categorized based on which receptors can be stimulated or blocked.

1. **Sympathomimetics** (or adrenergic agonists) produce symptoms of the fight-or-flight response and stimulate the sympathetic nervous system.
2. Parasympathomimetics (or cholinergic agonists) produce symptoms of the rest-and-relaxation response and stimulate the parasympathetic nervous system.
3. Adrenergic blockers produce actions opposite to sympathomimetics and inhibit the sympathetic nervous system.
4. Anticholinergics (or cholinergic blockers) produce actions opposite to parasympathomimetics and inhibit the parasympathetic nervous system.

Focus on Natural Products

Essential Fatty Acids

Essential fatty acids, which cannot be manufactured by the body, are most commonly found in polyunsaturated vegetable oils. Both Omega 3 and omega-6 fatty acids are converted in the body to powerful hormone-like substances (prostaglandins) that affect almost every biologic function, including regulation of smooth muscle and autonomic reflexes. omega-6 fatty acids are present in food sources, and it is important to balance their intake with omega-3 fatty acids, found in fish and flaxseed oil. Adding one tablespoon of flaxseed oil to the daily diet is beneficial.

ADRENERGIC AGONISTS OR SYMPATHOMIMETIC DRUGS

The adrenergic agonists are categorized as catecholamines and noncatecholamines. The catecholamines include norepinephrine, which is released at the nerve terminals; epinephrine, from the adrenal medulla; and dopamine, from sites in the brain, kidneys, and gastrointestinal (GI) tract. These types of drugs can be made synthetically to produce the same effects as those of the naturally secreted neurotransmitters. The noncatecholamines have somewhat similar actions to the catecholamines, but are more selective of receptor sites, are not quite as fast-acting, and have a longer duration. The medications of the adrenergic agonist class mimic the sympathetic nervous system and are also called *sympathomimetics* or *adrenergic agonists*. Classifications of sympathomimetic drugs are listed in Table 15-2 ■.

Table 15-2 ■ Classifications of Sympathomimetic Drugs

GENERIC NAME	TRADE NAME	PRIMARY USE
Catecholamines		
dopamine	Intropin (α_1 and β_1)	Shock
epinephrine	Adrenalin, Primatene (α and β)	Asthma, cardiac arrest
isoproterenol	Isuprel (β_1 and β_2)	Asthma, dysrhythmias, heart failure
norepinephrine	Levarterenol, Levophed (α and β)	Shock
Alpha$_1$ Agonists		
methoxamine	Vasoxyl	Maintain blood pressure during anesthesia
midodrine	Pro Amatine	Orthostatic hypotension
oxymetazoline	Afrin	Nasal congestion
phenylephrine	Neo-Synephrine	Nasal congestion
xylometazoline	Otrivin, Neo-Synephrine	Nasal congestion
Alpha$_2$ Agonists		
apraclonidine	Iopidine	Operative eye pressure, glaucoma
clonidine	Catapres (in CNS)	Hypertension
guanabenz	Wytensin	Hypertension
guanfacine	Tenex	Hypertension
methyldopa	AdoMet (in CNS)	Hypertension
Beta$_1$ Agonists		
Dobutamine	Dobutrex	Cardiac stimulant
Beta$_2$ Agonists		
albuterol	Ventolin	Asthma
metaproterenol	Alupent	Asthma
ritodrine	Yutopar	Slowing uterine contractions
salmeterol	Serevent	Decongestant
terbutaline	Brethine	Asthma
Miscellaneous Adrenergic Agonists		
amphetamine	Generic	Narcolepsy, ADD, obesity
ephedrine	Generic	Allergies, asthma, narcolepsy
methylphenidate	Ritalin	Attention deficit–hyperactivity disorder (ADHD), obesity
pemoline	Cylert	ADHD
pseudoephedrine	Sudafed (α and β)	Rhinitis, coryza, sinusitis

As previously discussed, there are two principal types of adrenoreceptors, alpha (α) and beta (β) These receptors have been further subdivided into the main subtypes of α_1, α_2, β_1, and β_2. The activation of alpha and beta receptors through the administration of adrenergic agonists produces effects consistent with sympathetic (fight-or-flight) stimulation.

Alpha₁-Receptor Agonists

Alpha₁ receptors are located on blood vessels and influence both blood pressure and blood flow into the tissues (called *tissue perfusion*). Resistance to blood flow is determined by the diameter of the vessels. Alpha₁ receptors are also found on the muscles of the iris; on smooth muscle of the GI tract and male and female reproductive tracts; and in liver cells, sweat glands, and sphincters of the urinary bladder.

How do they work?
Stimulation of α_1 receptors causes vasoconstriction of blood vessels, dilation of pupils (mydriasis), decreased GI motility, contraction of the external sphincter of the bladder, decreased bile secretion, and stimulation of sweat glands.

How are they used?
Alpha₁-receptor agonists are used to treat hypotension, nasal congestion, and subconjunctival hemorrhage (red eye).

What are the adverse effects?
The common adverse effects of α_1-receptor agonists are hypertension, blurred vision, constipation, urine retention, gooseflesh, and sweating.

What are the contraindications and interactions?
Alpha₁-receptor agonists are contraindicated for severe coronary or cardiovascular disease, glaucoma, hypovolemia (within 2 weeks of taking monoamine oxidase [MAO] inhibitors), acute kidney disease, urine retention, pheochromocytoma (adrenal tumor), thyrotoxicosis (hyperthyroidism or Graves' disease), sensitivity to adrenergic substances, supine hypertension (that is, when lying down), ventricular tachycardia, and for pregnant, lactating, or very young patients. Drug interactions occur with digoxin, doxazosin, ephedrine, guanethidine, halothane, methyldopa, oxytocin, phentolamine, phenothiazines, phenylpropanolamine, prazosin, pseudoephedrine, reserpine, alpha blockers, beta blockers, atropine, MAO inhibitors, terazosin, tricyclic antidepressants, vasopressin, and ergot alkaloids.

What are the important points patients should know?
Instruct patients taking α_1-receptor agonists to inform the health-care provider if they have high blood pressure, thyroid disease, an enlarged prostate, glaucoma, or are breastfeeding. Also instruct patients to inform the doctor of other prescriptions they are taking, such as antihypertensive medicines, thyroid medications, other decongestants, and tricyclic antidepressants. Caution them against taking more than the prescribed dosage or of combining these medications with over-the-counter drugs without consulting their health-care provider.

Alpha₂-Receptor Agonists

Alpha₂ receptors are believed to be located on the presynaptic neurons, and they seem to function as controllers of neurotransmitter release by the presynaptic neurons. They are often used in reducing blood pressure.

How do they work?
These agonists stimulate alpha₂ adrenergic receptors in the CNS to inhibit sympathetic vasomotor centers. They reduce plasma concentrations of norepinephrine, decrease systolic blood pressure and heart rate, and inhibit renin release from the kidneys.

How are they used?
These agonists are used to treat hypertension, either alone or with diuretic or other hypertensive agents. They are also used epidurally as adjunct therapy for severe pain.

What are the adverse effects?

Adverse effects of these agonists include hypotension, peripheral edema, dry mouth or eyes, constipation, drowsiness, dizziness, rash, pruritus, impotence, nausea and vomiting, hepatitis, hallucinations, depression, and recurrent herpes simplex.

What are the contraindications and interactions?

These agonists are contraindicated in pediatric, pregnant, or lactating patients; hypertension that is associated with toxemia of pregnancy; polyarteritis nodosa (swollen or damaged arteries); scleroderma (skin hardening); hepatitis; cirrhosis; pheochromocytoma; and blood dyscrasias. Interactions include alcohol and other CNS depressants, amphetamines, tricyclic antidepressants, ephedrine, haloperidol, levodopa, lithium, MAO inhibitors, methotrimeprazine, opiate analgesics, phenothiazines, phenoxybenzamine, digoxin, calcium channel blockers, or beta blockers.

What are the important points patients should know?

Instruct patients with hypertension that excessive sodium leads to fluid retention and to avoid foods that are high in sodium, including canned, frozen, or dehydrated soup, processed cheese, salted biscuits, potato chips, and pretzels.

Beta$_1$-Receptor Agonists

Beta$_1$ receptors are located on the myocardium, adipocytes (fat cells), sphincters and smooth muscle of the gastrointestinal tract, and renal arterioles.

How do they work?

Beta$_1$-receptor agonists increase the rate and force of contraction of the heart, increase lipolysis in adipose tissue, decrease digestion and gastrointestinal motility, and increase glomerular filtration.

How are they used?

Beta$_1$-receptor agonists are used to treat circulatory shock, hypotension, and cardiac arrest. Two important drugs represent this group: dobutamine (Dobutrex), a selective β_1-receptor agonist, and isoproterenol (Isuprel), a nonselective β_1-receptor agonist.

What are the adverse effects?

The common adverse effects of β_1-receptor agonists include hypertension, tachycardia, and constipation.

What are the contraindications and interactions?

Beta$_1$-receptor agonists are contraindicated in patients with a history of hypersensitivity to other sympathomimetic amines (nitrogen compounds); in those with ventricular tachycardia; in pediatric, pregnant, or lactating patients; or following an acute MI. Interactions can occur with general anesthetics (especially cyclopropane and halothane), beta-adrenergic blocking agents such as metoprolol and propranolol, MAO inhibitors, and tricyclic antidepressants.

What are the important points patients should know?

Alert patients that sputum and saliva may turn pink after inhalation of isoproterenol. Warn patients not to breast feed when taking these agents. Patients should not increase, decrease, or omit doses or change intervals between doses. Advise patients to immediately report anginal pain to the health-care provider.

Beta$_2$-Receptor Agonists

These adrenoreceptors are distributed on the smooth muscle of the bronchioles; skeletal muscle; and blood vessels supplying the brain, heart, kidneys, and skeletal muscle; the uterus; and in liver cells.

How do they work?

Stimulation of β_2 receptors results in bronchodilation; increased skeletal muscle excitability; vasodilation of blood vessels to the brain, heart, kidneys, and skeletal muscle; and relaxation of the uterus in pregnancy.

How are they used?

Beta$_2$-receptor agonists are used in patients with chronic obstructive airway disease, circulatory shock, premature labor, and peripheral vascular disease.

What are the adverse effects?

The common adverse effects of β_2-receptor agonists include muscle tremor (in the hands), increased muscle tension, and feelings of warmth. These agents also cause hyperglycemia (increased blood glucose).

What are the contraindications and interactions?

Beta$_2$-receptor agonists are contraindicated in pediatric, pregnant, or lactating patients; in those sensitive to other sympathomimetic agents; in patients with cardiac arrhythmias associated with tachycardia or digitalis intoxication, hyperthyroidism, preeclampsia (hypertension during pregnancy), eclampsia (coma and convulsions related to pregnancy), intrauterine infection, hypertension, diabetes mellitus, hypovolemia (decrease in volume of circulating blood), thyrotoxicosis, asthma that is treated with beta-mimetics, hypersensitivity, coronary artery disease (within 14 days of MAO inhibitor therapy), and angle-closure glaucoma. Interactions can occur with beta-adrenergic blockers, corticosteroids, epinephrine, other sympathomimetic bronchodilators, MAO inhibitors, and tricyclic antidepressants.

What are the important points patients should know?

Instruct patients about using the inhaler correctly and have them demonstrate the technique for you. Warn patients not to change the dose or frequency of doses. Patients should know that these drugs may cause dizziness (albuterol) or tremor (metaproterenol), so advise them to change positions slowly. They should not take other OTC drugs or breast feed without first consulting the health-care provider. Advise patients to report if the drug fails to reduce symptoms.

Focus on Pediatrics

Stress and Childhood Asthma

Stress caused by major events such as the birth of a sibling, the death of a family member, or moving to a new home can quadruple a child's risks of an asthma attack within 2 days of the events. The asthma attack often reoccurs about 6 weeks later. The autonomic nervous system of a child together with hormones and brain chemicals can trigger both immediate and delayed stress-related effects. Other events that may relate to asthma attacks are departures of family members, illnesses, hospital visits, separations, and changes in family relationships.

ADRENERGIC ANTAGONISTS OR SYMPATHOLYTICS

Like sympathomimetic agents, sympatholytics can act either directly or indirectly. Direct-acting sympatholytics are antagonists that have affinity for a receptor, but block the normal response. Adrenergic antagonists can show specificity for one receptor or subtype. Indirect-acting agents block adrenergic nerve transmission, usually by inhibiting the release of neurotransmitters or depleting the stores of transmitters. Table 15-3 ■ lists the common adrenergic antagonists.

Table 15-3 ■ Adrenergic Antagonists

GENERIC NAME	TRADE NAME	AVERAGE ADULT DOSE	ROUTE OF ADMINIS-TRATION	PRIMARY USE
Alpha-Receptor Antagonists				
doxazosin	Cardura	Start 1 mg at bedtime and titrate up to max of 16 mg/d in 1–2 divided doses	PO	Hypertension
phenoxybenzamine	Dibenzyline	5–10 mg bid; may increase by 10 mg/d at 4–d intervals to desired response	PO	Pheochromocytoma
phentolamine	Regitine	2–5 mg as needed	IV, IM	Hypertensive episode during surgery
prazosin	Minipress	Start 1 mg at bedtime; then 1 mg bid or tid; may increase to 20 mg/d in divided doses	PO	Hypertension
terazosin	Hytrin	Start 1 mg at bedtime; then 1–5 mg/d (max: 20 mg/d)	PO	Hypertension, urinary obstruction
Beta-Receptor Antagonists (Nonselective)				
labetalol	Normodyne	100 mg bid (max: 2,400 mg/d)	PO	Hypertension
		20 mg slowly (max: 300 mg total dose)	IV	Hypertension
nadolol	Corgard	40 mg/d (max: 320 mg/d in 1–2 divided doses)	PO	Hypertension, angina
pindolol	Visken	5 mg bid (max: 60 mg/d in 2–3 divided doses)	PO	Hypertension
		15–40 mg/d in 3–4 divided doses	PO	Angina pectoris
propranolol	Inderal	10–40 mg bid (max: 480 mg/d)	PO	Hypertension, angina, acute MI, and dysrhythmias
timolol	Betimol	10–45 mg in bid–tid/d (max: 60 mg/d in 2 divided doses)	PO	Hypertension, angina
Beta-Receptor Antagonists (Selective)				
acebutolol	Sectral	200–800 mg per d in 1–2 divided doses (max: 1200 mg/d)	PO	Hypertension, dysrhythmias
atenolol	Tenormin	25–50 mg/d (max: 100 mg/d)	PO	Hypertension, angina pectoris
		5 mg q5min × 2 doses	IV	MI
esmolol	Brevibloc	25–50 mg/d (max: 100 mg/d)	IV	Supraventricular tachydysrhythmias
metoprolol	Lopressor	50–100 mg/d in 1–2 divided doses (max: 450 mg/d)	IV	Hypertension
		100 mg/d in 2 divided doses (max: 400 mg/d)	PO	Angina pectoris
		5 mg q2min × 3 doses; then PO therapy	PO	MI
		50 mg q6h for 48 h; then 100 mg bid	PO	MI

Alpha-Receptor Antagonists

Alpha-receptor antagonists can work in a reversible or an irreversible manner. Some are nonselective and antagonize α_1 and α_2 receptors. Others are highly selective for α_1 receptors. All antagonize the effects of endogenous catecholamines.

How do they work?
These antagonists selectively inhibit the actions of alpha adrenoreceptors, producing vasodilation in arterioles and veins, with the result that both peripheral vascular resistance and blood pressure are reduced.

How are they used?
Applications for alpha-receptor antagonists include the control of hypertension, and the treatment of peripheral vascular disease, adrenal medulla tumor (pheochromocytoma), and urinary retention.

What are the adverse effects?
The common adverse effects of alpha-receptor antagonists include nasal congestion and stuffiness, postural hypotension (which occurs on sitting or standing), inhibition of ejaculation, and lack of energy.

What are the contraindications and interactions?
A contraindication for use of alpha-receptor antagonists is known hypersensitivity to any of these drugs. Interactions can occur with diuretics, ephedrine, epinephrine, methoxamine, norepinephrine, other hypotensive agents, NSAIDs, and phenylephrine.

What are the important points patients should know?
Because these drugs may cause dizziness, advise patients to change positions slowly. Patients should avoid driving for at least 12 hours after taking the first dose to determine side effects. Patients should not breast feed while taking these drugs, or take OTC drugs for coughs, colds, or allergies without discussing with the health-care provider.

Beta-Receptor Antagonists

These antagonists work against the effects of catecholamines at beta adrenoreceptors. Beta-blocking drugs reduce receptor occupancy by beta agonists. Most of these agents are pure antagonists and occupy beta receptors, causing no activation of the receptors.

How do they work?
Beta blockade by these antagonists results in vasodilation, decreased peripheral resistance, and orthostatic hypotension. These agents work primarily on cardiac muscle, competitively blocking beta-adrenergic receptors within the heart.

How are they used?
These agents are used in the management of hypertension, sometimes with a thiazide diuretic, for patients who have failed to respond to diet, exercise, and weight reduction. They are also used to treat cardiac arrhythmias, myocardial infarction, tachyarrhythmias, hypertrophic subaortic stenosis (thickening of the ventricular septum or wall), angina pectoris, pheochromocytoma, and hereditary essential tremor.

What are the adverse effects?
Common adverse effects of beta-receptor antagonists are dizziness, lethargy, insomnia, and diarrhea.

What are the contraindications and interactions?

Beta-blockers are contraindicated in patients with known hypersensitivity, heart block, severe heart failure, cardiogenic shock, and other severe circulatory disorders. These agents should be avoided in patients with a history of asthma or chronic obstructive airway disease, unless no alternative is available. Interactions can occur with phenothiazines, beta-adrenergic agonists, atropine, tricyclic antidepressants, diuretics and other hypotensive agents, tubocurarine, cimetidine, and antacids.

What are the important points patients should know?

Teach patients to take their heart rate and blood pressure and to report a decrease in either. Because these drugs may cause dizziness, advise patients to change positions slowly. Patients should avoid driving for at least 12 hours after taking the first dose to determine side effects. Patients should not breast feed while taking these drugs, or take OTC drugs for coughs, colds, or allergies without discussing with the health-care provider. Warn patients not to discontinue these drugs suddenly. Advise patients to check with the health-care provider before taking OTC medications.

Parasympathomimetics or Cholinergic Agonists

Cholinergic agonists (also called *parasympathomimetics* or *cholinomimetics*) stimulate the parasympathetic nervous system because they mimic the parasympathetic neurotransmitter acetylcholine. This neurotransmitter is located at the ganglions and the parasympathetic terminal nerve endings. It stimulates the receptors in tissues, organs, and glands. There are two types of cholinergic receptors: (1) **muscarinic receptors** (which innervate smooth muscle and slow the heart rate) and (2) **nicotinic receptors** (which affect the skeletal muscles). Many cholinergic drugs are nonselective and can therefore affect both the muscarinic and the nicotinic receptors. However, selective cholinergic drugs for the muscarinic receptors do not affect the nicotinic receptors.

How do they work?

The rapid destruction of systemically administered acetylcholine by cholinesterases makes the endogenous (self-produced) neurotransmitter of limited clinical value. Clinically useful cholinomimetic drugs are either cholinergic agonists that are resistant to the hydrolytic (water-eliminating) action of cholinesterases or agents that inhibit cholinesterases. Based on their mechanisms of action, cholinomimetic drugs may be classified as direct-acting agents (agonists) and indirect-acting agents (anticholinesterases).

How are they used?

Pilocarpine (Isopto-Carpine) is a direct-acting cholinergic drug that is used most commonly in ophthalmology to reduce elevated intraocular pressure in glaucoma and induce miosis. Specific muscarinic agonist drugs that are nonspecific may be used in the treatment of constipation that is due to lack of muscle tone (called *atonic*), congenital megacolon, and postoperative and postpartum intestinal ileus (that is, an obstructed bowel). Bethanechol (Urecholine) has been used to increase the tone of the lower esophageal sphincter in the treatment of reflux esophagitis. In the genitourinary tract, muscarinic agonists are useful in the treatment of postoperative and postpartum nonobstructive urine retention and neurogenic urinary bladder with retention. The primary use of the drug in the cardiovascular field is in the diagnosis of atrial tachycardia. In pulmonary practice, the hypersensitivity of asthmatic patients to bronchiolar constriction induced by cholinomimetics makes methacholine useful in the diagnosis of asthma. Muscarinic agonists are also known to increase secretion of the salivary and lacrimal glands. They are used to treat symptoms of dry mouth caused by radiotherapy for cancer of the head and neck. The most common cholinomimetic drugs are summarized in Table 15-4 ■.

What are the adverse effects?

Adverse effects produced by the cholinomimetics can be predicted based on the pharmacodynamic activity of the drugs. Thus, undesirable effects may include flushing, sweating, abdominal cramps, difficulty in visual accommodation, headache, and convulsions at high doses. Specific GI adverse effects include nausea, vomiting, diarrhea, and abdominal pain. Other adverse effects are bronchospasm, excessive salivation, and urinary frequency.

What are the contraindications and interactions?

Muscarinic drugs are contraindicated in the presence of atrioventricular arrhythmias, coronary insufficiency, hyperthyroidism, asthma, and peptic ulcer. Interactions can occur with ambenonium, neostigmine, and other cholinesterase inhibitors, mecamylamine, procainamide, quinidine, atropine, epinephrine, beta-adrenergic agonists, and parasympathomimetic drugs.

What are the important points patients should know?

Advise patients to inform the health-care provider of any other drugs they are taking. Because these drugs may cause dizziness, caution patients to change positions slowly. Warn patients not to breast feed without the health-care provider's approval. Explain to patients that they may experience increased sweating and urinary frequency.

Table 15-4 ■ Cholinergic Agents

GENERIC NAME	TRADE NAME	AVERAGE ADULT DOSE	ROUTE OF ADMINISTRATION	PRIMARY USE
Direct-Acting Cholinergic Agonists				
bethanechol	Duvoid	10–50 mg qid (max: 120 mg/d)	Subcutaneously	Nonobstructive urine retention
	Urabeth	2.5–5 mg; repeat at 15–30 min intervals PRN	PO	
carbachol	Miostat	1–2 drops q4–8h; 0.5 mL injected	Intraocular; topical	Glaucoma
cevimeline	Evoxac	30 mg tid	PO	Dry mouth from Sjögren's syndrome
pilocarpine	Pilocar	1–2 gtt in eye 1–6 times/d	Ocular	Glaucoma
Indirect-Acting Cholinergic Agonists				
ambenonium	Mytelase	5–75 mg qid	PO	Myasthenia gravis
edrophonium	Enlon, Tensilon	2 mg injected over 15–30 sec; if no reaction, inject 8 mg after 45 sec	IV	Diagnosis of myasthenia gravis
neostigmine	Prostigmin	15–375 mg/d in 3–6 divided doses	PO	Myasthenia gravis, urine retention
pyridostigmine	Mestinon	60 mg–1.5 g/d; 180–540 mg 1–2 times/d, sustained release	PO	Myasthenia gravis
tacrine	Cognex	10–40 mg/d (max: 160 mg/d)	PO	Alzheimer's disease

Cholinergic Blockers

Drugs that inhibit the actions of acetylcholine by occupying the acetylcholine receptors are called cholinergic antagonists or **cholinergic blockers** (also called **anticholinergics** or **parasympatholytics**). The major body tissues and organs affected by the cholinergic-blocking agents include the heart, respiratory tract, urinary bladder, eyes, GI tract, and the sweat glands.

ATROPINE

Atropine (Atropair, AtroPen) is a classic anticholinergic or muscarinic antagonist drug. Atropine sulfate was first derived from the belladonna plant. Scopolamine was the second belladonna alkaloid produced. Atropine and scopolamine act on the muscarinic receptor, but they have little effect on the nicotinic receptor.

How does it work?

Atropine acts by selectively blocking all muscarinic responses to acetylcholine, whether excitatory or inhibitory. Selective depression of the CNS relieves rigidity and tremor of Parkinson's syndrome.

How is it used?

Atropine is used adjunctively to treat the symptoms of GI disorders; to treat ophthalmic disorders, various cardiac conditions, bronchial conditions, chronic obstructive airway disease, and upper respiratory infections; to counteract mushroom poisoning; and is used in preoperative situations.

What are the adverse effects?

The common adverse effects of atropine and atropine-like drugs include dry mouth, decreased perspiration, blurred vision, tachycardia, constipation, and urine retention. Other adverse effects are nausea, headache, dry skin, abdominal distention, hypotension or hypertension, impotence, photophobia, and coma.

What are the contraindications and interactions?

Atropine is contraindicated for patients with hypersensitivity to belladonna alkaloids, with angle-closure glaucoma, parotitis (inflammation of the saliva glands), obstructive uropathy, intestinal atony (muscular weakness), paralytic ileus, GI obstructions, severe ulcerative colitis, toxic megacolon, tachycardia, acute hemorrhage, myasthenia gravis (muscle weakness brought on by movement), and in pregnant or lactating patients. Interactions include amantadine, antihistamines, tricyclic antidepressants, quinidine, disopyramide, procainamide, levodopa, methotrimeprazine, and phenothiazines.

What are the important points patients should know?

Encourage patients receiving atropine to use frequent mouth rinses, chew gum, or suck on sugarless sourball candy to relieve dry mouth. Meticulous dental hygiene should be encouraged. Caution patients to avoid driving. Warn patients not to breast feed while taking this drug. Tell patients to report a fast heartbeat or palpitations.

Focus Point

Ecstasy and the Autonomic Nervous System

Ecstasy is an illegal drug known as *3,4 methylenedioxymethamphetamine* (MDMA). Other names for MDMA are *Adam, XTC, Doves,* or just *E*. Originally patented as an appetite suppressant, data now shows that MDMA may be toxic to the brain. This drug is a serious problem in the United States because of its trendiness among teenagers, who may be unaware of its harmful effects. Studies have shown a 20 to 60% reduction in healthy serotonin cells in the brains of MDMA users, damaging their ability to remember and to learn. Tests on the brains of monkeys showed brain damage that remained visible 7 years after the monkeys were given MDMA.

✳ Apply Your Knowledge 15.3

The following questions focus on what you have just learned about drug effects on the autonomic nervous system. *See Appendix E for the correct answers.*

MATCHING
Match the lettered trade name to the numbered generic name.

GENERIC NAME	TRADE NAME
1. _____ clonidine	a. Serevent
2. _____ albuterol	b. Sudafed
3. _____ pseudoephedrine	c. Levarterenol
4. _____ salmeterol	d. Afrin
5. _____ guanabenz	e. Catapres
6. _____ norepinephrine	f. Wytensin
7. _____ dopamine	g. Ventolin
8. _____ oxymetazoline	h. Intropin

FILL IN THE BLANK
Select terms from your reading to fill in the blanks.

1. Alpha$_1$-receptor agonist drugs are used for _____, _____, and _____.

2. Beta$_1$-receptor agonists are located on the myocardium, fat cells, sphincters, and _____ of the gastrointestinal tract, and renal arterioles.

3. Applications for alpha antagonists include pheochromocytoma, urinary retention, and _____.

4. Common adverse effects of β antagonists are _____, _____, _____, and _____.

5. Pilocarpine is a direct-acting cholinergic drug that is used most commonly in _____.

6. Atropine is a classic _____.

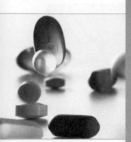

Chapter Capsule

This section repeats the objectives from the beginning of the chapter and then provides a summary of the most important concepts for that objective. Use this section as a quick review and to check your knowledge.

Objective 1: List the two divisions of the nervous system and their subdivisions.

- Central nervous system (CNS): brain and spinal cord
- Peripheral nervous system (PNS)
  - Autonomic nervous system
    - Motor neurons
      - Sympathetic nervous system
      - Parasympathetic nervous system
    - Sensory neurons

Objective 2: Explain the basic functional unit cell of the nervous system.

- Neurons—carry nervous system signals throughout body

Objective 3: Define the terms *cholinergic* and *adrenergic*.

- Cholinergic—liberating or activated by the neurotransmitter acetylcholine
- Adrenergic—liberating or activated by norepinephrine, epinephrine, or dopamine

Objective 4: Describe the fight-or-flight response.

- The body's reaction to a sudden threat or source of stress, such as trauma, fear, hypoglycemia, cold, or exercise
- Activates the sympathetic nervous system during emergencies

Objective 5: List the two main adrenergic receptors and what they respond to.

- Alpha receptor—responds to adrenaline
- Beta receptor—responds to norepinephrine and epinephrine

Objective 6: Explain the actions of adrenergic agonists.

- Mimic the sympathetic nervous system
- Produce fight-or-flight symptoms

Objective 7: Explain the actions of receptor agonists.

- Alpha-receptor agonists—influence both blood pressure and tissue perfusion
- Beta-receptor agonists—work against catecholamines, reducing receptor occupancy by beta agonists

Objective 8: Define adrenergic antagonists.

- Block adrenergic nerve transmission (usually by inhibiting the release of neurotransmitters or depleting the stores of transmitters)

Objective 9: List the two types of cholinergic receptors.

- Muscarinic receptors—innervate smooth muscle and slow the heart rate
- Nicotinic receptors—affect skeletal muscle

Objective 10: Discuss the source of atropine and how it works.

■ Original source—the belladonna plant

■ Selectively blocks all muscarinic responses to acetylcholine (whether excitatory or inhibitory); works on the muscarinic receptor, with little effect on the nicotinic receptor

Internet Sites of Interest

■ Search **http://faculty.washington.edu/chudler/ehceduc.html** for recent research and a great site called Neuroscience for Kids that explains and uses great graphics to illustrate the concepts of neurotransmitters, the autonomic nervous system, and more.

■ Go to the American Heart Association's Web site (**www.americanheart.org**) and search on "autonomic nervous system." You'll find information on how the system works in relation to the cardiovascular system. Learn, too, how the ANS impacts blood pressure.

■ Search for "autonomic nervous system" on Medline Plus at **http://www.nlm.nih.gov/medlineplus/**.

Chapter 16

Chapter

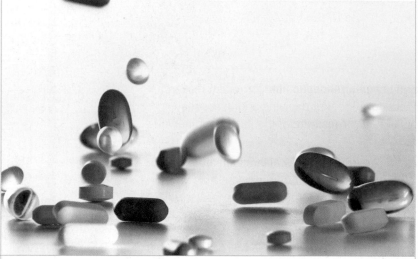

Anesthetic Agents

PRACTICAL SCENARIO

A nurse reports she was reprimanded for being late in giving a preanesthetic medication. She administered the drug 10 minutes before the patient was taken to surgery. The patient was placed under general anesthesia for the surgical procedure. Several hours after the surgery, the patient suffered complications and reported that no one told him ahead of time what to expect in the recovery room.

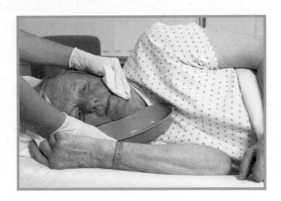

Critical Thinking Questions

1. Why is it important to administer the preanesthetic medication at the proper time prior to surgery?

2. When the nurse realized she was delayed in giving the preanesthetic, what should she have done?

3. In what way did the nurse neglect her responsibilities toward the patient?

Introduction

It was not until the 1840s that surgical anesthesia became possible with the introduction of three agents in quick succession: chloroform, ether, and nitrous oxide. These three agents, when inhaled quickly, led to unconsciousness, and surgical anesthesia was produced. Today, the patient having surgery receives medication before, during, and after surgery to achieve specific therapeutic outcomes. Usually, all other medication orders are withheld when the patient goes to surgery.

General **anesthetics** normally are used to produce loss of consciousness before and during surgery. However, for certain minor procedures, an anesthetic may be given in small amounts to relieve anxiety or pain without causing unconsciousness. These are called *local anesthetics*. They numb small areas of tissue where a minor procedure is to be done and are commonly used in dentistry and for minor surgery. **Regional anesthesia** affects a larger (but still limited) part of the body and is often used in obstetrics (labor and delivery). It does not make the person unconscious. Spinal and epidural anesthesia are examples of regional anesthesia.

The ideal anesthetic agent should possess the following characteristics:

✳ Rapid and pleasant induction and withdrawal from **anesthesia** (loss of sensation and/or consciousness)

✳ Skeletal muscle relaxation

✳ **Analgesia** (pain relief while still conscious)

✳ High potency

✳ A wide therapeutic index

✳ Nonflammability

✳ Chemical inertness with regard to anesthetic delivery devices

In practice, however, it is common to employ a variety of drugs because no one agent meets all these criteria.

Stages of Anesthesia

Before patients reach surgical anesthesia, they go through four stages: analgesia, excitement (delirium), surgical anesthesia, and medullary paralysis.

STAGE 1: Analgesia Pain is the first sense to be abolished, and consciousness is still retained. This type of anesthesia is often used in childbirth and in trauma, in the form of Entonox, which is a mixture of nitrous oxide and oxygen. The patient inhales the gas until pain recedes, but does not inhale enough to reach the unconscious state, thus maintaining some control over the situation. The sense of hearing is often enhanced in this stage.

STAGE 2: **Excitement** This stage may not be a pleasant time of anesthesia. The patient, more or less unconscious, can suffer from shaking and become violent. A sense of extreme fear may be felt, which can produce a phobic response to any suggestion of anesthetics in the future. It is important that the passage from Stage 1 to Stage 3 be attained as quickly as possible. Sudden death can occur during Stage 2, possibly due to vagal nerve inhibition (the vagus nerve extends from the cranium to the abdomen).

STAGE 3: **Surgical Anesthesia** This stage is characterized by progressive muscular relaxation. Muscle relaxation is important during many surgical procedures because reflex movements can occur when a scalpel slices through the tissues. This muscular relaxation ends in respiratory paralysis and, unless the patient is on a respirator, death may ensue fairly quickly. These reflexes are abolished with high delivery rates of gaseous anesthetics, but the dividing line between the desired state and respiratory paralysis is narrow. Early anesthetists used various reflexes of the body, such as corneal reflexes and pupillary size, to help them determine when to reduce the amount of anesthetic given to maintain surgical anesthesia, but not so much as to return to Stage 2. To prevent the danger of respiratory depression, the use of a respirator during surgical procedures is usually obligatory. An endotracheal tube is passed into the trachea, which is connected to the respirator. Unfortunately, the laryngeal reflex (gag reflex) is one of the last reflexes to disappear before Stage 4 is reached.

STAGE 4: **Medullary Paralysis** This stage begins with respiratory failure and can lead to circulatory collapse. Through careful monitoring, this stage is avoided. If it is reached, it is called an *anesthetic accident.* In the induction of anesthesia with intravenous anesthetic agents, stages 1 to 3 merge so quickly into one another that they are not apparent.

Focus on Geriatrics

Respiratory Apnea

During the recovery period, the patient must be observed for underventilation by monitoring for respiratory apnea. It is very important to watch elderly patients and those with preexisting respiratory insufficiency.

Preoperative Medications as Adjuncts to Surgery

The surgical patient usually is given preoperative medications, called **preanesthetics**, 45 to 70 minutes before the scheduled surgery. Any delay in administration should be reported promptly to the surgical department.

A combination of preoperative drugs may be ordered to achieve the desired outcomes with minimal side effects. Such outcomes include sedation, reduced anxiety, amnesia to minimize unpleasant surgical memories, increased comfort during preoperative procedures, reduced gastric acidity and volume, increased gastric emptying, decreased nausea and vomiting, and reduced incidence of aspiration by drying oral and respiratory secretions. Table 16-1 ■ lists commonly prescribed preoperative medications.

Table 16-1 ■ Preoperative Medications as Adjuncts to Surgery

GENERIC NAME	TRADE NAME	AVERAGE ADULT DOSAGE	ROUTE OF ADMINISTRATION
Benzodiazepines			
diazepam	Valium	2–10 mg bid–qid or 15–30 mg/d sustained release	PO
		2–10 mg, repeat if needed in 3–4h	IM, IV
lorazepam	Ativan	2–4 mg at least 2 h before surgery	IM
		0.044–2 mg/kg 15–20 min before surgery	IV
midazolam	Versed	Premedicated: 0.15–0.25 mg/kg over 20–30 sec; allow 2 min for effect	IV
		Nonpremedicated: 0.3–0.35 mg/kg over 20–30 sec; allow 2 min for effect	IV
Opioid Analgesics			
meperidine	Demerol	50–150 mg 30–90 min before surgery	IM, subcutaneous
morphine	DepoDur	10–15 mg as single dose 30 min before surgery (max: 20 mg)	Epidural
Antacids			
sodium citrate	Bicitra	15–30 mL	PO
H$_2$-Receptor Antagonists			
cimetidine	Tagamet	300 mg	IM, IV, or PO
famotidine	Pepcid	20 mg	IV
ranitidine	Zantac	50 mg	IM, IV, or PO
Gastric Acid Pump Inhibitors (See Chapter 27 for a complete list.)			
lansoprazole	Prevacid	15–60 mg	PO
omeprazole	Prilosec	20–40 mg	PO
Antiemetics			
droperidol	Inapsine	2.5–10 mg 30–60 min before surgery	IM, IV
metoclopramide	Reglan	10 mg administered over 1–2 min	IM, IV
Anticholinergics			
atropine sulfate	Atropisol	0.4–0.6 mg	IM, IV
glycopyrrolate	Robinul	0.1–0.3 mg	IM, IV
scopolamine hydrobromide	Hyoscine	0.5–1 mg	IM, IV, subcutaneous

✳ Apply Your Knowledge 16.1

The following questions focus on what you have just learned about the types of anesthesia and the use of preoperative medications as adjuncts to surgery. *See Appendix E for the correct answers.*

FILL IN THE BLANK

Select terms from your reading to fill in the blanks.

1. The ideal anesthetic agent should possess the following characteristics: _____ and _____ induction and _____, _____ _____ relaxation, and a wide _____ _____.

2. Regional anesthesia affects a larger part of the body (compared with local anesthesia). It does not make the patient _____.

3. Local anesthetics are used in _____ and for _____ surgery.

4. Stage 4 anesthesia is termed an _____ _____.

5. In stage _____ anesthesia the patient is still conscious, but in stage _____ the patient is unconscious.

MATCHING

Match the lettered trade name to the numbered generic name. Be sure to review the text and tables before completing this exercise.

GENERIC NAME	TRADE NAME
1. _____ ranitidine	a. Pepcid
2. _____ lorazepam	b. Prilosec
3. _____ meperidine	c. Demerol
4. _____ famotidine	d. Zantac
5. _____ omeprazole	e. Ativan

General Anesthetics

General anesthesia affects the entire body and makes the patient unconscious by depressing the central nervous system (CNS). The unconscious patient is completely unaware of what is going on and does not feel pain from the surgery or procedure. Skeletal muscles relax and reflexes diminish as well.

The advantages of general anesthesia include rapid excretion of the anesthetic agent and prompt reversal of its effects when desired. In addition, general anesthesia can be used with all age groups and in any type of surgical procedure.

An ideal anesthetic drug would induce anesthesia smoothly and rapidly while allowing for prompt recovery after its administration is discontinued. The drug would also possess a wide margin of safety and be devoid of adverse effects. No single anesthetic agent is capable of achieving all of these desirable effects without some disadvantages when used alone. For this reason, modern anesthesiology practice commonly uses combinations of intravenous and inhaled drugs, taking advantage of each drug's individual favorable properties while attempting to minimize any potential for adverse reactions.

Focus Point

Choosing Appropriate Anesthesia

The choice of anesthetic drug depends on many factors, including the patient's general physical condition; the area, organ, or body system being operated on; and the anticipated length of the surgical procedure.

The anesthetic technique varies depending on the proposed type of diagnostic, therapeutic, or surgical intervention. For minor procedures, conscious sedation is used, employing oral or parenteral sedatives in conjunction with local anesthetics. These techniques provide profound analgesia, but retain the patient's ability to maintain his or her own airway and to respond to verbal commands. For more extensive surgical procedures, anesthesia frequently includes the use of preoperative benzodiazepines, induction of anesthesia with intravenous thiopental or propofol, and maintenance of anesthesia with a combination of inhaled and intravenous anesthetic drugs.

Focus on Geriatrics

Adverse Drug Reactions

Older adults are more likely to experience adverse drug reactions than will younger adults because, in general, they take more prescription medications. These adverse reactions may be drug–drug interactions, drug–disease interactions (in which a drug may adversely affect a patient with a certain condition), or drug–food interactions.

TYPES OF GENERAL ANESTHETICS

General anesthetics are usually given by inhalation or by intravenous injection.

Inhalation Anesthetics

Drugs given to induce or maintain general anesthesia are given either as gases or vapors (inhalation anesthetics) or injections (intravenous anesthetics). Most commonly, these two forms are combined, although it is possible to deliver anesthesia solely by inhalation or injection.

Inhalation anesthetic agents are either **volatile liquids** (easily vaporized) or gases and are usually delivered using an anesthesia machine. These machines allow mixtures of anesthetic agents with oxygen. Anesthetics and ambient air are delivered to the patient who is monitored along with the machine's parameters. Liquid anesthetics are vaporized in the machine.

Many compounds have been used for inhalation anesthesia, but only a few are still in widespread use. Today, desflurane (Suprane) and sevoflurane (Ultane) are the most widely used volatile anesthetics. They are often combined with nitrous oxide (Entonox). Older, less popular volatile anesthetics include isoflurane (Forane), halothane (Fluothane, Somnothane), enflurane (Ethrane), and methoxyflurane (Penthrane). The major inhalation anesthetics are listed in Table 16-2 ∎.

Table 16-2 ■ General Anesthetics Used by Inhalation

GENERIC NAME	TRADE NAME	PHYSICAL STATE AT ROOM TEMPERATURE
desflurane	Suprane	Volatile liquid
enflurane	Ethrane	Volatile liquid
halothane	Fluothane, Somnothane	Volatile liquid
isoflurane	Forane	Volatile liquid
methoxyflurane	Penthrane	Volatile liquid
nitrous oxide (laughing gas)	Entonox	Gas
sevoflurane	Ultane	Volatile liquid

Focus Point

The Dangers of Malignant Hyperthermia

Malignant hyperthermia is a life-threatening, acute pharmacogenetic disorder, that develops during or after anesthesia. This is a disorder that presents itself in some patients undergoing anesthesia and, in some cases, in the postoperative care unit. Hyperthermia is characterized by a rapid increase in body temperature, unexplained tachycardia, unstable blood pressure, muscle rigidity, and cyanosis. The body temperature may rise to above 115°F (46°C).

Intravenous Anesthetics

Injectable anesthetics are used for induction and maintenance of a state of unconsciousness. Anesthetists prefer to use intravenous injections because they are faster, less painful, and more reliable than intramuscular or subcutaneous injections. Among the most widely used drugs (Table 16-3 ■) are propofol (Diprivan); etomidate (Amidate); barbiturates, such as methohexital (Brevital) and thiopental (Pentothal); benzodiazepines, such as midazolam (Versed) and diazepam (Valium); and ketamine (Ketalar).

How do they work?

The mechanism of action of most of the intravenous agents is principally confined to the CNS. A common property of all general anesthetics is that they are all very **lipophilic** (able to dissolve much more easily in lipids than in water). This property is essential because the drug must cross the blood–brain barrier to be effective. Cell membranes are, by nature, both lipophilic and hydrophilic, depending on the site in the membrane. When the lipophilic anesthetic enters the lipid membrane, the whole membrane is slightly distorted and closes the sodium channels, causing a marginal blockage, which prevents neural conduction (Figure 16-1 ■).

How are they used?

Volatile anesthetics are rarely used as the sole agents for both induction and maintenance of anesthesia. Most commonly, intravenous and volatile anesthetics are combined in regimens of so-called balanced anesthesia. Of the inhaled anesthetics, nitrous oxide (Entonox), desflurane (Suprane), sevoflurane (Ultane), and isoflurane (Forane) are the most commonly used in the United States. Use of the more soluble volatile anesthetics has declined during the last decade because more surgical procedures are being performed on an outpatient or *short-stay* basis. Both desflurane (Suprane) and sevoflurane (Ultane) allow a more rapid recovery and produce fewer postoperative adverse effects than halothane (Fluothane, Somnothane) or isoflurane (Forane). Although halothane (Fluothane, Somnothane) is still used in pediatric anesthesia, sevoflurane (Ultane) is rapidly replacing halothane in this setting.

In the last two decades, there has been increasing use of intravenous drugs in anesthesia, both as adjuncts to inhaled anesthetics and in techniques that do not include inhaled anesthetics. Intravenous drugs such as thiopental (Pentothal), etomidate (Amidate), ketamine (Ketalar), and propofol (Diprivan) have a faster onset of anesthetic action than the fastest of the inhaled gaseous agents such as desflurane (Suprane) and sevoflurane (Ultane). Therefore, intravenous agents are commonly used for induction of anesthesia.

What are the adverse effects?

Because intravenous (and inhaled) anesthetics affect the CNS, patients may feel drowsy, weak, or tired for as long as a few days after having general anesthesia. Fuzzy thinking, blurred vision, and coordination problems are also possible. For these reasons, anyone who has had general anesthesia should not drive, operate machinery, or perform other activities that could endanger themselves or others for at least 24 hours, or longer if necessary.

After general anesthesia, patients may also complain of headache, shivering, muscle pain, mental or mood changes, nausea or vomiting, sore throat, and nightmares.

What are the contraindications and interactions?

Intravenous anesthetics are contraindicated in patients who have received monoamine oxidase (MAO) inhibitors within 14 days. Those who are intolerant to benzodiazepines or have hypersensitivity, myasthenia gravis, acute narrow-angle glaucoma, increased intracranial pressure, impaired cerebral circulation, acute alcohol intoxication, intraarterial injection, a history of paradoxic excitation, status asthmaticus, and acute intermittent or other hepatic porphyrias should not receive general anesthetics. They are contraindicated in shock and coma, and during obstetric procedures, labor and delivery, and lactation. They must be used carefully during pregnancy and in children younger than age 12. Interactions occur with alcohol and other CNS depressants, MAO inhibitors, anticonvulsants, cimetidine (Tagamet), levodopa (Larodopa), phenytoin (Dilantin), phenothiazines, and in patients who smoke. The general anesthetic propofol (Diprivan) interacts with alfentanil (Alfenta). Midazolam (Versed) and thiopental (Pentothal) both interact with the herbal supplements kava-kava and valerian.

What are the important points patients should know?

Because these drugs can interact with medications administered in the perioperative period, ask the patient about the use of over-the-counter (OTC) medications, including herbal supplements. Instruct the patient in deep breathing and coughing, which reopens the lung alveoli and helps to clear secretions from the lower respiratory tract. Encourage the patient to perform these maneuvers as soon as possible after emergence from deep sedation or general anesthesia.

Focus on Natural Products

Stopping Herbal Medications Before Surgery

The recent increased use of natural products has been an issue raised by the American Society of Anesthesiologists concerning anesthesia. It is recommended that patients stop taking herbal medications at least two to three weeks before surgery to decrease the risk of adverse effects resulting from an enhancement or prolongation of anesthetic effects.

Table 16-3 ■ General Anesthetics Commonly Given by Injection

GENERIC NAME	TRADE NAME	AVERAGE ADULT DOSAGE	ROUTE OF ADMINISTRATION
etomidate	Amidate	0.3 mg/kg over 30–60 sec	IV
fentanyl	Sublimaze	Up to 150 mcg/kg PRN	IV
ketamine	Ketalar	100 mg	IM
methohexital sodium	Brevital Sodium	5–12 mL of 1% solution at a rate of 1 mL q5min; then 2–4 mL q4–7 min PRN	IV
midazolam	Versed	Premedicated: 0.15–0.25 mg/kg over 20–30 sec; allow 2 min for effect Nonpremedicated: 0.3–0.35 mg/kg over 20–30 sec; allow 2 min for effect	IV
propofol	Diprivan	2–2.5 mg/kg q10 sec until induction onset	IV
thiopental	Pentothal	Test dose: 25–75 mg; then 50–75 mg at 20–40 sec intervals; additional 50 mg may be given if needed	IV

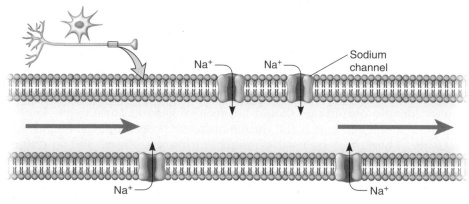

A Normal nerve conduction

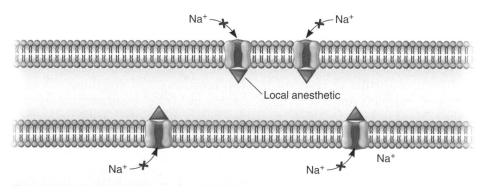

B Local anesthetic blocking sodium channels

Figure 16-1 ■ Mechanism of action of anesthetics: (A) normal nerve conduction; (B) anesthetic blocking sodium channels.

Focus Point

Diabetes and Surgery

The stress of surgery in diabetic patients may increase (rather than decrease) blood glucose level. Insulin injections and/or hypoglycemic medications should be coordinated with the patient, surgeon, and anesthesiologist.

✳ Apply Your Knowledge 16.2

The following questions focus on what you have just learned about general anesthetics. *See Appendix E for the correct answers.*

FILL IN THE BLANK

Select terms from your reading to fill in the blanks.

1. The mechanism of action of inhaled anesthetics is principally confined to the _____ _____.

2. _____ is the most widely used inhalation anesthetic today.

3. The advantages of intravenous anesthetic agents include greater _____, _____ action, and _____ pain.

4. The mechanism of action of inhaled anesthetics is principally confined to the _____.

5. The anesthetic technique varies depending on the proposed type of _____, _____, or _____ intervention.

MATCHING

Match the lettered trade name to the numbered generic name. Be sure to review the text and tables before completing this exercise.

GENERIC NAME	TRADE NAME
1. _____ methoxyflurane	a. Amidate
2. _____ halothane	b. Diprivan
3. _____ desflurane	c. Forane
4. _____ ketamine	d. Ethrane
5. _____ propofol	e. Sublimaze
6. _____ fentanyl	f. Ketalar
7. _____ enflurane	g. Versed
8. _____ isoflurane	h. Somnothane
9. _____ midazolam	i. Penthrane
10. _____ etomidate	j. Suprane

TYPES OF LOCAL ANESTHETICS

Local anesthesia is used to provide regional or topical anesthesia to relieve pain and to provide localized nerve block for surgical procedures without loss of consciousness. Generally, local anesthesia is safer than general anesthesia and allows for more rapid recovery. Local anesthetics are divided into two groups: esters and amides.

Ester-Type Agents

Ester-type local anesthetics have been in use longer than amides. Esters tend to have a rapid onset and short duration of activity (except tetracaine [Pontocaine]). Esters are associated with a higher incidence of allergic reactions due to one of their metabolites, para-amino benzoic acid (PABA). PABA is structurally similar to methylparaben. Ester-type agents include benzocaine, cocaine, procaine, propoxycaine, chloroprocaine, and tetracaine. Because of these possible hypersensitivity reactions, many manufacturers have reformulated some of their products to eliminate methylparaben.

Generally, they are used topically. Procaine 2% (Novocain) is still marketed for use with epinephrine (Adrenalin), but is rarely used. Tetracaine (Pontocaine) is most efficacious as a topical anesthetic, but also is 10 times more toxic than procaine. However, amides are often recommended over esters. They are safer and can be used for topical applications as well.

Amide-Type Agents

The most commonly recognized drug in the class of amides is lidocaine (Xylocaine), which was synthesized in 1943. The amides have several advantages over the esters. Amide local anesthetics do not undergo metabolism to PABA as esters do, and therefore, hypersensitivity to amide local anesthetics is rare. Also, they can undergo repeated high-temperature sterilization without losing potency. Most of the local anesthetics in common use today belong to the amide class. These include (in addition to lidocaine) bupivacaine (Marcaine, Sensorcaine), mepivacaine (Carbocaine), etidocaine (Duranest), prilocaine (Citanest), and the most recent, ropivacaine (Naropin).

Lidocaine is supplied in many formulations including an ointment, a water-soluble jelly, and a 4% solution for topical use; a 5% solution with dextrose for spinal administration; and 0.5%, 1%, 1.5%, and 2% solutions for injection. It is also widely available in a 1% multidose vial and pre-prepared with epinephrine (Adrenalin). The most common local anesthetics are summarized in Table 16-4 ■.

How do they work?

Local anesthetics appear to work by inhibiting the movement of sodium through channels in the membrane of a neuron, which, in turn, inhibits the transmission of nerve impulses. The action of the local anesthetics is dosedependent. The more drug present, the more the inhibition, until a complete block is produced.

Local anesthetics can also affect sodium channels in other parts of the body, such as the conduction system of the heart. This can lead to an abnormal heartbeat; thus, systemic distribution of local anesthetics is best kept to a minimum.

How are they used?

Local anesthesia is useful in a wide variety of clinical situations. It increases patient comfort and facilitates patient cooperation during procedures. As a diagnostic aid, it helps localize or identify the source of pain. Local anesthesia is warranted for any clinical procedure with a potential for pain, such as incision and drainage of abscesses, laceration repair, biopsy, wart treatment, vasectomy, neonatal circumcision, and dental procedures. Local anesthesia is also used during labor and delivery, and for diagnostic procedures such as gastrointestinal endoscopy. Occasionally, local anesthetics are used to relieve pain associated with pathologic conditions.

What are the adverse effects?

True allergic reactions to local anesthetics are rare and usually involve ester agents. Allergic reactions are seldom caused by amide anesthetics. There is no cross-reactivity between amide and ester agents.

It is important to keep track of the total anesthetic dose given because toxic effects are dose related. Adverse effects are related to the CNS and, to a lesser degree, the cardiovascular system. Symptoms of toxicity include light-headedness, dizziness, nystagmus (rhythmical oscillation of the eyeballs), restlessness, disorientation, and psychosis. Slurred speech and tremors often precede seizures. Hypotension, bradycardia, and cardiac arrest may occur.

What are the contraindications and interactions?

Local anesthetics are contraindicated in older adults and debilitated patients and should be used cautiously in children younger than 14 years. They should not be used during pregnancy, labor, or lactation. They are contraindicated in patients who are hypersensitive to these agents; and who have sepsis, acidosis, heart or spinal block, severe hemorrhage, hypotension and shock, hypertension, cerebrospinal deformities or diseases, blood dyscrasias, supraventricular dysrhythmias, untreated sinus bradycardia, or bowel pathology. They should not be used concurrently with long-term ophthalmic preparations, bupivacaine or chloroprocaine, obstetrical paracervical anesthesia, spinal anesthesia, or topical or IV regional anesthesia. Avoid use on infected application or injection sites, on a perforated eardrum or ear discharge, or on large areas. They are contraindicated in patients with a history of malignant hyperthermia or during severe trauma. These drugs interact with sulfonamides, epinephrine (Adrenalin), MAO inhibitors, antihypertensive agents, isoproterenol (Isuprel), ergonovine (Ergotrate Maleate), tricyclic antidepressants, phenothiazines, other local anesthetics, barbiturates, cimetidine (Tagamet), beta blockers, quinidine (Quinidex), phenytoin (Dilantin), and procainamide (Procan, Pronestyl).

What are the important points patients should know?

Instruct patients who have received local anesthetics to report symptoms such as lightheadedness, dizziness, disorientation, or slurred speech, and to avoid driving or operating heavy machinery.

Table 16-4 ■ Local Anesthetics

GENERIC NAME	TRADE NAME	AVERAGE ADULT DOSAGE	ROUTE OF ADMINISTRATION
Esters			
benzocaine	Americaine, Benzocol, Oracin	Lowest effective dose	Topical
cocaine	None	1–10% solution (use greater than 4% solution with caution) (max: single dose of 1 mg/kg)	Topical
procaine	Novocain	0.25–0.5% solution	Subcutaneous
tetracaine	Xylocaine	1–2 drops of 0.5% solution diluted with equal volume of 10% dextrose	Topical
Amides			
bupivacaine	Marcaine, Sensorcaine	0.25–0.75% solution	IM local infiltration, sympathetic block, lumbar epidural, caudal block, peripheral nerve block, retrobulbar block
etidocaine	Duranest	0.5–1.5% solution (max: 300 mg, 400 mg if given with epinephrine)	Percutaneous infiltration, peripheral nerve block (caudal), central neural block
lidocaine	Xylocaine	0.5–5% solution, solution w/glucose (spinal), solution with dextrose (saddle block), jelly/ointment/cream/solution (topical)	Infiltration, nerve block, epidural, caudal, spinal, saddle block, topical
mepivacaine	Carbocaine	1–2% solution	Infiltration, nerve block, caudal and lumbar epidural
ropivacaine	Naropin	5–250 mg (0.5–1% solution)	Epidural, nerve block

Focus on Pediatrics

Dose-Related Toxicity

In infants and young children, it is essential to administer the appropriate total anesthetic dose because the toxicity of these agents is dose-related.

✳ Apply Your Knowledge 16.3

The following questions focus on what you have just learned about local anesthesia. *See Appendix E for the correct answers.*

FILL IN THE BLANK
Select terms from your reading to fill in the blanks.

1. True allergic reactions to local anesthetics usually involve _____ _____.

2. Write five indications for local anesthesia: (1) _____, (2) _____, (3) _____, (4) _____, and (5) _____.

3. It is important to keep track of the total anesthetic dose given because _____ _____ are dose-related.

4. Local anesthetics are divided into two groups: _____ and _____.

5. Most of the local anesthetics in common use today belong to the _____ _____ class.

MATCHING
Match the lettered trade name to the numbered generic name.

GENERIC NAME	TRADE NAME
1. _____ tetracaine	a. Novocain
2. _____ bupivacaine	b. Marcaine
3. _____ mepivacaine	c. Duranest
4. _____ lidocaine	d. Xylocaine
5. _____ etidocaine	e. Carbocaine
6. _____ procaine	f. Pontacaine
7. _____ ropivacaine	g. Naropin

SPECIFIC APPLICATIONS

Several local anesthetics can be used with different techniques or specific applications. They include topical anesthesia, infiltration anesthesia, field block anesthesia, nerve block anesthesia, spinal anesthesia, and epidural anesthesia. Techniques for applying local anesthesia are illustrated in Figure 16-2 ■.

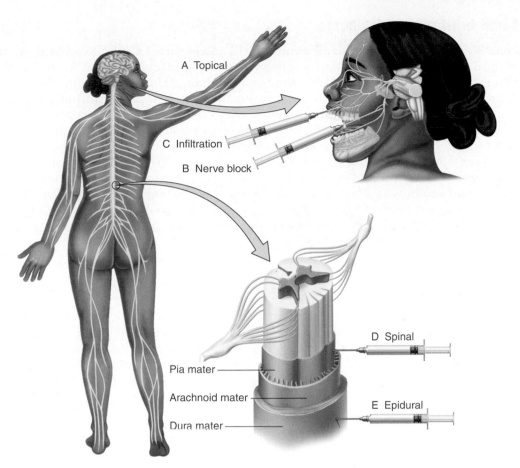

Figure 16-2 ■ Techniques for applying local anesthesia: (A) topical; (B) nerve block; (C) infiltration; (D) spinal; and (E) epidural.

Topical Anesthesia

Topical anesthesia involves the placement of a nerve conduction-blocking agent onto a tissue layer (skin or mucous membrane). This method is used to provide anesthesia on mucous membranes of the urethra, vagina, rectum, and skin. The tissue affected is limited to the area in contact with the topical anesthetic. Topical anesthesia is usually administered by the physician and is achieved with either the use of **cryoanesthesia** or a pharmacological agent.

Cryoanesthesia involves the reduction of nerve conduction by localized cooling. This may be accomplished with ice or by the use of a cryoanesthesia machine to produce the cooling action. Reduced skin temperature may also be a result of a pharmaceutical agent sprayed onto the skin, such as ethyl chloride. Lidocaine (Xylocaine) and cocaine are examples of topical anesthetic agents. Although the amount of agent applied is limited, the patient must be monitored for toxic reactions.

Focus Point

Contact with Topical Anesthetics

Patients should be advised that when using topical anesthetics for skin conditions, they must not touch their eyes. Also, topical medications should never be applied to areas where there is an open lesion or cut.

Local Infiltration Anesthesia

Local infiltration anesthesia, which works by blocking nerves, is produced by injection of local anesthetic solution directly into an area that is painful or about to be operated upon. Local infiltration is probably the most common route used to administer local anesthetics and is the simplest form of regional anesthesia. Local infiltration is used primarily for minor surgical procedures, such as the removal of superficial skin lesions, suturing of a wound, or slightly more invasive surgeries, such as insertion of chest tubes. In this technique, a local anesthetic agent is injected into superficial tissues to produce a small area of analgesia and anesthesia. When a local anesthetic is to be administered by infiltration, epinephrine may be added to it in order to decrease its dosage and prolong its duration of action. However, epinephrine (Adrenalin) should not be used to anesthetize fingers, toes, and other tissues with end arteries. Lidocaine (Xylocaine) is a popular choice for infiltration anesthesia, but bupivacaine (Marcaine, Sensorcaine) is used for longer procedures.

Field Block Anesthesia

Field block anesthesia affects a single nerve, a deep plexus, or a network of nerves. Field block anesthesia and nerve block are forms of regional anesthesia. For example, a radial nerve block may be used to anesthetize the structures innervated by the radial nerve, including portions of the forearm and hand. Intraorbital block is often used for ocular surgery. A local anesthetic is administered in a series of injections to form a wall of anesthesia encircling the operative field.

Spinal Anesthesia

During **spinal anesthesia**, an anesthetic agent is injected into the **subarachnoid** space (beneath the arachnoid membrane or between the arachnoid and pia mater, and filled with cerebrospinal fluid) through a spinal needle. Spinal anesthesia can be used for many procedures but is most often used for gynecological, obstetrical, orthopedic, and genitourinary surgery. Spinal anesthesia may cause marked vasodilation (hypotension), headaches, and respiratory depression. Lidocaine (Xylocaine), tetracaine (Xylocaine), or bupivacaine (Marcaine, Sensorcaine) are often used for spinal anesthesia.

Epidural Anesthesia

Epidural anesthesia involves injection of the local anesthetic into the epidural (lumbar or caudal) space via a catheter that allows repeated infusions. After injection, the anesthetic agent is very slowly absorbed into the cerebrospinal fluid. This is popular for labor and delivery. High concentrations of local anesthetic can get into the blood circulation and may increase risk of systemic toxicity. Therefore, they can cause cardiac depression and neurotoxicity in the mother and neonate. Highly lipid-soluble locals such as lidocaine (Xylocaine) tend to get into the blood more than the less lipid-soluble agents such as bupivacaine (Marcaine, Sensorcaine).

Focus Point

Alleviating Headache After Spinal Block

Patients should be advised to lay flat for approximately 12 hours following a spinal block or epidural to prevent the leakage of cerebrospinal fluid, which may increase the risk of a postanesthetic headache.

Apply Your Knowledge 16.4

The following questions focus on what you have just learned about specific applications of anesthesia. *See Appendix E for the correct answers.*

MATCHING

Match the lettered term to the numbered description.

DESCRIPTION

1. _____ May cause marked hypotension, headaches, and respiratory depression.
2. _____ Can relieve pain caused by oral, nasal, or rectal disorders.
3. _____ This type of local anesthesia is popular for labor and delivery.
4. _____ Intraorbital anesthesia is an example of this type of local anesthesia.
5. _____ Is probably the most common route used to administer local anesthetics.

TERM

a. Epidural anesthesia
b. Infiltration anesthesia
c. Topical anesthesia
d. Spinal anesthesia
e. Field block anesthesia

Chapter Capsule

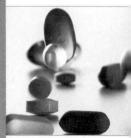

This section repeats the objectives from the beginning of the chapter and then provides a summary of the most important concepts for that objective. Use this section as a quick review and to check your knowledge.

Objective 1: Outline the stages of anesthesia.

- Stage 1—Analgesia: pain is abolished; consciousness is retained; sense of hearing is often enhanced
- Stage 2—Excitement: may be unpleasant; patient can suffer from shaking and become violent, or feel extreme fear; passage from Stage 1 to Stage 3 must be attained as quickly as possible, as sudden death can occur during Stage 2, possibly due to vagal nerve inhibition
- Stage 3—Surgical Anesthesia: characterized by progressive muscular relaxation, which must be controlled to avoid respiratory paralysis; various body reflexes, corneal reflexes, and pupillary size are helpful indicators; patients are usually put on a respirator during this stage
- Stage 4—Medullary Paralysis: begins with respiratory failure; can lead to circulatory collapse; through careful monitoring, this stage is avoided

Objective 2: Define the importance of premedications before anesthesia.

■ Premedications, also known as *preoperative medications* or preanesthetics help to:

- ❑ Achieve sedation
- ❑ Reduce anxiety
- ❑ Induce amnesia (to minimize unpleasant surgical memories)
- ❑ Increase comfort during preoperative procedures
- ❑ Reduce gastric acidity and volume
- ❑ Increase gastric emptying
- ❑ Decrease nausea and vomiting
- ❑ Reduce incidence of aspiration by drying oral and respiratory secretions

Objective 3: Explain the action of anesthetics within the central nervous system.

■ Depresses the CNS to cause unconsciousness

■ Creates unawareness of surroundings and blocks pain from surgery or procedure

■ Relaxes patients' skeletal muscles and diminishes reflexes

Objective 4: List the effects of general anesthetics.

■ Loss of consciousness before and during surgery

■ Relief of anxiety or pain without causing unconsciousness

Objective 5: Describe the common local anesthetics and their uses.

■ Ester-type agents—generally used topically

■ Amide-type agents—most commonly used; used to increase patient comfort, facilitate patient cooperation, as diagnostic aids, and for the following specific procedures:

- ❑ Incision and drainage of abscesses
- ❑ Laceration repair
- ❑ Biopsy
- ❑ Wart treatment
- ❑ Vasectomy
- ❑ Neonatal circumcision
- ❑ Dental procedures
- ❑ Labor and delivery
- ❑ Diagnostic procedures such as gastrointestinal endoscopy
- ❑ Pain relief associated with pathologic conditions

Objective 6: Compare ester and amide local anesthetics.

■ Ester-type agents—due to allergic reactions caused by PABA, these agents are generally not preferred; amide-type agents are often recommended instead

■ Amide-type agents—safer than ester-type agents with less allergic reaction potential; they are available in many forms including ointments, jellies, and solutions for injection

Objective 7: List the problems associated with the use of local anesthetics.

■ Allergic reactions involving the ester-type agents, due to the ingredient para-amino benzoic acid (PABA), are not uncommon

- Toxic effects are possible and dose related
- Light-headedness, dizziness, nystagmus, restlessness, disorientation, and psychosis may be experienced
- Slurred speech and tremors often precede seizures
- Hypotension, bradycardia, and cardiac arrest may occur

Objective 8: Explain the indications for spinal anesthesia.

- Gynecological, obstetrical, orthopedic, and genitourinary surgery

 Internet Sites of Interest

- The journal of the Anesthesia and Analgesia Organization can be searched at: **www.anesthesia-analgesia.org**
- Excellent patient information can be found at the Web site of the American Society of Anesthesiologists: **http://www.asahq.org/patientEducation.htm**
- Scientific America online offers an article titled "How does anesthesia work?" Search at: **http://www.sciam.com**
- Look up "anesthesia" at Health AtoZ's Web site: **http://www.healthatoz.com/healthatoz/Atoz/default.jsp** to find information on general and local anesthesia.

Chapter 17

Effects of Drugs on Skin Disorders

PRACTICAL SCENARIO

A 45-year-old woman who has spent more than 20 summers at the beaches of Florida and goes to the tanning salon three times a week notices that a small spot has appeared on her arm. It is a different color than the surrounding skin and has a bumpy surface. She assumes that it is a skin infection or bite and applies an over-the-counter antibiotic ointment for several weeks. Finally, she calls her physician's office and speaks to you, wondering if she should schedule an office visit for such a small matter.

Critical Thinking Questions

1. What questions might you ask the patient about the skin spot?
2. What should you tell the patient to do about scheduling an office visit?
3. Once the patient has been seen by the physician and treated, what patient education can you provide to her?

Introduction

The integumentary system is the largest of all organs in the human body. It consists of the skin, hair, nails, sweat glands, and oil glands. The skin forms a barrier between ourselves and our environment and, as such, is fundamental to the functioning of all other organs. The skin is vital in maintaining homeostasis. In addition to providing a protective covering, the skin helps regulate body temperature, retards water loss from deeper tissues, houses sensory receptors, synthesizes various biochemicals, and excretes small quantities of wastes.

The Skin

The skin consists of two distinct layers (Figure 17-1 ■). The outer layer is called the epidermis. The inner layer, or dermis, is thicker than the epidermis. Beneath the dermis are masses of loose connective and adipose tissues that bind the skin to the underlying organs. These tissues form the subcutaneous layer, which lies beneath the skin but is not a true layer of skin.

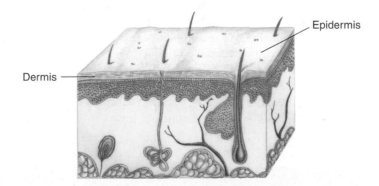

Epidermis

Dermis

Figure 17-1 ■ The two layers of the skin.

EPIDERMIS

The epidermis has either four or five sublayers. The outermost sublayer is the *stratum corneum* (horny layer). The deepest layer of epidermal cells, called the *stratum basale* or *stratum germinativum,* is close to the dermis and is nourished by dermal blood vessels. As the cells of this layer divide and grow, the older epidermal cells are pushed away from the dermis toward the skin surface. The farther the cells move, the poorer their nutrient supply becomes, and in time, they die. Specialized cells in the epidermis called *melanocytes* produce melanin, a dark pigment that provides skin color. Melanin absorbs ultraviolet (UV) radiation in sunlight, preventing mutations in the DNA of skin cells and other damaging effects. Melanocytes lie in the deepest portion of the epidermis.

DERMIS

The dermis binds the epidermis to underlying tissues. It is largely composed of dense, irregular connective tissue that gets its name from its irregular arrangement of thick protein fibers.

Dermal blood vessels supply nutrients to all skin cells. These vessels also help regulate body temperature. Nerve cell processes are scattered throughout the dermis. The dermis also contains hair follicles, oil glands, and sweat glands. Embedded in the skin are structures called *appendages,* such as the nails, hair follicles, and sweat and sebaceous glands, all of which are subject to disease.

SUBCUTANEOUS LAYER

The subcutaneous layer (hypodermis), beneath the dermal layer of the skin, consists of loose connective and adipose tissues. The adipose tissue of the subcutaneous layer insulates, helping to conserve body heat and impede the entrance of heat from the outside. The subcutaneous layer also contains the major blood vessels that supply the skin and underlying adipose tissue.

Disorders of the Skin

Disruptions in skin integrity may be precipitated by trauma, abnormal cellular function, infection and inflammation, and systemic diseases. Many of these diseases are caused by infections, and most of the drugs used to treat such infections are dealt with in Chapters 9 and 10. Other common diseases of the skin are due to inflammatory conditions resulting from allergies.

ECZEMA AND MISCELLANEOUS INFLAMMATORY DISORDERS

The most common inflammatory disorder of the skin is **eczema,** a response of the skin caused by endogenous and exogenous agents; it is often considered synonymous with **dermatitis** (inflammation of the skin). Endogenous eczemas include dermatitis and seborrheic dermatitis. Exogenous eczemas include irritant dermatitis and allergic contact dermatitis. Eczematous dermatitis is characterized by **erythema** (skin redness caused by capillary dilation), vesicles, scales, and itching.

The mainstay of treatment of acute or chronic inflammatory disorders is topical or oral corticosteroids. Systemic corticosteroids were discussed in other chapters. Only topical corticosteroids are discussed here (Table 17-1 ■).

Focus on Pediatrics

Eczema Common in Pediatric Patients

Atopic dermatitis (eczema) is common in pediatric patients. Eczema in some infants is believed to be traceable to sensitivity to milk, orange juice, or certain other foods.

Table 17-1 ■ Selected Topical Corticosteroids

GENERIC NAME	TRADE NAME	AVERAGE ADULT DOSAGE	ROUTE OF ADMINISTRATION
alclometasone	Aclovate	Apply 0.05% cream or ointment sparingly bid– tid.	Topical
amcinonide	Cyclocort	Apply thin film bid–tid.	Topical
betamethasone dipropionate	Diprolene, Diprosone	Apply thin film bid–tid.	Topical
betamethasone valerate	Betatrex, Psorion (cream), Valisone (scalp lotion)	Apply sparingly bid.	Topical
desoximetasone	Topicort	Apply thin layer bid.	Topical
dexamethasone sodium phosphate	Decaderm	Apply thin layer tid–qid.	Topical
diflorasone diacetate	Florone, Maxiflor	Apply thin layer of ointment 1–3 times/d or cream 2–4 times/d.	Topical
fluocinolone acetonide	Fluonid, Flurosyn	Apply thin layer bid–qid.	Topical
fluocinonide	Lidex	Apply thin layer bid–qid.	Topical
flurandrenolide	Cordran	Apply thin layer bid–tid; apply tape 1–2 times/d q12h.	Topical
hydrocortisone	Aeroseb-HC, Alphaderm	Apply a small amount to affected area 1–4 times/d.	Topical
triamcinolone	Aristocort, Atolone	Apply sparingly bid–tid.	Topical

Topical Corticosteroids

The corticosteroids are potent anti-inflammatory agents. Topical administration goes directly to the site of inflammation. These drug preparations are available as lotions, creams, and aerosols in various concentrations.

How do they work?
Topical corticosteroids prevent accumulation of inflammatory cells at sites of infection and inhibit phagocytosis. When applied to inflamed skin, they reduce itching, redness, and swelling.

How are they used?
Topical corticosteroids are used for treatment of skin disorders such as eczema, dermatitis, psoriasis, insect bite reactions, and burns (first- and second-degree). Topical corticosteroids are the primary agents used to treat dermatitis. Potency depends on the type of drug formulation and on whether it is packaged as a cream, lotion, solution, or gel.

What are the adverse effects?
Common localized adverse effects may include dryness, redness, itching, irritation, or burning of the skin. Topical corticosteroids may also produce secondary infections.

What are the contraindications and interactions?

Topical corticosteroids are contraindicated in bacterial skin infections. They must not be used in patients with known hypersensitivity. Topical corticosteroids should be used cautiously in pregnant or lactating women. Drug interactions are not significant when administered as directed.

What are the important points patients should know?

Advise patients to follow the directions of their physician regarding covering the treated area or leaving it exposed to air. The effectiveness of certain drugs depends on keeping the area covered or leaving it open. Instruct patients to not apply medications to areas other than those specified by their physician and to use the drug as directed (for example, a thin layer or apply liberally, and so forth). Topical corticosteroids must be kept away from the eyes (unless use in or around the eyes has been recommended).

✳ Apply Your Knowledge 17.1

The following questions focus on what you have just learned about the skin, disorders of the skin, and medications used to treat these disorders. *See Appendix E for the correct answers.*

MULTIPLE CHOICE

Choose the correct answers from choices a–d.

1. All of the following are important functions of the skin, except:
   a. Retarding water loss from deeper tissues
   b. Excreting small quantities of wastes
   c. Housing sensory receptors
   d. Housing motor nerve control

2. Specialized cells in the epidermis produce a dark pigment that provides skin color and is known as:
   a. Melanin
   b. Melatonin
   c. Bilirubin
   d. Keratin

3. Which of the following disorders is an example of eczema?
   a. Impetigo
   b. Seborrheic dermatitis
   c. Hay fever
   d. Shingles

4. The subcutaneous layer is also called:
   a. Dermis
   b. True skin
   c. Fibroderm
   d. Hypodermis

5. The subcutaneous layer consists of adipose tissues and contains:
   a. Melanocytes
   b. Melanin
   c. Major blood vessels
   d. Hair follicles

PSORIASIS

Psoriasis is a chronic, relapsing inflammatory skin disorder that occurs at any age. The onset usually occurs by 20 years of age. The cause of psoriasis is unknown, but it has a hereditary component. The disorder is marked by a greatly increased rate of cellular proliferation, which leads to thickening of the dermis and epidermis. It is characterized by rounded plaques, covered by silvery white, scaly patches. The skin lesions of psoriasis are variably pruritic. External factors may exacerbate psoriasis, including infections, stress, and medications such as lithium, beta blockers, and antimalarials.

The most common areas for psoriasis to occur are the elbows, knees, gluteal cleft, and scalp. Involvement tends to be symmetric. There is no cure for this disease yet, but remissions can often be produced by the available therapies, which include the use of UV light either alone or in combination with drugs, and topical and systemic treatments.

Focus Point

Preventing Recurrence of Psoriasis

Keeping the skin moist and lubricated, avoiding cold and dry climates, avoiding stress and anxiety, limiting alcohol intake, and not scratching the skin help to prevent recurrence of psoriasis.

Topical Antipsoriatics

Treatment is related to reducing epidermal cell turnover and immunomodulations. Mild lesions are usually treated with **emollients** (skin-softening agents), **keratolytic** agents (those that separate or loosen the horny layer of the epidermis), and topical corticosteroids. Systemic medications are used for moderate to severe lesions, which may respond to methotrexate (Amethopterin), acitretin (vitamin A), and vitamin D analogues. Sometimes, for the treatment of psoriasis, various techniques are used with or without other antipsoriasis medications (Table 17-2 ■). There are various forms of tar treatments (coal tar) and a material called *anthralin*. UV light (phototherapy) is used in cases of severe psoriasis.

How do they work?

The mechanism of action of acitretin (Soriatane), ammoniated mercury, and anthralin (Psoriatec) are unknown. Calcipotriene (Dovonex) is a synthetic vitamin D_3 that controls psoriasis by inhibiting proliferation of **keratinocytes** (epidermal cells that produce keratin) and decreasing the number of epithelial cells. Methoxsalen (Oxsoralen) is a psoralen derivative with strong photosensitizing effects. Methoxsalen (which causes photodamage) inhibits rapid and uncontrolled epidermal psoriasis.

How are they used?

Antipsoriatic agents are used for the treatment of moderate to severe forms of psoriasis in adults.

What are the adverse effects?

The major adverse effects associated with acitretin are alopecia, skin peeling, dry skin, **pruritus** (itching), rash, skin atrophy, and abnormal skin odor. The adverse effects of calcipotriene include facial dermatitis, burning, stinging, erythema, and itching. Methoxsalen may cause severe edema, erythema, burning, peeling, and thinning of the skin.

What are the contraindications and interactions?

Topical antipsoriatics are contraindicated in hypersensitivity to these agents. Patients with hypercalcemia or vitamin D toxicity should not use calcipotriene. The antipsoriatics are also contraindicated in pregnancy or lactating women.

What are the important points patients should know?

Instruct patients to avoid additional exposure to UV light for at least 8 hours after oral drug ingestion and UVA exposure. Warn patients against mixing calcipotriene with any other topical medicines. Advise patients to discontinue the drug and immediately report visual problems.

Table 17-2 ■ Antipsoriatic Drugs

GENERIC NAME	TRADE NAME	AVERAGE ADULT DOSAGE	ROUTE OF ADMINISTRATION
acitretin	Soriatane	10–50 mg/d with main meal	PO
azelaic acid	Azelex	Apply twice daily.	Topical
calcipotriene	Dovonex	Apply twice daily.	Topical
methoxsalen	Oxsoralen, Uvadex	Give 1.5–2 h before exposure to UV light 2–3 times/wk (amounts to use range from 10 mg to 70 mg based on weight of patient).	PO

ACNE

Acne vulgaris is an inflammatory disorder of the sebaceous glands that commonly occurs during puberty. The incidence of acne tends to decline with age and is unusual in adults, although it can persist for many years. Sebaceous glands secrete sebum, the natural oil of the skin. Testosterone is partially responsible for the secretion of sebum, and it may be that acne is caused by an increased responsiveness of the sebaceous glands to varying levels of this hormone during puberty. When too much sebum is produced, the duct of the gland may become blocked, and bacteria can become trapped beneath the sebum plug. The bacteria then grow in the duct, leading to a small abscess.

Focus on Natural Products

Use Caution in Treating Acne with Zinc

A variety of natural products are used to treat acne. The most common of these are zinc, niacinamide gel, and tea tree oil. It is important to note that zinc can be toxic at high dosages, primarily because it causes copper deficiency.

Antiacne Agents

Major drugs for acne-related disorders are listed in Table 17-3 ■. Benzoyl peroxide is a powerful oxidizing agent, which at least partially relieves some cases of acne by having bacterial action, and is the main over-the-counter (OTC) drug used for this purpose. Azelaic acid (Azelex) is a naturally occurring dicarboxylic acid. Topical antibiotics such as clindamycin (Cleocin) and erythromycin (Eryc) are also prescribed.

How do they work?

The antimicrobial action of these agents may be attributable to inhibition of microbial cellular protein synthesis. A normalization of **keratinization** (keratin formation or development of a horny layer) of some of these agents, such as azelaic acid and benzoyl peroxide, may also contribute to their clinical effectiveness.

How are they used?

These agents are used for mild to moderate inflammatory acne vulgaris. Topical applications of clindamycin are used in the treatment of acne vulgaris, and vaginal applications are used in the treatment of bacterial vaginosis in nonpregnant women.

What are the adverse effects?

Topical antiacne drugs may cause pruritus, burning, erythema, and stinging. Benzoyl peroxide can produce allergic dermatitis, excessive drying, peeling, erythema, and stinging. Topical clindamycin and erythromycin also produce dryness, burning, and excessive oil in the skin. In rare cases, clindamycin may cause bloody diarrhea and abdominal pain.

What are the contraindications and interactions?

These agents are avoided in patients with known hypersensitivity. Topical antiacne drugs are contraindicated during pregnancy and lactation.

What are the important points patients should know?

Instruct patients that proper application of these creams and gels is essential. Warn them to avoid contact with the eyes or mucous membranes, and to wash out the eyes with large amounts of water if contact with the medication occurs. Advise patients to avoid breastfeeding while using these agents or to consult their physician.

Table 17-3 ■ Major Drugs Used to Treat Acne

GENERIC NAME	TRADE NAME	AVERAGE ADULT DOSAGE	ROUTE OF ADMINISTRATION
adapalene	Differin	Apply once daily to affected areas (in the evening).	Topical
azelaic acid	Azelex	Apply twice daily.	Topical
benzoyl peroxide	BenzaClin, Benzamycin	Apply 1–2 times/d.	Topical
clindamycin, hydrochloride	Cleocin	Apply to affected areas bid.	Topical
doxycycline hyclate	Doryx, Vibramycin	100 mg q12h on Day 1; then 100 mg/d.	PO
tetracycline hydrochloride	Achromycin	Oral: 500–1,000 mg/d in 4 divided doses.	PO
		Topical: Apply to cleansed areas bid.	Topical
tretinoin	Retin-A	Apply once daily at bedtime.	Topical

Keratoses

Keratoses are characterized by a thickening of the keratin layer of the skin. Keratoses are benign lesions that are usually associated with aging or skin damage. *Seborrheic keratoses* result from proliferation of epidermis, leading to an oval elevation that may be smooth or rough and is often dark in color. *Actinic keratoses* occur on skin (especially fair skin) exposed to UV radiation. The lesion appears as a pigmented, scaly patch. Actinic keratoses may develop into skin cancer.

Keratolytic Agents

Keratolytic agents promote shedding of the horny layer of the epidermis and softening of scales. The most commonly used keratolytic agents are salicylic acid (Fostex), resorcinol, and sulfur. Selected keratolytic medications are summarized in Table 17-4 ■.

How do they work?

Keratolytics act by breaking down the protein structure of the keratin layer, thereby permitting easier removal of compacted cellular material.

How are they used?

Keratolytic agents are used in the treatment of corns, calluses, and plantar warts. Some of these medications (such as sulfur and ammonium lactate) are used in the treatment of acne, eczema, psoriasis, and seborrheic dermatitis.

What are the adverse effects?

The adverse effects of keratolytic agents include burning, local irritation, rash, dry skin, and scaling.

What are the contraindications and interactions?

Keratolytic drugs must be avoided in patients with known hypersensitivity. They are contraindicated on moles, warts with hair growing from them, genital or facial warts, birthmarks, or infected skin. Salicylic acid may cause salicylate toxicity (see Chapter 12) with prolonged use. These agents must be used cautiously during pregnancy and lactation.

What are the important points patients should know?

Instruct patients that keratolytic agents are for external use only. Tell them to avoid contact with the eye, face, mucous membranes, and normal skin around warts. Advise the patient to soak the area in warm water for 5 minutes prior to application to enhance the effect of the medication.

Table 17-4 ■ Selected Keratolytic Agents

GENERIC NAME	TRADE NAME	AVERAGE ADULT DOSAGE	ROUTE OF ADMINISTRATION
diclofenac sodium	Solaraze	Apply to affected area bid for 60–90 d.	Topical
masoprocol cream	Actinex	Apply to lesions bid for 14–28 d.	Topical
salicylic acid	Fostex, Mediplast	Apply enough medicine to cover affected area and rub in gently, or apply patch as directed.	Topical
salicylic acid with podophyllum	Podocon-25, Podofin	Apply enough medicine to cover affected area and rub in gently, or apply patch as directed.	Topical

Focus Point

Corns and Calluses

Corns and calluses are extremely common, localized hyperplastic areas of the stratum corneum layer of the epidermis.

✳ Apply Your Knowledge 17.2

The following questions focus on what you have just learned about psoriasis, acne, and keratoses and medications that are used to treat them. *See Appendix E for the correct answers.*

FILL IN THE BLANK

Select terms from your reading to fill in the blanks.

1. A chronic, relapsing inflammatory skin disorder that occurs at any age is known as _____.

2. After taking antipsoriatics, patients should avoid exposure to _____.

3. An inflammatory disorder of the sebaceous glands that commonly occurs during puberty is known as _____.

4. The main OTC drug used to treat acne is known as _____.

5. Keratoses are characterized by a thickening of the keratin layer of the skin, and these conditions include _____, _____, and _____.

6. The mechanism of action of acitretin (Soriatane) is _____.

7. Systemic medications are used for moderate to severe lesions and may include methotrexate, _____, and _____.

8. Seborrheic keratoses result from proliferation of _____.

Bacterial Skin Infections

Cutaneous infections are common forms of skin disease. Most bacterial infections of the skin are caused by local invasion by pathogens. Staphylococci and beta-hemolytic streptococci are the common causative microorganisms. Examples of skin and hair bacterial infections include impetigo, cellulites, and folliculitis. These infections generally remain localized, although serious complications can occur. Impetigo is a common superficial bacterial infection of skin caused by either *Streptococcus* or *Staphylococcus aureas*. The primary lesion is a superficial pustule that ruptures and forms a characteristic yellow-brown crust. Lesions caused by staphylococci may be tense, clear bullae, and this less common form of the disease is called *bulbous impetigo*. Treatment of impetigo involves gentle debridement of adherent crusts, which is facilitated by the use of soaks and topical antibiotics in conjunction with appropriate oral antibiotics. Topical antibiotic drugs are listed in Table 17-5 ■. Systemic antibiotics were discussed in Chapter 9.

Table 17-5 ■ Topical Antibiotic Drugs

GENERIC NAME	TRADE NAME	AVERAGE ADULT DOSAGE	ROUTE OF ADMINISTRATION
azelaic acid	Azelex	Apply thin film to clean and dry area bid.	Topical
bacitracin	Baciguent	Apply thin layer of ointment bid–tid as solution of 250–1,000 units/mL in wet dressing.	Topical
benzoyl peroxide	Benzac, Loroxide	Apply 1–2 times/d.	Topical
clindamycin, topical	Clcocin T, Dalacin C	Apply to affected areas bid.	Topical

(*continued*)

Table 17-5 ■ Topical Antibiotic Drugs (*continued*)

GENERIC NAME	TRADE NAME	AVERAGE ADULT DOSAGE	ROUTE OF ADMINISTRATION
gentamicin sulfate	Garamycin	1–2 drops of solution in eye q4h up to 2 drops q1h or small amount of ointment bid–tid.	Topical
metronidazole	MetroGel, MetroLotion	Apply thin film to affected area bid.	Topical
mupirocin	Bactroban	Apply to affected area tid; if no response in 3–5 d, reevaluate (usually continue for 1–2 wk).	Topical
neomycin sulfate	Myciguent	Apply 1–3 times/d.	Topical
sulfacetamide sodium	Sebizon	Apply thin film to affected area 1–3 times/d.	Topical

FUNGAL INFECTIONS

Dermatophytes are fungi that infect skin, hair, and nails. Infection of the foot (tinea pedis) is most common and is often chronic. It is characterized by variable erythema and edema, scaling, pruritus, and occasionally vesiculation. Involvement may be widespread or localized, but almost invariably the web space between the fourth and fifth toes is affected. Infection of the nails (tinea unguium) occurs in many patients with tinea pedis and is characterized by opacified, thickened nails, and subungual debris.

The groin is the next most commonly involved area (tinea cruris), with men affected much more often than women. Dermatophyte infection of the scalp (tinea capitis) produces an inflammatory or relatively noninflammatory condition that may present with either well-defined or irregular, diffuse areas of mild scaling and hair loss.

Candidiasis is also a fungal infection caused by a related group of yeasts, mostly *Candida albicans*. This organism is a normal flora of the gastrointestinal (GI) tract, but it may overgrow (usually because of broad-spectrum antibiotic therapy) and cause disease at a number of skin sites. Other predisposing factors include diabetes mellitus, oral contraceptive use, and cellular immune deficiency. Candidiasis is a very common infection in HIV-infected individuals. The oral cavity (the tongue or buccal mucosa) is usually involved, and this type of infection is also known as *thrush*. Candida infection may involve vulvovaginal candidiasis, which is very common in women of reproductive age.

Antifungal Agents

Both topical and systemic therapies may be used to treat dermatophyte infections. Treatment depends on the site involved and the type of infection (Table 17-6 ■). Systemic therapies for fungal disorders were discussed in Chapter 10.

SCABIES AND PEDICULOSIS

Scabies is a group of dermatologic conditions caused by mites that burrow into the skin, causing intense itching. Scabies may be found anywhere on the trunk or extremities. Pediculosis is a lice infestation. Lice primarily affect hairy areas of the body, including the top of the head, eyebrows, eyelids, underarms, chest, and pubic area. Lice can infest just the head or the entire body. Another species, pubic lice, is commonly referred to as *crabs*. Lice feed on human blood and lay their eggs, called *nits*, on hair shafts. When a louse has its blood meal, irritation may be produced, which can eventually lead to a severe inflammatory reaction. The condition is highly contagious and requires treatment with specially formulated insecticides.

Table 17-6 ■ Topical Antifungal Drugs

GENERIC NAME	TRADE NAME	AVERAGE ADULT DOSAGE	ROUTE OF ADMINISTRATION
amphotericin B	Fungizone	100 mg swish and swallow qid.	PO
ciclopirox	Loprox, Penlac Nail	Massage cream into affected area and surrounding skin bid (morning and evening).	Topical
		Paint affected nails under the surface and on the nail bed once daily at bedtime (at least 8 h before washing) After 7 d, remove lacquer with alcohol and remove or trim away unattached nail. Continue for 48 wk.	Nail lacquer
		Wet hair and apply approx. 1 tsp to scalp (up to 10 mL for long hair); leave on for 3 min, then rinse. Repeat twice/wk × 4 wk, with a min of 3 d between applications.	Topical on scalp
econazole nitrate	Spectazole	Apply sufficient amount of 1% cream to affected areas 1–2 times/d (morning and evening).	Topical
haloprogin	Halotex	Apply liberally to affected area bid for 2–3 wk.	Topical
miconazole nitrate	Fungoid-HC	Apply cream sparingly to affected areas bid, and once daily for tinea versicolor, for 2 wk (improvement expected in 2–3 d; tinea pedis is treated for 1 mo to prevent recurrence).	Topical
		Insert suppository or vaginal cream at bedtime for 7 d (100 mg) or 3 d (200 mg).	Intravaginal
naftifine	Naftin	Apply cream once daily, or apply gel bid; may use up to 4 wk.	Topical
nystatin	Mycostatin, Nystex	Apply 100,000 units/g cream, ointment, and powder, or 1–2 tablets daily for 2 wk.	Intravaginal
oxiconazole	Oxistat	Apply to affected area once daily in the evening.	Topical
terbinafine hydrochloride	Lamisil	Apply 1–2 times/d to affected and immediately surrounding areas until clinical signs and symptoms are significantly improved (1–7 wk).	Topical
tolnaftate	Aftate, Tinactin	Apply 0.5–1 cm (1/4–1/2 in.) of cream or 3 drops of solution bid in morning and evening; powder may be used prophylactically in normally moist areas.	Topical

Antilice Drugs

Scabicides are pharmacologic drugs that kill mites; **pediculicides** kill lice. However, either treatment may be effective for both types of parasites. The choice of drug depends on where the infestation has occurred. Table 17-7 ■ summarizes the most commonly used agents.

How do they work?

The mechanism of action of antilice drugs is related to their direct absorption by parasites and ova (nits). They stimulate the nervous system of the parasites, resulting in seizures and death.

How are they used?

These agents are used topically in the treatment of *Pediculus humanus* infestations.

What are the adverse effects?

The adverse effects include irritation with repeated use, causing pruritus, burning, stinging, numbness, erythema, edema, and rash.

What are the contraindications and interactions?

Lindane (Kwell) is contraindicated in premature neonates and patients with known seizure disorders. It should not be applied to the eyes, face, mucous membranes, or open cuts. The use of pyrethrins with dyes is contraindicated. These drugs should be avoided in acute inflammation of the scalp and in pregnant or lactating women. They should be used cautiously in children younger than 2 years. There are no clinically significant interactions established with these topical agents.

What are the most important points patients should know?

Instruct patients and their families that these agents are highly toxic drugs if used in excess or if they are swallowed or inhaled. Warn patients to keep these agents out of the reach of children. Advise patients to use a fine-toothed comb (infused with medication) to remove dead lice and remaining nits or nit shells when hair is dry. Regular shampooing should be resumed after treatment; residual deposit of drug on the hair is not reduced. Warn patients not to share combs, brushes, or other grooming equipment with other people. Instruct female patients to avoid breastfeeding while using these drugs without consulting their physician.

Table 17-7 ■ Drugs Used to Treat Lice

GENERIC NAME	TRADE NAME	AVERAGE ADULT DOSAGE	ROUTE OF ADMINISTRATION
crotamiton	Eurax	Apply directly from neck to toes; apply a second layer 24 h later. Bathe 48 h after last application to remove drug.	Topical
lindane	Kwell, Scabene	Apply to all body areas except the face; leave lotion on 8–12 h, then rinse off; leave shampoo on 5 min, then rinse thoroughly. Do NOT repeat in less than 1 wk.	Lotion, shampoo
permethrin	Acticin, Nix	Apply sufficient volume to clean, wet hair to saturate the hair and scalp; leave on 10 min; then rinse hair thoroughly.	Cream, lotion
pyrethrins	Pyrinate, Pyrinyl	Apply to affected areas and leave on 10 min; then rinse thoroughly. Reapply only as directed.	Topical

✳ Apply Your Knowledge 17.3

The following questions focus on what you have learned about skin infections, scabies, and pediculosis. *See Appendix E for the correct answers.*

MULTIPLE CHOICE

Choose the correct answers from choices a–d.

1. Scabies may be found in which of the following parts of the body?
   a. Eyebrows
   b. Head
   c. Underarms
   d. Anywhere

2. Which of the following microorganisms is one of the most common causes of bacterial infections of the skin?

    a. *Hemophilus influenzae*

    b. *Salmonella typhosa*

    c. Streptococci

    d. *Proteus mirabilis*

3. Fungi that affect nails, hair, and skin are known as:

    a. Dermatophytes

    b. Dermatographism

    c. Impetigo

    d. Inflammation

4. A fungal infection caused by a related group of yeasts is known as:

    a. Impetigo

    b. Crabs

    c. Candidiasis

    d. Scabies

5. Pediculosis, which involves infestation by lice, may affect:

    a. Hairy areas of the body

    b. Hairless areas of the body

    c. Only children and adolescents

    d. Patients who are allergic to milk

Chapter Capsule

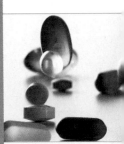

This section repeats the objectives from the beginning of the chapter and then provides a summary of the most important concepts for that objective. Use this section as a quick review and to check your knowledge.

Objective 1: Describe the top two layers of the skin.

■ Epidermis—outer layer with four or five sublayers; contains specialized cells in the called *melanocytes,* which produce melanin, a dark pigment that provides skin color.

■ Dermis—inner layer; thicker than the epidermis. Beneath the dermis are masses of loose connective and adipose tissues that bind the skin to the underlying organs.

Objective 2: List five different skin disorders.

■ Eczema

■ Dermatitis

■ Psoriasis

■ Acne

■ Keratoses

Objective 3: Identify the mainstay of treatment for acute or chronic inflammatory disorders of the skin.

■ Topical or oral corticosteroids

Objective 4: Describe the mechanism of action of topical corticosteroids.

■ Prevent accumulation of inflammatory cells at sites of infection and inhibit phagocytosis; when applied to inflamed skin, they reduce itching, redness, and swelling.

Objective 5: Identify the drugs used to treat psoriasis.

■ Emollients
■ Keratolytic agents
■ Topical corticosteroids
■ Systemic medications
■ Tar treatments
■ Anthralin
■ UV light (phototherapy)

Objective 6: List the drugs used to treat acne.

■ Benzoyl peroxide
■ Azelaic acid
■ Clindamycin
■ Erythromycin

Objective 7: Explain the action and uses of keratolytics.

■ Keratolytics—promote shedding of the horny layer of the epidermis and soften scales
■ Used in the treatment of corns, calluses, and plantar warts; some (such as sulfur and ammonium lactate) used in the treatment of acne, eczema, psoriasis, and seborrheic dermatitis

Objective 8: Describe the treatments for scabies and pediculosis.

■ Scabicides—pharmacologic drugs that kill mites
■ Pediculicides—kill lice
■ Both treatments may be effective for both types of parasites; choice of drug depends on where the infestation has occurred

Internet Sites of Interest

- Dermatology A to Z, sun safety, and consumer information can be found at the American Academy of Dermatology's Web site: **www.aad.org**

- A detailed discussion of eczema, its triggers, and its treatments can be found at this Web site of the Joint Council for Allergy, Asthma and Immunology: **www.jcaai.org/param/Eczema/Treat.htm**

- The About.com Web site includes an article on the use of corticosteroids in skin disorders such as acne. The article is written by a physician. See **http://dermatology.about.com/cs/medications/a/steroidswork.htm**

- Medline Plus offers a discussion of scabies, including photos, treatments, and an interactive tutorial at: **www.nlm.nih.gov/medlineplus/scabies.html**

Chapter 18

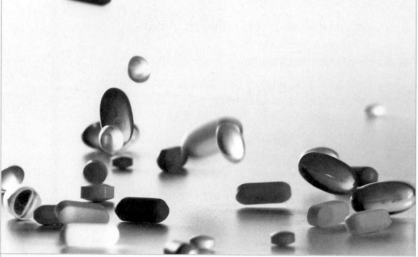

Effects of Drugs on the Cardiovascular System

Chapter Objectives

After completing this chapter, you should be able to:

1. Identify the electrical conduction system of the heart.
2. Name the three layers of the heart and the four heart valves.
3. Define three types of angina pectoris.
4. Name the mainstays of angina therapy.
5. Describe the action of vasodilation.
6. Define calcium channel blockers.
7. Explain myocardial infarction.
8. Identify the classifications of antidysrhythmic drugs and explain their actions.
9. Describe the adverse reactions of quinidine.
10. Identify the mechanism of action of lidocaine.
11. List the adverse effects of phenytoin.

Key Terms

Angina pectoris (an-JIE-nuh pek-TORE-iss) (page 382)

Atrioventricular node (AY-tree-oh-ven-TRI-kyoo-ler node) (page 383)

Atrium (AY-tree-um) (page 383)

Automaticity (aw-toe-muh-TIH-sih-tee) (page 395)

Bradycardia (bray-dee-KAR-dee-uh) (page 390)

Bundle of His (page 384)

Dysrhythmia (dis-RITH-mee-uh) (page 391)

Electrocardiogram (ECG/EKG) (ee-lek-tro-KAR-dee-oh-gram) (page 385)

Endocardium (en-do-KAR-dee-um) (page 383)

Epicardium (ep-ih-KAR-dee-um) (page 383)

Fibrillation (fib-rih-LAY-shun) (page 393)

Flutter (page 393)

Gingival hyperplasia (JIN-jih-vul hi-per-PLAY-zhuh) (page 395)

Hypertension (HI-per-ten-shun) (page 381)

Hypotension (HI-poe-ten-shun) (page 387)

Insomnia (in-SOM-nee-uh) (page 388)

Ischemia (is-KEE-mee-uh) (page 385)

Myocardial infarction (my-oh-KAR-dee-ull in-FARK-shun) (page 381)

Myocardium (my-oh-KAR-dee-um) (page 381)

Nystagmus (nis-TAG-mus) (page 395)

Platelets (PLATE-lets) (page 394)

Prophylaxis (pro-fih-LAK-sis) (page 388)

Purkinje fibers (pur-KIN-jee) (page 385)

Refractory (ree-FRAK-tor-ee) (page 397)

Sinoatrial node (syn-oh-AY-tree-ull node) (page 383)

Somnolence (SAHM-no-lents) (page 395)

Sympathetic (sim-puh-THEH-tik) (page 388)

Syndrome (SIN-drome) (page 390)

Tachycardia (tak-ee-KAR-dee-uh) (page 387)

Vasodilation (vass-oh-dy-LAY-shun) (page 389)

Vasospasms (VAY-soh-spah-zims) (page 387)

Ventricles (VEN-trih-kuls) (page 383)

Vertigo (VER-tih-go) (page 395)

PRACTICAL SCENARIO

A 60-year-old man called emergency medical services, complaining of severe angina and dizziness. He told the paramedic that he had been prescribed nitroglycerin for angina pectoris and was taking it as needed. He stated that he always kept a little envelope of the drug in his breast pocket and the rest in his car, in case he needed more. About 2 hours earlier, he reported, he had finished a large meal preceded by a cocktail and accompanied by wine. When he felt the pain begin, he slipped a nitroglycerin tablet under his tongue. When it had no effect after 10 minutes, he took another, waited, and then took another. Nothing stopped the pain, and now he was afraid he was having a heart attack. His ECG was negative for a myocardial infarction. The paramedic realized why the nitroglycerin did not alleviate his angina.

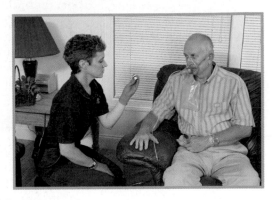

Critical Thinking Questions

1. What were the "clues" that helped the paramedic figure out why the nitroglycerin did not alleviate the man's angina?
2. Why did dizziness accompany the man's angina?
3. What important advice should be given to patients taking nitroglycerin?

Introduction

The circulatory system is often referred to as the cardiovascular system and is composed of the heart and blood vessels (vasculature). Cardiovascular disease (CVD) is the most common cause of death in the United States and can result from coronary artery disease (CAD) (blockage of the arteries that supply the heart muscle itself), which can lead to **myocardial infarction** (MI), or a heart attack. An MI occurs when part of the heart is deprived of its blood supply to such an extent that the cells of the myocardium die. Another term for CAD is *coronary heart disease (CHD)*; the terms may be used interchangeably. Other related cardiovascular conditions that can lead to or result from CAD or MI include dysrhythmias (also called *arrhythmias*), congestive heart failure (CHF), hyperlipidemia, and **hypertension** (blood pressure that is elevated above the normal limits). A stroke, also known as *cerebral vascular accident (CVA)* or *brain attack,* may be thought of as analogous to an MI, except the vasculature affected is in the brain and the resulting damage occurs to brain cells.

To understand the drug therapies used to treat CVD, the health-care professional must have a solid understanding of the anatomy, physiology, and electrical properties of the heart as well as the vasculature. The medications in current use can produce their effects on the **myocardium** (the middle layer and most important structure of the heart; it contains the heart muscles that regulate cardiac output), the conduction system, and the coronary and other blood vessels (Figure 18-1 ■).

Focus on Geriatrics

Lifestyle and Cardiovascular Disease

Cardiovascular disease is most prevalent in older, sedentary individuals who are overweight or obese. With the aging of the "Baby Boom" generation, many of whom grew up on a diet of fast food rich in salt and fats, the prevalence of heart disease in the United States is increasing significantly.

Angina pectoris is a common form of ischemic heart disease and often precedes and accompanies MI. It has been described as chest pain and a squeezing pressure that can radiate to the jaw and arm. Related components of CVD and their manifestations, including CHF, hypertension, hyperlipidemia, and stroke, will be discussed in Chapter 19.

Cardiac drugs to be discussed in this chapter are broadly classified according to their effects on certain parts of the cardiovascular system. These drugs can affect (1) the rate of the heart; (2) the rhythm of the heartbeat; (3) the amount of blood output; or (4) the strength of contraction.

The Cardiovascular System

The cardiovascular system begins its activity when the fetus is barely 4 weeks old and is the last system to cease activity at the end of life. This body system is so vital that it helps define the presence of life.

The heart, arteries, veins, and lymphatic system form the cardiovascular network that serves as the body's transport system. This system brings life-supporting oxygen and nutrients to cells, removes metabolic waste products, and carries hormones from one part of the body to another.

The cardiovascular, or circulatory, system is divided into two branches: pulmonary circulation and systemic circulation. In pulmonary circulation, blood picks up oxygen and liberates the waste product, carbon dioxide. In systemic circulation (which includes coronary circulation), blood carries oxygen and nutrients to all active cells and transports waste products to the kidneys, liver, and skin for excretion.

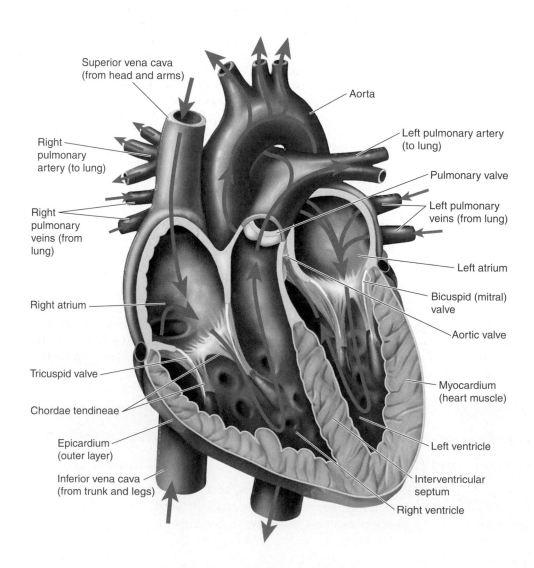

Figure 18-1 ■ Anatomy of the heart.

Circulation requires normal heart function, to propel blood through the system by continuous rhythmic contractions of the heart. Blood circulates through three types of vessels: arteries, veins, and capillaries.

The heart is a muscular pump located within the mediastinum of the thorax. It consists of three layers:

1. The **endocardium**, which is the thin membrane lining the inside of the cardiac muscle
2. The cardiac muscle, which is called the *myocardium*
3. The **epicardium**, which is a thin membrane lining the outside of the myocardium

The heart is comprised of four compartments that maintain the body's blood circulation. The two smaller upper chambers are the receiving chambers, called the left **atrium** and the right atrium; together they are known as *atria*. The two lower chambers are called the left and right **ventricles** (the chambers that pump blood out of the heart). The upper and lower chambers are divided by a septum.

The four valves of the heart—tricuspid, pulmonary, mitral, and aortic—are located at the entrance and exit of each ventricle. Blood pumps through the four chambers of the heart with the help of the valves, which open and close via flaps, to allow blood to flow in only one direction.

The electrical conduction system contains all the wiring to initiate and maintain rhythmic contraction of the heart (Figure 18-2 ■). The system consists of:

Sinoatrial (SA) node. Located just beneath the epicardium, in the right atrium, near the opening of the superior vena cava, this small, elongated mass of specialized cardiac muscle tissue initiates one impulse after another. Because it generates the heart's rhythmic contractions, it is known as the "pacemaker."

Atrioventricular (AV) node. Located in the inferior portion of the septum, which separates the atria, and just beneath the endocardium, the AV node provides the only normal conduction pathway between the atrial and ventricular syncytia, and its fibers delay impulse transmission. This delay allows more time for the atria to completely contract, so that they empty all of their blood into the ventricles before ventricular contraction occurs.

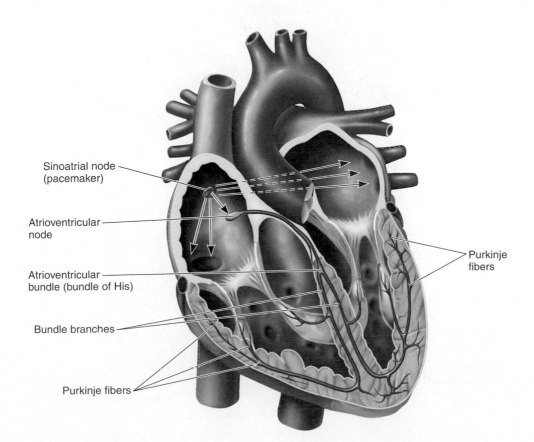

Sinoatrial node
(pacemaker)

Atrioventricular
node

Atrioventricular
bundle (bundle of His)

Bundle branches

Purkinje fibers

Purkinje
fibers

Figure 18-2 ■ Electrical conduction system of the heart.

Bundle of His. Located between the AV node and the Purkinje fibers, and also known as the *atrioventricular bundle*, the bundle of His consists of a large group of fibers that enter the upper part of the intraventricular septum and are divided into right and left bundle branches lying just beneath the endocardium.

Right and left bundle branches. Located in the heart's lower chambers (ventricles), the bundle branches divide at the bundle of His and form the right and left

✳ Apply Your Knowledge 18.1

The following questions focus on what you have just learned about the anatomy and physiology of the cardiovascular system. *See Appendix E for the correct answers.*

FILL IN THE BLANK
Select terms from your reading to fill in the blanks.

1. The cardiovascular system functions in the transport of _____ and _____ to cells.

2. The heart is pocketed within a space contained by the thoracic cavity, which is called the _____. It is surrounded by an outer membrane, which is known as the _____.

3. The thin membrane lining the inside of the cardiac muscle is called the _____.

4. The three types of blood vessels are _____, _____, and _____.

5. The cardiovascular network is formed by the _____, _____, _____, and _____.

LABELING
Label the anatomy of the heart.

    Bicuspid valve

    Myocardium

    Inferior vena cava

    Right atrium

    Epicardium

    Left ventricle

    Aorta

    Aortic valve

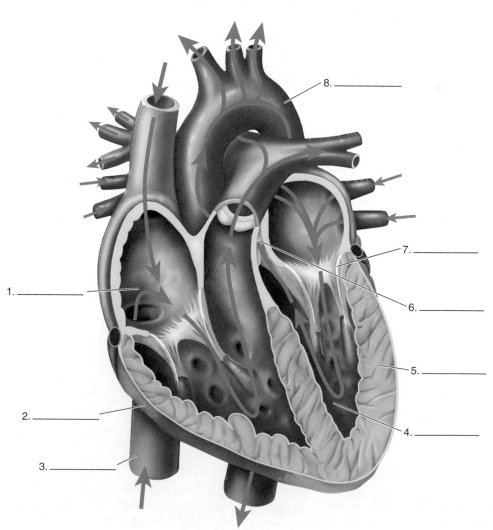

bundle branches. An electrical impulse travels down the right and left bundle branches at the same speed and causes the left and right ventricles to contract at the same time.

Purkinje fibers. Located about halfway down the septum, the Purkinje fibers spread from the interventricular septum into the papillary muscles toward the apex of the heart. Along this pathway, the Purkinje fibers give off many small branches, which become continuous with cardiac muscle fibers.

An **electrocardiogram** (ECG or EKG) is a tracing of the heart's electrical activity. It measures electrical activity across the myocardium. Each electrical impulse takes less than one quarter of a second to occur. An ECG provides a visual means of examining the electrical impulses of the heart, which are labeled in a series of letters known as P, QRS, and T. An ECG graphs the atrial depolarization, ventricular depolarization, and ventricular repolarization of each electrical impulse of the heart.

Coronary Heart Disease (CHD)

When the delivery of oxygen to the myocardium is inadequate to meet the heart's oxygen consumption needs, myocardial **ischemia** (insufficient blood flow to the myocardium) occurs. One of the major causes of ischemia is CAD, including atherosclerosis (blockage of an artery) and arteriosclerosis (hardening of an artery).

Angina pectoris is an episodic, reversible oxygen insufficiency. Oxygen demand is directly related to the strength of contraction, heart rate, and resistance to blood flow. Angina pectoris may result from obstruction or narrowing of coronary arteries (by fatty deposits or clots), arterial spasm, pulmonary hypertension, and cardiac hypertrophy (enlargement of the heart).

Antianginal drugs are used primarily for the treatment of angina pectoris. There are several types of angina: classical (stable), variant (vasospastic), and unstable.

✳ *Classical (stable) angina* is the most common form and often occurs during exertion, emotional stress, or indigestion due to excessive eating or a meal rich in fats and proteins. It usually causes chest discomfort, which is relieved by rest, nitroglycerin, or both. The pain typically radiates to the jaw, neck, shoulder, and left arm. Stable angina is characteristically due to a fixed obstruction in a coronary artery.

✳ *Variant* or *vasospastic angina* is the result of a coronary artery spasm that reduces blood flow. It usually occurs at rest rather than with exertion or emotional stress.

✳ *Unstable angina* is caused by significant CAD. It occurs at rest for the first time and decreases in response to rest or nitroglycerin. It often portends myocardial infarction.

THERAPEUTIC AGENTS FOR CHD

Antianginal drugs are used primarily to dilate coronary blood vessels. The mainstays of treatment include the following three classes of drugs:

✳ Organic nitrates

✳ Beta-adrenergic blockers (also called beta-blockers)

✳ Calcium channel blockers

Although nitrates and calcium channel blockers dilate coronary arteries, this dilation makes a minimal contribution to their antianginal effects, except in vasospastic angina.

Organic Nitrates

The oldest and most frequently prescribed drugs for the different types of angina are organic nitrates, administered to stop an acute angina attack. Inhaled amyl nitrate, translingual spray, or sublingual nitrates have a rapid onset of action and are effective for short periods. A variety of dosage forms of organic nitrates is seen in Table 18-1 ■.

Table 18-1 ■ Organonitrates and Other Anginal Medications

GENERIC NAME	TRADE NAME	USUAL DOSE FOR ADULT	ROUTES OF ADMINISTRATION
Nitrates			
nitroglycerin	Nitrolingual	0.4–0.8 mg PRN	Translingual spray
	Nitrostat	0.15–0.6 mg PRN	Sublingual
	Nitro-Bid	2.5–6.5 mg tid or qid	PO
isosorbide dinitrate	Isordil, Sorbitrate, Dilatrate-SR	2.5–40 mg tid	Sublingual
isosorbide mononitrate	Imdur, ISMO	20 mg bid	PO
erythrityl tetranitrate	Cardilate	10–30 mg tid	PO
pentaerythritol tetranitrate	Peritrate, Duotrate	10–20 mg tid or qid	30-80 mg/d
Beta-Adrenergic Blockers			
atenolol	Tenormin	25–50 mg/d, may increase to 100 mg/d	PO
propranolol	Inderal	10–90 mg bid or qid	PO
	Vascor	200–400 mg/d	PO
Calcium Channel Blockers (See Table 17-3 Class IV for other calcium channel blockers used as antidysrhythmics.)			
verapamil	Calan, Calan SR, Covera-HS, Isoptin, Isoptin SR, Verelan, Verelan PM	80 mg q6–8h, may increase up to 320–480 mg/d in divided doses (Covera-HS must be given once daily at bedtime.)	PO

NITROGLYCERIN

The classic organic nitrate, nitroglycerin (Nitrostat, Nitrobid), was once the drug of choice for the treatment of angina pectoris. Nitroglycerin is effective, inexpensive, and fast acting.

How does it work?

Nitroglycerin directly affects vascular smooth muscle to dilate blood vessels. It decreases cardiac oxygen demand in stable angina, whereas in variant angina, it relaxes the spasms and increases oxygen supply.

How is it used?

Nitroglycerin preparations are administered using a variety of routes, producing similar responses but differing in the time of onset and duration. Some of these preparations are rapidly effective (1 to 5 minutes) and last about 60 minutes, whereas for others the effect is slower in onset but lasts several hours. Only a few medications have a rapid onset and long duration of action. They can be used to relieve acute anginal pain or prophylactically to prevent angina attack with extended-release forms.

Sublingual nitroglycerin is effective rapidly, lasts about 1 hour, and is an ideal preparation for acute anginal pain. By this route of administration, it avoids hepatic first-pass metabolism. If one dose is not sufficient, one or two additional doses should be taken at 5-minute intervals. The medication bottle should not be opened unless it is needed, because its shelf life is longer in a dark and tightly closed container.

Transdermal nitroglycerin can release its reservoir slowly for absorption through the skin. These patches should be applied once a day to a hairless site of skin. The patch sites should be rotated daily to prevent local irritation. The patch should not be worn for more than 10 to 12 hours per day; this so-called off period is necessary to prevent the development of a tolerance to the drug and allows for continued therapeutic efficacy.

Nitroglycerin is also available as a topical ointment that must be measured on a paper provided with the prescription to ensure proper dosage. See Chapter 4 for the application of percutaneous medications.

Discontinuation of nitroglycerin should take place over time because discontinuation of long-acting nitroglycerin preparations can cause **vasospasms** (spasms of the blood vessels) and angina.

What are the adverse effects?

The most common adverse effects include headache, **hypotension** (an abnormal condition in which the blood pressure is not adequate for full oxygenation of the tissues), and **tachycardia** (an abnormally fast heartbeat). The dizziness and lightheadedness of hypotension are better tolerated with time.

What are the contraindications and interactions?

Nitroglycerin's contraindications include obstructive hypertrophic cardiomyopathy, pronounced hypovolemia (a decrease in the volume of circulating blood), inferior MI with right ventricular involvement, raised intracranial pressure (ICP), and cardiac tamponade (blockage in the heart). It should not be stopped abruptly after long therapy because there is a rebound risk of more frequent angina pectoris. Nitroglycerin (Nitrostat, Nitro-Bid) reinforces the hypotensive effect of antihypertensive agents. If combined with alcohol, a sudden drop in blood pressure can occur. Nitroglycerin increases the bioavailability of dihydroergotamine. In smokers, nicotine antagonizes the coronary dilating effect of nitroglycerin. Nitroglycerin is also contraindicated in pregnancy and lactation.

What are the important points patients should know?

Advise patients that nitroglycerin should not be carried close to the body because heat from the body can deactivate it. Tell patients to store the medication in a cool, dark place, and keep it in the original container. Advise patients to avoid alcoholic beverages when taking nitroglycerin, and to take one tablet sublingually every 5 minutes, not exceeding three tablets. Tell patients that if chest pain continues, they should seek emergency medical attention. Advise patients to discard unused tablets after 6 months.

Focus Point

Nitroglycerin

Nitroglycerin may cause severe low blood pressure (marked by dizziness or lightheadedness), especially if an individual is in an upright position or has just gotten up from sitting or lying down. The heart rate can slow and chest pain can increase. People taking diuretic medication, or those who have low systolic blood pressure (less than 90 mm Hg), should use nitroglycerin with caution.

ISOSORBIDE DINITRATE AND ISOSORBIDE MONONITRATE

Isosorbide dinitrate (Cedocard Retard, Isordil, Sorbid SA) and isosorbide mononitrate (Elantan, Imdur, Ismo) are other forms of organic nitrates that provide a longer duration of action than nitroglycerin. These agents are effective in the treatment of all types of angina pectoris and are available in sublingual and chewable tablet forms. The most common complaint by users is headache. Both agents should be given cautiously to patients with glaucoma (see Chapter 27). The advantage of isosorbide mononitrate over isosorbide dinitrate is that there is no first-pass metabolism.

ERYTHRITYL TETRANITRATE

The principal use of another form of organic nitrate, erythrityl tetranitrate (Cardilate), is in the **prophylaxis** (prevention) of angina pectoris in acute situations in which an attack can be anticipated. Adverse effects include tachycardia, headache, flushing, dizziness, syncope (loss of consciousness and body tone; fainting), and nausea. It also should be given cautiously to patients with glaucoma.

PENTAERYTHRITOL TETRANITRATE

Pentaerythritol tetranitrate (Peritrate, Duotrate) is a long-acting organic nitrate. It is used in the prophylaxis of angina pectoris, but not in the management of the acute attack. Transient headache and nausea may accompany its use. It should be given cautiously to patients with glaucoma.

Beta-Adrenergic Blockers

Beta-adrenergic blockers (propranolol, atenolol), known as *beta-blockers* or *β-blockers*, reduce the heart's oxygen demand by decreasing the heart rate. In the heart, **sympathetic** stimulation causes increased rate and force, as well as increased oxygen use. (*Sympathetic* relates to the sympathetic part of the autonomic nervous system, or the *fight or flight* response.) Beta-blockers prevent the development of myocardial ischemia and pain. Propranolol (Inderal) is often used for the treatment of angina, and it may be used in combination with nitrates for control of angina. Beta-blockers should be used with caution or avoided in patients with asthma because of the potential for bronchospasm, and they may mask hypoglycemia in patients with diabetes mellitus. Beta-blockers may produce **insomnia** (inability to sleep normally), bizarre dreams, and depression. See Table 18-1 for dosages and routes of transmission. Beta-blockers are discussed in more depth later in this chapter.

Focus on Natural Products

Food and Drug Interactions

Many natural substances (including food) interact with pharmaceuticals; for example, warfarin sodium (Coumadin) interacts with foods such as beef liver, broccoli, Brussels sprouts, cabbage, spinach, and other green, leafy vegetables. These foods contain large amounts of vitamin K, which decreases the effect of the drug.

Calcium Channel Blockers

Calcium channel blockers (for example, verapamil, bepridil) interfere with the movement of calcium ions through cell membranes. These drugs can affect the heart itself or the peripheral vasculature. They are used to treat the pain of angina pectoris and to lower blood pressure. Contraction of vascular smooth muscle depends on calcium movement from extracellular to intracellular sites. The prevention of calcium action inhibits this contraction. Therefore, it decreases vascular tone and causes **vasodilation** (dilation of blood vessels; this action relaxes the smooth muscle of the peripheral arterioles). These agents are prescribed for vasospastic angina. Calcium channel blockers are used for the treatment of angina, dysrhythmia, and hypertension (see Table 18-1 and Table 18-3 ■ for dosages and routes of delivery). Bepridil (Vascor) is a calcium channel blocker used specifically for angina pectoris. It slows the heart rate and has antidysrhythmic properties. The common adverse effects are dizziness, hypotension, fatigue, headache, and constipation. Calcium channel blockers are discussed in detail in a later section of this chapter.

✱ Apply Your Knowledge 18.2

The following questions focus on what you have just learned about coronary heart disease (CHD) and therapeutic agents to treat CHD. *See Appendix E for the correct answers.*

FILL IN THE BLANK
Select terms from your reading to fill in the blanks.

1. Episodic, reversible oxygen insufficiency is called _____.

2. The most common form of angina is _____.

3. The type of angina that usually occurs at rest, rather than with exertion or emotional stress, is _____.

4. The main purpose of using antianginal drugs is to _____.

5. _____ was once the drug of choice for the treatment of angina pectoris.

6. Isosorbide dinitrate and isosorbide mononitrate should be given cautiously to patients with _____.

7. Beta blockers prevent the development of _____ and _____.

MATCHING
Match the lettered term to the numbered description.

DESCRIPTION	TERM
1. _____ Should be avoided in patients with asthma	a. nitroglycerin
2. _____ Prevents angina	b. propranolol
3. _____ Treats angina	c. organic nitrates
4. _____ Has common adverse effect of hypotension	d. atenolol
5. _____ Lower blood pressure	e. calcium channel blockers
6. _____ Have common adverse effect of headache	f. beta-blockers
7. _____ Cause vasodilation	
8. _____ Decrease the heart rate	

Myocardial Infarction (MI)

Acute myocardial infarction (AMI) occurs when a part of the myocardium suffers a severe and prolonged restriction of oxygenated coronary blood. Nearly 40% of all patients experiencing AMI die before reaching acute care health centers. An AMI can occur when an area of the heart muscle dies through lack of sufficient oxygen. AMI is the leading cause of death in industrialized nations, possibly because of a diet high in cholesterol and fat and a sedentary lifestyle. The insufficient oxygen supply to the myocardium is the result of (1) a decreased flow of oxygen-rich blood to the heart muscle and (2) an increased demand for oxygen by the myocardium that exceeds what the circulation can supply. CAD, clot formation in the coronary artery or spasm of these arteries, stress, heavy exertion, and an abrupt increase in blood pressure are the main causes of AMI.

Focus on Pediatrics

AMI in Children

AMI is rare in childhood. Adults usually develop coronary artery disease from the lifelong buildup of atheroma (a yellow-tinted swelling of the arteries, characteristic of atherosclerosis) and plaque, which causes coronary artery spasm and thrombosis. Pediatric patients with AMI usually have either an acute inflammatory condition of the coronary arteries or an anomalous origin of the left coronary artery.

THERAPEUTIC AGENTS FOR MI

The goal of treatment in AMI is to limit damage to the myocardium, thereby preserving enough myocardial function to sustain life. In addition to intravenous fluids, pharmacotherapeutics are used as the first line of treatment for AMI. Treatment is designed to relieve distress, reverse ischemia, limit the size of infarct (the amount of tissue death related to lack of arterial or venous blood), reduce cardiac work, and prevent and treat complications. AMI is an acute medical emergency, and outcome is significantly influenced by rapid diagnosis and treatment. Fifty percent of deaths from AMI occur within 3 to 4 hours of onset of the clinical **syndrome** (a collection of signs and symptoms that, together, signify a specific disease). The outcome can be influenced by early treatment.

Nitroglycerin is administered to decrease the heart's workload and increase blood supply to the heart muscle. Aspirin and thrombolytic drugs are most effective if given within the first few minutes and hours after onset of MI. The greatest risk of thrombolytic therapy is hemorrhage (bleeding), specifically inside the brain. Anticoagulants are discussed in Chapter 20.

Morphine sulfate, 2 to 4 mg IV, repeated as needed, is a critical adjunct to nitroglycerin. Morphine is highly effective for the pain of MI. Potential side effects of morphine are depression of respiration and reduction of myocardial contractility. Hypotension and **bradycardia** (an abnormally slow heartbeat) secondary to morphine can usually be overcome by prompt elevation of the lower extremities. Beta-blockers, such as metoprolol (Toprol, Lopressor) and atenolol (Tenormin), reduce the heart's oxygen demand by decreasing the heart rate. Calcium channel blockers such as nifedipine (Procardia, Aldalat) and diltiazem (Cardizem, Dilacor) decrease myocardial oxygen demand and increase oxygen supply. Oxygen is also reasonably administered via 40% mask or nasal prongs at 4 to 6 L/min for the first few hours.

* Apply Your Knowledge 18.3

The following questions focus on what you have just learned about myocardial infarction (MI) and its therapeutic agents. *See Appendix E for the correct answers.*

FILL IN THE BLANK

Select terms from your reading to fill in the blanks.

1. An AMI can occur when a part of the heart muscle dies because of insufficient _____.

2. The first-line treatment for AMI consists of pharmacotherapeutics and _____.

3. The greatest risk of thrombolytic therapy is _____.

4. Nearly _____ of all patients experiencing AMI die before reaching acute care health centers.

5. The goal of treatment of MI is to reduce myocardial _____.

6. _____ is a critical adjunct to nitroglycerin to reduce the pain of MI.

7. Potential side effects of morphine are depression of _____ and reduction of _____.

8. Nitroglycerin is administered to decrease the heart's _____ and increase _____ to the heart muscle.

Dysrhythmias

The rate of heartbeat and rhythm of the heart are controlled by the sinoatrial (SA) node (sometimes termed the *pacemaker*) in the right atrium. This node generates tiny electrical impulses to the adjacent muscle of the atrium, causing the atria to contract and pump blood into the ventricles. The impulses sent out by the SA node are received by the atrioventricular (AV) node, travel down the bundle of His, and are transported to the ventricular muscles by a network of nerves. The SA node, as well as the AV node, receives autonomic innervation that controls the rate of the heart to a certain extent.

Any deviation from the normal orderly sequence of impulses is a disturbance of the rhythm and is called a **dysrhythmia** or an *arrhythmia*. Sometimes an area of muscle in one of the atria becomes more excitable than the SA node and fires more rapid impulses. The rest of the heart then responds to this new pacemaker, and the resulting dysrhythmia is known as *atrial tachycardia*. Dysrhythmias may be benign (as in atrial tachycardia) or malignant (as in ventricular tachycardia). Benign abnormalities generally have a low risk of sudden death. Malignant abnormalities have a moderate risk of sudden death. Malignant arrhythmias indicate an immediate risk for heart disease. Table 18-2 ■ summarizes different arrhythmias and beats per minute.

lidocaine

Table 18-2 ■ Various Dysrhythmias

ARRHYTHMIA	BEATS PER MINUTE
Bradycardia	Less than 60
Tachycardia	150–250
Atrial flutter	200–350
Atrial fibrillation	More than 350
Ventricular fibrillation	Variable
Premature atrial contraction	Variable
Premature ventricular contraction	Variable

ANTIDYSRHYTHMIC AGENTS

Dysrhythmias can occur from heart disease or from chronic drug therapy. Dysrhythmias can also be caused by the drugs used to regulate dysrhythmia, because they create an alteration of the heart's electrical impulse. When severe dysrhythmia occurs, especially in ventricular disorders, the patient can be experiencing a medical emergency requiring hospital care.

Antidysrhythmic drug therapy is the mainstay of management for most important dysrhythmias. There is no universally effective drug. All of these agents have important safety limitations and can aggravate or promote arrhythmias. Drug selection is difficult and often involves trial and error (Table 18-3 ■).

Table 18-3 ■ Antidysrhythmic Medications

GENERIC NAME	TRADE NAME	USUAL DOSE FOR ADULTS	ROUTES OF ADMINISTRATION
Class Ia			
quinidine	Cardioquin	200–600 mg tid-qid	PO
procainamide	Pronestyl, Procan-SR	1 g followed by 250–500 mg q3h	PO
		0.5–1 g q4–6h until able to take PO	IM
		100 mg q5min at a rate of 25–50 mg/min (up to 1 g)	IV
disopyramide	Norpace	400–800 mg/d in divided doses	PO
Class Ib			
lidocaine	Xylocaine	1–1.5 mg/kg; may repeat 0.5–1.5 mg/kg q5–10 min to total of 3 mg/kg	IV
		4.3 mg/kg	IM
mexiletine	Mexitil	200–400 mg q8h	PO
phenytoin	Dilantin	100 mg q5min	PO
Class Ic			
flecainide	Tambocor	Initially, 100 mg q12h; increase in 50-mg increments twice daily q4d until effective	PO
propafenone	Rythmol	450 mg/d; increase dosage slowly, if needed, up to 900 mg/d	PO
moricizine	Ethmozine	600–900 mg/d	PO
Class II			
esmolol	Brevibloc	50–500 mcg/min	IV
propranolol	Inderal	10–30 mg 3–4 times/d before meals and at bedtime	PO
		1–3 mg initially; repeated if necessary in 2 min	IV
metoprolol	Lopressor	100 mg/d in 2 divided doses	PO
		5 mg q2min for 3 doses, followed by PO	IV
acebutolol	Sectral	Initially, 200 mg bid. Dose is increased gradually until optimal response is obtained.	PO

Table 18-3 ■ Antidysrhythmic Medications

GENERIC	TRADE NAME	USUAL DOSE FOR ADULTS	ROUTES OF ADMINISTRATION
Class III			
amiodarone	Cordarone	400–1600 mg/d	PO
		150 mg over 10 min followed by 360 mg over next 6h	IV loading dose
sotalol	Betapace	80–320 mg/d	PO
dofetilide	Tikosyn	125–250 mcg bid	PO
ibutilide	Corvert	Weight <60 kg, 0.01 mg/kg (0.1mL/kg) injection.	IV
		Weight >60 kg, 1 mg (10 mL)	IV
bretylium	Bretylol	5–10 mg/kg by infusion	IM
Class IV			
verapamil	Calan	240–480 mg/d divided into 3–4 doses	PO
		Initially, 5–10 mg as IV bolus over 2 min	IV
diltiazem	Cardizem, Tiazac	60–120 mg sustained released bid	PO
		0.25 mg/kg IV bolus over 2 min	IV

Antidysrhythmic drug actions based on cellular electrophysiologic effects have been classified into four groups. This classification is recognized internationally and provides a general logic for grouping drugs. Classifications of antidysrhythmic drugs are seen in Table 18-3.

Class I—Drugs that Bind to Sodium Channels

Class I drugs are sodium channel blockers, including older antidysrhythmic drugs (for example, quinidine). These drugs reduce the maximal rate of contraction of the myocardium and slow conduction. Class I drugs are subclassified into three classes:

Class Ia—drugs with intermediate onset and offset

Class Ib—drugs with short effects

Class Ic—drugs with prolonged effects

QUINIDINE (CLASS IA)

Quinidine (Quinidex, Duraquin) is approved for atrial **fibrillation** (very rapid, irregular contractions or twitching of the individual muscular fibers of the atria or ventricles) and **flutter** (rapid, regular atrial contractions that often produce "sawtooth" waves in an ECG, or rapid ventricular tachycardia that appears as a regular, undulating pattern in an ECG, without QRS and T waves as would normally be found). Quinidine is related to quinine and has been used in cardiac conditions since the 1920s.

How does it work?

Quinidine depresses the myocardium and the conduction system, decreasing the contractile force of the heart and slowing the heart rate.

How is it used?

If an initial test dose of quinidine sulfate (Quinidex) is tolerated, the maintenance dosage is usually 200 to 400 mg orally every 4 to 6 hours. A salt form of quinidine gluconate is also available in IM and IV forms. Sustained-release forms are also available for the sulfate and gluconate salts.

What are the adverse effects?

Adverse reactions include diarrhea, flatulence, and abdominal pain. Fever, reduced **platelets** (megakaryocyte fragments important in the clotting of blood), and liver function abnormalities can occur. Quinidine syncope (sudden ventricular fibrillation in patients taking quinidine) is potentially dangerous and can be life threatening.

What are the contraindications and interactions?

Quinidine is contraindicated in pregnancy, lactation, bacterial endocarditis, and myasthenia gravis. Quinidine has the potential to double digoxin (Lanoxin) levels in the blood. Potentially fatal interactions can occur when quinidine is given with digoxin. Quinidine also interacts with amiodarone (Cordarone) and verapamil (Calan).

What are the important points patients should know?

Tell patients to immediately report any chest pain or change in heart rhythm to the health-care provider. Advise patients to take quinidine with food to avoid gastric upset, although this may delay absorption of the drug. A diet high in citrus fruits, vegetables, and milk may delay excretion of the drug, so advise patients not to increase their intake of these foods beyond their normal diet. Advise the patient to report diarrhea to the health-care provider.

PROCAINAMIDE (CLASS IA)

Procainamide (Pronestyl, Procan-SR) is an antidysrrhythmic drug approved for life-threatening ventricular dysrhythmias. It is related to procaine and has much less effect than quinidine on refraction (resistance to disease treatment). The usual oral dosage is 250 to 625 mg every 3 to 4 hours. Fever, arthralgia (joint pain), and pleural effusions (increased amounts of fluid accumulating in the areas surrounding the lungs) are adverse reactions of procainamide.

DISOPYRAMIDE (CLASS IA)

Disopyramide (Norpace) decreases cardiac excitability and is a cardiac depressant. Oral dosing is usually 100 to 150 mg every 6 hours. Adverse effects are dry mouth, constipation, visual disturbances, and urine retention.

LIDOCAINE (CLASS IB)

Lidocaine (Xylocaine) can suppress the ventricular arrhythmias that complicate MI and reduce the incidence of primary ventricular fibrillation when given prophylactically in early AMI. Its mechanism of action appears to be the blocking of both activated and inactivated sodium channels, with a great effect on depolarized or ischemic tissues. Adverse effects are neurologic, such as tremor and convulsions, rather than cardiac. Drowsiness, delirium, and paresthesias (abnormal burning, pricking, tickling, or tingling) may occur with too-rapid administration. Mexiletine (Mexitil) and tocainide (Tonocard) are chemically and therapeutically related to lidocaine (Xylocaine). These two drugs have been modified for oral administration so that they can be used in ambulatory care. Lidocaine (Xylocaine) has noted drug interactions with cimetidine (Tagamet).

MEXILETINE (CLASS IB)

Mexiletine (Mexitil) has an action similar to lidocaine. It is prescribed for ventricular tachycardia but is more effective when used with another antidysrhythmic agent. Adverse effects are neurologic and gastrointestinal symptoms, and increased liver enzyme levels.

PHENYTOIN (CLASS IB)

Phenytoin (Dilantin) was used extensively for dysrhythmia management, particularly for suppressing the ventricular dysrhythmias of digitalis toxicity, until the advent of newer drugs and the decline of digoxin toxicity. Now, phenytoin is most commonly used for epilepsy. The common adverse effects are **gingival hyperplasia** (an increase in the number of cells in the gums of the mouth, causing them to have a swollen appearance), blurred vision, **vertigo** (a sensation of revolving, either of the patients themselves or of their environment), and **nystagmus** (a constant, involuntary movement of the eye). Phenytoin has noted drug interactions with cimetidine (Tagamet), disulfiram (Antabuse), dopamine (Dopastat or Entropion), and fluconazole (Diflucan).

FLECAINIDE (CLASS IC)

Flecainide (Tambocor) is an antidysrhythmic with electrophysiologic properties similar to those of other class Ic antidysrhythmic drugs. It is used for treatment of life-threatening ventricular dysrhythmias. Adverse effects include dizziness, headache, fatigue, chest pain, and blurred vision. Flecainide may also produce nausea, constipation, and a change in taste perception.

PROPAFENONE (CLASS IC)

Propafenone (Rythmol) is another class Ic antidysrhythmic drug with a direct stabilizing action on myocardial membranes. It is used for treatment and management of ventricular dysrhythmias. Adverse effects include blurred vision, dizziness, fatigue, **somnolence** (sleepiness, dullness, or a deadening sensation), vertigo, and headache. It may also cause hypotension, nausea, abdominal discomfort, constipation, vomiting, dry mouth, and taste alterations.

MORICIZINE (CLASS IC)

Moricizine (Ethmozine) is an antidysrhythmic agent with potent local anesthetic effects. It is prescribed for the treatment of ventricular tachycardia and ventricular premature depolarization (change in direction, destruction, or neutralization of polarity). Adverse effects include dizziness, lightheadedness, anxiety, euphoria, and headache. The other adverse effects may be nausea, diarrhea, dry mouth, and abdominal discomfort.

Class II—Beta-Adrenergic Blockers

Beta-blockers may be the least toxic and most powerful drugs available, yet their antidysrhythmic effects are often overlooked. Relatively few dysrhythmias are caused primarily by sympathetic overactivity; most are regulated by autonomic tone (which is the firmness of muscles as controlled by the autonomic nervous system).

Overactivity of the sympathetic nerves releases norepinephrine and epinephrine. These agents increase heart rate, heart excitability, conduction velocity, and **automaticity** (the heart impulse's automatic, spontaneous initiation), particularly of the ventricles. In general, beta-blockers are well tolerated, but they may depress left ventricular function, particularly in antirrhythmic doses. They are contraindicated in asthma. Gastrointestinal disturbances, insomnia, and nightmares may occur. Beta-adrenergic blockers will be discussed in Chapter 18.

PROPRANOLOL (CLASS II)

Propranolol (Inderal) is the most common beta-blocker used as an antidysrhythmic. Prior to 1978, it was the only beta-blocker approved to treat dysrhythmias. Since then, several other beta-blockers have been approved to treat dysrhythmias, but propranolol is still the mainstay of treatment.

How does it work?

Propranolol affects both types of beta receptors; because of this, it is considered a nonselective beta-blocker. It reduces or slows the heart rate and lowers blood pressure. In addition to its beta-blocking effect, it also causes quinidine-like depression of the myocardium.

How is it used?

Propranolol is often combined with other cardiovascular drugs such as digoxin (Lanoxin) and quinidine (Quinidex) to treat cardiovascular disease. It is most effective for tachycardia, but it is also approved to treat a broad range of other disorders, such as hypertension, angina, and prevention of myocardial infarction. It is prescribed in oral form and is also administered by IV. Sustained-release forms are also available.

What are the adverse effects?

Hypotension and bradycardia are the most common side effects. Patients with other cardiac disorders such as heart failure must be carefully monitored because propranolol can slow heart rate. Side effects such as diminished sex drive and impotence can also occur.

What are the contraindications and interactions?

Propranolol is contraindicated in bronchial asthma or bronchospasm, severe chronic obstructive airway disease, allergic rhinitis during pollen season, and pregnancy. Propranolol interacts with clonidine (Catapres), cimetidine (Tagamet), epinephrine, and insulin.

What are the important points patients should know?

Propranolol should not be abruptly discontinued because it may cause myocardial infarction or severe dysrhythmias. Tell the patient to take his or her pulse on a regular basis; if the pulse is less than 60 beats per minute, the patient's health-care provider should be notified immediately. Because of propranolol's potential to cause hypotension, advise the patient to rise from a lying or sitting position slowly.

Class III—Drugs that Interfere with Potassium Outflow

Class III antidysrhythmic agents, potassium channel blockers, interfere with potassium channels to alter the repolarization phase of the heart's contraction. This prolongs the potential contraction duration of the Purkinje fibers and the muscle fibers of the ventricles. The prolonged period decreases the frequency of heart failure.

AMIODARONE

Amiodarone (Cordarone, Pacerone) is a powerful class III antidysrhythmic.

How does it work?

Amiodarone blocks potassium ion channels as well as sodium ion channels. This action prolongs the resting stage of the heart's contraction as well as the refractory period, which stabilizes atrial and ventricular dysrhythmias.

How is it used?

It is used to treat atrial dysrhythmias in patients with heart failure. Oral dosage forms may take several weeks to produce an effect. However, its effects can last 4 to 8 weeks after it is discontinued because of its extended half-life. An IV form is available, but that is usually reserved for serious ventricular dysrhythmias.

What are the adverse effects?

Amiodarone has few cardiovascular adverse effects, perhaps because of its modest vasodilator action, which produces little or no left ventricular depression. SA node activity is minimally affected. Amiodarone decreases automaticity, prolongs atrioventricular conduction, and can even block the exchange of sodium and potassium. Amiodarone (Cordarone, Pacerone) is too toxic for long-term use, except for serious ventricular dysrhythmias. Pulmonary fibrosis can occur in some patients treated with the drug for more than 5 years and could be fatal. Other significant potential adverse effects include changes in thyroid function (hypothyroidism or hyperthyroidism) and visual disturbances as a result of optic neuritis and/or corneal microdeposits. Common adverse effects that may be self-limiting include dizziness, nausea, vomiting, anorexia, bitter taste, weight loss, numbness of the fingers and toes. Weakness can also occur.

What are the contraindications and interactions?

Amiodarone is contraindicated in severe liver disease, pregnancy, children, and severe sinus bradycardia. Amiodarone interacts with many other drugs, including digoxin (Lanoxin) and phenytoin (Dilantin).

What are the important points patients should know?

Tell patients to notify the health-care provider immediately if shortness of breath, cough, or change in heart rate and rhythm occurs. Also instruct patients to immediately report any vision changes to the health-care provider. Advise patients to change positions slowly to avoid dizziness. Advise patients, especially elderly patients, to protect their skin and eyes from the sun.

SOTALOL

Sotalol (Betapace) has class II and III antidysrhythmic properties. Although measurable class III effects can be detected in clinical use, they largely are masked by the drug's beta-blocking properties. Sotalol is used for the treatment of documented ventricular arrhythmias that, in the judgment of the physician, are life threatening.

DOFETILIDE

Dofetilide (Tikosyn) is a class III antidysrhythmic agent that prolongs the cardiac action potential by blocking the potassium channels. It is used for treatment of symptomatic atrial fibrillation and flutter. Adverse effects on the body as a whole include flu-like syndrome and back pain. The most common adverse effects of dofetilide are headache, dizziness, insomnia, nausea, diarrhea, and abdominal pain.

IBUTILIDE

Ibutilide (Corvert) is a newly approved class III drug that differs markedly from amiodarone and sotalol. It achieves its effect by activating a slow, inward sodium current rather than by blocking outward potassium currents. Injecting ibutilide can acutely terminate atrial fibrillation and atrial flutter, particularly in patients with recent onset of dysrhythmia.

BRETYLIUM

Bretylium (Bretylo) also has antisympathetic class III action. It may cause marked hypotension and is indicated only for the management of potentially lethal **refractory** ventricular tachyarrhythmias. (*Refractory* means the period during repolarization when cells cannot respond normally to a second stimulus.) Bretylium usually is effective within 30 minutes of injection.

Class IV—Calcium Channel Blockers

Class IV drugs are termed *calcium channel blockers* because they decrease the entry of calcium into the cells of the heart and blood vessels. The SA and AV nodes require calcium for normal activity and normal sinus rhythm. Reducing calcium decreases the rate of the SA node and the conduction velocity of the AV node, and it is effective in the treatment of supraventricular tachycardia. Class IV drugs can decrease the ability of the heart to produce forceful contractions, leading to congestive heart failure. These medications also relax smooth muscle and cause vasodilation. Therefore, these agents are useful for angina and hypertension.

Focus on Geriatrics

Heart Failure and Surgery

The chance of having heart failure increases as we age. One in 15 elderly patients between the ages of 75 and 84 (men more often than women) is diagnosed with some type of heart failure. Coronary heart disease, heart failure, and clinically significant dysrhythmias require in-depth evaluation and control before any type of elective, noncardiac surgery is performed.

VERAPAMIL

Verapamil (Calan, Isoptin) was the first calcium channel blocker approved by the FDA.

How does it work?

Verapamil acts principally on the AV node, slowing conduction. Therefore, it causes depression of myocardial contractibility and dilation of coronary arteries. These effects lead to decreased cardiac work and decreased cardiac energy consumption in patients with vasospastic angina. This effect increases delivery of oxygen to myocardial cells.

How is it used?

Verapamil is used to stabilize dysrhythmias. It is also approved for use in hypertension and angina. For dysrhythmias, it is prescribed in oral forms, but sustained-release and IV forms are also available.

What are the adverse effects?

The adverse effects are dizziness, vertigo, emotional depression, sleepiness, headache, peripheral edema, hypotension, nausea, and constipation.

What are the contraindications and interactions?

Verapamil (Calan, Isoptin) is contraindicated in patients with allergy to this agent, hypotension, pregnancy, lactation, and congestive heart failure. Verapamil interacts with carbamazepine, lithium, cyclosporine, and calcium salts. It may also increase blood levels of digoxin (Lanoxin).

What are the important points patients should know?

Instruct patients to take their blood pressure prior to taking verapamil. They should contact their health-care provider if their blood pressure is below 90/60 mm Hg. Advise patients to notify their health-care provider if they experience any breathing difficulty or change in heart rhythm. Also advise patients to take verapamil with food to avoid stomach upset, and to increase their intake of fiber to avoid constipation.

Focus Point

Top 10 Prescribed Cardiovascular Drugs

1. atorvastatin (Lipitor)
2. amlodipine (Norvasc)
3. lisinopril (Zestril)
4. digoxin (Lanoxin)
5. simvastatin (Zocor)
6. enalapril (Vasotec)
7. warfarin sodium (Coumadin)
8. pravastatin (Pravachol)
9. quinapril (Accupril)
10. diltiazem (Cardizem CD)

DILTIAZEM

Diltiazem (Cardizem, Dilacor) is less potent than verapamil in decreasing heart rate but is more potent as a vasodilator. It is used for essential hypertension, angina pectoris due to coronary artery spasm, and dysrhythmias such as atrial fibrillation, atrial flutter, and supraventricular tachycardia. Adverse effects include headache, fatigue, dizziness, nervousness, insomnia, and confusion. It also may cause edema, flushing, hypotension, nausea, vomiting, and impaired taste. Diltiazem has noted drug interactions with cyclosporine (Nedral).

Focus Point

Look-Alike and Sound-Alike Drugs

Drug Name and Purpose	Looks Like/ Sounds Like
amiodarone (antidysrhythmic)	amrinone (cardiac inotropic agent)
dopamine (heart stimulant)	dobutamine (sympathetic A and B agonist)
metoprolol (beta-blocker)	misoprostol (prostaglandin analog for ulcer therapy)
Lanoxin (digoxin-cardiac glycoside)	Lasix (diuretic)
pindolol (beta-blocker)	Parlodel (dopaminergic agonist inhibitor of prolactin)
Propulsid (stimulator of GI function)	propranolol (beta-blocker)

✳ Apply Your Knowledge 18.4

The following questions focus on what you have just learned about dysrhythmias (arrhythmias) and their therapeutic agents. *See Appendix E for the correct answers.*

FILL IN THE BLANK

Select terms from your reading to fill in the blanks.

1. Arrhythmias may be benign or malignant; this type of arrhythmia, _____, is most often fatal.

2. Class _____ antidysrhythmic drugs may be the least toxic. They are also known as _____.

3. Which subclass of class I antidysrhythmics has short effects? _____.

4. Which class Ia drug has been used since the 1920s in cardiac conditions? _____.

5. If used in early acute MI, which drug can reduce the incidence of primary ventricular fibrillation? _____.

6. Which class Ib drug is also used for epilepsy? _____

7. Which drug is the most common beta-blocker used as an antidysrhythmic? _____

8. Which class III drug is too toxic for long-term use, except for serious arrhythmias? _____

9. Which calcium channel blocker acts principally on the AV node and slows conduction? _____

10. Which drug activates a slow inward sodium current rather than blocking outward potassium currents? _____

LABELING

Answer the following drug labeling questions using the label depicted below. You may need to use your drug guide or the *Physicians' Desk Reference* to answer some of the questions.

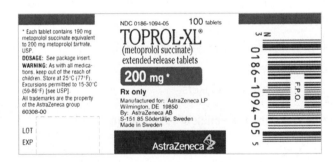

Courtesy of Astra Zeneca Pharmaceuticals LP.

1. Generic name: _____

2. Drug class: _____

3. Form of drug: _____

4. Drug schedule (use "Rx" if not a scheduled drug): _____

5. Adult dosage: _____

6. Typical use: _____

7. Body system that this drug targets: _____

8. Manufacturer: _____

9. Storage requirements: _____

10. Pregnancy category: _____

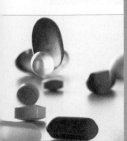

Chapter Capsule

This section repeats the objectives from the beginning of the chapter and then provides a summary of the most important concepts for that objective. Use this section as a quick review and to check your knowledge.

Objective 1: Identify the electrical conduction system of the heart.

- Sinoatrial (SA) node
- Atrioventricular (AV) node
- Bundle of His
- Right and left bundle branches
- Purkinje fibers

Objective 2: Name the three layers of the heart and the four heart valves.

- Layers of the heart—endocardium, myocardium, epicardium
- Heart valves—tricuspid, pulmonary, mitral, aortic

Objective 3: Define three types of angina pectoris.

- Classical or stable angina—due to a fixed obstruction in a coronary artery and brought on by exertion, emotional stress, or indigestion; usually causes chest discomfort (with pain radiating to the jaw, neck, shoulder, and left arm) that is relieved by rest and/or nitroglycerin; the most common form
- Variant or vasospastic angina—due to coronary artery spasm that reduces blood flow; usually occurs at rest rather than with exertion or emotional stress
- Unstable angina—due to significant coronary artery disease; occurs at rest for the first time and decreases in response to rest or nitroglycerin; often portends myocardial infarction

Objective 4: Name the mainstays of angina therapy.

- Beta-blockers
- Calcium channel blockers

Objective 5: Describe the action of vasodilation.

- Increases the size of blood vessels to improve circulation of the blood

Objective 6: Define calcium channel blockers.

- Drugs that decrease vascular tone and cause vasodilation by interfering with the movement of calcium ions through cell membranes, inhibiting the contraction of vascular smooth muscle
- Can affect the heart and/or peripheral vasculature
- Used to treat dysrhythmias, the pain of angina pectoris, vasospastic angina, and hypertension

Objective 7: Explain myocardial infarction.

- Occurs when part of the myocardium suffers prolonged restriction of oxygenated coronary blood
- Requires rapid diagnosis and treatment for a good outcome
- Is the leading cause of death in industrialized nations

Objective 8: Identify the classification of antidysrhythmic drugs and explain their actions.

- Four classes (I to IV) of drugs are used to treat arrhythmias

- Class I includes subtypes a, b, and c
- Class I drugs bind to sodium channels, reducing the maximal rate of contraction of the myocardium and slowing conduction
- Class II drugs—beta-adrenergic blockers reduce the heart's oxygen demand by decreasing heart rate and preventing development of myocardial ischemias and angina
- Class III drugs—interfere with potassium channels to alter the repolarization phase; prolong the potential contraction duration of the Purkinje fibers and the muscle fibers of the ventricles, decreasing the frequency of heart failure
- Class IV drugs—calcium channel blockers decrease vascular tone and cause vasodilation by interfering with the movement of calcium ions through cell membranes, thereby inhibiting the contraction of vascular smooth muscle

Objective 9: Describe the adverse reactions of quinidine.

- Diarrhea, flatulence, abdominal pain, and fever
- Reduced platelets
- Liver function abnormalities
- Quinidine syncope

Objective 10: Identify the mechanism of action of lidocaine.

- Blocks both activated and inactivated sodium channels, affecting depolarized or ischemic tissues

Objective 11: List the adverse effects of phenytoin.

- Gingival hyperplasia
- Blurred vision
- Vertigo
- Nystagmus

 Internet Sites of Interest

- At the IntelHealth Web site, experience an interactive look at the heart and its functions: **www.intelihealth.com**. Click on "Interactive Tools" on the left and choose "Heart Basics."
- Search for "heart and circulatory disorders" at: **www.intelihealth.com**

Chapter 19

Effects of Drugs on the Vascular System

Chapter Objectives

After completing this chapter, you should be able to:

1. Describe primary and secondary hypertension.
2. Identify the different types of antihypertensive agents and their actions.
3. Explain the effects of angiotensin converting enzyme (ACE) inhibitors.
4. Describe the newest and oldest drugs that are used for congestive heart failure.
5. Explain the most common side effects of digitalis.
6. Describe disorders that are related to hyperlipidemia.
7. Define statin drugs (HMG-CoA reductase inhibitors).
8. Identify the adverse effects of niacin.

Key Terms

Blood pressure (page 404)

Blood volume (page 404)

Cardiac output (page 404)

Congestive heart failure (CHF) (page 403)

Connective tissue (page 404)

Cutaneous flush (kew-TAY-nee-us) (page 424)

Diastole (dye-AH stoh-lee) (page 404)

Hypercholesterolemia (hy-per-koh-les-ter-rawl-LEE-mee-uh) (page 421)

Hypertensive crisis (page 405)

Peripheral resistance (page 404)

Primary hypertension (page 404)

Steatorrhea (stee-at-oh-REE-ah) (page 423)

Stroke volume (page 404)

Systole (SIS-toh-lee) (page 404)

PRACTICAL SCENARIO

The husband of an elderly woman, who had become incoherent over the past day, called emergency medical services (EMS). When they arrived at the house and asked the woman's husband for her history, he told them that his wife had had diabetes and hypertension for many years. Before calling EMS, he had checked her medicines, and based on the number of pills still left in the bottle, he estimated that she had not been taking her antihypertensive medication for about 2 weeks. On examination, the EMS team found that she was afebrile, her pulse rate was 112 beats per minute, respirations were 24 breaths per minute, and her blood pressure was 230/160 mm Hg.

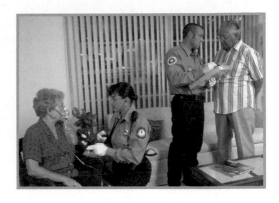

Critical Thinking Questions

1. What might be the results of this patient stopping her antihypertensive medications so abruptly?

2. What consequences could a long-term blood pressure of 230/160 mm Hg have for this patient?

3. What questions would you ask the patient and her family to help guide ongoing treatment and adherence to the medication regimen?

Introduction

It is estimated that there are nearly 60 million people in the United States who have hypertension (signified by a systolic blood pressure more than 140 mm Hg and diastolic above 90 mm Hg, or those taking antihypertensive medication). *Prehypertension* is classified as 120/80 mm Hg to 140/90 mm Hg, whereas *normal* blood pressure is 119/79 mm Hg or less. Hypertension, the most common of the cardiovascular diseases, occurs more often in black than in white adults, and morbidity and mortality are greater in blacks. Men experience more hypertension than women. The actual level of pressure that can be considered hypertensive is difficult to define; it depends on a number of factors, including the patient's age, gender, race, and lifestyle.

Uncontrolled hypertension can damage small blood vessels, causing narrowing of the arteries, which can result in kidney failure, strokes, and cardiac arrest. Chronic hypertension causes the heart to work harder pumping blood to organs and tissues and can result in **congestive heart failure (CHF)**, which develops when plasma volume increases and fluid accumulates in the lungs, abdominal organs (especially the liver), and peripheral tissues.

Hyperlipidemia, an elevation of lipoprotein levels in the plasma, is also a strong risk factor for cardiovascular disease (CVD). The major plasma lipids are cholesterol and the triglycerides that are bound to proteins and transported as macromolecular complexes called *lipoproteins*. These help to form the fatty material (plaque) that builds up in the lining of blood vessels and can cause angina, stroke, and myocardial infarction (MI). Hyperlipidemias are linked to specific genetic mutations, and most have a multifactorial basis that can respond to lifestyle changes and/or drug therapy.

Lifestyle changes, such as reduction of body weight; decreased intake of dietary total fat, cholesterol, saturated fatty acids, and salt; smoking cessation; increased exercise; and stress management can be effective for minor hypertension and hyperlipidemias. Pharmacologic methods combined with healthy lifestyle habits are usually necessary to treat chronic hypertension and serious hyperlipidemias.

The Vascular System

Circulatory pressure within the vascular system is divided into three components: (1) arterial pressure, (2) capillary pressure, and (3) venous pressure. **Blood pressure**, which commonly means arterial pressure, is created by the pumping action of the heart and varies from one vessel to another within the systemic circuit. Systemic pressures are highest in the aorta, peaking at around 120 mm Hg, and lowest at the venae cavae, averaging about 2 mm Hg. Blood pressure in large and small arteries rises and falls, rising during ventricular **systole** (when the ventricles of the heart contract and eject blood) and falling during ventricular **diastole** (when the ventricles relax and the heart stops ejecting blood).

Three main factors affect blood pressure.

1. **Cardiac output:** the volume of blood pumped per minute, which is determined by heart rate and **stroke volume** (amount of blood pumped by a ventricle in one contraction). The higher the cardiac output, the higher the blood pressure.

2. **Peripheral resistance:** the friction in the arteries as blood flows through the vessels. The smooth muscle in artery walls can constrict, causing the inside diameter of the artery to narrow, creating more resistance and higher pressure.

3. **Blood volume:** the total amount of blood in the vascular system; more blood creates added pressure on the artery walls, increasing blood pressure.

Many of the drugs used to treat hypertension target one of these three factors.

The body regulates blood pressure through the vasomotor center, a cluster of neurons in the medulla oblongata, that signal the smooth muscle of the arteries to constrict (raising blood pressure) or relax (lowering blood pressure). Baroreceptors, one type of clusters of neurons in the aorta and internal carotid artery, sense pressure within the large vessels of the vascular system and send this information to the vasomotor center. Another type, chemoreceptors, send information to the vasomotor center about levels of oxygen, carbon dioxide, and the acidity or pH of the blood. The vasomotor center raises or lowers blood pressure based on the information it receives.

The walls of arteries and veins contain three distinct layers (Figure 19-1 ■):

1. Tunica interna: the innermost layer of blood vessels that includes the endothelial lining of the vessel and an underlying layer of **connective tissue** (elastic fibers).

2. Tunica media: the middle layer that contains smooth muscle tissue in a framework of collagen and elastic fibers.

3. Tunica externa: the outer layer, which is a sheath of connective tissue around the vessel.

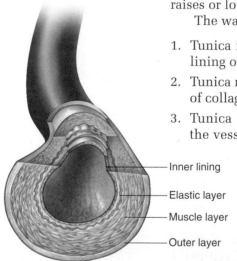
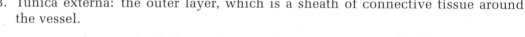

Inner lining

Elastic layer

Muscle layer

Outer layer

These multiple layers give arteries and veins considerable strength, and the muscular and elastic components permit controlled alterations in diameter as blood pressure or blood volume changes. Under normal circumstances, blood flow is equal to cardiac output. When cardiac output goes up, so does capillary blood flow; when cardiac output declines, blood flow is reduced. Two factors—pressure and resistance—affect the flow rates of blood through the capillaries.

Figure 19-1 ■ The structure of an artery, showing the outer protective layer, muscle layer, elastic layer, and inner lining.
© Dorling Kindersley.

Hypertension

Hypertension is the most prevalent cardiovascular disorder in the United States and is the result of chronically elevated pressure throughout the vascular system. Atherosclerosis, arteriosclerosis, renal disease, and any condition that creates increased vascular pressure causes the heart to work harder as it pumps against the increased resistance. The cause of **primary hypertension** (also called *essential hypertension*), which accounts for 90% of cases, is unknown. Heredity is a predisposing factor, but the exact mechanism is unclear. Environmental factors such as dietary sodium, obesity, and stress seem to act only in genetically susceptible people. *Secondary hypertension* is associated with renal disease such as chronic glomerulonephritis, pyelonephritis, polycystic renal disease, or endocrine disorders, which include Cushing's syndrome, pheochromocytoma, and myxedema. It may also be associated with the use of excessive alcohol, oral contraceptives, corticosteroids, and cocaine. Table 19-1 ■ summarizes classifications of blood pressure in adults.

Table 19-1 ■ Classification of Blood Pressure in Adults

CLASSIFICATION	SYSTOLIC (mm HG)		DIASTOLIC (mm HG)
Normal	< 120	and	< 80
Prehypertension	120–139	or	80–89
Stage I hypertension	140–159	or	90–99
Stage II hypertension	≥ 160	or	≥ 100

Hypertension is a major cause of cerebrovascular accident, cardiac disease, and renal failure. The prognosis is good if this disorder is detected early and treatment begins before complications develop. Severely elevated blood pressure (**hypertensive crisis**) may be fatal.

The values shown in Table 19-1 should not be considered as absolutes, but they are representative as models for treatment of hypertension. In general terms, hypertension can be defined as the level of blood pressure at which there is risk. The ultimate judgment concerning the severity of hypertension in any given patient must also include a consideration of factors other than diastolic or systolic pressure, such as age and comorbid conditions.

✱ Apply Your Knowledge 19.1

The following questions focus on what you have just learned about the vascular system and hypertension. *See Appendix E for the correct answers.*

FILL IN THE BLANK
Select terms from your reading to fill in the blanks.

1. Two factors, _____ and _____, affect the flow rate of blood through the capillaries.

2. Circulatory pressure is often divided into three components: _____ pressure, _____ pressure, and _____ pressure.

3. Systemic pressures are highest in the _____.

4. The most prevalent cardiovascular disorder in the United States is _____.

5. Severely elevated blood pressure, also known as _____, may be fatal.

6. The etiology of essential hypertension is _____.

7. Secondary hypertension may be associated with the use of excessive alcohol, oral contraceptives, _____, or _____.

8. Stage I hypertension occurs when diastolic pressure is _____ to _____ mm Hg, or systolic pressure is _____ to _____ mm Hg.

(continued)

Apply Your Knowledge 19.1 (continued)

MATCHING

Match the lettered term to the numbered description.

DESCRIPTION	TERM
1. _____ Regulates blood pressure by signaling smooth muscle of arteries to constrict or relax	a. Cardiac output
2. _____ Constitutes 90% of all hypertension cases	b. Peripheral resistance
3. _____ Associated with renal disease or endocrine disorders	c. Blood volume
4. _____ Volume of blood pumped per minute	d. Stroke volume
5. _____ Total amount of blood in the vascular system	e. Vasomotor center
6. _____ Amount of blood pumped by a ventricle in one contraction	f. Primary hypertension
7. _____ Friction in the arteries as blood flows through	g. Secondary hypertension

ANTIHYPERTENSIVE AGENTS

Antihypertensive agents are used to reduce blood pressure to within the normal levels. If the cause of hypertension is known, such as secondary hypertension, therapy is directed toward correction of the etiology. Unfortunately, the cause of about 90% of cases of hypertension is unknown.

Primary hypertension has no cure, but treatment can modify its course. The basic approach for antihypertensive therapy starts with changes in lifestyle. These changes include controlling weight by diet and exercise, stopping smoking, decreasing alcohol intake, decreasing sodium intake, exercising on a regular basis, resting and avoiding stress, and taking prescribed medications. Long-term therapy is essential to prevent the morbidity and mortality associated with uncontrolled hypertension. Drug therapy used in the treatment of hypertension includes diuretics (to reduce circulating blood volume), beta-adrenergic blockers (to slow the heartbeat and dilate vessels), vasodilators (to dilate vessels), calcium channel blockers (to slow the heartbeat, reduce conduction irritability, and dilate vessels), and angiotensin-converting enzyme (ACE) inhibitors (to produce vasodilation and increase renal blood flow.) These medications may be prescribed singly or in combination. Administration of drug therapy is designed to fit each patient's needs and response. Noncompliance is associated with poor prognosis, whereas compliance with an individualized regimen is associated with good prognosis. Table 19-2 ■ lists the most commonly used agents for hypertension.

Diuretics

Diuretics reduce circulating blood volume by blocking the reabsorption of sodium and chloride, which results in more water being retained in the kidney and the excretion of excess fluid. Diuretics are mainstays of hypertensive therapy and can be used alone or in combination with other antihypertensive agents. The four major groups of diuretics include thiazide diuretics, thiazide-like diuretics, loop diuretics, and potassium-sparing diuretics. These agents will be discussed in more detail in Chapter 21.

Table 19-2 ■ Most Commonly Prescribed Antihypertensive Agents

GENERIC NAME	TRADE NAME	AVERAGE ADULT DOSAGE	ROUTE OF ADMINISTRATION
Diuretics (see Table 19-3)			
Beta-blockers			
acebutolol	Sectral	200–800 mg bid	PO
atenolol	Tenormin	25–100 mg/d	PO
betaxolol	Kerlone	10–20 mg/d	PO
bisoprolol	Zebeta	2.5–20 mg/d	PO
carteolol	Cartrol	2.5–10 mg/d	PO
metoprolol	Lopressor	50–450 mg/d	PO
nadolol	Corgard	40–320 mg/d	PO
penbutolol	Levatol	20–80 mg/d	PO
pindolol	Visken	up to 60 mg/d	PO
propranolol	Inderal	10–240 mg/d	PO
timolol	Blocadren	20–60 mg/d	PO
Alpha- and Beta-blockers			
labetalol	Normodyne	100–400 mg PO bid (max: 1,200–2,400 mg/d)	PO
		20 mg slowly over 2 min, with 40–80 mg q10min if needed (max: 300 g total dose)	IV
Centrally Acting Blockers			
clonidine	Catapres	0.1–0.8 mg bid	PO
		Apply patch q7d	Transdermal
guanabenz	Wytensin	4–32 mg bid	PO
guanfacine	Tenex	1–3 mg bid	PO
methyldopa	Aldomet	250 mg bid–tid (max: 3 g/d in divided doses)	PO
		250–500 mg q6h increased up to 1 g q6h	IV
Peripherally Acting Blockers			
doxazosin	Cardura	1–16 mg/d	PO
guanadrel	Hylorel	10–75 mg/d	PO
guanethidine	Ismelin	10–50 mg/d	PO
prazosin	Minipress	1–20 mg/d	PO
reserpine	Serpalan, Serpasil	0.1–0.25 mg/d	PO
terazosin	Hytrin	1–20 mg/d	PO

(*continued*)

Table 19-2 ■ **Most Commonly Prescribed Antihypertensive Agents** (*continued*)

GENERIC NAME	TRADE NAME	AVERAGE ADULT DOSAGE	ROUTE OF ADMINISTRATION
Calcium Channel Blockers			
amlodipine with benazepril	Norvasc	5–10 mg/d	PO
diltiazem	Cardizem	80–120 mg tid	PO
felodipine	Plendil	5–10 mg/d	PO
isradipine	DynaCirc	1.25–10 mg bid	PO
nicardipine	Cardene	20–40 mg tid	PO
nifedipine	Procardia, Adalat	10–20 mg tid	PO
nisoldipine	Nisocor, Sular	10–20 mg tid	PO
verapamil	Calan, Verelan	40–80 mg tid	PO
Angiotensin II Receptor Blockers			
bisoprolol	Zebeta	2.5–5 mg/d (max: 20 mg/d)	PO
candesartan	Atacand	8–32 mg/d	PO
eprosartan	Teveten	400–800 mg/d	PO
irbesartan	Avapro	150–300 mg/d	PO
losartan	Cozaar	25–50 mg 1–2 times/d	PO
olmesartan	Benicar	20–40 mg/d	PO
valsartan	Diovan	80–160 mg/d	PO
telmisartan	Micardis	40–80 mg/d	PO
ACE Inhibitors			
benazepril	Lotensin	4–50 mg/d	PO
captopril	Capoten	25/100 mg/d	PO
enalapril	Vasotec	5–40 mg/d	PO
fosinopril	Monopril	10–40 mg/d	PO
lisinopril	Prinivil, Zestril	10–40 mg/d	PO
moexipril	Univasc	7.5–30 mg/d	PO
perindopril	Aceon	2.5–20 mg/d	PO
quinapril	Accupril	2–8 mg/d	PO
ramipril	Altace	2.5–5 mg/d	PO
trandolapril	Mavik	1–4 mg/d	PO
Vasodilators			
fenoldopam	Corlopam	0.025–0.3 mcg/kg/min by continuous infusion for up to 48h	IV

Table 19-2 ■ Most Commonly Prescribed Antihypertensive Agents

GENERIC NAME	TRADE NAME	AVERAGE ADULT DOSAGE	ROUTE OF ADMINISTRATION
hydralazine	Apresoline	10–50 mg qid	PO
		10–50 mg q4–6h	IM
		10–20 mg q4–6h	IV
minoxidil	Loniten, Rogaine	5 mg/d, increased q3–5d up to 40 mg/d in single or divided doses as needed (max: 100 mg/d)	PO

Diuretic drugs, either alone or in combination with other agents are frequently used in the management of mild to moderate hypertension. Diuresis and restriction of salt intake are often sufficient for many hypertensive patients except those with severe, malignant, or complicated hypertension. Table 19-3 ■ lists commonly used diuretics.

Table 19-3 ■ Diuretics

GENERIC NAME	TRADE NAME	AVERAGE ADULT DOSAGE	ROUTE OF ADMINISTRATION
Thiazide Diuretics			
chlorothiazide	Diuril, Duragen	500 mg 1–2 times/d	PO
hydrochlorothiazide	Esidrix, HydroDIURIL	25–100 mg/d	PO
indapamide	Lozol	2.5–5 mg/d	PO
polythiazide	Renese	1–4 mg/d	PO
hydroflumethiazide	Diucardin	25–200 mg 1–2 times/d	PO
Thiazide-like Diuretics			
chlorthalidone	Hygroton	12.5–25 mg/d (max: 100 mg/d)	PO
indapamide	Lozol	1.25–5 mg/d	PO
metolazone	Zaroxolyn	5–20 mg/d	PO
quinethazone	Hydromox	50 mg 1–2 times/d	PO
Loop Diuretics			
furosemide	Lasix	20–80 mg/d, up to 600 mg/d	PO
		20–40 mg in 1 or more divided doses (max: 600 mg/d)	IM, IV
ethacrynic acid	Edecrin	50–100 mg 1–2 times/d	PO
		0.5–1 mg/kg or 50 mg up to 100 mg	IV
torsemide	Demadex	5–20 mg/d, up to 200 mg/d	PO, IV

(continued)

Table 19-3 ■ Diuretics (*continued*)

GENERIC NAME	TRADE NAME	AVERAGE ADULT DOSAGE	ROUTE OF ADMINISTRATION
bumetanide	Bumex	0.5–2 mg/d, may repeat at 4–5-h intervals (max: 10 mg/d)	PO
		0.5–1 mg over 1–2 min, repeated q2–3h PRN (max: 10 mg/d)	IM, IV
Potassium-sparing Diuretics			
amiloride	Midamor	5 mg/d	PO
spironolactone	Aldactone	50–100 mg bid	PO
triamterene	Dyrenium	50–100 mg bid	PO

Beta-Adrenergic Blockers

The beta-blockers are very popular antihypertensive drugs. They competitively antagonize the responses to catecholamines that are mediated by beta receptors. (See Chapter 18 for a detailed discussion of beta-adrenergic blockers.)

Alpha- and Beta-Blockers

Alpha- and beta-blockers are indicated for severe hypertension. Alpha- and beta-blocking actions contribute to the blood pressure–lowering effect.

How do they work?

Alpha- and beta-blockers act as adrenergic-receptor blocking agents that combine selective alpha activity and nonselective beta-adrenergic blocking actions. Both actions contribute to blood pressure reduction.

How are they used?

Alpha- and beta-blockers, such as labetalol (Normodyne), are used in the treatment of mild, moderate, and severe hypertension. They may be used alone or in combination with other antihypertensive agents, especially thiazide diuretics.

What are the adverse effects?

The adverse effects include postural hypotension, dizziness, vertigo, headache, bronchospasm, and dyspnea. Alpha-receptor blockade causes vasodilation and decreased peripheral vascular resistance that is added to the beta-blocking mechanisms (see Table 19-2).

What are the contraindications and interactions?

Alpha- and beta-blockers are contraindicated in bronchial asthma, uncontrolled cardiac failure, cardiogenic shock, and severe bradycardia. Safe use during pregnancy, lactation, or in children is not established.

Labetalol should be used cautiously in patients with impaired liver function, jaundice, and diabetes mellitus. Cimetidine (Tagamet) may increase the effects of labetalol, and glutethimide (Doriglute) decreases its effects.

What are the important points patients should know?

Inform patients who are taking alpha- and beta-blockers that hypotension may occur. Instruct them to make all position changes slowly and in stages, particularly from a lying to an upright position. Advise patients to avoid driving or engaging in other potentially hazardous activities until their responses to the drug are known.

Focus on Geriatrics

Alpha- and Beta-Blocker Use in Older Adults

Older adults are especially sensitive to the hypotensive effects of alpha- and beta-blockers. They must be careful not to engage in any activity that could be especially dangerous because of low blood pressure.

Centrally Acting Adrenergic Blockers

Centrally acting adrenergic blockers, such as clonidine hydrochloride (Catapres) and methyldopa (Aldomet), are not regarded as first-line therapies in hypertension. These drugs tend to be used in cases in which the affected person has not responded to other therapies.

How do they work?

These agents are able to reduce the hyperactivity in the medulla oblongata of the brain. Sympathetic outflow from the medulla is diminished, and, as a result, either systemic vascular resistance or cardiac output is decreased.

How are they used?

Centrally acting adrenergic blockers are used for management of hypertension, especially in combination with a diuretic.

What are the adverse effects?

The adverse effects include drowsiness, sedation, headache, nightmares, anxiety, orthostatic hypotension, and CHF (see Table 19-2). Centrally acting agents may also cause peripheral edema, tachycardia, bradycardia, flushing, and hepatitis.

What are the contraindications and interactions?

Centrally acting blockers are contraindicated in pregnancy, lactation, hepatitis, cirrhosis of the liver, and blood dyscrasias. These agents should be used cautiously in kidney disease, angina pectoris, and history of mental depression.

What are the important points patients should know?

Advise patients to avoid potentially hazardous tasks such as driving until response to these drugs is known. Instruct them to check with their physician before taking OTC medications. Tell women that they should not breast feed while taking these drugs without consulting their physician.

Peripherally Acting Adrenergic Blockers

Peripherally acting adrenergic blockers, such as doxazosin (Cardura), phenoxybenzamine (Dibenzyline), and reserpine (Serpalan), lower blood pressure in supine or standing individuals, with the most pronounced effect on diastolic blood pressure.

How do they work?

Peripherally acting blockers are antihypertensive in that their effects depend on inhibition of norepinephrine release and depletion of norepinephrine from nerve terminals. These drugs reduce blood pressure by reducing vascular tone, primarily in the veins and the arteries.

How are they used?

Peripherally acting adrenergic blockers are used for severe hypertension or as adjunctive therapy with other antihypertensive agents in the more severe form of hypertension.

What are the adverse effects?

The adverse effects of these drugs are drowsiness, fatigue, headache, confusion, palpitation, dry mouth, dyspnea, nausea, and vomiting (see Table 19-2).

What are the contraindications and interactions?

Contraindications include hypersensitivity to reserpine (Serpalan), history of mental depression, acute peptic ulcer, and ulcerative colitis. Safe use during pregnancy, lactation, or in children is not established. Peripherally acting adrenergic blockers should be used cautiously in patients with diabetes mellitus, impaired renal or hepatic function, coronary disease with insufficiency, and recent heart attack. Alcohol intensifies orthostatic hypotension and sedation. Reserpine may enhance the action of epinephrine (Bronkaid Mist), norepinephrine (Levarterenol), and antidepressants.

What are the important points patients should know?

Inform patients about the possibility of orthostatic hypotension and advise them to have assistance getting out of bed during initial dosage adjustment. Tell them to take the drug at the same time(s) each day, in relation to a daily routine activity. OTC drugs for treatment of colds, allergy, asthma, or appetite suppressants should not be used without consulting the physician or pharmacist.

Angiotensin-Converting Enzyme Inhibitors

Angiotensin-converting enzyme (ACE) inhibitors, such as enalapril maleate (Vasotec) and ramipril (Altace), are drugs that prevent ACE from producing angiotensin II. ACE inhibitors are used to treat hypertension and CHF.

How do they work?

ACE inhibitors decrease the formation of angiotensin II, which lowers blood volume and blood pressure. Renin is an enzyme that is secreted by the kidneys in response to reduced renal blood circulation or lower sodium in the blood. The renin–angiotensin system controls blood pressure and fluid balance and is one of the body's primary homeostatic mechanisms. Figure 19-2 ■ shows the renin–angiotensin system.

How are they used?

ACE inhibitors are a very popular class of drugs for the treatment of severe hypertension. They are becoming the drugs of choice in the treatment of primary hypertension. These agents are also used to treat CHF.

What are the adverse effects?

Although ACE inhibitors as a group are relatively free of side effects in the majority of patients, they do occur, and some can be life threatening. The adverse effects include loss of taste, photosensitivity, severe hypotension, hyperkalemia, renal impairment, blood dyscrasias, dizziness, and angioedema. ACE inhibitors are contraindicated in angioedema, pregnant women, renal impairment, scleroderma, and lupus erthytomatosis.

What are the contraindications and interactions?

ACE inhibitors are contraindicated in patients with hypersensitivity to these agents. Safety during pregnancy, lactation, or in children is not established. ACE inhibitors should be used cautiously in renal impairment and renal-artery stenosis, and in patients with hypovolemia, receiving diuretics, undergoing dialysis, with hepatic impairment, or with diabetes mellitus.

Potassium-sparing diuretics may increase the risk of hyperkalemia. Aspirin and other NSAIDs may antagonize hypotensive effects. ACE inhibitors may increase lithium (Eskalith) levels and toxicity.

What are the important points patients should know?

Instruct patients who are using ACE inhibitors to consult their physician promptly if vomiting or diarrhea occur. OTC medications should be used only with the approval of their physician. Advise patients to inform surgeons or dentists that they are taking ACE inhibitors.

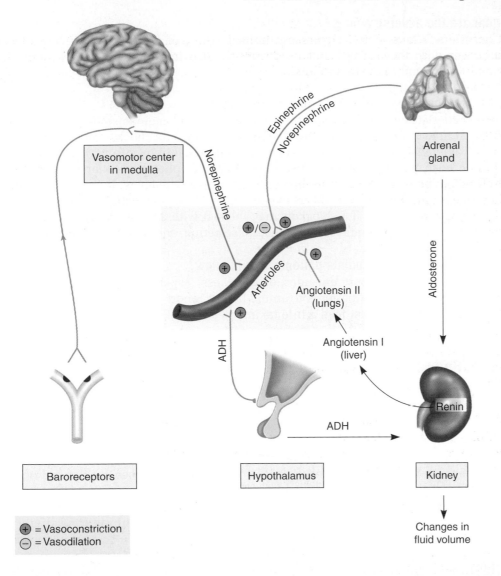

Figure 19-2 ■ The renin–angiotensin system.

Focus Point

ACE Inhibitors and Diabetes

ACE inhibitors can produce hypoglycemia in diabetic patients. Monitoring blood glucose is important during the first few weeks of therapy.

Angiotensin II Receptor Blockers

Angiotensin receptor blockers antagonize the effects of angiotensin II.

How do they work?

Angiotensin II receptor blockers inhibit the binding of angiotensin II to the angiotensin I receptor in vascular smooth muscle. By blocking these receptors, angiotensin II cannot raise blood pressure. This action blocks the vasoconstriction and aldosterone secretion stimulated by angiotensin II.

How are they used?

These agents have beneficial effects on patients with CHF. Angiotensin II receptor blockers have been one of the fastest growing groups of agents for the management of hypertension. The most common angiotensin II receptor blockers are listed in Table 19-2.

What are the adverse effects?

The adverse effects of these drugs are similar to those of ACE inhibitors. One effect that is absent with these drugs, but present with ACE inhibitors, is a persistent cough, which can be annoying to patients.

What are the contraindications and interactions?

These drugs are contraindicated in known sensitivity to angiotensin II receptor blockers, bilateral artery stenosis, overt cardiac failure, cardiogenic shock, pregnancy, and lactation. Angiotensin II receptor blockers must be used cautiously in patients with asthma, chronic obstructive pulmonary disease (COPD), peripheral vascular disease, diabetes mellitus, hyperthyroidism, and renal or hepatic insufficiency.

Angiotensin II receptor blockers may interact with amiodarone (Cordarone) and cause significant bradycardia. Beta-blockers may interact with angiotensin II receptor blockers and reduce glucose tolerance, inhibit insulin secretion, and produce hypertension.

What are the important points patients should know?

Advise patients to report episodes of dizziness, especially when making position changes. Inform female patients to immediately report pregnancy to their physician. Women should not breast feed while taking these drugs.

Vasodilators

Vasodilators (listed in Table 19-2) are agents that cause blood vessels to expand, increasing blood flow and lowering blood pressure in the affected area.

How do they work?

Vasodilators produce a direct relaxation of vascular smooth muscle, and these actions result in vasodilation. This effect is called *direct* because it does not depend on the innervation of vascular smooth muscle and is not mediated by receptors. The vasodilators decrease total peripheral resistance and thus correct primary hypertension. Unlike many other antihypertensive agents, the vasodilators do not inhibit the activity of the sympathetic nervous system; therefore, orthostatic hypotension and impotence are not problems. In addition, most vasodilators relax arterial smooth muscle to a greater extent than venous smooth muscle, thereby further minimizing postural hypotension.

How are they used?

The vasodilators are generally inadequate as the sole therapy for hypertension and produce many side effects. However, administration of beta-blockers and diuretics is more useful than vasodilators alone.

What are the adverse effects?

The main adverse effects of vasodilators include headache, dizziness, tachycardia, nausea, and vomiting. The specific adverse effects of fenoldopam (Corlopam), a commonly prescribed vasodilator, include insomnia, nervousness, flushing, postural hypotension, bradycardia, and heart failure.

What are the contraindications and interactions?

Vasodilators are contraindicated in patients with hypersensitivity to these agents. Fenoldopam (Corlopam) should be avoided if beta-blockers are being used. Hydralazine (Apresoline) is contraindicated in coronary artery disease, mitral valvular rheumatic heart disease, and myocardial infarction. Safety during pregnancy or lactation for vasodilators has not been established.

Vasodilators should be used cautiously in cerebrovascular accident, advanced renal impairment, and coronary artery disease. Drug interactions occur with epinephrine (Bronkaid Mist) and norepinephrine (Levarterenol), which can cause excessive cardiac stimulation. These agents, if used with guanethidine (Ismelin), cause profound orthostatic hypotension.

What are the important points patients should know?
Instruct patients to monitor their weight, check for edema, make position changes slowly, and avoid standing still. Advise them to avoid excessive alcohol intake and driving or engaging in other potentially hazardous activities until their responses to these drugs are known. Female patients should not breast feed while taking these drugs without consulting their physicians.

✳ Apply Your Knowledge 19.2 ▬▬▬

The following questions focus on what you have just learned about antihypertensive agents. *See Appendix E for the correct answers.*

MULTIPLE CHOICE
Select the correct answers from choices a–d.

1. The cause of about 90% of cases of hypertension is:
   a. Unknown
   b. Cholesterol
   c. Diuretics
   d. Being underweight

2. Which of the following is NOT one of the four major groups of diuretics?
   a. Loop
   b. Calcium-sparing
   c. Thiazide-like
   d. Potassium-sparing

3. Patients taking beta-blockers should be careful when making position changes, so that they may avoid:
   a. Vomiting
   b. Postural hypertension
   c. Edema
   d. Postural hypotension

4. Which of the following reduce blood pressure by reducing vascular tone?
   a. Diuretics
   b. Calcium channel blockers
   c. Peripherally acting adrenergic blockers
   d. Centrally acting adrenergic blockers

5. Which of the following are becoming the drugs of choice in the treatment of primary hypertension?
   a. ACE inhibitors
   b. Diuretics
   c. Vasodilators
   d. Calcium channel blockers

MATCHING
Match the lettered trade name to the numbered generic drug name.

GENERIC NAME	TRADE NAME
1. _____ labetalol	a. Apresoline
2. _____ reserpine	b. Monopril
3. _____ fenoldopam	c. Corlopam
4. _____ hydralazine	d. Normodyne
5. _____ fosinopril	e. Serpalan

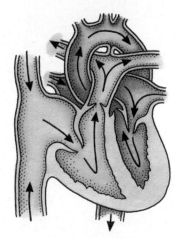

Figure 19-3 ■ Human heart with atrium and ventricles highlighted to illustrate the flow of blood through the chambers and pulmonary blood vessels. Arrows depict the path of blood through the open valves.

© Dorling Kindersley.

Congestive Heart Failure and Treatment

Heart failure is defined as an inability of the heart, under normal filling conditions, to pump blood at a rate sufficient to meet the metabolic demands of the tissues. The inability to pump blood can be due to various abnormalities in the myocardium. When the heart pumps blood at an insufficient rate, the kidneys retain salt and water, and fluid accumulates in interstitial spaces. Thus, the term *congestive heart failure* (CHF) is used to describe this condition. Figure 19-3 ■ shows normal blood flow through the heart.

Congestive heart failure occurs when the heart pumps less blood than it receives, which results in blood accumulating in the heart chambers and the stretching of the heart walls. CHF is accompanied by abnormal increases in blood volume and interstitial fluid; the heart, veins, and capillaries are generally dilated with blood. As a result of CHF, organs receive less blood circulation. Therefore, less oxygen reaches the kidneys and water is retained, increasing blood volume. Edema of the lower limbs is a common symptom. Other symptoms include pulmonary congestion with left heart failure and peripheral edema with right heart failure. The underlying causes of CHF include arteriosclerotic heart disease, hypertensive heart disease, valvular heart disease, dilated cardiomyopathy, and congenital heart disease. Left systolic dysfunction secondary to coronary artery disease is the most common cause of heart failure. Figure 19-4 ■ shows signs and symptoms of the patient with heart failure.

w/ pulmonary congestion

edema of lower limbs

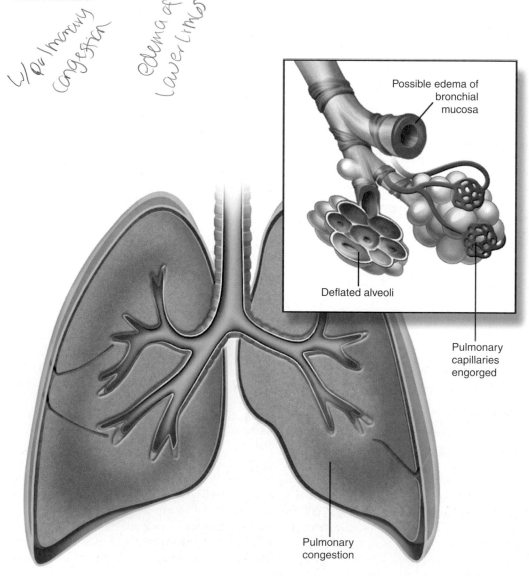

Possible edema of bronchial mucosa

Deflated alveoli

Pulmonary capillaries engorged

Pulmonary congestion

Figure 19-4 ■ Signs of congestive heart failure with pulmonary congestion.

The therapeutic goal for CHF is to increase cardiac output. Three classes of drugs have been shown to be clinically effective in reducing symptoms and prolonging life: inotropic, diuretics, and vasodilators. Treatment of CHF may include combinations of inotropic drugs, diuretics, and vasodilators that include ACE inhibitors. Table 19-4 ■ lists the main classes of drugs used for CHF.

Table 19-4 ■ Main Classes of Drugs Used for Congestive Heart Failure (CHF)

GENERIC NAME	TRADE NAME	AVERAGE ADULT DOSAGE	ROUTE OF ADMINISTRATION
Inotropic Drugs			
Cardiac Glycosides			
digitoxin	Crystodigin	150 mcg daily (max: 0.3 mg/d)	PO
digoxin	Lanoxin	10–15 mcg/kg in divided doses over 24–48 h; then 0.1–0.375 mg/d	PO
		10–15 mcg/kg in divided doses over 24 h; then 0.1–0.375 mg/d	IV
Beta-adrenergic Agonists			
propranolol	Inderal	40 mg bid (usually need 160–480 mg/d in divided doses)	PO
Phosphodiesterase Inhibitors			
inamrinone lactate	Inocor	0.75 mg/kg bolus given slowly over 2–3 min; then start infusion at 5–10 mcg/kg/min; may repeat bolus in 30 min (max: 10 mg/kg/d)	IV
milrinone lactate	Primacor	Loading dose: 50 mcg/kg over 10 min; maintenance dose: 0.375–0.75 mcg/kg/min	IV
Diuretics (see Table 19-3)			
Vasodilators (see Table 19-2)			

Inotropic Drugs

Inotropic agents increase the cardiac muscle's strength of contraction. These drugs relieve the symptoms of cardiac insufficiency but do not reverse the underlying pathologic condition. Knowledge of the physiology of heart muscle contraction is essential to an understanding of the compensatory responses evoked by the failing heart, as well as the actions of drugs used to treat CHF.

Inotropic drugs act by different mechanisms; in each case, the inotropic action is the result of an increased cell calcium concentration that enhances the contractility of cardiac muscle. Inotropic drugs include cardiac glycosides, and beta-adrenergic agonists (see Table 19-4). Cardiac glycosides, such as digitoxin (Crystodigin) and digoxin (Lanoxin) are obtained from the plant leaves of *Digitalis pupurea* and *Digitalis lanata*. They all are derived from natural sources whose medicinal qualities have been recognized for centuries. The cardiac glycosides are popular and effective drugs for the treatment of CHF. They act by exerting a positive inotropic action on the heart that increases the force of myocardial contraction, thereby improving the mechanical efficiency of the heart as a blood-pumping organ. This ultimately results in reduced heart size and increased blood flow to the kidneys.

How do they work?

Cardiac glycosides act by increasing the force and velocity of myocardial systolic contraction and decreasing conduction velocity through the atrioventricular node. Cardiac glycosides inhibit the enzyme *ATPase*, which is associated with the sodium pump, and the exchange between sodium and calcium is impaired. Stores of calcium within the myocardium are released, and the membrane becomes more permeable to this ion. As a result, intracellular calcium levels are elevated. Because calcium is necessary for normal muscle contraction, the elevated calcium levels result in a stronger force of contraction (Figure 19-5 ■).

How are they used?

Digoxin (Lanoxin) is the most commonly prescribed digitalis preparation for treating CHF. It is used for rapid digitalization and maintenance therapy in congestive heart failure, as well as for atrial fibrillation and flutter. Digoxin and digitoxin (Crystodigin), the two primary cardiac glycosides, are similar in efficacy. The main difference between the two drugs is digitoxin's more prolonged half-life.

What are the adverse effects?

Common adverse effects of cardiac glycosides include fatigue, muscle weakness, headache, mental depression, visual disturbances, anorexia, nausea, vomiting, and diarrhea.

What are the contraindications and interactions?

Cardiac glycosides are contraindicated in patients with digitalis hypersensitivity, ventricular fibrillation, and ventricular tachycardia (unless it is due to CHF). These drugs should be used cautiously in patients with renal insufficiency, hypokalemia, advanced heart disease, acute myocardial infarction, hypothyroidism, pregnancy, and lactation, and in older adults.

Antacids, cholestyramine (LoCholest), and colestipol (Colestid) decrease digoxin absorption. Diuretics, corticosteroids, amphotericin B (Amphocin), and laxatives may cause hypokalemia.

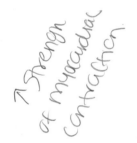

↑ Strength of myocardial contraction

What are the important points patients should know?

Advise patients who are taking digoxin (Lanoxin) for atrial fibrillation to report to their physician a pulse rate that falls below 60 or rises above 110 beats per minute (bpm). Inform patients of the occurrence of anorexia, nausea, vomiting, diarrhea, or visual disturbances, because these adverse effects may be due to toxicity. They must report these adverse effects to their physician.

Digoxin must be taken exactly as prescribed and at the same time each day; be sure to tell patients to not skip or double a dose, or change dose intervals. Patients should not take OTC medications, especially those for coughs, colds, allergies, GI upset, or obesity without the prior approval of their physician.

Focus on Natural Products

Foxglove and Digoxin

The cardiac drug digoxin is derived from foxglove, a purple flowering plant, and has been described in medical literature for more than 200 years as a treatment for heart disease. English physician William Withering is credited with discovering in 1775 that the foxglove plant could help those suffering from a condition of abnormal fluid buildup, which, at that time, was called *dropsy*. In 1930 the glycosides of the woolly foxglove, *Digitalis lanata,* were isolated and the drug digoxin was born. Like foxglove, other plants such as oleander and lily of the valley also have cardiac glycoside properties. Patients must be aware of taking digoxin and these herbs together, because they may receive a toxic dose. Reports of digoxin toxicity are often linked with extracts and teas containing the foxglove, oleander, and lily of the valley herbs.

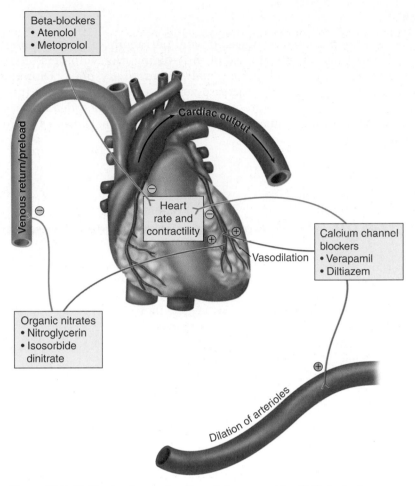

Figure 19-5 ■ Mechanisms of action of drugs used for CHF, including cardiac glycosides.

Focus Point

Cardiac Glycosides and Low Pulse

If the apical pulse falls below a set parameter in a patient taking cardiac glycosides, administration of the drug should be withheld and the physician notified.

Beta-adrenergic Agonists

Beta-adrenergic stimulation improves cardiac performance by positive inotropic effects and vasodilation (see Chapter 25 for a detailed discussion of beta-adrenergic agonists). See Table 19-4 for beta-adrenergic agonists.

Phosphodiesterase Inhibitors

Phosphodiesterase inhibitors, such as amrinone (Inocor) and milrinone lactate (Primacor), increase the force of the heart's contraction and cause vasodilation. They work by blocking the enzyme phosphodiesterase in cardiac and smooth muscle, resulting in a positive inotropic response and vasodilation. They are commonly used for the short-term control of acute heart failure, and they have high toxicity.

Diuretics

Diuretics relieve the pulmonary congestion and peripheral edema common in congestive heart failure. These agents are useful in reducing the symptoms of volume overload, including orthopnea and paroxysmal nocturnal dyspnea. Diuretics decrease plasma volume and subsequently decrease venous return to the heart (preload). This decreases the cardiac workload and oxygen demand. Diuretics also decrease afterload by reducing plasma volume, thus decreasing blood pressure. Diuretics are discussed in detail in Chapter 21.

✳ Apply Your Knowledge 19.3

The following questions focus on what you have just learned about CHF and its treatment. *See Appendix E for the correct answers.*

MULTIPLE CHOICE

Select the correct answers from choices a–d.

1. Which of the following is the therapeutic goal of CHF treatment?

    a. Decreased cardiac output

    b. Decreased blood in the myocardium

    c. Increased cardiac output

    d. Increased kidney retention of salt and water

2. The cardiac glycosides inhibit the enzyme associated with which of the following?

    a. Sodium pump

    b. Potassium pump

    c. Calcium and potassium pump

    d. Sodium and potassium pump

3. Digoxin is prescribed for all of the following disorders, except:

    a. CHF

    b. Ventricular fibrillation

    c. Atrial fibrillation

    d. Flutter

4. As a result of CHF, organs receive:

    a. And retain smaller amounts of water

    b. Increased blood circulation

    c. More oxygen

    d. Less blood circulation

5. The most commonly prescribed digitalis preparation for treating CHF is:

    a. Diazepam

    b. Diazoxide

    c. Digoxin

    d. Diltiazem

MATCHING

Match the lettered trade name to the numbered generic drug name.

GENERIC NAME	TRADE NAME
1. _____ atorvastatin	a. Crystodigin
2. _____ digoxin	b. Primacor
3. _____ digitoxin	c. Inderal
4. _____ propranolol	d. Lanoxin
5. _____ milrinone lactate	e. Lipitor

Hyperlipidemia and Related Disorders

Hyperlipidemia is characterized by an increase in both plasma cholesterol and/or triglycerides containing lipoprotein particles. These particles, which are key to the development of atherogenesis, are initially synthesized by the intestinal mucosa and the liver and undergo extensive metabolism in the plasma. They also play an essential role in the transport of lipids between tissues. The lipoproteins differ in density and are referred to as very-low-density lipoprotein (VLDL), low-density lipoprotein (LDL), high-density lipoprotein (HDL), and chylomicrons. Each lipoprotein includes different amounts of triglycerides and cholesterol in the core. The size of the core varies with the size of the lipoprotein. When carried as circulating lipoprotein, cholesterol is the predominant core of LDL and HDL. Chylomicrons produced by the intestines transport dietary cholesterol and triglycerides. Triglycerides are the predominant makers of chylomicrons and the VLDL secreted by the liver.

A patient with high serum cholesterol and increased LDL is at risk for atherosclerotic coronary disease, myocardial infarction, and hypertension. Disorders of hyperlipidemia are characterized by an elevation in triglycerides and an elevation of cholesterol. Elevated triglycerides can produce life-threatening pancreatitis.

Although **hypercholesterolemia** (higher-than-normal levels of cholesterol in the blood) are linked to specific genetic mutations, most have a multifactorial basis that can respond to lifestyle changes. These changes include reduction of body weight; decreased dietary total fat, cholesterol, and saturated fatty acids; increased exercise; and stress management.

There are several different types of hypercholesterolemia. *Type IIa* is associated with high levels of both cholesterol and LDL in the blood. Ischemic heart disease is common in this type. The condition may be hereditary and is then termed *familial hypercholesterolemia*.

Type IIb is associated with high VLDL and LDL, and therefore, high triglycerides and cholesterol blood levels. Ischemic heart disease may result. This type may be related to high alcohol intake, obesity, diabetes mellitus, and overeating. Dietary modification is usually all that is required, but drugs may be necessary in resistant cases.

Type IV is characterized by high VLDL and hypertriglyceridemia. Causes are similar to that of type IIb, but peripheral vascular disease, and ischemic heart disease can be found in sufferers. Treatment is the same as for type IIb.

ANTIHYPERLIPIDEMICS

Antihyperlipidemic medications should be used if diet modification and exercise programs fail to lower LDL to normal levels. When medications are started, diet therapy must continue. Some of the antihyperlipidemic drugs decrease production of the lipoprotein carriers of cholesterol and tricylycerol, whereas others increase lipoprotein degradation. Still others directly increase cholesterol removal from the body. These drugs may be used singly or in combination, but are always accompanied by the requirement that dietary lipid intake be significantly low, especially cholesterol and saturated fats, and the caloric content of diet must be closely monitored. The major drugs for reduction of LDL cholesterol levels are bile acid sequestrants and nicotinic acid. The fibric acid derivatives such as clofibrate are less effective in reducing LDL cholesterol. The most effective drugs for lowering plasma LDL levels are the HMG-CoA reductase inhibitors, or statins. Antihyperlipidemic drugs are listed in Table 19-5 ∎.

Table 19-5 ∎ Antihyperlipidemic Drugs

GENERIC NAME	TRADE NAME	AVERAGE ADULT DOSAGE	ROUTE OF ADMINISTRATION
Bile Acid Sequestrants			
cholestyramine resin	LoCholest, Questran	4–6 g/d	PO
colestipol	Colestid	15–30 g/d	PO
HMG-CoA Reductase Inhibitors (Statins)			
atorvastatin	Lipitor	10–80 mg qid	PO
fluvastatin	Lescol	20–40 mg/d	PO
lovastatin	Altoprev, Mevacor	20–80 mg/d	PO
pravastatin	Pravachol	10–40 mg/d	PO
rosuvastatin	Crestor	5–40 mg/d	PO
simvastatin	Zocor	10–80 mg/d	PO
simvastatin/ezitimibe	Vytorin	10/10 mg/d to 10/80 mg/d (ezitimibe is 10 mg)	PO
Miscellaneous Drugs			
nicotinic acid (niacin)	Niac, Nicobid	1–2 g bid–tid	PO
Fibric Acid Derivatives			
clofibrate	Atromid-S	2 g/d	PO
gemfibrozil	Lopid	1,200 mg/d	PO
dextrothyroxine	Choloxin	4–8 mg/d	PO

Focus Point

Alcohol and Cholesterol

Moderate alcohol intake increases HDL cholesterol (the "good" cholesterol) but does not reduce LDL cholesterol (the "bad" cholesterol).

Bile Acid Sequestrants

Bile acid sequestrants, such as cholestyramine resin (LoCholest, Questran) and colestipol (Colestid), are drugs that chemically combine with bile acids in the intestine, causing these bile acids to be excreted from the body.

How do they work?
Bile acid sequestrants are used for their cholesterol-lowering effect. They *bind* with bile salts in the intestinal tract to form an insoluble complex that is excreted in the feces, thus reducing circulating cholesterol and increasing serum LDL removal rates.

How are they used?

Bile acid sequestrants are nonabsorbable drugs prescribed for decreasing serum cholesterol. Lowering the bile acid concentration causes the liver to increase conversion of cholesterol to bile acids, resulting in a replenished supply of these compounds, which are essential components of the bile. Because the bile acids are lost in feces, LDLs and serum cholesterol are reduced. The bile acid binding resins are prescribed for primary hyperlipidemias.

What are the adverse effects?

The adverse effects of bile acid sequestrants include constipation, nausea, flatulence, *[Liver failure]* and impaired absorption of fat-soluble vitamins.

What are the contraindications and interactions?

Bile acid sequestrants should be avoided in patients with bowel obstruction, and their safety is not established for patients with dysphagia, swallowing disorders, and major GI tract surgery. Safety during pregnancy and lactation or in children younger than 6 is not established. These agents should be used cautiously in patients with bleeding disorders, hemorrhoids, peptic ulcer, and malabsorption states such as **steatorrhea** (elimination of large amounts of fat in the stool).

Cholestyramine resin and colestipol interfere with the intestinal absorption of many drugs, for example, tetracycline (Achromycin), phenobarbital (Barbital), digoxin (Lanoxin), warfarin (Coumadin), aspirin, and thiazide diuretics.

What are the important points patients should know?

Advise patients to report promptly to their physician if they develop severe gastric distress with nausea and vomiting, unusual weight loss, black stools, severe hemorrhoids, and sudden back pain. A high-bulk diet with adequate fluid intake is an essential adjunct to resolve constipation.

HMG-CoA Reductase Inhibitors (Statin Drugs)

This powerful group of antihyperlipidemic agents includes the most effective drugs for reducing LDL and cholesterol levels. They share the generic name of *statin*, and are described as *the statins*.

How do they work?

Statin drugs reduce LDL and total triglyceride production. These agents are inhibitors of reductase (HMG-CoA), which is essential to hepatic production of cholesterol. *[prevent heart attack (myoccardial infarction)]*

How are they used?

The statins are the most widely used drugs for lowering hyperlipidemia. Lovastatin (Altoprev), simvastatin (Zocor), pravastatin (Pravachol), and fluvastatin (Lescol) are completely effective in inhibiting HMG-CoA reductase, which is the enzyme needed in cholesterol production. These drugs are often given in combination with other antihyperlipidemic drugs. It should be noted that in spite of the protection afforded by cholesterol lowering, about one fourth of the patients treated with these drugs still present with coronary events. Thus, additional strategies such as diet, exercise, or additional agents may be warranted.

What are the adverse effects?

Some patients may have muscle pain. A severe, but rare, adverse effect is life-threatening rhabdomyolysis (degeneration of skeletal muscle tissue with possible renal failure). Other adverse effects may include abdominal pain, flatulence, constipation, dyspepsia, headache, and cramping. Liver function and serum transaminase levels must be measured periodically. If there is muscle pain, creatine kinase levels should be monitored to rule out rhabdomyolysis. The HMG-CoA reductase inhibitors may increase coumarin levels. Thus, it is important to evaluate prothrombin times frequently.

What are the contraindications and interactions?

Statins are contraindicated for patients who are hypersensitive to these agents, and in myopathy, active liver disease, unexplained persistent transaminase elevations, and during pregnancy and lactation. Statin drugs may increase levels of digoxin (Lanoxin), norethindrone (Micronor), and the oral contraceptive ethinyl estradiol (Estinyl).

What are the important points patients should know?
Instruct patients that they cannot interrupt, increase, decrease, or omit dosage without the advice of their physicians. They should notify their physicians promptly about muscle tenderness or pain, especially if accompanied by fever or malaise. Alcohol consumption should be avoided or reduced. Advise women that they should not breast feed while taking these drugs without consulting their physicians.

Focus on Pediatrics

Statin Drugs and Children

Statin drugs should not be prescribed for children or teenagers. The safety and effectiveness of these drugs in children and adolescents has not been established.

Focus on Natural Products

Food Interactions and Statins

Grapefruit and grapefruit juice should be avoided by patients who are taking the statin drug simvastatin (Zocor). Regular consumption of the fruit or juice can lead to high levels of the drug in the blood. This is not true of other statin drugs.

MISCELLANEOUS ANTIHYPERLIPIDEMIC DRUGS

Some other antihyperlipidemic drugs lower serum lipids in both primary and secondary hyperlipidemias. Nicotinic acid (Niac) and the fibrates, such as clofibrate (Atromid-S) and gemfibrozil (Lopid), are included in this category.

Nicotinic Acid (Niacin)

Nicotinic acid, or niacin (Niac), has a broad lipid-lowering ability, but its clinical use is limited because of its unpleasant side effects. Derivatives of this drug, which are not available in the United States, appear to have fewer adverse effects.

How does it work?
Niacin (Niac) appears to reduce the level of the VLDL, LDL, and total cholesterol. Combination drug therapy, such as nicotinic acid, bile acid binding sequestrants, and a statin, may decrease LDL cholesterol levels by 70% or more. Niacin causes a decrease in liver triacylglycerol synthesis, which is required for VLDL production. LDL is derived from VLDL in the plasma. Therefore, a reduction in the VLDL concentration also results in a decreased plasma LDL concentration.

How is it used?
Niacin (Niac) is used in adjuvant treatment of hypercholesterolemias in patients who do not respond adequately to diet or weight loss. It is the most potent antihyperlipidemic agent for raising plasma HDL levels.

What are the adverse effects?
The most common adverse effects of niacin therapy are an intense **cutaneous flush** (skin reddening) and pruritus. Administration of aspirin prior to taking niacin decreases the flush. Some patients also experience nausea and abdominal pain, syncope, nervousness, and blurred vision. Hyperuricemia, gout, impaired glucose tolerance, and hepatotoxicity have been reported.

What are the contraindications and interactions?

Niacin is contraindicated in patients with hypersensitivity to this agent. It must be avoided in hepatic impairment, severe hypotension, active peptic ulcer, pregnancy, lactation, and in children younger than 16.

Niacin should be used cautiously in patients with a history of gallbladder disease, liver disease, and peptic ulcer, glaucoma, coronary artery disease, and diabetes mellitus. Niacin is able to potentiate hypotensive effects of antihypertensive agents.

What are the important points patients should know?

Alert patients to the possibility of feeling warm and flushed in the face, neck, and ears within the first 2 hours after oral ingestion and immediately after parenteral administration. This may last for several hours. Effects are usually transient and subside as therapy continues. Instruct patients to sit or lie down, avoiding sudden posture changes if they feel weak or dizzy. These symptoms, as well as persistent flushing, should be reported to their physician. Relief may be obtained by reducing the dosage, increasing subsequent doses in small increments, or changing to a sustained-release formulation. Alcohol and large doses of niacin cause increased flushing and sensations of warmth. Tell patients to avoid exposure to direct sunlight until lesions have entirely cleared if they have skin manifestations. Women should not breast feed while taking niacin.

Fibric Acid Derivatives

Gemfibrozil (Lopid) and clofibrate (Atromid-S) are derivatives of fibric acid that lower triglycerides and VLDL and increase HDL.

How do they work?

Both drugs cause a decrease in plasma triglyceride levels by blocking lipolysis of stored triglycerides in adipose tissue and inhibiting hepatic uptake of fatty acids. In addition to inhibiting the breakdown of fats into triglycerides, liver production of triglycerides is inhibited.

How are they used?

Fibric acid derivatives are approved for use in hypertriglyceridemia patients who do not respond to diet—those in whom triglyceride levels can exceed 1000 mg/dL (normal is 10 to 190 mg/dL). They can also be prescribed in combination with other drugs to facilitate a reduction in triglycerides that complements the cholesterol-lowering action of the antihyperlipidemic agent. These agents are also used for severe familial hypercholesterolemia (type IIa or IIb) that develops early in childhood and has failed to respond to dietary control or to other cholesterol-lowering drugs.

What are the adverse effects?

The most common adverse effects are mild gastrointestinal disturbances, dizziness, and blurred vision. Gemfibrozil (Lopid) may increase cholesterol excretion into the bile, leading to gallstone formation. Treatment with clofibrate (Atromid-S) has resulted in significant occurrences of cancer. Inflammation of the skeletal muscle can occur with both drugs; thus, muscle weakness or tenderness should be evaluated.

What are the contraindications and interactions?

Fibric acid derivatives are contraindicated in patients with gallbladder disease, biliary cirrhosis, hepatic or severe renal dysfunction, and during pregnancy and lactation. Safety and efficacy in children younger than age 18 are not established. These drugs should be used cautiously in patients with diabetes mellitus, hypothyroidism, renal impairment, and *cholelithiasis* (gallstones).

Fibric acid derivatives may potentiate hypoprothrombinemic effects of oral anticoagulants. Lovastatin (Altoprev) increases the risk of myopathy and rhabdomyolysis and may increase repaglinide (Prandin) levels and duration of action.

What are the important points patients should know?

Instruct patients to notify their physicians promptly if unexplained bleeding occurs. This includes easy bruising, epistaxis (nosebleed), and hematuria (blood present in the urine).

✱ Apply Your Knowledge 19.4

The following questions focus on what you have just learned about hyperlipidemia and the medications used to treat it and related disorders. *See Appendix E for the correct answers.*

FILL IN THE BLANK

Select terms from your reading to fill in the blanks.

1. When carried as circulating lipoprotein, _____ is the predominant core of HDL and LDL.

2. Antihyperlipidemic medications should be used if _____ and _____ programs fail to lower _____ to normal levels.

3. The most effective drugs for lowering LDL and cholesterol levels are known as the _____.

4. Nicotinic acid has a broad lipid-lowering ability, is also known as _____, but has limited use due to its _____.

5. Fibric acid derivatives lower _____ and _____.

MATCHING

Match the lettered trade name to the numbered generic drug name.

GENERIC NAME	TRADE NAME
1. _____ gemfibrozil	a. Questran
2. _____ pravastatin	b. Zocor
3. _____ niacin	c. Lopid
4. _____ simvastatin	d. Niac
5. _____ cholestyramine resin	e. Pravachol

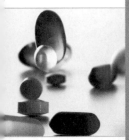

Chapter Capsule

This section repeats the objectives from the beginning of the chapter and then provides a summary of the most important concepts for that objective. Use this section as a quick review and to check your knowledge.

Objective 1: Describe primary and secondary hypertension.

- Primary (essential) hypertension—unknown etiology; heredity is a predisposing factor, but the exact mechanism is unclear; environmental/lifestyle factors (dietary sodium, obesity, stress) seem to act only in genetically susceptible people

- Secondary hypertension—associated with renal disease such as chronic glomerulonephritis, pyelonephritis, polycystic renal disease, or endocrine disorders, which include Cushing's syndrome, pheochromocytoma, and myxedema; may also be associated with the use of excessive alcohol, oral contraceptives, corticosteroids, and cocaine

Objective 2: Identify the different types of antihypertensive agents and their actions.

- Diuretics (reduce circulating blood volume)
- Beta-adrenergic blockers (slow the heartbeat and dilate vessels)
- Vasodilators (dilate vessels)
- Calcium channel blockers (slow the heartbeat, reduce conduction irritability, and dilate vessels)
- Angiotensin-converting enzyme (ACE) inhibitors (produce vasodilation and increase renal blood flow)

Objective 3: Explain the effects of angiotensin-converting enzyme (ACE) inhibitors.

- ACE inhibitors decrease the formation of angiotensin II, which lowers blood volume and blood pressure

■ The renin–angiotensin system controls blood pressure and fluid balance and is one of the body's primary homeostatic mechanisms; renin is an enzyme that is secreted by the kidneys in response to reduced renal blood circulation or lower sodium in the blood

Objective 4: Describe the newest and oldest drugs used for congestive heart failure.

■ Combinations of inotropic drugs, diuretics, and vasodilators that include ACE inhibitors are the newest treatments

■ Cardiac glycosides, derived from natural plant sources, have been recognized for centuries for their medicinal qualities

Objective 5: Explain the most common side effects of digitalis.

■ Fatigue, muscle weakness, headache, mental depression, visual disturbances, anorexia, nausea, vomiting, diarrhea

Objective 6: Describe disorders that are related to hyperlipidemia.

■ Atherosclerotic coronary disease

■ Myocardial infarction

■ Hypertension

■ Pancreatitis due to elevated triglycerides

Objective 7: Define statin drugs (HMG-CoA reductase inhibitors).

■ Inhibitors of reductase (HMG-CoA), which is essential to hepatic production of cholesterol

■ Most effective drugs for reducing LDL and cholesterol levels

■ Reduce LDL and total triglyceride production

Objective 8: Identify the adverse effects of niacin.

■ Intense cutaneous flush (skin reddening) and pruritus (very common)

■ Nausea and abdominal pain, syncope, nervousness, blurred vision (less common)

■ Hyperuricemia, gout, impaired glucose tolerance, hepatotoxicity (uncommon)

Internet Sites of Interest

■ The American Heart Association at: **http://www.americanheart.org/** is one of the best sites of information for patients and professionals on all topics related to heart diseases, as well as medications and lifestyle changes to treat or prevent them. Take a look around the site.

■ A site dedicated to heart disease in women is Heart Healthy Women at: **http://www.hearthealthywomen.org/** where information for patients and professionals can be found.

■ Cardiovascular Physiology Concepts offers information about secondary hypertension at: **www.cvphysiology.com**. Click on "Hypertension" in the left column.

■ Everything you have always wanted to know about hypertension is available at: **www.hypertension-facts.org**

■ MedicineNet.com, a pharmacists' Web site, discusses ACE inhibitors at: **www.medicinenet.com/ace_inhibitors/article.htm**

■ MedlinePlus, a service of the NIH and National Library of Medicine presents an in-depth look at digitalis drugs at: **http://www.nlm.nih.gov/medlineplus**. Click the "Drugs and Supplements" tab and search for "digitalis."

■ ADAM Healthcare Center of About.com offers information about high blood cholesterol and triglycerides at: **http://adam.about.com/encyclopedia**. Search for "cholesterol."

Checkpoint Review 4

Select the best answer for the following questions.

1. Which of the following neurotransmitters is released by the preganglionic sympathetic neuron?

   a. Norepinephrine
   b. Acetylcholine
   c. Dopamine
   d. Serotonin

2. Which of the following neurotransmitters is released by the parasympathetic postganglionic neurons?

   a. Serotonin
   b. Norepinephrine
   c. Dopamine
   d. Acetylcholine

3. Sympathomimetics are also called:

   a. Cholinergic antagonists
   b. Cholinergic agonists
   c. Adrenergic agonists
   d. Adrenergic antagonists

4. The "pacemaker," or SA node, is located in which of the following chambers of the heart?

   a. Left atrium
   b. Right atrium
   c. Right ventricle
   d. Left ventricle

5. Which of the following are class I antidysrhythmic drugs?

   a. Beta-adrenergic blockers
   b. Drugs that bind to sodium channels
   c. Drugs that interfere with potassium outflow
   d. Calcium channel blockers

6. Which of the following drugs has antisympathetic class III action?

   a. bretylium (Bretylo)
   b. verapamil (Calan)
   c. propranolol (Inderal)
   d. lidocaine (Xylocaine)

7. Alpha$_2$-receptor agonists are used to treat:

   a. Hypertension
   b. Hypotension
   c. Hepatitis
   d. Impotence

8. Sublingual nitroglycerin is rapidly effective and lasts for about:

   a. 15 minutes
   b. 30 minutes
   c. 1 hour
   d. 3 hours

9. Which of the following describes stage 2 of anesthesia?

   a. Surgical
   b. Analgesia
   c. Medullary paralysis
   d. Excitement

10. Beta$_2$-receptor agonists are used in patients with:

    a. Cardiac arrhythmias associated with digitalis intoxication
    b. Chronic obstructive airway disease
    c. Hypertension
    d. Thyrotoxicosis

11. The most common adverse effects of phenytoin (Dilantin) include which of the following?

    a. Nosebleed
    b. Asthma
    c. Bloody urine
    d. Gingival hyperplasia

12. Specialized cells in the epidermis called *melanocytes* produce:

    a. Melatonin
    b. Melanin
    c. Melanogen
    d. Melanotropin

13. Beta-receptor antagonists are used in the management of:

    a. Hypertension and weight reduction
    b. Cardiac arrhythmias
    c. Angina pectoris
    d. All of the above

14. Which of the following stages of anesthesia is called an *anesthetic accident*?

    a. Medullary paralysis
    b. Excitement
    c. Surgical anesthesia
    d. Analgesia

15. Pilocarpine is used most commonly in which of the following?

    a. Gynecology
    b. Ophthalmology
    c. Dermatology
    d. Cardiology

16. Cholinergic blockers are also called:

    a. Sympatholytics
    b. Sympathomimetics
    c. Parasympatholytics
    d. Parasympathomimetics

17. Which of the following is the cause of primary (essential) hypertension?

    a. Obesity
    b. Chronic glomerulonephritis
    c. Excessive alcohol
    d. Unknown

18. Discontinuation of nitroglycerin should take place over time, because the length of action of these drug preparations can cause:

    a. Hypertension
    b. Vasospasms
    c. Bradycardia
    d. Vomiting

19. Which of the following is/are the mechanism(s) of action of quinidine?

    a. Slowing of the heart rate
    b. Decreasing the contractile force of the heart
    c. Depressing the myocardium and the conduction system
    d. All of the above

20. General anesthetics are contraindicated in patients who have received monoamine oxidase (MAO) inhibitors within how many days?

    a. 2
    b. 4
    c. 7
    d. 14

21. Which of the following must patients do when taking nitroglycerin?

    a. Avoid food or liquids.
    b. Avoid alcoholic beverages.
    c. Avoid coffee or tea.
    d. Discard unused tablets after 5 minutes.

22. Which of the following is the mainstay of treatment for acute or chronic inflammatory disorders of the skin and may be topical or oral?

    a. Emollients (skin-softening agents)
    b. Keratolytic agents
    c. Antibiotics
    d. Corticosteroids

23. Which of the following drugs are mainstays of hypertensive therapy?

    a. Diuretics
    b. Statin drugs
    c. Beta-adrenergic blockers
    d. Centrally acting adrenergic blockers

24. Rhabdomyolysis (degeneration of skeletal muscle tissue) is a rare but life-threatening adverse effect of:

    a. Diuretics
    b. Angiotensin II receptor blockers
    c. Statins
    d. Fat-soluble vitamins

25. Parasympathomimetics (or cholinergic agonists) produce symptoms of:

    a. Fight-or-flight
    b. Rest-and-relaxation
    c. Fight-and-rest
    d. Speed-and-rest

26. Acne vulgaris is an inflammatory disorder of which of the following glands?

    a. Sweat
    b. Sebaceous
    c. Bartholin
    d. Mammary

27. Dopamine is released from which of the following?

    a. Kidneys
    b. GI tract
    c. Brain
    d. All of the above

28. Which of the following is an example of a beta-adrenergic blocker?

    a. Verapamil
    b. Diltiazem
    c. Inderal
    d. Amiodarone

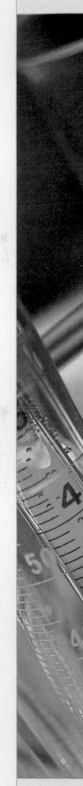

29. A chemical compound containing nitrogen that is derived from the amino acid tyrosine is called:

   a. Catecholamine
   b. Melanin
   c. Melatonin
   d. Cardiolipin

30. Which of the following agents are used in the treatment of corns, calluses, and plantar warts?

   a. Topical antibiotics
   b. Topical corticosteroids
   c. Keratolytics
   d. Emollients

31. Peripherally acting blockers are antihypertensive in that their effects depend on the inhibition of:

   a. Renin release
   b. Norepinephrine release
   c. Acetylcholine release
   d. Serotonin release

32. Beta$_1$-receptor agonists are used to treat which of the following?

   a. Cardiac arrest
   b. Circulatory shock
   c. Hypotension
   d. All of the above

33. Atropine acts by selectively blocking all muscarinic responses to:

   a. Dopamine
   b. Acetylcholine
   c. Norepinephrine
   d. Serotonin

34. Which of the following agents is a popular choice for infiltration anesthesia?

   a. Lidocaine
   b. Nitrous oxide
   c. Sevoflurane
   d. Cocaine

35. Which of the following is the trade name of lidocaine?

   a. Marcaine
   b. Carbocaine
   c. Novocaine
   d. Xylocaine

36. The primary use of bethanechol (Urecholine), which is a cholinergic agonist used in the cardiovascular field, is in the diagnosis of:

   a. Prolapse of the mitral valve
   b. Atrial tachycardia
   c. Myocardial infarction
   d. Hypertensive crises

37. During spinal anesthesia, the anesthetic agent is injected into which of the following spaces or parts of the spinal column?

   a. Pia mater
   b. Arachnoid
   c. Subarachnoid
   d. Epidural

38. Which of the following is the most commonly used route to administer local anesthetics?

   a. Local infiltration
   b. Topical anesthesia
   c. Spinal anesthesia
   d. Epidural anesthesia

39. Which of the following is the most frequent adverse effect associated with barbiturates?

   a. Blurred vision
   b. Thrombocytopenia
   c. Sedation
   d. Aplastic anemia

40. Stage 3 (surgical anesthesia) is characterized by progressive:

   a. Muscular contraction
   b. Circulatory collapse
   c. Muscular relaxation
   d. Dysfunction of the respiratory system, which can cause sudden death

41. Valproic acid is classified as an:

   a. Antipyretic
   b. Anticonvulsant
   c. Anticoagulant
   d. Antineoplastic

42. The trade name of ethosuximide is:

   a. Celontin
   b. Dilantin
   c. Ativan
   d. Zarontin

43. Cholinergic drugs exhibit effects similar to which of the following substances?

    a. Monoamine oxidase inhibitors
    b. Methotrimeprazine
    c. Acetylcholine
    d. Amphetamines

44. Stimulation of beta$_2$-receptors results in which of the following?

    a. Postural hypotension
    b. Nasal congestion
    c. Bronchoconstriction
    d. Bronchodilation

45. Which of the following is a cholinergic drug?

    a. Noradrenaline
    b. Dopamine
    c. Acetylcholine
    d. Any calcium channel blocker

46. Which of the following properties of general anesthetics is essential for the drug to cross the blood–brain barrier?

    a. Lipophilic
    b. Hydrophilic
    c. Proteinphilic
    d. None of the above

47. All of the following inhaled anesthetics are commonly used in the United States, except:

    a. Nitrous oxide
    b. Sevoflurane
    c. Diethyl ether
    d. Isoflurane

48. Which of the following drugs is in the group of ester-type local anesthetics?

    a. Bupivacaine
    b. Etidocaine
    c. Ropivacaine
    d. Benzocaine

49. Which of the following drugs is used to treat ophthalmic disorders and in preoperative situations?

    a. Niacin
    b. Atropine
    c. Alcohol
    d. Amantadine

50. Beta$_2$-receptor agonists are used in patients with all of the following, except:

    a. Premature labor
    b. Circulatory shock
    c. Anaphylactic shock
    d. Chronic obstructive airway disease

Select terms from your reading to fill in the blanks.

51. The space between each synapse is bridged by chemicals called _____.

52. Intraorbital block is often used for _____ surgery.

53. Atropine is a classic anticholinergic or _____ antagonist drug.

54. Neurons that release acetylcholine are termed _____.

55. Cryoanesthesia involves the reduction of nerve conduction by localized _____.

56. Alpha-receptor antagonists can be reversible or _____.

57. There are two types of cholinergic receptors, either muscarinic or _____.

58. Beta-blockers competitively antagonize the responses to _____ that are mediated by beta receptors.

59. Cholinergic blockers are also called _____.

60. Volatile anesthetics are combined with intravenous agents in regimens of so-called _____ anesthesia.

Chapter 20

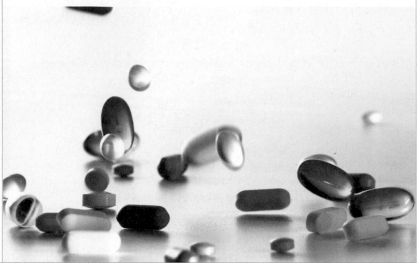

Anticoagulants

Chapter Objectives

After completing this chapter, you should be able to:

1. Explain hemostasis.
2. Explain the mechanisms of action of heparin and warfarin.
3. Describe the advantages of low-molecular-weight heparin (LMWH).
4. Name the class of drugs that can be used to induce bleeding or delay coagulation, and explain individual drug mechanisms of action.
5. Explain the mechanism of action of thrombolytic drugs, and list five drugs in this class.

Key Terms

Coagulation (ko-ag-yew-LAY-shun) (page 434)

Embolus (EM-bo-lus) (page 436)

Hemostasis (hee-mo-STAY-sis) (page 433)

Platelet plug (PLAY-tel-let) (page 433)

Serotonin (sayr-uh-TO-nin) (page 433)

Thrombi (THROM-beye) (page 437)

Thromboembolism (throm-bo-EM-bo-liz-im) (page 439)

PRACTICAL SCENARIO

A 65-year-old patient with a history of deep vein thrombosis (DVT) has been admitted to the hospital with chest pain. He is having trouble breathing. His physician orders an ECG, Doppler ultrasound, ventilation-perfusion scan, and a computed tomography scan. The diagnosis is a pulmonary embolus.

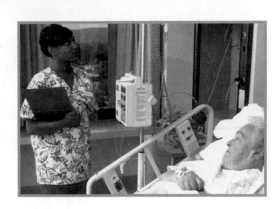

Critical Thinking Questions

1. What medicine will the physician likely immediately prescribe for this patient while he is hospitalized?

2. What teaching will you provide the patient and family about the reasons he is taking this medication and the precautions he needs to take during therapy?

3. Do you think the patient will be released from the hospital while taking this medication, or will his medication be switched? If the medication is changed when the patient is discharged, what is a likely alternative medicine that will be prescribed?

4. What teaching will you provide the patient when he leaves the hospital, especially regarding his medication?

Introduction

The blood transports blood cells, gases, hormones, immune cells, metabolic wastes, and nutrients. Normal blood clotting protects against excessive hemorrhaging, but the development of certain clots may obstruct the flow of blood and ultimately cause a myocardial infarction (MI), or stroke, and necrosis (death) of tissue. Hemorrhagic and thrombotic disorders may be treated with a variety of medications.

This chapter focuses on anticoagulant drug therapy, which is aimed at reducing the occurrences of thrombosis. Anticoagulants decrease the blood's ability to clot. There are two main types of anticoagulants: parenteral and oral. Often, both types are used together. Caution must be taken by health-care professionals because there are many conditions that cause an increased risk of hemorrhaging. Anticoagulants should not be used, or should be used only in severely limited quantities, in treating patients who have these types of conditions, such as hemophilia or thrombocytopenia (low-platelet count).

Hemostasis

Limited intravascular coagulation of blood occurs in normal physiologic conditions. The circulatory system has to be self-sealing; otherwise, continued blood loss from even the smallest injury would be life-threatening. Bleeding usually stops spontaneously when the injury is minor. A more serious bleeding episode, however, can be life-threatening and often requires medical intervention. Normally, all but the most catastrophic bleeding is rapidly stopped through a physiologic progression of several steps, known as **hemostasis** (Figure 20-1 ■).

Hemostasis involves three events:

1. Vascular Spasms. The platelets release the neurotransmitter, **serotonin**, which causes the blood vessel to go into spasms. The spasms decrease blood loss until clotting can occur.

2. Formation of a Platelet Plug. When a blood vessel is torn, the inner lining of the vessel stimulates, or activates, the platelets. The platelets become sticky and adhere to the inner lining of the injured vessel and to each other. By sticking together, they form a **platelet plug**. Over several minutes, the plug is invaded by activated blood-clotting factors, and eventually evolves into a stable and strong blood clot.

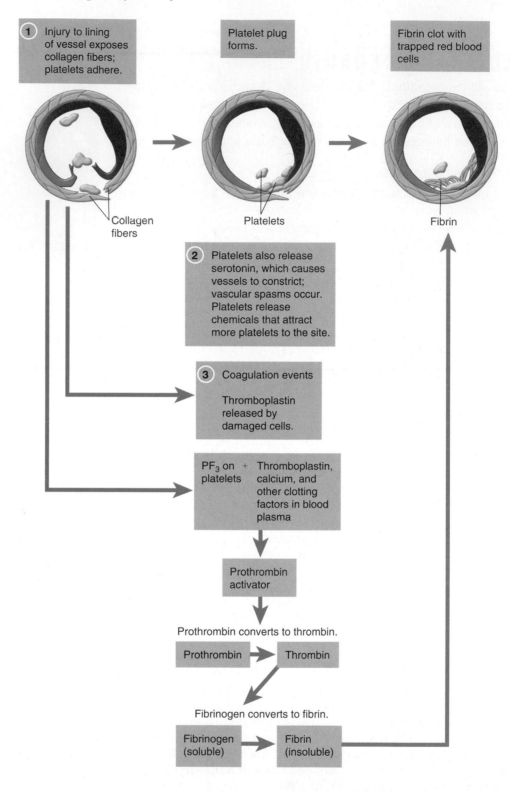

Figure 20-1 ■ Hemostasis begins when a blood vessel is damaged and ends when the fibrin threads trap blood cells, forming a clot that seals the injured vessel.

3. Blood Clotting. Vascular spasm and a platelet plug alone are not sufficient to prevent the bleeding caused by a larger tear in a blood vessel. With a more serious injury to the vessel wall, bleeding stops only if a blood clot forms. Blood clotting, or **coagulation**, is the third event in the process of hemostasis. A blood clot is formed by a series of chemical reactions that result in the formation of a netlike structure. The net is composed of protein fibers called *fibrin,* which seals off the opening in the injured blood vessel and stops the bleeding. The three basic steps of hemostasis are shown in Figure 20-2 ■.

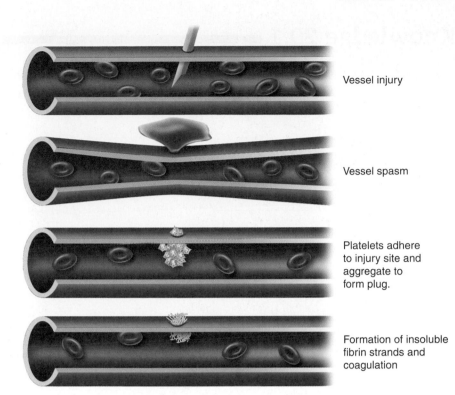

Vessel injury

Vessel spasm

Platelets adhere
to injury site and
aggregate to
form plug.

Formation of insoluble
fibrin strands and
coagulation

Figure 20-2 ■ Basic steps
of hemostasis.

HEMOSTASIS MECHANISM OF ACTION

The mechanism of action of hemostasis is complex and involves 11 different plasma
proteins called *clotting factors*. The process of blood clotting occurs in a series of sequential steps that are referred to as a *cascade*.

Normal coagulation cannot occur unless the plasma contains the necessary clotting
factors. Most of the circulating clotting proteins are synthesized by the liver. The
injured vessel releases a chemical called *prothrombin activator* (prothrombinase).
Prothrombin activator converts the clotting factor *prothrombin* to an enzyme called
thrombin. Thrombin then converts *fibrinogen* to *fibrin*. Normal blood clotting occurs in about 6 minutes. The primary steps in the coagulation cascade are shown in
Figure 20-3 ■.

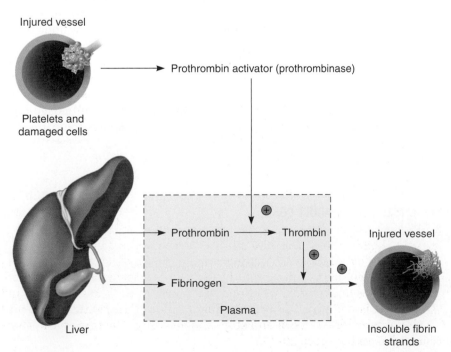

Injured vessel

Platelets and
damaged cells

Prothrombin activator (prothrombinase)

Prothrombin → Thrombin

Fibrinogen

Plasma

Liver

Injured vessel

Insoluble fibrin
strands

Figure 20-3 ■ The steps in
the coagulation cascade.

✳ Apply Your Knowledge 20.1

The following exercises focus on what you have just learned about the physiology of hemostasis. *See Appendix E for the correct answers.*

FILL IN THE BLANK

Select terms from your reading to fill in the blanks.

1. Normal blood clotting protects against _____.
2. A protein called _____ forms a mesh that traps the red blood cells.
3. A process of stoppage of blood flow is known as _____.
4. The platelets release a neurotransmitter called _____.
5. When a blood vessel is torn, the inner lining of the vessel stimulates or activates the _____.
6. Bleeding usually stops spontaneously when an _____ is minor.

MATCHING

Match the lettered term to the numbered description.

DESCRIPTION	TERM
1. _____ Decrease the blood's ability to clot	a. Circulation system
2. _____ Is self-sealing	b. Serotonin
3. _____ Involves vascular spasms, platelet plug formation, and blood clotting	c. Activated clotting factors
4. _____ Causes blood vessels to spasm	d. Hemostasis
5. _____ Invade platelet plugs to form a stable clot	e. Anticoagulants
6. _____ Is term for sequential steps in hemostatis	f. Cascade

Anticoagulant Agents

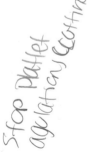

Stop platelet aggregation (clotting)

Anticoagulants are medications used to prolong bleeding time; therefore, they help to prevent harmful clots from forming in the blood vessels. These medications are sometimes called *blood thinners,* although they do not actually thin the blood. Anticoagulants do not dissolve clots that have already formed, but they may prevent the clots from becoming larger and causing more serious problems. They are often used as treatment for certain cardiovascular (CV) and lung conditions, such as MI, venous thrombosis, peripheral arterial **embolus** (an abnormal particle circulating in blood, such as an air bubble or blood clot), and pulmonary emboli. Anticoagulants have been used to prevent transient ischemic attacks and to reduce the risk of recurrent MI. There are two main groups of anticoagulants: (1) drugs that are administered orally and (2) drugs that are administered parenterally. Warfarin (Coumadin) is an example of an oral anticoagulant, and heparin is an anticoagulant only given parenterally. Table 20-1 ■ lists the primary anticoagulants.

Table 20-1 ■ Anticoagulants

GENERIC NAME	TRADE NAME	ADULT DOSE	ROUTE OF ADMINISTRATION
heparin sodium*	Hep-Lock	15,000–20,000 units bid	IV infusion
		5,000–40,000 units/d subcutaneously	Subcutaneous
pentoxifylline	Trental	400 mg tid	PO
warfarin sodium	Coumadin	2–15 mg/d	PO

*For low-molecular-weight heparins, see Table 20-2.

Drugs that dissolve preformed clots (thrombolytic agents, or tissue plasminogen activators [tPAs]), including streptokinase (Streptase, Kabikinase) and urokinase (Abbokinase), are not referred to as anticoagulants.

Focus on Geriatrics

Anticoagulants in Elderly Patients

Older adults are more susceptible to the effects of anticoagulants. Signs of overdose include nosebleeds, blood in stool or urine, excessive bruising, and prolonged bleeding from the gums after brushing or from cutting the face while shaving. Elderly patients, especially, should limit use of alcohol to only 1 drink per day while using anticoagulants.

HEPARIN

Heparin is an anticoagulant and a protein. Two types of heparin are used clinically. The first and older of the two, standard (unfractionated) heparin, is an animal extract (from pork). The second and newer type, called *low-molecular-weight heparin (LMWH),* is derived from unfractionated heparin. The two classes are similar, but not identical, in their actions and pharmacokinetic characteristics. Standard heparin (heparin sodium) is produced by and can be released from mast cells located throughout the body. It is especially abundant in the liver, lung, and intestines.

How does it work?

Heparin, like other anticoagulants, is a drug that increases the length of clotting time and prevents thrombi from forming or growing larger. The anticoagulation action of heparin depends on the inhibition of **thrombi** (blood clots that form within a blood vessel and attach to the site of formation) and clot formation by blocking the conversion of prothrombin to thrombin, and fibrinogen to fibrin, which is the final step in the clotting process. Figure 20-4 ■ shows the mechanisms of action of anticoagulants.

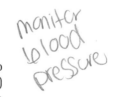

How is it used?

Heparin is prescribed as a treatment for certain CV and lung disorders. It is also used to prevent blood clotting during open-heart surgery, coronary artery bypass graft (CABG) surgery, and dialysis. Heparin is measured on a unit (international unit) rather than milligram basis. The dose must be determined on an individual basis. Heparin is not absorbed after oral administration and therefore must be given parenterally. Intravenous administration results in an almost immediate anticoagulant effect.

What are the adverse effects?

The major adverse effect resulting from heparin therapy is hemorrhage. Bleeding can occur in the urinary or gastrointestinal (GI) tract. Other types of hemorrhages and related conditions that may occur include subdural hematoma (bleeding into the areas below the dura mater, which encases the brain and central nervous system), acute hemorrhagic pancreatitis, hemarthrosis (blood in a joint), and ecchymosis (blood that has pooled in the skin). Additional adverse effects of heparin treatment include hypersensitivity reactions, fever, alopecia, osteoporosis, and ostealgia.

What are the contraindications and interactions?

Absolute contraindications include serious bleeding and intracranial bleeding. Heparin is also contraindicated in severe liver or kidney disease, as well as malignant hypertension. It has not been shown to cause birth defects or bleeding problems in infants. It does not pass into breast milk.

Drugs that inhibit platelet function (for example, aspirin) or produce thrombocytopenia increase the risk of bleeding when heparin is administered. Other drugs that interact with heparin include nonsteroidal anti-inflammatory drugs (NSAIDs), anesthetics, valproic acid, sulfinpyrazone, cefamandole, cefoperazone, cefotetan, plicamycin, methimazole, propylthiouracil, probenecid, and various thrombolytics.

What are the most important points patients should know?

Teach patients how to correctly administer heparin subcutaneously, if they are discharged from the hospital while on heparin. Advise patients to protect themselves from injury (for instance, by using an electric shaver instead of a razor). Warn patients against taking aspirin or other over-the-counter (OTC) medications. Instruct them to notify the health-care provider if urine is pink, red, dark brown, or cloudy; if vomitus is red or dark brown; or if stools are red or black. Also instruct patients to report bleeding gums or oral mucosa; bruising; hematoma; epistaxis; bloody sputum; chest, abdominal, lumbar, or pelvic pain; an unusual increase in menstrual flow; and severe or continuous headache, faintness, or dizziness.

Focus Point

Heparin

Overdosage of heparin can be treated by the administration of a slow infusion of 1% protamine sulfate solution. A dose of 0.5–1 mg of protamine is required to antagonize the action of each 100 unit of heparin.

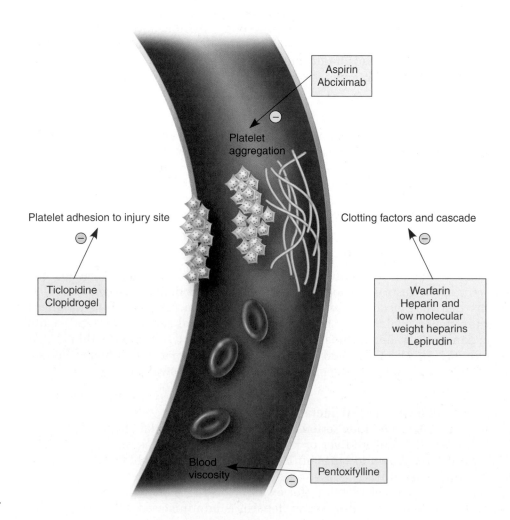

Figure 20-4 ■ Mechanism of action of anticoagulants.

LOW-MOLECULAR-WEIGHT HEPARIN (LMWH)

LMWH is a relatively new class of anticoagulant that has been used in Europe and is now being used more often in the United States.

How do they work?

LMWHs are derived from standard heparin (hence, from pork). Low-molecular-weight fragments have greater bioavailability (the proportion of a drug's dose that is absorbed into the bloodstream) than standard heparin, longer-lasting effect, and dose-independent clearance pharmacokinetics.

How are they used?

LMWHs are more effective than standard heparin in preventing and treating venous **thromboembolism** (blockage of blood vessel by a part of a thrombus that has broken away from its formation site and is circulating in the blood), such as deep venous thrombosis (DVT). The incidence of thrombocytopenia after administration of LMWHs is lower than with standard heparin. They can be given according to body weight once or twice daily without laboratory monitoring. LMWHs are superior for preventing venous thrombosis in patients undergoing hip replacement. They are administered by subcutaneous injection, and they offer the option of treatment on an outpatient basis for patients with DVT. The clinical advantages of LMWHs include predictability, dose-dependent plasma levels, a long half-life, and less bleeding for a given antithrombotic effect. Standard treatment of DVT with IV heparin administered in the hospital offers no advantages over LMWH administered in the outpatient setting.

What are the adverse effects?

Adverse effects like those caused by standard heparin have been seen during therapy with LMWH, and overdose is treated with protamine. The most common LMWHs are shown in Table 20-2 ■.

What are the contraindications and interactions?

Though safer than regular heparin, LWMHs are contraindicated for use in children and in patients with unstable angina, allergy to heparin or pork, active bleeding, and thrombocytopenia. Drug interactions occur with oral anticoagulants, antiplatelets, and thrombolytics.

What are the most important points patients should know?

The points to teach patients who are taking LMWHs are the same as those for regular heparins. See the previous section on patient teaching.

Table 20-2 ■ Common Low-Molecular-Weight Heparins

GENERIC NAME	TRADE NAME	PROPHYLACTIC DOSING	ROUTE OF ADMINISTRATION
ardeparin	Normiflo	50 international units/kg on evening of day of surgery or following morning; then q12h for 14 d or until ambulatory	Subcutaneous
dalteparin	Fragmin	2,500 international units 1–2 h before surgery; then 2,500 international units/d for 5–10 d	Subcutaneous
danaparoid	Orgaran	750 international units 1–4 h before surgery; then 750 units q12h for 7–10 d	Subcutaneous
enoxaparin	Lovenox	30 mg q12h or 40 mg/d for 7–10 d depending on type of surgery; therapy should begin postoperatively	Subcutaneous
tinzaparin	Innohep	175 international units/kg/d	Subcutaneous

Focus Point

Low-Molecular-Weight Heparin

LMWH is associated with less bleeding and fewer episodes of heparin-induced thrombocytopenia than unfractionated heparin.

WARFARIN

Orally effective anticoagulant drugs are fat-soluble derivatives of coumarin or indandione, and they resemble vitamin K. Warfarin (Coumadin) is the oral anticoagulant of choice. It is the most widely used anticoagulant drug because of its potency and reliable bioavailability. It is the fourth most prescribed CV agent and, overall, the eleventh most prescribed drug in the United States, with annual sales of approximately $500 million. The indandione anticoagulants have greater toxicity than the coumarin drugs. Table 20-1 lists the primary anticoagulants.

How does it work?

Warfarin interferes with the hepatic synthesis of vitamin K–dependent clotting factors (factors II [prothrombin], VII, IX, and X), resulting in their eventual depletion and prolongation of clotting times. Warfarin is rapidly and almost completely absorbed after oral administration (its onset of action is from 12 hours to 3 days), and it is bound extensively to plasma proteins. Although these drugs do not cross the blood–brain barrier, they can cross the placenta and may cause teratogenicity (the capability of producing malformations) and hemorrhage in the fetus. Therefore, warfarin carries a strong warning against its use during pregnancy.

How is it used?

Warfarin is used both on an inpatient and outpatient basis when long-term anticoagulant therapy is indicated. Warfarin is administered in conventional doses or mini-doses to reduce bleeding. The dose range is adjusted to provide the desired endpoint. The duration of action of warfarin is 2 to 5 days.

What are the adverse effects?

The major adverse effect of warfarin is hemorrhage that occurs at a predisposing abnormality, such as ulcer or tumor. Prolonged therapy with the coumarin-type anticoagulants is relatively free of untoward effects. Bleeding may occur in the skin, mucous membranes, GI tract, kidneys, brain, liver, uterus, or lungs. However, close monitoring of the degree of anticoagulation is important. Practitioners are advised to keep treatment periods at a minimum to reduce risks. Rare adverse effects include diarrhea, urticaria (eruption of itching hives), alopecia, skin necrosis, and dermatitis.

What are the contraindications and interactions?

Oral anticoagulants are ordinarily contraindicated in the presence of active or past GI ulceration, hepatic or renal disease, malignant hypertension, bacterial endocarditis, chronic alcoholism, and pregnancy. Warfarin is an antagonist of vitamin K, a necessary element in the synthesis of clotting factors II, VII, IX, and X. Drug interactions occur with hepatic enzyme inhibitors, aspirin, NSAIDs, and thrombolytics.

What are the most important points patients should know?

Instruct patients to report signs of bleeding, including blood in urine, red or black tarry stools, vomiting of blood, bleeding with toothbrushing, blue or purple spots on skin or mucous membranes, pinpoint purplish red spots, nosebleed, and bloody sputum. Chest, abdominal, lumbar, and pelvic pain should also be reported. Advise patients to stop the drug immediately if they have signs of hepatitis (dark urine, itchy skin, jaundice, light stools, and abdominal pain) or hypersensitivity reaction. Instruct patients to avoid changing brands of warfarin and to take the same dose of drug at the same time each day. Advise female patients to use a barrier contraceptive to avoid pregnancy. Breastfeeding is not advised.

Focus on Natural Products

Anticoagulants and Natural Products

Dietary or supplemental intake of vitamin K can potentiate or inhibit the actions of oral anticoagulants. The top five leafy green food sources that contain vitamin K are Swiss chard, kale, parsley, brussel sprouts, and spinach. Mineral oil and other laxatives may reduce the absorption of warfarin.

Focus Point

Warfarin

Approximately 5 days are required for the antithrombotic effects of warfarin to occur. It should not be used in patients who must undergo dental procedures.

✳ Apply Your Knowledge 20.2

The following exercises focus on what you have just learned about anticoagulant agents. *See Appendix E for the correct answers.*

FILL IN THE BLANK
Select terms from your reading to fill in the blanks.

1. Anticoagulants _____ bleeding time.

2. Anticoagulants do not _____ clots, but prevent clots from becoming _____.

3. Warfarin is an _____ anticoagulant.

4. Streptokinase and urokinase are _____.

5. _____ is produced by and released from mast cells throughout the body.

6. LMWHs have greater _____ than standard heparins and longer lasting _____.

MULTIPLE CHOICE
Choose the correct answer from choices a–d.

1. Which of the following is a thrombolytic agent?
   a. Heparin
   b. Warfarin
   c. Urokinase
   d. Fibrinogen

2. Standard heparin is also called:
   a. Low-molecular-weight heparin (LMWH)
   b. Unfractionated heparin
   c. Eptifibatide
   d. Ardeparin

3. The trade name of enoxaparin is:
   a. Lovenox
   b. Hep-Lock
   c. Innohep
   d. Coumadin

4. The major adverse effect of heparin therapy is:
   a. Hypertension
   b. Hemorrhage
   c. Fever
   d. Osteoporosis

5. An absolute contraindication for heparin therapy is:
   a. Breastfeeding
   b. Shaving
   c. Infancy
   d. Intracranial bleeding

6. LMWHs are more effective than standard heparins in treating:
   a. DVT
   b. MI
   c. CABG
   d. Dialysis

Antiplatelet Agents

Antiplatelets are medications that help to prevent the formation of blood clots by keeping platelets from binding together, a process called *platelet aggregation*. Unlike the anticoagulants, which are used primarily to prevent thrombosis in veins, antiplatelet drugs are used to prevent clot formation in arteries. Antiplatelet drugs include aspirin, ticlopidine (Ticlid), clopidogrel (Plavix), abciximab (ReoPro), eptifibatide (Integrilin), and tirofiban (Aggrastat) (Table 20-3 ■).

How do they work?

The role platelets play in blood clotting is essential when the body has been cut. Without platelets to stop the bleeding, a person would bleed to death. There are times, however, when blood clotting is harmful. The size and location of blood clots may increase the person's risk of an MI or stroke. Therefore, antiplatelets may be prescribed for patients with heart disease to reduce the likelihood that the platelets will aggregate and form potentially harmful blood clots.

Aspirin in low doses inhibits platelet aggregation and prolongs bleeding time. It remains the first choice in antiplatelet therapy. Aspirin is useful in preventing coronary thrombosis in patients with unstable angina, in serving as an adjunct to thrombolytic therapy, and in reducing recurrence of thrombotic stroke.

Ticlopidine (Ticlid) and clopidogrel (Plavix) are structurally related drugs that irreversibly inhibit platelet activation, leading to inhibition of platelet aggregation. Clopidogrel is preferred to ticlopidine because of its better safety profile and its lack of the serious life-threatening side effects (leukopenia and thrombocytopenia) that can occur with ticlopidine. Clopidogrel is also more potent, is better tolerated, and can be administered as a loading dose.

Abciximab (ReoPro), eptifibatide (Integrilin), and tirofiban (Aggrastat), which interrupt the interaction of fibrinogen with clotting factors, are capable of inhibiting the aggregation of platelets activated by a wide variety of stimuli. Abciximab is used in conjunction with angioplasty and stent procedures, and it is an adjunct to fibrinolytic therapy. Eptifibatide is approved for treatment of acute coronary disease and for use in patients undergoing percutaneous transluminal coronary angioplasty (PTCA), commonly known as *stenting*.

How are they used?

Drugs that inhibit platelet function are administered for the relatively specific prophylaxis of arterial thrombosis and for the prophylaxis or therapeutic management of MI and stroke. The antiplatelet drugs are administered as adjuncts to thrombolytic therapy, along with heparin, to maintain perfusion (blood flow per unit volume of tissue) and to limit the size of MI. Recently, antiplatelet drugs have found new importance in preventing thrombosis in PCTA. Administration of an antiplatelet drug increases the risk of bleeding.

What are the adverse effects?

Antiplatelet agents may be associated with epigastric pain, heartburn, nausea, diarrhea, and major or minor bleeding events. Abciximab may also be associated with cardiac arrhythmias, abnormal thoughts, and dizziness.

What are the contraindications and interactions?

Antiplatelet drugs are generally contraindicated in patients with a history of past gastrointestinal (GI) ulceration, hypertension, asthma, allergies, and nasal polyps. Patients should consult their physicians before taking any other medication (either prescription or OTC), nutritional supplements, or herbal remedies. Some of these substances can interact with antiplatelets. Interactions occur with anticoagulants, platelet aggregation inhibitors, thrombolytic agents, dextran, abciximab, anagrelide, and dipyridamole.

What are the most importants points patients should know?

Instruct patients to report nausea, diarrhea, rash, sore throat, or infection; signs of bleeding; and yellow skin, dark urine, and clay-colored stools. Advise patients to not take aspirin or antacids and to keep appointments for blood tests.

Table 20-3 ■ Antiplatelet Agents

GENERIC NAME	TRADE NAME	ADULT DOSE	ROUTE OF ADMINISTRATION
abciximab	ReoPro	0.25 mg/kg initially over 5 min; then 10 mcg/min for 12 h	IV
aspirin	Bayer and others	80 mg/d–650 mg bid	PO
clopidogrel	Plavix	75 mg/d	PO
dipyridamole	Persantine	75–100 mg qid	PO
eptifibatide	Integrilin	180 mcg/kg initial bolus over 1–2 min; then 2 mcg/kg/min for 24–72 h	IV
ticlopidine	Ticlid	250 mg bid	PO
tirofiban	Aggrastat	0.4 mcg/kg/min for 30 min; then 0.1 mcg/kg/min for 12–24 h	IV

Focus on Natural Products

Garlic as an Anticoagulant

Garlic has long been studied as a natural alternative to antiplatelet drugs because it has been shown to decrease platelet aggregation. Proponents of garlic claim that it can reduce heart disease and incidence of stroke. Garlic is also used by many people to treat colds, coughing, infections, bronchitis, arteriosclerosis, high blood cholesterol levels, and hypertension. It is wise to alert patients that use of garlic concomitantly with anticoagulants may cause bleeding complications.

Focus Point

Antiplatelets During Pregnancy

Taking antiplatelets in the last 2 weeks of pregnancy may cause bleeding problems in the baby, both before and after delivery. When taken in the last 3 months of pregnancy, antiplatelets may prolong the length of the pregnancy and the delivery.

✳ Apply Your Knowledge 20.3

The following exercises focus on what you have just learned about antiplatelet agents. *See Appendix E for the correct answers.*

FILL IN THE BLANK
Select terms from your reading to fill in the blanks.

1. Drugs that inhibit platelet function are administered for the relatively specific prophylaxis of _____.
2. Ticlopidine and clopidogrel are structurally related drugs that irreversibly inhibit _____.
3. Antiplatelet drugs are generally contraindicated in patients with a history of past _____.
4. Aspirin in low doses inhibits platelet aggregation and prolongs _____.
5. The role _____ play in blood clotting is essential when the body has been cut.

(continued)

Apply Your Knowledge 20.3 (continued)

MATCHING

Match the lettered generic drug name to its numbered trade name.

TRADE NAME	GENERIC NAME
1. _____ Ticlid	a. clopidogrel
2. _____ Aggrastat	b. abciximab
3. _____ Integrilin	c. ticlopidine
4. _____ ReoPro	d. tirofiban
5. _____ Plavix	e. eptifibatide

Thrombolytic Agents

Thrombolytic agents (also called *thrombolytics*) are the small group of drugs used to prevent and treat excessive bleeding from surgical sites. There are five thrombolytic drugs available: streptokinase (Streptase, Kabikinase), alteplase (Activase), urokinase (Abbokinase), reteplase (Retavase), and anistreplase (Eminase). These drugs are prescribed in a hospital setting. Table 20-4 ■ lists thrombolytic drugs.

How do they work?

Thrombolytics facilitate conversion of plasminogen to plasmin, which subsequently hydrolyzes fibrin to dissolve blood clots, or thrombi, that have already formed. Thrombolytic agents are plasminogen activators. The ideal thrombolytic drug is one that can be administered intravenously to produce clot-selective fibrinolysis without activating plasminogen to plasmin in plasma. Newer thrombolytic agents bind to fibrin and activate fibrinolysis (breakdown of fibrin) more than fibrinogenolysis (breakdown of fibrinogen).

How are they used?

Thrombolytic drugs are indicated for the management of severe pulmonary embolism, DVT, and arterial thromboembolism; they are especially important for therapy after MI and acute ischemic stroke. Thrombolysis must be accomplished quickly after MI or cerebral infarction because clots become more difficult to dissolve (or lyse) as they age. Adjunctive anticoagulant and antiplatelet drugs may contribute to bleeding during thrombolytic therapy.

What are the adverse effects?

The principal adverse effect associated with thrombolytic therapy is bleeding caused by fibrinogenolysis or fibrinolysis at the site of vascular injury. The incidence of bleeding occurs at a similar rate for all agents. Life-threatening intracranial bleeding may necessitate stopping therapy.

What are the contraindications and interactions?

The contraindications to the use of thrombolytic drugs are similar to those for anticoagulant drugs. Absolute contraindications include active bleeding, pregnancy, lactation, intracranial trauma, vascular disease, and cancer.

Anticoagulants and aspirin can cause interactions with thrombolytics and increase risk of bleeding. Herbs such as feverfew, galling, ginger, and ginkgo may increase risk of bleeding.

What are the most important points patients should know?

Instruct patients to immediately report signs of bleeding (blood in urine, tarry stools, or oozing from cuts) or changes in consciousness to their health-care provider. Advise women to not breast feed while taking urokinase.

Table 20-4 ■ Thrombolytics

GENERIC NAME	TRADE NAME	ADULT DOSE	ROUTE OF ADMINISTRATION
alteplase recombinant	Activase	Begin with 60 mg and then infuse 20 mg/h over next 2 h.	IV
anistreplase	Eminase	30 units over 2–5 min	IV
reteplase recombinant	Retavase	10 units over 2 min; repeat dose in 30 min	IV
streptokinase	Streptase, Kabikinase	250,000–1.5 million units over a short period	IV
urokinase	Abbokinase	4,400–6,000 units administered over several min to 12 h	IV

Focus Point

Thrombocytopenia

Platelet deficiency (thrombocytopenia) is the most common cause of abnormal bleeding. The term *hemophilia* applies to several different hereditary bleeding disorders that result from a lack of any of the factors needed for clotting.

Focus Point

Top 5 Prescribed Anticoagulants

1. warfarin (Coumadin, Panwarfin)
2. clopidogrel (Plavix)
3. ticlopidine (Ticlid)
4. alteplase (Activase)
5. dipyridamole (Persantine)

✳ Apply Your Knowledge 20.4

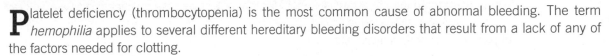

The following exercises focus on what you have just learned about thrombolytic agents. *See Appendix E for the correct answers.*

FILL IN THE BLANK

Select terms from your reading to fill in the blanks.

1. Thrombolytic drugs are used to prevent and treat excessive bleeding from _____.
2. Thrombolytics facilitate conversion of _____ to _____, which subsequently hydrolyzes _____ to dissolve _____ that have already formed.
3. The major adverse effect associated with thrombolytic therapy is _____.
4. Two herbal agents that may interact with thrombolytic drugs are _____ _____.
5. Newer thrombolytic agents bind to fibrin and activate _____ more than _____.
6. For female patients, absolute contraindications to thrombolytic therapy include _____ and _____.
7. Clots are more difficult to _____ as they age.

(continued)

Apply Your Knowledge 20.4 (continued)

MATCHING

Match the following lettered trade name to its numbered generic name.

GENERIC NAME	TRADE NAME
1. _____ reteplase	a. Eminase
2. _____ alteplase	b. Abbokinase
3. _____ urokinase	c. Retavase
4. _____ streptokinase	d. Activase
5. _____ anistreplase	e. Streptase

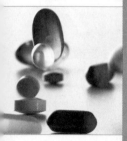

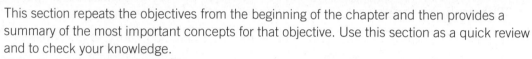

Chapter Capsule

This section repeats the objectives from the beginning of the chapter and then provides a summary of the most important concepts for that objective. Use this section as a quick review and to check your knowledge.

Objective 1: Explain hemostasis.

- Hemostasis encompasses three events that occur in a cascade:
  - ❑ Blood vessel spasm
  - ❑ Formation of platelet plug
  - ❑ Blood clotting

Objective 2: Explain the mechanisms of action of heparin and warfarin.

- Heparin (parenteral anticoagulant)—increases length of clotting time and prevents thrombi from forming or growing larger; action depends on inhibition of thrombus and clot formation by blocking conversion of prothrombin to thrombin, and fibrinogen to fibrin

- Warfarin (oral anticoagulant)—interferes with hepatic synthesis of vitamin K–dependent clotting factors (factors II [prothrombin], VII, IX, and X), resulting in eventual depletion and prolongation of clotting times

Objective 3: Describe the advantages of low-molecular-weight heparin (LMWH).

- Greater bioavailability and longer-lasting effect than standard heparins, and dose-independent clearance pharmacokinetics

Objective 4: Name the class of drugs that can be used to induce bleeding or delay coagulation, and explain individual drug mechanisms of action.

- Antiplatelets:
  - ❑ aspirin (Bayer, and others)—inhibits platelet aggregation and prolongs bleeding time
  - ❑ ticlopidine (Ticlid) and clopidogrel (Plavix)—structurally related to aspirin; irreversibly block platelet activation, leading to inhibition of platelet aggregation
  - ❑ abciximab (ReoPro), eptifibatide (Integrilin), and tirofiban (Aggrastat)—interrupt interaction of fibrinogen with clotting factors and inhibit aggregation of platelets activated by a wide variety of stimuli

Objective 5: Explain the mechanism of action of thrombolytic drugs, and list five drugs in this class.

■ Facilitate conversion of plasminogen to plasmin, which subsequently hydrolyzes fibrin to dissolve blood clots that have already formed; they are plasminogen activators that include:

- ❑ alteplase recombinant (Alteplase)
- ❑ anistreplase (Eminase)
- ❑ reteplase recombinant (Retavase)
- ❑ streptokinase (Streptase, Kabikinase)
- ❑ urokinase (Abbokinase)

 ## Internet Sites of Interest

■ The American Heart Association Web site contains a brief discussion of anticoagulants at: **http://www.americanheart.org/**. Search for "anticoagulants." Additional links to policy statements regarding the use of anticoagulants are available from this site, as is information on coronary heart disease and stroke.

■ HealthCenter Online offers a discussion and illustrations of thrombus formation with patient information on anticoagulants and antiplatelets at: **http://heart.healthcentersonline.com/bloodclot/anticoagulants.cfm**. Considerations for use of these drugs in children, pregnant women, and elderly patients are included. Also available is a list of questions that patients can ask their health-care provider.

■ A discussion of coronary heart disease is available on WebMD at: **http://www.webmd.com/heart-disease/antiplatelet-drugs**. The site offers information on many drug therapies for heart disease, including anticoagulants and antiplatelets. You will also find information on this site about the drug classes that were discussed in Chapter 18.

■ MedicineNet explains DVT and pulmonary embolism at: **http://www.medicinenet.com/**. Search for "DVT" for symptoms, diagnosis, treatment, and lifestyle considerations.

Chapter 21

Effects of Drugs on Fluid and Electrolyte Balance

Chapter Objectives

After completing this chapter, you should be able to:

1. Describe the structure of the nephron and the processes involved in the formation of urine.
2. Explain the processes of urine formation.
3. List the ways that electrolytes are lost from the body.
4. Describe how antidiuretic hormone and aldosterone levels influence the volume and concentration of urine.
5. Explain the indications for use of diuretics in various conditions and disorders of the human body.
6. Classify the five major types of diuretics.
7. Describe the mechanism of action of osmotic diuretics.
8. List the major adverse effects of potassium-sparing diuretics.

Key Terms

Anions (AN-eye-ons) (page 457)

Antidiuretic hormone (ADH) (page 453)

Cations (KAT-eye-ons) (page 457)

Creatinine (kree-AT-tih-neen) (page 450)

Dehydration (dee-hy-DRAY-shun) (page 459)

Diuretics (dy-yoo-REH-tiks) (page 458)

Edema (eh-DEE-muh) (page 458)

Glomerular capsule (glah-MAYR-yoo-lar KAP-sool) (page 450)

Glomerular filtration (page 451)

Glomerulus (glo-MAYR-yoo-lus) (page 450)

Hyperkalemia (hi-per-kah-LEE-mee-uh) (page 464)

Hypokalemia (hi-po-kah-LEE-mee-uh) (page 460)

Hyponatremia (hi-po-nuh-TREE-mee-uh) (page 460)

Loop of Henle (loop of HEN-lee) (page 450)

Nephrons (NEH-fronz) (page 450)

Osmolality (oz-moh-LAL-ih-tee) (page 455)

Renal corpuscle (REE-nul KOR-pus-sul) (page 450)

Renal tubule (REE-nul TOO-byool) (page 450)

Renin (REE-nin) (page 449)

Total body water (page 451)

Tubular reabsorption (TOO-byoo-lar ree-ab-SORP-shun) (page 452)

Tubular secretion (TOO-byoo-lar seh-KREE-shun) (page 452)

Urea (yoo-REE-uh) (page 450)

Uric acid (YOO-rik) (page 450)

Water deficit (page 455)

Water of metabolism (page 455)

PRACTICAL SCENARIO

A middle-aged man who is being treated with hydrochlorothiazide for control of mild edema presents to the physician complaining of malaise, fatigue, muscular weakness, and muscle cramps. In response to the physician's questions about how he is taking his medication, he reports that he takes the medication daily, but it causes constipation. Therefore, he has been taking laxatives. The physician orders an ECG and blood tests to check the patient's levels of creatinine, blood urea nitrogen, uric acid, and electrolytes.

Critical Thinking Questions

1. What do you think might be the result of the man's use of diuretics and laxatives together?
2. Why do you think the physician ordered the ECG and blood tests, and what is he looking for?
3. What blood test results do you expect to find?
4. When providing patient education for this man, what would you tell him?

Introduction

The primary function of the kidneys is to maintain a stable internal environment for optimal cell and tissue metabolism. The kidneys accomplish these life-sustaining tasks by balancing solute and water transport, excreting metabolic waste products, conserving nutrients, and regulating acids and bases. The kidneys also have an endocrine function and secrete the hormones **renin** (a hormone that converts angiotensinogen to angiotensin I), erythropoietin, and vitamin D_3 for regulation of blood pressure, red blood cell (RBC) production, and calcium metabolism, respectively. The formation of urine is achieved through the process of filtration, reabsorption, and secretion by the glomeruli and tubules within the kidneys. The bladder stores the urine that is received from the kidneys by way of the ureters. Urine is then removed from the body through the urethra. Figure 21-1 ■ illustrates the urinary system.

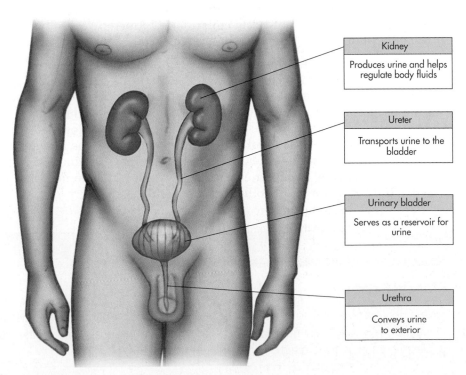

Kidney
Produces urine and helps regulate body fluids

Ureter
Transports urine to the bladder

Urinary bladder
Serves as a reservoir for urine

Urethra
Conveys urine to exterior

Figure 21-1 ■ The urinary system.

Kidney Structure and Functions

The kidneys include two distinct regions: an inner medulla and an outer cortex. The renal *cortex* is the superficial portion of the kidney. The renal *medulla* consists of 6 to 18 distinct triangular structures called *renal pyramids*. The base of each pyramid faces the cortex, and the tip of each pyramid, a region known as the *renal papilla*, projects into the renal sinus. The basic unit of the kidney is the nephron. The main function of the kidneys is to regulate the volume, composition, and pH of body fluids. The kidneys remove metabolic wastes from the blood and excrete them to the outside.

NEPHRONS

Each kidney contains about 1 million functional units called **nephrons**. Nephrons are located in the renal cortex. Each nephron consists of a **renal corpuscle** and a **renal tubule**. A renal corpuscle consists of a filtering unit composed of a cluster of blood capillaries called a **glomerulus** and a surrounding thin-walled, sac-like structure called a **glomerular capsule**. The renal tubule leads away from the glomerular capsule and becomes highly coiled. This coiled portion of the tubule is the *proximal convoluted tubule*. Following the proximal convoluted tubule is the *nephron loop* (**loop of Henle**). The ascending limb of this loop becomes highly coiled again and is called the *distal convoluted tubule*. This portion of the nephron then forms a *collecting duct* (collecting tubule), which is technically not part of the nephron (Figure 21-2 ■).

PRINCIPLES OF RENAL PHYSIOLOGY

The aim of urine production is to maintain homeostasis by regulating the volume and composition of blood. This process involves the excretion of solutes—specifically, metabolic waste products. Three organic waste products are very important: urea, creatinine, and uric acid.

✳ **Urea** is the most abundant organic waste. Each person generates about 21 grams of urea each day, which results in the breakdown of amino acids.

✳ **Creatinine**, a chemical waste molecule, is produced in skeletal muscle tissue by the breakdown of *creatine phosphate*, a high-energy compound that plays an important role in muscle contraction. The body generates roughly 1.8 grams of creatinine each day, and virtually all of it is excreted in urine.

✳ **Uric acid**, another type of waste molecule, is formed by recycling nitrogenous base from RNA molecules. Humans produce approximately 480 mg of uric acid each day.

These waste products are dissolved in the bloodstream and can be eliminated only while dissolved in the bloodstream or urine. As a result, their removal is accompanied by an unavoidable water loss. The kidneys are usually capable of producing more than four times the amount of concentrated urine than plasma. If the kidneys were not able to concentrate the filtrate produced by glomerular filtration, losses of fluid would lead to fatal dehydration in a matter of hours. At the same time, the kidneys ensure that the fluid lost does not contain potentially useful organic substances that are present in blood plasma, such as sugars or amino acids. These valuable materials must be reabsorbed and retained for use by other tissues.

Focus on Geriatrics

Diuresis in Elderly People

Older adults have a decreased ability to concentrate urine and are less able to tolerate dehydration or water loads because they have fewer nephrons. In older adults, drugs eliminated by the kidneys can accumulate in the plasma, causing toxic reactions.

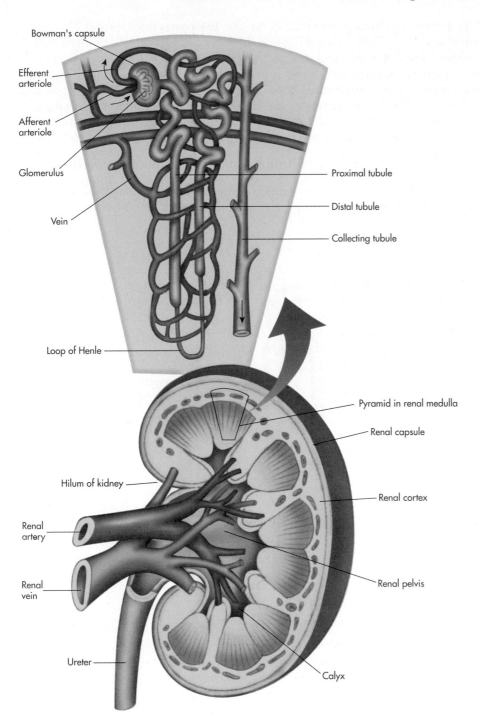

Figure 21-2 ■ The kidney with an expanded view of the nephron.

URINE FORMATION

The main function of the nephrons is to control the composition of the body fluids and remove wastes from the blood. The product is urine, which is excreted from the body. It contains wastes, excess water, and electrolytes.

Urine formation begins with filtration of plasma by the glomerular capillaries, a process called **glomerular filtration**. However, glomerular filtration produces 180 liters of fluid, which is more than four times the amount of **total body water** (total water content of the body), every 24 hours. Glomerular filtration could not continue for very long unless most of this filtered fluid was returned to the internal environment.

The kidneys return filtered fluid to the internal environment through **tubular reabsorption**, selectively reclaiming just the right amounts of substances that the body requires, such as water, electrolytes, and glucose. Waste products and excess substances are processed out of the body. Some substances that the body must eliminate, such as hydrogen ions and certain toxins, are removed even faster than through filtration alone by the process of **tubular secretion** (the cells of the tubules remove certain substances from the blood and deposit them into the fluid in the tubules). In other words, the following relationship determines the volume of substances excreted in the urine:

Urinary excretion = glomerular filtration + tubular secretion − tubular reabsorption

The final product of these processes is urine. The kidneys contribute to homeostasis by maintaining composition of the internal environment (see Figure 21-3 ■).

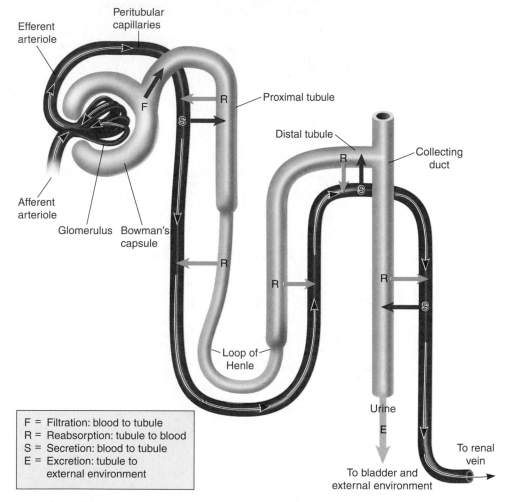

F = Filtration: blood to tubule
R = Reabsorption: tubule to blood
S = Secretion: blood to tubule
E = Excretion: tubule to
    external environment

Figure 21-3 ■ Sites of resorption and secretion in a nephron.

Focus on Pediatrics

Fluid Imbalances in Children

The urine of infants and children is more dilute than that of adults because of pediatric higher blood flow and shorter loops of Henle. Pediatric patients are more affected by fluid imbalances resulting from diarrhea, infection, or improper feeding because their systems have limited ability to quickly regulate changes in pH or osmotic pressure.

CONTROL OF URINE VOLUME

Urine volume is regulated by controlling the reabsorption of water. Water is reabsorbed by osmosis in the proximal convoluted tubule and the descending limb of the loop of Henle, a long, U-shaped part of the *renal tubule* extending through the *medulla* from the end of the *proximal convoluted tubule* to the beginning of the *distal convoluted tubule* (DCT). The ascending limb of the loop of Henle is impermeable to water. The DCT and collecting duct are also impermeable to water, except in the presence of **antidiuretic hormone** (ADH). ADH is a hormone (also called *vasopressin*) that is released from the posterior lobe of the pituitary gland. The higher the circulating levels of ADH, the greater water permeability of these segments of the urinary system. In the absence of ADH, water is not reabsorbed in the DCT or the collecting system. Therefore, large amounts of very dilute urine are produced, which can cause diabetes insipidus. Failure of the posterior pituitary to produce ADH, or hypophysectomy (removal of the pituitary gland), may cause diabetes insipidus.

[handwritten margin note: which hormone controls water reabsorption]

Focus Point

Medications and Urine Retention

Several medications cause urine retention and require careful consideration of use in certain patients. These include:

- Anticholinergic and antispasmodic medications, such as atropine and papaverine
- Antidepressant and antipsychotic agents, such as phenothiazines and monoamine oxidase (MAO) inhibitors
- Antihistamine preparations, such as pseudoephedrine (Sudafed and Actifed)
- Antihypertensives, such as hydralazine (Apresoline) and methyldopa (Aldomet)
- Beta-adrenergic blockers, such as propranolol (Inderal)
- Opioids, such as hydrocodone (Vicodin)

✳ Apply Your Knowledge 21.1

The following questions focus on what you have just learned about urine formation and control of urine volume. *See Appendix E for the correct answers.*

MULTIPLE CHOICE
Choose the correct answer from choices a–d.

1. The majority of nephrons are located in which of the following parts of the kidney?
   a. Pelvis
   b. Cortex
   c. Medulla
   d. Pyramid

2. Which of the following substances is the most abundant organic waste?
   a. Creatinine
   b. Creatine phosphate
   c. Uric acid
   d. Urea

(continued)

Apply Your Knowledge 21.1 (continued)

3. Which of the following hormone insufficiencies may result in diabetes insipidus?
   a. Vasopressin
   b. Aldosterone
   c. Insulin
   d. Prolactin

4. Which of the following is NOT one of the main functions of the kidneys?
   a. To regulate composition of urine
   b. To regulate pH of body fluids
   c. To regulate the volume of body fluids
   d. To control blood sugar

5. Urine formation begins with which of the following processes?
   a. Tubular reabsorption
   b. Tubular secretion
   c. Glomerular filtration
   d. Urinary excretion

FILL IN THE BLANK

Select terms from your reading to fill in the blanks.

1. The three distinct processes involved in the production of urine are _____, _____, and _____.

2. The primary functional unit of the urinary system is the _____.

3. The renal medulla consists of 6 to 18 distinct triangular structures called _____.

4. The distal convoluted tubule is located between the ascending limb of Henle and the _____.

5. Antidiuretic hormone can affect the _____ and _____.

6. When the quantities entering the body equal the quantities leaving it, this is called _____.

7. Approximately 10% of water is a by-product of the oxidative metabolism of nutrients and is called _____.

Fluid and Electrolyte Balance

The term *balance* suggests a state of equilibrium, and in the case of water and electrolytes, it means that the quantities entering the body equal the quantities leaving it. Maintaining such a balance requires mechanisms to ensure that lost water and electrolytes are replaced and that any excesses are excreted. As a result, the levels of water and electrolytes in the body remain relatively stable at all times.

It is important to remember that water balance and electrolyte balance are interdependent because electrolytes are dissolved in the water of body fluids. Consequently, anything that alters the concentrations of the electrolytes alters the concentration of the water by adding solutes to it or by removing solutes from it. Likewise, anything that changes the concentration of the water changes the concentrations of the electrolytes by concentrating or diluting them.

Focus on Pediatrics

Threat of Dehydration in Infants

At birth, total body water (TBW) represents about 75 to 80% of body weight and decreases to about 67% during the first year of life. Infants are particularly susceptible to significant changes in TBW because of a high metabolic rate and greater body surface area. Renal mechanisms of fluid and electrolyte conservation may not be mature enough to counter losses, thereby allowing dehydration to occur.

Focus Point

Water Deficit

Dehydration describes water deficit but also is commonly used to indicate both sodium and water loss. Pure water deficits are rare because most people have access to water. Patients who are comatose or paralyzed have insensible water loss through the skin and lungs, with minimal obligatory formation of urine, and must be monitored closely for water deficit.

WATER BALANCE

Water balance exists when water intake equals water output. Homeostasis requires control of both water intake and water output. Ultimately, maintenance of the internal environment depends on thirst centers in the brain to vary water intake and on the kidneys' ability to vary water output. Water balance is regulated by the secretion of ADH and the perception of thirst. Thirst stimulates water drinking and is experienced when water loss equals 2% of an individual's body weight, or when there is an increase in **osmolality** (concentration of particles in plasma). ADH is secreted when plasma osmolality increases or when circulating blood volume decreases and blood pressure drops. Increased plasma osmolality occurs with **water deficit** (low levels of water in the body) or sodium excess in relation to water.

Focus on Geriatrics

Fluctuating Total Body Water Content in Elderly Patients

The decline in the percentage of total body water (TBW) content in elderly patients results, in part, because of increased body fat and decreased muscle, as well as the kidney's reduced ability to regulate sodium and water balance. Kidneys are less efficient in producing concentrated urine, and sodium-conserving responses are sluggish. With stress, or when disease is present, this normal decrease in TBW can become life threatening.

Water Intake: The volume of water gained each day varies among individuals (Table 21-1 ■). An average adult living in a moderate environment takes in about 2,500 milliliters. Approximately 60% is obtained from drinking water or other beverages, and another 30% comes from moist foods. The remaining 10% is a by-product of the oxidative metabolism of nutrients, which is called **water of metabolism**.

Table 21-1 ■ Normal Water Gains and Losses*

DAILY INTAKE	(mL)	DAILY OUTPUT	(mL)
Drinking	1,400–1,800	Urine	1,400–1,800
Water in food	700–1,000	Stool	100
Water of oxidation	300–400	Skin	300–500
		Lungs	600–800
Total	**2,000–3,200**	**Total**	**2,400–3,200**

*Based on a 70-kg adult man.

Maintaining Fluid and Electrolyte Balance

Remind patients of the following points to promote fluid and electrolyte balance:

- Consume six to eight glasses of water daily.
- Avoid excess amounts of foods or fluids high in salt, sugar, and caffeine.
- Eat a well-balanced diet.
- Limit alcohol intake because it has a diuretic effect.
- Increase fluid intake before, during, and after strenuous exercise.
- Maintain normal body weight.

Water Output: Water normally enters the body only through the mouth, but it can be lost by a variety of routes. These include obvious losses in urine (the largest amount), feces, and sweat, as well as evaporation from the skin and from the lungs during breathing (insensible water loss).

If an average adult takes in 2,500 milliliters of water each day, then 2500 milliliters must be eliminated to maintain water balance. Of this volume, perhaps 60% will be lost in urine, 6% in feces, and 6% in sweat. About 28% will be lost by evaporation from the skin and lungs. These percentages vary with such environmental factors as temperature and relative humidity, or with physical exercise. Therefore, the primary means of regulating water output is control of urine production.

ELECTROLYTE BALANCE

An *electrolyte* is any compound that, in solution, conducts electricity or is decomposed by it. An electrolyte balance exists when the quantities of electrolytes (molecules that release ions in water) gained and lost are equal (Figure 21-4 ■).

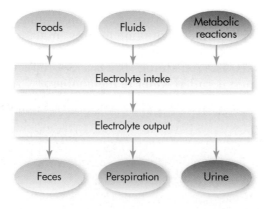

Figure 21-4 ■ Electrolyte balance. Electrolyte intake occurs through ingestion of foods and fluids and through metabolic reactions. Electrolyte output occurs through excretion of feces, sweat, and urine.

Electrolyte Intake: The electrolytes of greatest importance to cellular functions release sodium, potassium, calcium, magnesium, chloride, sulfate, phosphate, bicarbonate, and hydrogen ions. These electrolytes are primarily obtained from foods, but they may also be found in drinking water and other beverages. In addition, some electrolytes are by-products of metabolic reactions.

Electrolyte Output: The body loses some electrolytes by perspiring (sweat has about half the solute concentration of plasma). The quantities of lost electrolytes vary with the amount of perspiration. More electrolytes are lost in sweat on warmer days and during strenuous exercise. Varying amounts of electrolytes are lost in the feces. The greatest electrolyte output occurs because of kidney function and urine production. The kidneys alter renal electrolyte losses to maintain the proper composition of body fluids.

The concentrations of positively charged ions, such as sodium (Na^+), potassium (K^+), and calcium (Ca^{+2}), are particularly important. For example, certain concentrations of these ions are vital for nerve impulse conduction, muscle fiber contraction, and maintenance of cell membrane permeability. Potassium is especially important in maintaining the resting potential of nerve and cardiac muscle cells, and abnormal potassium levels may cause these cells to function abnormally.

Sodium ions account for nearly 90% of the **cations** (positively charged ions) in extracellular fluids. Primarily, the kidneys and the hormone aldosterone regulate these ions. Aldosterone, which the adrenal cortex secretes, increases sodium ion reabsorption in the distal convoluted tubules and collecting ducts of the nephrons. A decrease in sodium ion concentration in the extracellular fluid stimulates aldosterone secretion.

Aldosterone also regulates potassium ions. An important stimulus for aldosterone secretion is a rising potassium ion concentration, which directly stimulates cells of the adrenal cortex. This hormone enhances the renal tubular reabsorption of sodium ions and, at the same time, stimulates renal tubular secretion of potassium ions.

Generally, the regulatory mechanisms that control positively charged ions secondarily control the concentrations of **anions** (negatively charged ions). For example, chloride ions (Cl^-), the most abundant negatively charged ions in the extracellular fluids, are passively reabsorbed from the renal tubules in response to the active reabsorption of sodium ions. That is, the negatively charged chloride ions are electrically attracted to the positively charged sodium ions and accompany them as they are reabsorbed. The main electrolytes in the body are listed in Table 21-2 ■.

Table 21-2 ■ The Main Electrolytes in the Body

CATIONS	IONS	ANIONS	IONS
calcium	Ca^{++}	phosphate	PO^{4-} or HPO^{4-}
magnesium	Mg^{++}	sulfate	SO^{4-}
potassium	K^+	bicarbonate	HCO_3^-
sodium	Na^+	chloride	Cl^-

Focus on Geriatrics

Threats to Fluid and Electrolyte Imbalance in Elderly Patients

Certain changes related to aging cause elderly people to be at higher risk for serious problems with fluid and electrolyte imbalance if homeostatic mechanisms are compromised. Some of these changes include:

- Decreased thirst sensation
- Decreased ability of the kidneys to concentrate urine
- Decreased intracellular fluid and total body water
- Decreased response to body hormones that help regulate fluid and electrolytes
- Increased use of diuretics for hypertension and heart disease
- Decreased fluid and food intake

✳ Apply Your Knowledge 21.2

The following questions focus on what you have just learned about fluid and electrolyte balance. *See Appendix E for the correct answers.*

FILL IN THE BLANK

Select terms from your reading to fill in the blanks.

1. Anything that changes the concentration of body water will change the concentrations of the _____ by concentrating or diluting their levels.

2. An average adult living in a moderate environment takes in about _____ of water.

3. About 60% of water is lost from the human body in _____.

4. The electrolytes of greatest importance to cellular functions include _____, _____, _____, _____, _____, _____, and _____ ions.

5. The positively charged ions in extracellular fluids are called _____.

6. Increased sodium ion reabsorption in the kidneys depends on the hormone _____.

MATCHING

Match the lettered drug class to the numbered description.

DESCRIPTION

1. _____ This group includes mannitol (Osmitrol) and glycerin (Osmoglyn)

2. _____ The drugs of choice in acute pulmonary edema of congestive heart failure

3. _____ Acetazolamide (Diamox) is the best example.

4. _____ The most commonly used diuretic drugs

5. _____ Aldosterone antagonists

DRUG CLASS

a. Loop diuretics

b. Thiazide diuretics

c. Potassium-sparing diuretics

d. Osmotic diuretics

e. Carbonic anhydrase inhibitors

DIURETICS

Diuretics are a group of drugs that promote water loss from the body into the urine. As urine formation takes place in the kidneys, it is not surprising that diuretics have their principal action at the level of the nephrons. Diuretics remove the excess extracellular fluid from the body that can result in **edema** (abnormal fluid accumulation) of the tissues; ascites; and hypertension. These conditions occur in diseases of the heart, kidneys, and liver.

Each human kidney has a million nephrons. More than 120 mL of ultrafiltrate is formed per minute, but only 1 mL of urine is produced. Thus, more than 99% of ultrafiltrate is reabsorbed. Diuretics increase the rate of urine flow. Clinically useful diuretics increase the rate of excretion of sodium (Na^+) and chloride (Cl^-).

NaCl is the major determinant of the extracellular fluid volume; therefore, most clinical applications of diuretics are directed toward reducing extracellular fluid volume by decreasing total body NaCl content. Sustained positive Na^+ balance causes volume overload with pulmonary edema. Sustained negative Na^+ balance causes volume depletion and cardiovascular collapse. There are five major classes of diuretics:

1. Osmotic diuretics
2. Carbonic anhydrase inhibitors

3. Thiazide diuretics
4. Loop diuretics
5. Potassium-sparing diuretics

Focus Point

Contraindications of Diuretics in Pregnancy

Diuretics during pregnancy are not recommended because they may interfere with normal expansion of fluid that occurs during pregnancy and disrupt neurodevelopment of the fetus. Diuretic use increases the fetus's risk of conditions such as schizophrenia, jaundice, blood problems, and potassium depletion. Most diuretics pass into breast milk and can cause dehydration in nursing babies.

Osmotic Diuretics

The capacity of the renal tubule to reabsorb various electrolytes and nonelectrolytes is limited and varies for each ionic species. If large amounts of these substances are administered to an individual, their concentration in the body fluids, and subsequently, in the glomerular filtrate exceeds the reabsorption capacity of the tubules. The excess then appears in the urine, accompanied by an increased volume of water.

Generally, substances that increase urine formation in this manner are called *osmotic diuretics*. This group of diuretics includes osmotic electrolytes (potassium and sodium salts), osmotic nonelectrolytes (urea, glycerin, and mannitol), and acid-forming salts (ammonium chloride) (Table 21-3 ■).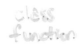

How do they work?
Osmotic agents may have multiple sites of action. Nevertheless, their major component is a decrease in solute content resulting in less water reabsorption from the descending loop of Henle and collecting duct, and less sodium chloride reabsorption in the proximal tubule and ascending limb of Henle.

How are they used?
Osmotic diuretics are highly effective treatments for cerebral edema and are used primarily for this purpose.

What are the adverse effects?
The major adverse effects of osmotic diuretics are related to the amount of solute administered and the effect on the volume and distribution of body fluids. They may cause headache, tremor, convulsions, dizziness, hypotension or hypertension, and thrombophlebitis. They may also produce blurred vision, dry mouth, nausea, vomiting, chills, fever, and allergic reactions.

What are the contraindications and interactions?
Osmotic diuretics are contraindicated in patients with anuria, marked pulmonary congestion or edema, severe congestive heart failure (CHF), metabolic edema, organic CNS disease, intracranial bleeding, shock, severe **dehydration** (excessive loss of body water), history of allergy, pregnancy, and lactation.

What are the important points patients should know?
Advise patients to report thirst, muscle cramps or weakness, paresthesia, dyspnea, or headache and to keep follow-up appointments for lab tests. Instruct female patients to avoid breastfeeding while taking these drugs.

Table 21-3 ■ Osmotic Diuretics

GENERIC NAME	TRADE NAME	AVERAGE ADULT DOSAGE	ROUTE OF ADMINISTRATION
glycerin	Osmoglyn	1–2 g/kg	PO
isosorbide	Ismotic	1–3 mg/kg bid–qid	PO
mannitol	Osmitrol	50–100 g as 10–20% solution over 2–6h	IV for edema or ascites
urea	Ureaphil	1.0–1.5 g/kg/d	IV

Carbonic Anhydrase Inhibitors

Carbonic anhydrase inhibitors stop the conversion of carbon dioxide to carbonic acid and bicarbonate ions. They are generally used to treat glaucoma and epilepsy, and to lessen the effects of high altitudes on the body (Table 21-4 ■).

How do they work?

The enzyme carbonic anhydrase catalyses the conversion of carbon dioxide into bicarbonate ions and vice versa, according to the following equation:

$$CO_2 + H_2O \; H_2CO_3^- \leftrightarrow H_2CO_3 \; H^+ + HCO_3^-$$

This reaction occurs in the kidneys as well as other parts of the body. In the kidneys, the reaction occurs mainly in the proximal tubule, and because it involves bicarbonate loss, it affects acid-base balance. The tubular cells are not very permeable to bicarbonate ions or carbonic acid, but they are very permeable to carbon dioxide. Under normal conditions, carbonic anhydrase in the tubular cell converts the carbonic acid into carbon dioxide and water, which are promptly reabsorbed. If the enzyme is inhibited, there will be a net loss of bicarbonate from the body with a consequent loss of water. The drug acetazolamide (Diamox) is a noncompetitive inhibitor of this enzyme and has been used as a diuretic.

How are they used?

Carbonic anhydrase inhibitors are used in the treatment of absence, generalized tonic-clonic, and focal seizures. They can also be used for reduction of intraocular pressure in glaucoma (see Chapter 27) and to treat acute high-altitude sickness.

What are the adverse effects?

The adverse effects of carbonic anhydrase inhibitors include anorexia, nausea, vomiting, weight loss, dry mouth, thirst, diarrhea, and bone-marrow depression. Other adverse effects are fatigue, dizziness, drowsiness, hyperglycemia, exacerbation of gout, and hepatic dysfunction.

What are the contraindications and interactions?

Carbonic anhydrase inhibitors are contraindicated in patients with hypersensitivity to sulfonamides and derivatives such as thiazides. They should be avoided in marked renal and hepatic dysfunction, Addison's disease or other types of adrenocortical insufficiency, **hyponatremia** (an abnormally low concentration of sodium ions in blood), **hypokalemia** (an abnormally low concentration of potassium ions in blood), or hypochloremic acidosis. Safety during pregnancy and lactation is not established.

Carbonic anhydrase inhibitors should be used cautiously in patients with a history of hypercalciuria, diabetes mellitus, gout, obstructive pulmonary disease, and respiratory acidosis, and in those patients receiving digitalis. Carbonic anhydrase inhibitors such as acetazolamide (Diamox) may cause renal excretion of amphetamines, ephedrine, quinidine, and procainamide. They may decrease the effects of tricyclic antidepressants. Renal excretion of lithium is increased. Excretion of phenobarbital may be increased. Amphotericin B and corticosteroids may accelerate potassium loss.

What are the important points patients should know?
Instruct patients taking carbonic anhydrase inhibitors to avoid driving or operating heavy machinery if drowsiness or dizziness occurs.

Table 21-4 ■ Carbonic Anhydrase Inhibitors

GENERIC NAME	TRADE NAME	AVERAGE ADULT DOSAGE	ROUTE OF ADMINISTRATION
acetazolamide	Diamox Sequels,	250 mg/d 1–4 times/d; 500 mg sustained release bid	PO
	Diamox Parenteral	500 mg, may repeat in 2–4 h	IV, IM
dichlorphenamide	Daramide, Oratrol	100–200 mg followed by 100 mg q12h until desired response is obtained	PO
methazolamide	Neptazane	50–100 mg bid–tid	PO

Focus Point

The Threat of Hypokalemia

Hypokalemia is a potentially life-threatening condition that occurs most often as a side effect of diuretic therapy or prolonged diarrhea. Hypokalemia may be caused by inappropriate or excessive use of drugs such as corticosteroids, penicillin, aminoglycosides, cardiac glycosides, laxatives, and vitamin B_{12} therapy.

Thiazide and Thiazide-Like Diuretics

Thiazides are a group of drugs that are chemically similar. The thiazide-like drugs are chemically dissimilar from the thiazides, but have an identical mode of action. Thiazides are the most commonly used diuretic drugs influencing function of the urinary tract (Table 21-5 ■).

How do they work?
The thiazide diuretics increase urinary excretion of sodium and water by inhibiting sodium reabsorption on the distal convoluted tubules and collecting ducts. They also increase excretion of chloride, potassium, and bicarbonate ions.

How are they used?
The thiazide drugs are commonly used in the treatment of hypertension and can add to the effectiveness of other antihypertensive drugs, reversing fluid retention caused by some of these agents.

Thiazide diuretics are also used as adjunctive therapy in edema associated with CHF, hepatic cirrhosis, and corticosteroids or estrogen therapy, as well as edema due to acute glomerulonephritis, and chronic renal failure.

What are the adverse effects?
The common adverse effects of thiazide diuretics include anorexia, gastric irritation, nausea, vomiting, cramping, diarrhea, constipation, jaundice, hypokalemia, and pancreatitis. Other adverse effects are headache, dizziness, vertigo, leukopenia, aplastic anemia, orthostatic hypotension, fever, respiratory distress, anaphylactic reactions, and hyperglycemia.

All Diuretics cause hypokalemia.

except

Potassium Sparing Diuretics cause hypokalemia

What are the contraindications and interactions?

Thiazide diuretics are contraindicated in patients with diabetes, a history of gout, severe renal disease, and impaired liver function, and in elderly patients. Thiazide diuretics are not recommended for use by nursing mothers. Drug interactions may occur with corticosteroids, lithium, probenecid, and antidiabetic agents.

What are the important points patients should know?

Instruct patients with diabetes to monitor their blood glucose levels with extra care because thiazide, loop, and potassium-sparing diuretics can cause hyperglycemia.

Table 21-5 ■ Thiazides and Thiazide–Like Diuretics

GENERIC NAME	TRADE NAME	AVERAGE ADULT DOSAGE	ROUTE OF ADMINISTRATION
Thiazide Diuretics			
chlorothiazide	Diuril, Duragen	250–500 mg 1–2 times/d	PO
cyclothiazide	Anhydron	2 mg/d	PO
hydrochlorothiazide	HydroDIURIL, Esidrix	12.5–100 mg/d	PO
hydroflumethiazide	Diucardin, Saluron	25–100 mg 1–2 times/d	PO
methyclothiazide	Aquatensen, Enduron	2.5–10 mg/d	PO
polythiazide	Renese	1–4 mg/d	PO
Thiazide–Like Diuretics			
chlorthalidone	Hygroton	50–100 mg/d	PO
indapamide	Lozol	2.5–5 mg/d	PO

Focus on Natural Products

Gossypol and Diuretics

Gossypol (an herbal supplement used as a vaginal spermicide, to induce labor and delivery, and to treat dysmenorrhea), when used concomitantly with diuretics, may result in hypokalemia.

Loop Diuretics

The loop diuretics are sometimes referred to as high-ceiling diuretics. In high doses, loop diuretics can increase urine output astronomically, leading to severe hypovolemia (decreased blood volume) and death (Table 21-6 ■).

How do they work?

Loop diuretics act directly on the loop of Henle in the kidneys to inhibit sodium and chloride reabsorption. Potent diuretics, such as furosemide (Lasix), bumetanide (Bumex), and ethacrynic acid (Edecrin) are not thiazides, but act in a similar way to increase excretion of water, sodium, chloride, and potassium. Their action is more rapid and effective than that of thiazides, with greater diuresis.

How are they used?

The loop diuretics are the drugs of choice in acute pulmonary edema of CHF. Because of their rapid onset of action, the drugs are useful in emergencies such as acute pulmonary edema. They are also useful in treating hypercalcemia because they stimulate tubular calcium ion secretion. Loop diuretics are used in hypertension when other diuretics and other antihypertensives do not result in satisfactory response. In edema of nephrotic syndrome, only loop diuretics are capable of reducing edema.

What are the adverse effects?

The adverse effects of the loop diuretics include abnormalities of fluid and electrolyte balance, hyponatremia, hypotension, circulatory collapse, thromboemboli, and hepatic encephalopathy. They may cause hypokalemia (which may induce cardiac dysrhythmias in patients taking glycosides), and hypocalcemia (which can lead to tetany).

Loop diuretics are toxic to the ear, particularly when used in conjunction with the aminoglycosides (antibiotics). Ethacrynic acid (Edecrin) is the most ototoxic. Irreversible damage may result with continued treatment. Furosemide (Lasix) and ethacrynic acid compete with uric acid for the renal and biliary secretory systems. This results in the blocking of secretions, resulting in hyperuricemia and causing gout attacks. Other adverse effects of loop diuretics may be skin rashes, photosensitivity, hypotension, shock, cardiac arrhythmias, and bone-marrow depression.

What are the contraindications and interactions?

Loop diuretics are contraindicated in patients with hypersensitivity to these drugs. They are not recommended for use in infants or lactating women. They should be avoided in patients with severe diarrhea, dehydration, electrolyte imbalance, or hypotension.

Loop diuretics should be used cautiously in patients with hepatic cirrhosis, diabetes mellitus, pulmonary edema, pregnancy, and a history of gout. They may cause drug interactions with aminoglycosides, anticoagulants, lithium, propranolol, sulfonylureas, nonsteroidal anti-inflammatory drugs (NSAIDs), probenecid, and thiazide diuretics.

What are the important points patients should know?

Instruct patients to follow their physician's order to take diuretic medications early in the morning and not at bedtime. Advise women to avoid this drug when breastfeeding.

Table 21-6 ■ Loop Diuretics

GENERIC NAME	TRADE NAME	AVERAGE ADULT DOSAGE	ROUTE OF ADMINISTRATION
bumetanide	Bumex	0.5–2 mg/d	PO
		0.5–1 mg over 1–2 min, repeated q2–3h PRN (max: 10 mg/d)	IV, IM
ethacrynic acid	Edecrin	50–100 mg 1–2 times/day (max: 400 mg/d)	PO
		0.5–1 mg/kg	IV
furosemide	Lasix	20–80 mg/d in 1 or more divided doses (max: 600 mg/d)	PO
		20–40 mg in 1 or more divided doses up to 600 mg/d	IM, IV
torsemide	Demadex	4–20 mg/d	PO, IV

Potassium-Sparing Diuretics

The potassium-sparing diuretics include spironolactone (Aldactone), triamterene (Dyrenium), and amiloride (Midamor). The potassium-sparing diuretics are able to produce a mild diuresis without affecting blood potassium levels. The effects of these agents on urine electrolyte composition are similar in that they decrease potassium and hydrogen ion excretion. Despite this similarity, these agents actually compose two groups with respect to mechanism of action. Spironolactone, the prototype agent of the aldosterone antagonists, is a specific competitive inhibitor of aldosterone at the receptor site level; hence, it is effective only when aldosterone is present. The other two potassium-sparing diuretics, triamterene and amiloride, exert their effects independently of the presence or absence of aldosterone (Table 21-7 ■).

How do they work?

Spironolactone (Aldactone) is a synthetic aldosterone antagonist that competes with aldosterone for intracellular cytoplasmic receptor sites. The spironolactone receptor complex cannot translocate into the nucleus of the target cell. Therefore, this prevents sodium reabsorption in the distal tubule.

How are they used?

The potassium-sparing agents are used in the treatment of edema associated with CHF, hepatic cirrhosis with ascites, and the nephrotic syndrome. Because these diuretics have little antihypertensive action of their own, they are used mainly in combination with other drugs in the management of hypertension and to correct hypokalemia often caused by other diuretic agents. Spironolactone also is used in primary hyperaldosteronism.

What are the adverse effects?

Potassium-sparing diuretics may cause life-threatening **hyperkalemia** (an abnormally high amount of potassium ions in blood). The main adverse effects of these agents include hyperkalemia, acute renal failure, and kidney stones. Because spironolactone chemically resembles some of the sex steroids, it has minimal hormonal activity and may cause gynecomastia (development of mammary glands) in men and menstrual irregularities in women. At low doses, spironolactone can be used chronically with few adverse effects. Potassium-sparing diuretics may cause nausea, lethargy, headache, and mental confusion.

What are the contraindications and interactions?

Potassium-sparing diuretics are contraindicated in patients with anuria, acute renal insufficiency, impaired renal function, or hyperkalemia. They should be used cautiously in patients with cirrhosis of the liver or who are pregnant or lactating. Potassium supplements, NSAIDs, and lithium may interact with potassium-sparing diuretics.

What are the important points patients should know?

Teach patients taking potassium-sparing diuretics about the symptoms of hypokalemia, such as muscle cramps and weakness, lethargy, anorexia, irregular pulse, and confusion. Instruct them about the symptoms of hyperkalemia, such as thirst, dry mouth, and drowsiness. Caution patients to maintain normal potassium levels while on combination digoxin and diuretic therapy.

Table 21-7 ■ Potassium-Sparing Diuretics

GENERIC NAME	TRADE NAME	AVERAGE ADULT DOSAGE	ROUTE OF ADMINISTRATION
amiloride	Midamor	5–20 mg/d	PO
spironolactone	Aldactone	Up to 400 mg/d	PO
triamterene	Dyrenium	Up to 300 mg/d	PO

✳ Apply Your Knowledge 21.3

These questions focus on what you have just learned about diuretics and their effects on fluid and electrolyte balance. *See Appendix E for the correct answers.*

MULTIPLE CHOICE

Choose the correct answer from choices a–d.

1. Which class of diuretics is sometimes referred to as high-ceiling diuretics?

    a. Osmotic diuretics

    b. Carbonic anhydrase inhibitors

    c. Loop diuretics

    d. Thiazide diuretics

2. Which of the following is the trade name of acetazolamide?

    a. Mannitol

    b. Diamox

    c. Lasix

    d. Bumex

3. Which class of diuretics may cause gynecomastia?

    a. Potassium-sparing diuretics

    b. Loop diuretics

    c. Osmotic diuretics

    d. Carbonic anhydrase inhibitors

4. Which class of diuretics can be used for reduction of intraocular pressure in glaucoma?

    a. Loop diuretics

    b. Osmotic diuretics

    c. Thiazide and thiazide-like diuretics

    d. Carbonic anhydrase inhibitors

5. Which of the following loop diuretics is the most ototoxic?

    a. Edecrin

    b. Lasix

    c. Demadex

    d. Bumex

6. Which class of diuretics is most useful in treating cerebral edema?

    a. Osmotic

    b. Loop

    c. Thiazide

    d. Carbonic anhydrase inhibitors

(*continued*)

Apply Your Knowledge 21.3 (continued)

7. Which class of diuretics may cause life-threatening hyperkalemia if the dose is too high?

   a. Osmotic

   b. Thiazide

   c. Loop

   d. Potassium-sparing

8. Which class of diuretics is most likely to cause severe hypovolemia and death if given in high doses?

   a. Osmotic

   b. Thiazide

   c. Loop

   d. Potassium-sparing

MATCHING

Match the lettered trade name to the numbered generic name.

GENERIC NAME	TRADE NAME
1. _____ glycerin	a. Diuril
2. _____ mannitol	b. Osmitrol
3. _____ methazolamide	c. Lozol
4. _____ chlorothiazide	d. Lasix
5. _____ indapamide	e. Neptazane
6. _____ furosemide	f. Aldactone
7. _____ spironolactone	g. Osmoglyn

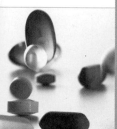

Chapter Capsule

This section repeats the objectives from the beginning of the chapter and then provides a summary of the most important concepts for that objective. Use this section as a quick review and to check your knowledge.

Objective 1: Describe the structure of the nephron and the processes involved in the formation of urine.

- Nephrons—consist of a renal corpuscle and renal tubule

  - The renal corpuscle has a filtering unit composed of a cluster of blood capillaries called a *glomerulus*, and a surrounding thin-walled, sac-like structure called a *glomerular capsule*

  - The renal tubule leads away from the glomerular capsule and becomes highly coiled (the proximal convoluted tubule)

  - Next is the loop of Henle, the ascending limb of which becomes highly coiled again (the distal convoluted tubule), forming a collecting duct (tubule)

  - Urinary excretion = glomerular filtration + tubular secretion − tubular reabsorption

Objective 2: Explain the processes of urine formation.

■ Urine formation—maintains homeostasis by regulating the volume and composition of blood

■ Involves excretion of solutes (specifically, metabolic waste products) such as urea, creatinine, and uric acid

■ Valuable materials, such as sugars or amino acids, are reabsorbed and retained for use by other tissues

Objective 3: List the ways that electrolytes are lost from the body.

■ Sweat, feces, urine

Objective 4: Describe how antidiuretic hormone and aldosterone levels influence the volume and concentration of urine.

■ ADH—controls water permeability; when absent, water is not reabsorbed in the DCT and the collecting system, producing large amounts of very dilute urine, which can cause diabetes insipidus

■ Aldosterone—increases sodium ion reabsorption in the distal convoluted tubules and collecting ducts of the nephrons

Objective 5: Explain the indications for use of diuretics in various conditions and disorders of the human body.

■ Diuretics are indicated for edema (cerebral, acute pulmonary edema of CHF), hepatic cirrhosis with or without ascites; use with corticosteroids or estrogen therapies; acute glomerulonephritis, hypercalcemia, nephrotic syndrome, and chronic renal failure); various seizures; for reduction of intraocular pressure in glaucoma; acute high-altitude sickness; and hypertension (including the reversal of fluid retention caused by some antihypertensive drugs)

Objective 6: Classify the five major types of diuretics.

■ Osmotic diuretics—affect the capacity of the renal tubule to reabsorb electrolytes and nonelectrolytes

■ Carbonic anhydrase inhibitors—stop conversion of carbon dioxide to carbonic acid and bicarbonate ions

■ Thiazide and thiazide-like diuretics—inhibit sodium reabsorption on distal convoluted tubules and collecting ducts

■ Loop diuretics—work on the loop of Henle to inhibit sodium and chloride reabsorption

■ Potassium-sparing diuretics—decrease potassium and hydrogen ion excretion

Objective 7: Describe the mechanism of action of osmotic diuretics.

■ Decrease solute content, resulting in less water reabsorption from the descending loop of Henle and collecting duct, and less sodium chloride reabsorption in the proximal tubule and ascending loop of Henle

Objective 8: List the major adverse effects of potassium-sparing diuretics.

■ Hyperkalemia, acute renal failure, and kidney stones

Internet Sites of Interest

- Answers to your questions about diuretics can be found at the HeartCenter Online at: **http://heart.healthcentersonline.com**. Search for "diuretics."

- A description of kidneys and how they work can be found on the National Kidney and Urologic Diseases (a service of National Institute of Diabetes and Digestive and Kidney Diseases [NIDDK]) Web site at: **http://kidney.niddk.nih.gov**. Search for "your kidneys."

- Medical tests to determine kidney function are explained on the NIDDK site at: **http://kidney.niddk.nih.gov**. Search for "medical tests kidneys."

Chapter Objectives

After completing this chapter, you should be able to:

1. Describe the main functions of a hormone.
2. Explain the endocrine functions of the hypothalamus.
3. List six types of hormones that are secreted from the anterior pituitary gland.
4. Describe the role of the thyroid gland and its replacement and antithyroid drugs.
5. Explain the pharmacotherapy of diabetes insipidus.
6. Identify the role of hypoglycemic medications in treating diabetes mellitus.
7. Describe the adverse effects of insulin and corticosteroids.
8. Identify the two major classes of steroids.

Chapter 22

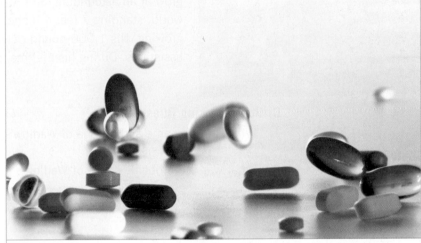

Effects of Drugs on the Endocrine System

Key Terms

Acromegaly (ak-roh-MEHG-uh-lee) (page 473)

Addison's disease (ADD-iss-uns) (page 477)

Adenohypophysis (ADD-eh-no-hy-PO-fih-sis) (page 472)

Cretinism (KREE-ten-izm) (page 476)

Cushing's disease (KUSH-ings) (page 473)

Cushing's syndrome (page 473)

Diabetes insipidus (dy-uh-BEE-tees in-SIP-uh-dus) (page 474)

Diabetes mellitus (dy-uh-BEE-tees MEL-uh-tiss) (page 482)

Dwarfism (DWARF-izm) (page 473)

Gestational diabetes mellitus (jeh-STAY-shuh-nul) (page 483)

Gigantism (jy-GANT-izm) (page 473)

Glucagon (GLOO-kuh-gon) (page 482)

Graves' disease (page 473)

Hyperglycemia (hi-per-GLI-seem-ee-uh) (page 484)

Hyperthyroidism (hy-per-THY-royd-izm) (page 476)

Hypoglycemia (hy-po-gli-SEE-mee-uh) (page 485)

Hypoparathyroidism (hy-po-par-uh-THY-royd-izm) (page 480)

Hypopituitarism (hy-po-pih-TOO-ih-tair-izm) (page 472)

Hypothyroidism (hi-po-THIE-royd-izm) (page 479)

Iatrogenic (eye-a-troh-JEH-nik) (page 494)

Islets of Langerhans (EYE-lits of LANG-ur-hans) (page 470)

Lithium (LITH-ee-um) (page 478)

Myxedema (mix-uh-DEEM-uh) (page 476)

Neurohypophysis (noor-oh-hy-PO-fih-sis) (page 472)

Oxytocin (awk-see-TOH-sin) (page 474)

Parafollicular cells (par-uh-fo-LIK-u-lur) (page 475)

Thyrotoxicosis (thy-ro-toks-ih-KOH-sis) (page 476)

Vasopressin (vaz-oh-PRESS-in) (page 474)

PRACTICAL SCENARIO

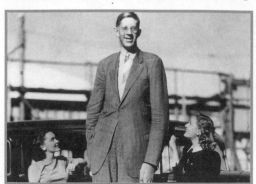

Perhaps the greatest example of an endocrine system run amuck was the case of Robert Wadlow (b. 2/22/1918, d. 7/15/1940), who attained the height of 8 feet 11.1 inches and a weight of 490 pounds. Though normal at birth, by 6 months of age he weighed 30 pounds, and continued to grow at an astounding rate. At age 13, he was the tallest Boy Scout in the world, standing 7 feet 4 inches high. At his death at age 22, he was still growing. His 1,000-pound casket required twelve pallbearers and eight assistants. During his lifetime, his condition was untreatable.

Critical Thinking Questions

1. What are the name and criteria of Wadlow's condition, and what part of the endocrine system was responsible for it?
2. What was the probable cause of Wadlow's condition?
3. How would physicians treat such a problem today?

Introduction

Hormones are chemical substances secreted directly into the blood by endocrine glands, generally in response to a change in the internal condition of the body and with the goal of maintaining homeostasis. This chapter focuses on hormones that regulate growth, blood glucose, and intermediary metabolism. The synthesis and secretion of many hormones are controlled by other hormones or changes in the concentration of essential chemicals or electrolytes in the blood. The interrelationships among the peptide hormones of the hypothalamus, the trophic hormones of the anterior pituitary, and other endocrine glands are examples of elegant feedback regulation, both positive feedback, in which one hormone stimulates the secretion of another, or negative feedback, in which one hormone turns off the action of the previous hormone. Drugs and diseases can modify hormone secretion, as well as specific hormone effects at target organs.

Pharmacologic preparations are used to detect and treat disorders involving any of the following glands: pituitary, thyroid, adrenal cortex, pancreas, or gonads. The effects of these drugs are derived from the physiological actions of the endogenous hormones that they stimulate, if they are activators (agonists), or block, if they are antagonists.

Endocrine System

The endocrine system secretes hormones that control the body by maintaining its internal environment within certain narrow ranges, which is known as *homeostasis*. The maintenance of homeostasis involves growth, maturation, reproduction, metabolism, and human behavior. Responsibility for homeostasis is shared by both the endocrine system and the nervous system, working in tandem in a unique partnership. The hypothalamus of the brain (a part of the nervous system) sends directions via chemical signals (the releasing of hormones) to the pituitary gland (a part of the endocrine system). It also controls the release of corticotropin-releasing hormone (CRH), growth hormone–releasing hormone (GHRH), gonadotropin-releasing hormone (GnRH), thyrotropin-releasing hormone (TRH), and anterior–pituitary hormones. The pituitary stimulates the other endocrine glands to secrete their hormones. The endocrine glands include the pituitary gland, the pineal gland, the thyroid gland, the parathyroid glands, the thymus gland, the adrenal glands, the **islets of Langerhans**

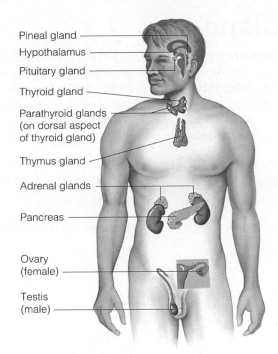
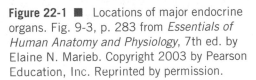

Figure 22-1 ■ Locations of major endocrine organs. Fig. 9-3, p. 283 from *Essentials of Human Anatomy and Physiology*, 7th ed. by Elaine N. Marieb. Copyright 2003 by Pearson Education, Inc. Reprinted by permission.

(small clusters of cells within the pancreas), the ovaries in women, and the testes in men (see Figure 22-1 ■). The ovarian and testicular hormones will be discussed in Chapter 23. Hormone secretion is precisely regulated by the hypothalamus, the anterior pituitary gland, and other groups of glands that respond to the hypothalamus and pituitary glands (see Figure 22-2 ■).

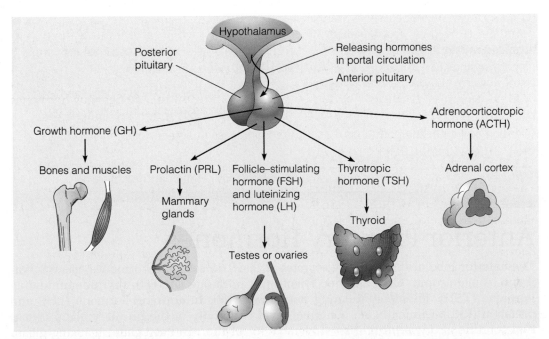

Figure 22-2 ■ Anterior pituitary hormones and their target organs. Fig. 9-4, p. 284 from *Essentials of Human Anatomy and Physiology*, 7th ed. by Elaine N. Marieb. Copyright 2003 by Pearson Education, Inc. Reprinted by permission.

Pituitary Gland

The pituitary gland, sometimes called the *master gland* because of its regulatory effects on the other endocrine glands, consists of an anterior lobe (**adenohypophysis**) and a posterior lobe (**neurohypophysis**) that are under the influence of hypothalamic hormones. The hypothalamic hormones control the secretion of specific trophic hormones; they in turn regulate other endocrine gland secretions and target tissues. Table 22-1 ■ lists the pituitary and other endocrine glands and their functions.

Table 22-1 ■ Endocrine Glands and Their Functions

GLAND	HORMONE	MAJOR FUNCTIONS
Anterior pituitary	Adrenocorticotropic hormone (ACTH)	Stimulates adrenal cortex to produce cortisol
	Follicle-stimulating hormone (FSH)	Stimulates follicular growth, secretion of estrogen, growth of testes; promotes development of sperm cells
	Growth hormone (GH)	Promotes growth of soft tissue and bone
	Luteinizing hormone (LH); in men, this is called *interstitial cell-stimulating hormone* (ICSH)	Causes development of corpus luteum at site of a ruptured ovarian follicle in women; also can stimulate secretion of testosterone in men
	Prolactin	Promotes breast development in women and stimulates milk secretion
	Thyroid-stimulating hormone (TSH)	Stimulates thyroid gland to produce thyroid hormones (T3 and T4)
Posterior pituitary (hormone storage site)	Oxytocin	Increases contractility of uterus and causes milk ejection postpartum
	Vasopressin (antidiuretic hormone)	Increases reabsorption of water in kidney tubules, and stimulates smooth muscle tissue in blood vessels to constrict
Thyroid	Calcitonin	Decreases plasma calcium concentrations
	Thyroid hormone (thyroxine [T4] and triiodothyronine [T3])	Increase metabolic rate; are essential for normal growth and nerve development
Parathyroid	Parathyroid hormone	Regulates exchange of calcium between blood and bones; increases calcium level in blood
Hypothalamus	Releasing and inhibiting hormones (CRH, GHRH, GnRH, TRH)	Control release of anterior pituitary hormones
Thymus	Thymosin	Enhances proliferation and function of T lymphocytes

Anterior Pituitary Hormones

The anterior lobe of the pituitary secretes at least six separate hormones: growth hormone (somatotropin, GH), adrenocorticotropin hormone (ACTH), thyroid-stimulating hormone (TSH), follicle-stimulating hormone (FSH), luteinizing hormone (LH), and prolactin (PRL). Clinically, an abnormal level of activity of the pituitary gland causes two conditions: *hyperpituitarism*—overactivity of the pituitary gland (causing gigantism or acromegaly)—and **hypopituitarism**—underactivity of the pituitary gland (causing dwarfism). The relationships between hypothalamic hormones, pituitary hormones, and target organs are shown in Table 22-2 ■.

Table 22-2 ■ Relationships Among Hypothalamic, Anterior Pituitary, and Target Organ Hormones

HYPOTHALAMIC HORMONE	PITUITARY HORMONE	TARGET ORGAN (HORMONE PRODUCT)
Stimulatory hormones		
CRH	ACTH	Adrenal cortex (glucocorticoids, mineralocorticoids, androgens)
GHRH	Somatotropin, GH	Liver (somatomedins)
GnRH	FSH, LH	Gonads (estrogen, progesterone, testosterone)
TRH	TSH	Thyroid (thyroxine)
Inhibitory hormones		
Dopamine	Prolactin (Prl)	Breast (none)
Somatostatin	GH	Liver (IGF)
		Pancreas (insulin)

GROWTH HORMONE

Growth hormone (GH, somatotropin) causes an increase in the weight and length of the body. The increase in length is especially prominent, due to bone growth, but its effect is manifested in nearly all of the tissues of the body. Excessive secretion of growth hormone before puberty, usually the result of a tumor of the anterior pituitary, causes gigantism (a condition in which the entire body or any of its parts is abnormally large). If excessive production of growth hormone occurs after puberty, it can result in acromegaly (a disorder in which the extremities, such as the hands, feet, and head, are greatly enlarged). Growth hormone insufficiency during childhood causes dwarfism (a condition in which the body is abnormally undersized).

THYROID-STIMULATING HORMONE

Thyroid-stimulating hormone (TSH), another hormone of the anterior lobe of the pituitary gland, controls the secretion of thyroid hormone, and is important for the growth and function of the thyroid gland. TSH stimulates the thyroid gland to increase the uptake of iodine and increase the synthesis and release of thyroid hormones.

In the absence of TSH, the thyroid gland atrophies, producing only small amounts of thyroid hormone, which can have numerous multisystem negative effects on the body. An excess of TSH causes hypertrophy and hyperplasia of the thyroid, and a severe form of hyperthyroidism called **Graves' disease** (an overactive thyroid condition characterized by numerous eye problems).

ADRENOCORTICOTROPIC HORMONE

Adrenocorticotropic hormone (ACTH) is released by the anterior lobe of the pituitary gland and by the placenta during pregnancy. It stimulates the growth of the adrenal gland cortex and the secretion of corticosteroids. Hypersecretion of ACTH can cause **Cushing's syndrome** (a condition that affects the trunk of the body, in which a pad of fat develops between the shoulders, producing a "buffalo hump," and the face becomes round and moon-shaped). Cushing's syndrome is called **Cushing's disease** when it is caused by a tumor in the pituitary gland.

GONADOTROPIC HORMONES

The gonadotropic hormones include follicle-stimulating hormone (FSH) and luteinizing hormone (LH), which are produced by gonadotroph cells in the anterior pituitary. These two hormones affect the target gonadal tissue in both men and women.

The principal function of FSH is to stimulate gametogenesis and follicular development in women, and spermatogenesis in men. LH is primarily responsible for regulation of gonadal steroid hormone production.

PROLACTIN

Prolactin (Prl) is a hormone with many different actions. By itself, prolactin does not cause breast development, but in concert with estrogens, progesterone, hydrocortisone, and insulin, it is mammotropic. In humans, it also stimulates milk secretion by the mammary glands. Other effects in humans include increase in testicular steroidogenesis and development of the male accessory sex organs. It is also involved in the regulation of gonadotropin release. Prolactin deficiency is associated with disorders of the hypothalamus or pituitary gland.

Posterior Pituitary Hormones

The posterior pituitary gland is also called the *neurohypophysis* and contains two peptide hormones, **vasopressin** and **oxytocin**. Neither is made in the posterior pituitary; rather, they are synthesized in neurons in the hypothalamus.

VASOPRESSIN

Vasopressin is also called *antidiuretic hormone* (*ADH*), which stimulates water reabsorption from the nephrons (collecting ducts) of the kidneys back into the bloodstream. It plays a significant role in concentrating urine in order to conserve water. When there is a defect in the hypothalamic–pituitary secretion of ADH, **diabetes insipidus** (chronic increased thirst and urination due to damage of the hypothalamus) results in a water diuresis. Vasopressin is used mainly for its antidiuretic effects in this disease rather than for its vasoconstrictor actions, from which the name vasopressin is derived.

OXYTOCIN

Oxytocin stimulates the contraction of smooth muscle in the uterus and alveoli of the lactating breast. The hormone enhances uterine contractions during labor and stimulates the release of milk during breastfeeding.

✳ Apply Your Knowledge 22.1

The following questions focus on what you have just learned about the endocrine system and the pituitary gland. *See Appendix E for the correct answers.*

MATCHING
Match the lettered term to the numbered description.

DESCRIPTION

1. _____ Also called "antidiuretic hormone"
2. _____ A mammotropic hormone
3. _____ Stimulates the growth of the adrenal cortex
4. _____ In excess causes a clinical picture resembling Graves' disease
5. _____ Stimulates gametogenesis
6. _____ Insufficiency of this hormone during childhood causes dwarfism
7. _____ Enhances uterine contractions
8. _____ Regulates gonadal steroids

TERM

a. Thyroid-stimulating hormone (TSH)
b. Growth hormone (GH)
c. Luteinizing hormone (LH)
d. Prolactin (Prl)
e. Adrenocorticotropic hormone (ACTH)
f. Oxytocin
g. Follicle-stimulating hormone (FSH)
h. Vasopressin

MULTIPLE CHOICE

Select the correct answers from choices a–d.

1. The anterior lobe of the pituitary secretes at least six separate hormones. Which of the following is not secreted by the pituitary gland?

    a. Thyroid-stimulating hormone (TSH)

    b. Adrenocorticotropic hormone (ACTH)

    c. Follicle-stimulating hormone (FSH)

    d. Corticotropin releasing factor (CRF)

2. Excessive production of growth hormone can result in:

    a. Acromegaly

    b. Graves' disease

    c. Addison's disease

    d. Cushing's syndrome

3. An excess of thyroid-stimulating hormone (TSH) can cause:

    a. Gigantism

    b. Cretinism

    c. Grave's disease

    d. Cushing's disease

4. Lack of the peptide hormone vasopressin can result in:

    a. Diabetes mellitus

    b. Cushing's syndrome

    c. Diabetes insipidus

    d. Addison's disease

5. Hypopituitarism can cause:

    a. Cretinism

    b. Dwarfism

    c. Acromegaly

    d. Chronic increased thirst and urination

Thyroid Gland

The thyroid gland lies in the neck, just below the larynx and in front of the trachea. It plays a vital role in regulating the body's metabolic processes.

THYROID HORMONES

Thyroid hormone is secreted from follicular cells in the thyroid gland and includes two different hormones: thyroxine (tetraiodothyronine, or T4) and triiodothyronine (T3). Iodine is vital for the synthesis of these hormones and is provided through the dietary intake of common iodized salt. Another hormone releases from **parafollicular**

cells in the thyroid gland, calcitonin, which is involved with calcium homeostasis. Calcitonin inhibits bone reabsorption and the release of calcium ions into the blood, while promoting the uptake of these ions back into bone. Its effects on blood calcium levels are rapid but short acting.

Focus on Geriatrics

Myxedema Coma

Myxedema coma is a medical emergency that is indicated by a diminished level of consciousness associated with severe hypothyroidism. Symptoms include hypothermia without shivering, hypoventilation, hypotension, and hypoglycemia. Older patients with severe vascular disease and moderate or untreated hypothyroidism are particularly at risk. Myxedema coma can be caused by overuse of narcotics or sedatives or, in hypothyroid patients, by an acute illness.

In the absence of the thyroid gland, and thus thyroid hormones, the basal metabolic rate is less than half its normal rate, and growth and development are impaired. In the presence of a hyperactive gland, the metabolic rate is much higher than normal, resulting in tachycardia, nervousness, and other symptoms. An enlargement of the thyroid gland is called a *goiter*. Simple (nontoxic) goiter results from a shortage of iodine in the diet. A goiter also can be caused by constant stimulation of an underactive or nonfunctioning thyroid to release more hormones.

The two most common thyroid disorders are Graves' disease and Hashimoto's thyroiditis of the immune system, an autoimmune disease that attacks the thyroid gland causing hypothyroidism. Graves' disease, an autoimmune disease in which antibodies overstimulate the thyroid gland, is characterized by **hyperthyroidism** (overactive thyroid), usually associated with an enlarged thyroid gland and exophthalmos (protrusion of the eyeballs). Graves' disease is also known as **thyrotoxicosis**.

Deficiency of thyroid hormones (hypothyroidism) during infancy causes **cretinism**, resulting in dwarfism and severe mental retardation. **Myxedema** is the most severe hypothyroidism, developing in the older child or adult. It is characterized by swelling of the hands, feet, and face (especially around the eyes) and can lead to coma and death. In older adults, severe hypothyroidism can cause myxedema coma.

Focus on Pediatrics

Thyroid Hormone Essential to Fetal Development

Congenital hypothyroidism is the absence of thyroid tissue during fetal development, or due to defects in hormone synthesis. Absence of the thyroid occurs more often in female infants, with permanent abnormalities in 1 of every 4,000 live births. Because thyroid hormone is essential for embryonic growth, particularly of brain tissue, the infant will be mentally retarded if there is no thyroxine during fetal life.

Antithyroid Drugs

Disorders of the thyroid gland are quite common, and treatment of these conditions indicates drug therapy. In the case of hyperthyroidism, a number of organic compounds inhibit the production of thyroid hormone by the thyroid gland. Iodine drugs, such as potassium iodide, radioactive iodine, and thioamide derivatives, are the drugs of choice for antithyroid therapy (see Table 22-3 ■) and are discussed here.

Table 22-3 ■ Common Thyroid and Antithyroid Agents

GENERIC NAME	TRADE NAME	AVERAGE ADULT DOSAGE	ROUTE OF ADMINISTRATION
Thyroid agents			
levothyroxine	Synthroid, Levothroid, Levoxyl	100–400 mcg/d	PO (Synthroid IV available)
liothyronine	Cytomel	25–75 mcg/d	PO
thyroid	Thyroid, Thyrar	60–180 mg/d	PO
Antithyroid agents			
methimazole	Tapazole	5–15 mg/d	PO
potassium iodide	Lugol's solution	0.1–1.0 mL tid	PO
propylthiouracil	PTU	100–150 mg tid	PO
radioactive iodide	^{131}I, Iodotope	0.8–150 millicurie (mCi)*	PO

* Based on radiation quantity; millicurie stands for 1/1,000 of a curie, a measurement of radiation intensity.

POTASSIUM IODIDE

Iodine drugs, such as potassium iodide (Pima, SSKI), may be administered to inhibit thyroid hormones by saturating the thyroid gland.

How does it work?

The exact mechanism of action is not clear, but excess iodide ions cause minimal change in thyroid gland mass. Conversely, when the thyroid gland is hyperplastic, excess iodide ions temporarily inhibit secretion of thyroid hormone.

How is it used?

Iodide is used alone for hyperthyroidism or in conjunction with antithyroid drugs and propranolol in treatment of thyrotoxic crisis. It is also prescribed for treatment of persistent or recurring hyperthyroidism that occurs in Graves' disease patients. Iodide can be administered as a radiation protectant.

What are the adverse effects?

Iodide may cause diarrhea, nausea, vomiting, and stomach pain. Fever, joint pain, lymph node enlargement, and weakness are also seen. Iodide can produce irregular heartbeat, mental confusion, productive cough, and pulmonary edema.

What are the contraindications and interactions?

Iodide is contraindicated in patients with hypersensitivity to this agent. It must be avoided in patients who are suffering from hypothyroidism, hyperkalemia (excessive potassium in the blood), and acute bronchitis. Safety during pregnancy, lactation, or in children under one year of age is not established. Iodide must be used cautiously in patients with renal impairment, cardiac disease, pulmonary tuberculosis, and **Addison's disease** (adrenocortical insufficiency caused by an autoimmune response to the adrenal gland).

Drug interactions include antithyroid drugs, **lithium** (a drug that reduces the activity of certain neurotransmitters and is used in the treatment of bipolar disorder), which may potentiate hypothyroid and goitrogenic actions, potassium-sparing diuretics, and potassium supplements, which increase the risk of hyperkalemia.

What are the important points patients should know?

Instruct patients about the effects of iodine and its presence in shellfish, iodized salt, and certain over-the-counter (OTC) cough preparations. Advise patients about the manifestations of hyperthyroidism and hypothyroidism, and about the fact that each of them can occur as a result of treatment for the other. Teach patients how to monitor pulse rate and to report any marked rise or fall.

Focus Point

Graves' Disease

Every year, approximately 5 in 10,000 people in the United States contract Graves' disease, which is related to hyperthyroidism. There are 4 to 8 times more female patients than male patients with Graves' disease. Most patients who contract this disease are between 20 and 45 years of age. Besides the prevalent eye problems, signs of Graves' disease also include rapid heartbeat, palpitations, nervousness, excitability, weight loss, profuse perspiration, and insomnia.

METHIMAZOLE

Methimazole (Tapazole) is an antithyroid drug that is approximately 10 times as potent as propylthiouracil and is faster in eliciting an antithyroid response.

How does it work?

Methimazole inhibits synthesis of thyroid hormones as the drug accumulates in the thyroid gland. It does not affect existing T3 or T4 levels.

How is it used?

Methimazole is used for hyperthyroidism and prior to surgery or radiotherapy of the thyroid. It may be used cautiously to treat hyperthyroidism in pregnancy.

What are the adverse effects?

The adverse effects of methimazole include hypothyroidism, pancytopenia (a blood disorder), aplastic anemia, arthralgia (joint pain), peripheral neuropathy, drowsiness, vertigo, rash, alopecia, and pruritus.

What are the contraindications and interactions?

Methimazole is contraindicated in pregnancy and lactation. It should be used cautiously with other drugs known to cause agranulocytosis. Methimazole can reduce the anticoagulant effects of warfarin (Coumadin). It may increase serum levels of digoxin and alter theophylline levels. Methimazole may require decreased doses of beta blockers.

What are the important points patients should know?

Instruct patients to take methimazole at the same time each day, preferably before breakfast. Food tends to inhibit the absorption rate.

PROPYLTHIOURACIL

Propylthiouracil (PTU) is an antithyroid agent that has no effect on hormone release, and the antithyroid action cannot be observed until the thyroid stores of T3 and T4 become depleted.

How does it work?

Propylthiouracil belongs in the thioamide family. It interferes with the use of iodine and blocks synthesis of T3 and T4. It does not interfere with the release and utilization of stored thyroid hormone. Therefore, antithyroid action of propylthiouracil is delayed days and weeks until preformed T3 and T4 are degraded.

How is it used?

Propylthiouracil is prescribed for hyperthyroidism, iodine-induced thyrotoxicosis, and hyperthyroidism associated with thyroiditis. It is also used to shrink the size of the thyroid prior to surgery.

What are the adverse effects?

Propylthiouracil may cause headache, vertigo, drowsiness, nausea, vomiting, diarrhea, loss of taste, and hepatitis. Other adverse effects include agranulocytosis, hypothyroidism, periorbital edema, puffy hands and feet, bradycardia, cool and pale skin, sleepiness, fatigue, mental depression, changes in menstrual periods, and unusual weight gain.

What are the contraindications and interactions?

Propylthiouracil is contraindicated in the last trimester of pregnancy and during lactation. It should not be concurrently administered with sulfonamides or coal tar derivatives, such as aminopyrine or antipyrine. Thyroid hormones can reverse the efficacy of amiodarone, potassium iodide, and sodium iodide.

What are the important points patients should know?

Remind patients with Graves' disease who are taking propylthiouracil about the drug's side effects. Patients taking propylthiouracil often complain of a sore throat and fever, but agranulocytosis is the most serious adverse effect of this drug. Stress the importance of reporting agranulocytosis symptoms to these patients. Instruct patients to avoid foods that can inhibit thyroid secretion, such as strawberries, peaches, pears, cabbage, turnips, radishes, peas, and spinach, and to take medication early in the day to prevent nighttime insomnia. Advise female patients to keep a record of menstruation because menstrual irregularities may occur.

Thyroid Drugs

Hypothyroidism (low or absent thyroid function) is a common disorder caused by deficient secretion of TSH or other thyroid hormones. Replacement therapy with natural or synthetic thyroid hormone is required. Periodic testing and adjustment of the drug level may be necessary.

LEVOTHYROXINE

Levothyroxine (Synthroid) is a commonly prescribed synthetic form of thyroxine (T4).

How does it work?

The actions of levothyroxine replicate those of natural thyroid hormone, which regulates the body's basal metabolic rate.

How is it used?

Levothyroxine is used in cases of low thyroid function. It generally is taken orally, and an IV form is also available.

What are the adverse effects?

Too high a dose level of levothyroxine can cause symptoms resembling hyperthyroidism, including tachycardia, weight loss, insomnia, anxiety, and intolerance of heat. Women can experience menstrual irregularities, and long-term use can cause osteoporosis. Serious adverse effects include chest pain (angina) and rapid or irregular heartbeat or pulse.

What are the contraindications and interactions?

People with allergies to povidone-iodine or tartrazine (a yellow dye in some processed foods and drugs) should inform their doctors, for levothyroxine contains these ingredients.

Patients taking amphetamines; anticoagulants such as warfarin (Coumadin); antidepressants or antianxiety agents; arthritis medicine; aspirin; beta-blockers such as metoprolol (Lopressor, Toprol), propranolol (Inderal), or timolol (Blocadren, Timoptic); cancer chemotherapy agents; diabetes medications (insulin); digoxin (Lanoxin); estrogens; iron; methadone; oral contraceptives; phenytoin (Dilantin); steroids; or theophylline (TheoDur) should inform their doctors. Caution should be used in prescribing the drug for women who are pregnant or may become pregnant or are breastfeeding.

What are the important points patients should know?

Instruct patients to see their physicians regularly so that their blood can be tested to be sure that the prescribed dose is therapeutic. There is a fine line between the proper dose and one that produces adverse effects, and periodic adjustment of dose level may be needed. Tell patients to take levothyroxine on an empty stomach with a full glass of water (first thing in the morning is generally best) and to not eat for an hour after. Antacids, calcium carbonate (Tums), cholestyramine (Questran), colestipol (Colestid), iron, sodium polystyrene sulfonate (Kayexalate), simethicone (Phazyme, Gas X), or sucralfate (Carafate) should be taken at least 4 hours before or 4 hours after taking levothyroxine. Advise patients to call their physician immediately if chest pain (angina) and rapid or irregular heartbeat or pulse are experienced.

PARATHYROID HORMONE

The four tiny parathyroid glands are located in the neck, behind the thyroid gland. Spontaneous atrophy or injury (as in thyroidectomy) of the parathyroid glands is followed by a decrease in the concentration of serum calcium and an increase in serum phosphorus. These changes can be reversed by the parenteral administration of suitably prepared extracts of the parathyroids of domestic animals. **Hypoparathyroidism** is a rare disorder in which the body produces little or no parathyroid hormone, resulting in an abnormally low level of blood calcium (hypocalcemia).

Secretion of parathyroid hormone (PTH) is stimulated by a fall in the free calcium ion concentration of the plasma. The hormone then acts to restore calcium concentration by:

✳ Increasing reabsorption of calcium and excretion of phosphate

✳ Decreasing the absorption of bicarbonate by the kidney

✳ Increasing reabsorption of bone, with release of calcium ions

✳ Increasing absorption of calcium and phosphate from the GI tract

The gastrointestinal (GI) tract mediates calcitriol (a metabolite of vitamin D_3), which may be considered a hormone. PTH is a tropin for renal synthesis of calcitriol. Vitamin D_2 (calciferol) can stimulate the hypercalcemic effect of PTH. Overdosage with any of these compounds can lead to dangerously high calcium concentrations in the blood, which may cause calcification of kidneys and blood vessels.

✳ Apply Your Knowledge 22.2

The following questions focus on what you have just learned about the thyroid hormones, parathyroid hormone, and antithyroid drugs. *See Appendix E for the correct answers.*

MULTIPLE CHOICE

Select the correct answers from choices a–d.

1. Iodide is used in conjunction with antithyroid drugs and propranolol in the treatment of:

   a. Hyperthyroidism

   b. Hypothyroidism

   c. Thyrotoxic crisis

   d. Renal impairment

2. Propylthiouracil is indicated for all of the following disorders, except:

   a. Hyperthyroidism associated with thyroiditis

   b. Hyperthyroidism

   c. Hypothyroidism

   d. Iodine-induced thyrotoxicosis

3. Parathyroid hormone acts to restore calcium concentration in the blood circulation by all of the following, except:

   a. Decreasing the absorption of bicarbonate by the kidneys

   b. Decreasing reabsorption of calcium and excretion of phosphate

   c. Increasing absorption of calcium and phosphate from the GI tract

   d. Increasing reabsorption of bone, with release of calcium ions

4. Which of the following vitamins can stimulate the hypercalcemic effect of parathyroid hormone?

   a. Calciferol

   b. Calcitonin

   c. Niacin

   d. Thiamin

5. Methimazole is an antithyroid drug that is 10 times as potent as:

   a. Levothyroxine

   b. Radioactive iodide

   c. Potassium iodide

   d. Propylthiouracil

6. Which of the following is the exact mechanism of action of potassium iodide?

   a. Inhibits synthesis of thyroid hormones

   b. Interferes with the use of iodine

   c. Blocks existing T3 or T4 levels

   d. Unknown

MATCHING

Match the lettered trade name to the numbered generic name.

GENERIC NAME	TRADE NAME
1. _____ methimazole	a. Cytomel
2. _____ propylthiouracil	b. Lodotope
3. _____ liothyronine	c. Lugol's solution
4. _____ levothyroxine	d. PTU
5. _____ potassium iodide	e. Synthroid
6. _____ radioactive iodide	f. Tapazole

Pancreas

The *pancreas* is found beneath the great curvature of the stomach and is connected by a duct to the duodenum of the small intestine. The pancreas is made up of clusters of glandular epithelial cells. One group of these clusters, the *islets of Langerhans*, form the endocrine portions of the gland (and are therefore part of the endocrine system), regulating blood glucose levels and playing a vital role in metabolism.

PANCREATIC HORMONES

Some of the islets of Langerhans cells consist of alpha cells that secrete the hormone **glucagon,** which is secreted when blood glucose levels are low. The function of glucagon is to maintain adequate levels of glucose in the blood between meals. Other clusters consist of beta cells that secrete the hormone *insulin,* which is essential for the maintenance of normal blood sugar. Insulin promotes the use of glucose in cells (so that it can used as fuel), thereby lowering the blood glucose level, and in the metabolism of carbohydrates, proteins, and fats. Dysregulation of beta cell function can lead to a disorder known as diabetes mellitus (see Figure 22-3 ■).

Diabetes mellitus (DM) is a serious endocrine disorder characterized by hyperglycemia (high glucose levels in the blood) and resulting from deficient insulin secretion or decreased sensitivity of insulin receptors on target cells. This condition affects approximately 17 million people in the United States. Diabetes mellitus exists in three forms: type 1, type 2, and gestational diabetes mellitus. Diabetes is more prevalent in the African American and Hispanic populations, and genetic predisposition may increase susceptibility (especially with type 2 diabetes).

Type 1 diabetes, also called insulin-dependent diabetes mellitus (IDDM) comprises about 10% of the diabetic population and is still sometimes referred to as juvenile-

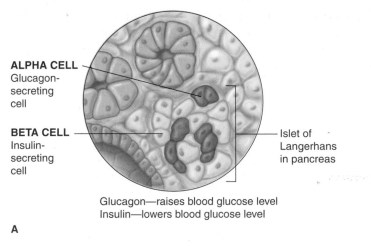

ALPHA CELL
Glucagon-
secreting
cell

BETA CELL
Insulin-
secreting
cell

Islet of
Langerhans
in pancreas

Glucagon—raises blood glucose level
Insulin—lowers blood glucose level

A

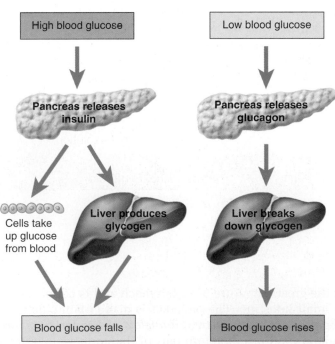

B

Figure 22-3 ■ (A) Diabetes mellitus can be caused by dysregulation of beta cell function. (B) Interaction of blood glucose levels, insulin, and glucagon.

onset diabetes despite the fact that a significant percentage of people are diagnosed with the disease after the age of 20. It results from a lack of insulin secretion by the pancreas, often occurs between the ages of 11 to 13, and has an abrupt onset. Within 5 to 10 years after diagnosis, the beta cells of the pancreas have been destroyed and even minute amounts of insulin are no longer produced. Treatment of type 1 diabetes involves drug therapy with insulin or other hypoglycemics, the goal being maintenance of proper blood glucose levels.

Focus on Pediatrics

Diabetes in Children

Chronic pathological conditions resulting from diabetes mellitus in children include diabetic neuropathy, retinopathy, nephropathy, stroke, coronary artery disease, and infection.

Type 2 diabetes is also called noninsulin-dependent diabetes mellitus (NIDDM), and makes up approximately 90% of all cases of diabetes mellitus. It occurs mainly in adults older than 40 years of age, although the incidence has been increasing in younger patients due to physical inactivity and obesity. The onset is gradual and often is diagnosed by a routine physical examination, with the patient unaware of any signs and symptoms. Type 2 diabetics may secrete small amounts of insulin, but the greater problem is that insulin receptors in the target cells have become resistant to the hormone. Type 2 diabetes mellitus can be treated through diet and exercise (which can sometimes increase the sensitivity of the receptors) and, if needed, through use of oral antidiabetic medications, or even insulin.

Gestational diabetes mellitus develops during pregnancy, and symptoms may be similar to type 2 diabetes. Generally temporary, it ends when the pregnancy is over. Treatment is through diet and exercise. In some cases, low doses of insulin are appropriate, but oral hypoglycemics are not given.

Complications from diabetes are a leading cause of suffering, disability, and premature death. The following disorders are associated with long-term diabetes, especially with poorly controlled hyperglycemia: retinopathy, nephropathy, depressed immune function, elevated blood lipid levels, and vascular disease. The consequences of these complications are blindness, renal impairment and kidney failure, neuropathic pain, opportunistic infections, wounds and sores that do not heal, loss of limbs, atherosclerosis, hypertension, and myocardial infarction.

Focus Point

Diabetes and Obesity

Seventeen million Americans have diabetes. Forty million are obese, a major cause of type 2 diabetes. These conditions are among the top public health problems in the United States today. Usually, type 2 diabetes affects people older than age 40, but due to increased obesity in children and other young patients, more of them than ever before are being diagnosed with this condition. African Americans have the highest rates of both obesity and diabetes compared with other ethnic groups. For good health, 30 minutes of moderate physical activity most days of the week are recommended, and 60 minutes are recommended to achieve significant weight loss.

HYPOGLYCEMIC DRUGS

The purpose of hypoglycemic drugs is to treat **hyperglycemia** (abnormally high blood glucose level) by lowering glucose levels in the blood. There are two types of hypoglycemic drugs; they are classified according to the manner in which they are administered: parenteral and oral. Insulin is the sole representative of the parenteral type.

Insulin Injection

Insulin is an antidiabetic hormone that lowers blood glucose levels by facilitating glucose uptake into body cells. Insulin cannot be taken orally because it is destroyed by digestive enzymes. Several types of insulin are available for subcutaneous or intramuscular injection (see Table 22-4 ■). Patient participation is an essential component of comprehensive insulin care.

Table 22-4 ■ Classifications of Insulin

GENERIC NAME	TRADE NAME	AVERAGE ADULT DOSAGE	ROUTE OF ADMINISTRATION
Rapid-Acting			
insulin lispro	Humalog	5–10 U 0–15 min ac	Subcutaneous
insulin aspart	NovoLog	0.25–0.7 U/kg/d 5–10 min ac	Subcutaneous
insulin (human recombinant)	Exubera	Individualized doses	Inhalation
Short-Acting			
insulin (regular)	Humulin R, Novolin R	5–10 U 15–30 min ac and at bedtime	Subcutaneous
insulin (regular) (from pork pancreas)	Iletin	5–10 U 15–30 min ac and at bedtime	Subcutaneous
Intermediate-Acting			
insulin isophane (NPH: neutral protamine hagedorn)	Humulin N, Novolin N	Individualized doses	Subcutaneous
insulin zinc suspension (lente)	Humulin L, Novolin L	Individualized doses	IM, Subcutaneous
Long-Acting			
insulin glargine	Lantus	If not taking insulin, give 10 U 1 time/d (usually at bedtime); if taking NPH or Ultralente insulin 1 time/d, give same dose daily (usually at bedtime); if taking NPH insulin 2 times/d, give 80% of total daily dose 1 time/d (usually at bedtime)	Subcutaneous
Extended Zinc Suspension			
insulin zinc suspension, extended	Humulin U Ultralente	Individualized doses	IM, Subcutaneous

Focus Point

Insulin Therapy

Insulin controls the level of blood glucose but does not cure diabetes. Therefore, insulin therapy is required long-term.

RAPID-ACTING INSULIN: LISPRO

Lispro insulin (Humalog) is one of this class that has a rapid onset (5 to 10 minutes) and short duration of effect (2 to 4 hours). It is used to achieve glycemic control if taken immediately before or after meals, which reduces the danger of **hypoglycemia** (abnormally low blood glucose level). Rapid-acting insulins must be used in combination with longer-acting preparations.

How does it work?

Lispro, human insulin of recombinant DNA origin, is a rapid-acting and glucose-lowering agent that increases peripheral glucose uptake, especially by skeletal muscle and fat tissue, by inhibiting the liver from changing glycogen to glucose.

How is it used?

Lispro is used in the treatment of diabetes mellitus.

What are the adverse effects?

Most adverse effects are related to hypoglycemia, which results from either an overdose of insulin or a mismatch in blood glucose levels with the appropriate dose of insulin. Lipodystrophy, allergic reactions, and insulin resistance are other complications of insulin therapy.

What are the contraindications and interactions?

Insulin is contraindicated during episodes of hypoglycemia or in patients sensitive to any ingredient in the formulation. It must be used cautiously in insulin-resistant patients; those with hyperthyroidism or hypothyroidism; renal or hepatic impairment; women who are lactating or pregnant; and in older adults. Safety and efficacy in children less than 3 years old is not established.

Alcohol, anabolic steroids, and salicylates may potentiate hypoglycemic effects. Corticosteroids, epinephrine, and dextrothyroxine may antagonize hypoglycemic effects.

What are the important points patients should know?

Instruct patients to recognize the manifestations of a hypoglycemic reaction (nervousness, sweating, tremors, rapid pulse, hunger, and weakness), as well as manifestations of a hyperglycemic reaction (thirst, sweating, a "fruity" breath odor, abdominal pain, increased urine output, nausea, and vomiting). Eating a sugary snack or taking glucose tablets, followed by a food containing complex carbohydrates (milk, crackers, fruit), will reverse a hypoglycemic reaction. However, if not treated, the result can be coma and even death.

Focus on Natural Products

Garlic and Ginseng

Garlic and ginseng may potentiate the hypoglycemic effects of insulin lispro (Humalog).

SHORT-ACTING INSULINS: REGULAR INSULIN

Regular (natural) insulin (Humulin R, Novolin R) is an example of a short-acting insulin that is injected prior to a meal. The onset is 30 to 60 minutes, and duration of action is 5 to 7 hours. Short-acting insulins are highly soluble, and their solutions have a clear appearance. Regular insulin may be administered either subcutaneously or intravenously.

How does it work?

Regular insulin lowers blood glucose levels by increasing peripheral glucose uptake, especially by skeletal muscle and fat tissue, and by inhibiting the liver from changing glycogen to glucose.

How is it used?

Regular insulin is used in emergency treatment of diabetic ketoacidosis or coma, to initiate therapy in patients with insulin-dependent diabetes mellitus, and in combination with intermediate-acting or long-acting insulins to provide better control of blood glucose concentrations in diabetic patients.

What are the adverse effects?

The most common adverse effects are hypoglycemic reactions, especially when diabetes is newly diagnosed and the correct insulin dosage, which is highly individualized for each patient, has not yet been established, or the patient is pregnant. Symptoms of hypoglycemia include headache, hunger, weakness, sweating, tachycardia, confusion, and emotional disturbances, as well as coma and death.

What are the contraindications and interactions?

Regular insulin is contraindicated in patients with hypersensitivity to any ingredient of the product and when a patient is hypoglycemic. Insulin is used cautiously during pregnancy and in patients with kidney or liver impairments. It should be avoided during lactation. Certain drugs such as contraceptives, corticosteroids, diuretics, epinephrine, lithium, niacin, thyroid hormones, albuterol, and dobutamine may interact with administration of insulin, and increase or decrease blood sugar.

What are the important points patients should know?

Advise patients to drink orange juice and sugar-containing drinks and foods when a hypoglycemic reaction occurs.

INTERMEDIATE-ACTING INSULINS

Insulin isophane, an NPH (neutral protamine hagedorn) insulin (Humulin N, Novolin N), and insulin lente, an insulin zinc suspension (Humulin L, Novolin L), are classified as intermediate-acting insulins. NPH insulin is a sterile suspension of zinc-insulin crystals and protamine sulfate in buffered water for injection. It is typically injected twice daily. NPH insulin has an onset of action of 1 to 2 hours, a peak of 6 to 14 hours, and duration of action of approximately 10 to 16 hours.

Lente insulin is a sterile suspension in buffered water for injection, modified by the addition of zinc chloride. Lente insulin is also an intermediate-acting insulin that is typically injected twice daily. It has an onset of action of 1 to 2 hours, a peak of 6 to 14 hours, and duration of action of approximately 10 to 16 hours.

How do they work?

The mechanism of action of intermediate-acting insulins is similar to that of rapid-acting insulins.

How are they used?

NPH insulin and other intermediate-acting insulins are used to control hyperglycemia in the diabetic patient. Mixtard and Novolin 70/30 are fixed combinations of purified regular insulin 30% and NPH 70%.

What are the adverse effects?

The adverse effects of intermediate-acting insulins occur in fewer than 1% of patients and are similar to rapid-acting insulins.

What are the contraindications and interactions?

Intermediate-acting insulins are contraindicated during episodes of hypoglycemia or in patients sensitive to any ingredient in the formulation. They must be used cautiously in insulin-resistant patients; those with hyperthyroidism or hypothyroidism; renal or hepatic impairment; women who are lactating or pregnant; and in older adults. Safety and efficacy in children younger than 3 years of age are not established. Drug interactions are similar to rapid-acting insulins.

What are the important points patients should know?

Teach patients how to check their blood glucose level using a blood glucose monitoring machine. These levels should be checked about 4 times daily. More frequent monitoring is required if levels are not within the normal range. Stress the importance of maintaining a well-balanced diet with the dietary restrictions specified by the health-care team. Delaying or missing a meal may lead to hypoglycemia. Advise patients to avoid alcohol.

LONG-ACTING INSULINS: INSULIN GLARGINE

Insulin glargine (Lantus) was introduced for use in the United States in 2001. It is a long-acting insulin, with a slow onset of effect but a very long duration of activity. The preparation made from beef pancreas is the longest-acting type. It has an onset of action of approximately 2 hours, and it has a duration of action of 24 hours. It is the only true 24-hour insulin available and must be administered subcutaneously.

How does it work?

The mechanism of action of insulin glargine is similar to that of other types of insulin, such as lispro insulin, in that it inhibits the liver from changing glycogen to glucose.

How is it used?

Insulin glargine is used in treatment of both type 1 and 2 diabetes. It should be administered subcutaneously, usually at bedtime, once daily.

What are the adverse effects?

The adverse effects of insulin glargine include allergic reactions, hypoglycemia, and hypokalemia. Other adverse effects are injection site reaction, lipodystrophy, pruritus, and rash.

What are the contraindications and interactions?

Insulin glargine is contraindicated in patients with prior hypersensitivity to this agent, or who have hypoglycemia. This agent should be used cautiously in patients with renal and hepatic impairment, or during pregnancy and lactation. Safety and efficacy in children under 6 years of age are not established.

What are the important points patients should know?

Advise patients to always carry a source of sugar when away from home.

EXTENDED INSULIN IN ZINC SUSPENSION

This type of suspension consists of sterile insulin (Humulin U) suspended in buffered water for injection, modified by the addition of zinc chloride. Large particle size and high zinc content delay absorption and prolong action. The brand name is Ultralente and it has an onset of action of 4 to 8 hours, a peak of 10 to 30 hours, and duration usually in excess of 36 hours. A theoretical advantage is that it is free of protamine and other foreign proteins, so the incidence of allergic reactions may be minimized. This type of insulin is obtained from pork pancreas.

How does it work?

The mechanism of action of extended-insulin zinc suspension is similar to other types of insulin (see "Rapid-Acting Insulin").

How is it used?

Ultralente is used for diabetes mellitus type 1. It is composed of 70% Ultralente and 30% Semilente (prompt-release) insulin.

What are the adverse effects?

The adverse effects of extended-insulin zinc suspension are similar to rapid-acting insulins.

What are the contraindications and interactions?

Extended-insulin zinc suspension is contraindicated during episodes of hypoglycemia or in patients sensitive to any ingredient in the formulation. Drug interactions and cautioned uses are similar to those of other types of insulin.

What are the important points patients should know?

Advise patients to recognize the manifestations of a hypoglycemic reaction, and instruct them to use orange juice and sugar-containing foods when a hypoglycemic reaction occurs. Educate patients with diabetes mellitus about nutrition, exercise, care of diabetes during illness, and medications to lower plasma glucose.

Focus Point

Patient Education about Diabetes

Patient education is a continuing process; regular visits are needed for reinforcement.

COMBINATION INSULIN PRODUCTS

Combinations of different types of insulins can increase the onset of effects while maintaining long duration of glycemic control. The following combination insulin products are examples:

✳ Insulin 70/30: 70% NPH and 30% Regular (Humulin 70/30, Novolin 70/30)

✳ Insulin 50/50: 50% NPH and 50% Regular (Humulin 50/50)

✳ Insulin 75/25: 75% Insulin Lispro Protamine (Intermediate-acting) and 25% Lispro (Humalog Mix 75/25)

Focus Point

Hypoglycemic Reactions

Patient participation is an essential component of comprehensive diabetes care. The patient with type 1 or type 2 diabetes who is receiving insulin should be taught to be cautious about hypoglycemic reactions. Signs and symptoms include hunger, nausea, pale and cool skin, and sweating.

ORAL ANTIDIABETIC DRUGS

Patients with type II diabetes mellitus have a defect in insulin secretion from the pancreas, inappropriate hepatic glucose production, tissue insulin resistance, or a combination of any of these as a major cause of glucose dysregulation. Drugs that improve insulin secretion, decrease hepatic glucose production, and improve insulin sensitivity at the tissue receptors are therefore effective in treating type 2 diabetes mellitus.

There are now four chemical categories of orally administered agents that act on lower blood sugar levels: (1) sulfonylureas, (2) biguanides, (3) thiazolidinediones, and (4) alpha-glucosidase inhibitors. The sulfonylureas and biguanides have been available the longest and are the traditional initial treatment choices for type 2 diabetes. Table 22-5 ■ lists common oral antidiabetic drugs.

Table 22-5 ■ Common Oral Antidiabetic Drugs

GENERIC NAME	TRADE NAME	AVERAGE ADULT DOSAGE	ROUTE OF ADMINISTRATION
Sulfonylureas: First Generation			
acetohexamide	Dymelor	250–750 mg/d	PO
chlorpropamide	Diabinese, Glucamide	100–250 mg/d	PO
tolazamide	Tolamide, Tolinase	100–500 mg bid	PO
tolbutamide	Orinase	250–1500 mg bid	PO
Sulfonylureas: Second Generation			
glimepiride	Amaryl	1–4 mg/d	PO
glipizide	Glucotrol	2.5–20 mg bid	PO
glyburide	DiaBeta, Micronase, Glynase	1.25–5 mg/d with breakfast	PO
Biguanides			
metformin	Glucophage, Fortamet	500–850 mg tid	PO
Thiazolidinediones			
pioglitazone	Actos	15–30 mg/d	PO
rosiglitazone	Avandia	4 mg/d	PO
Alpha-Glucosidase Inhibitors			
acarbose	Precose	25–100 mg tid	PO
miglitol	Glyset	25–100 mg tid	PO
Other			
pramlintide acetate	Symlin	Initially: 60 mcg before meals; insulin dose must be reduced. Increase to 120 mcg as directed by physician.	Subcutaneous
exenatide (incretin mimetic)	Byetta	Individual dosing according to size of meal and amount of exercise	Subcutaneous
sitagliptin (dipeptidyl peptidase inhibitor)	Januvia	100 mg/d in single dose	PO

Sulfonylureas

The sulfonylurea drugs have been available in the United States since 1954 and have been the mainstay of oral antidiabetic therapy for many years. They are classified as either first generation: acetohexamide (Dymelor), tolbutamide (Orinase), tolazamide (Tolamide, Tolinase), and chlorpropamide (Diabinese, Glucamide); or second generation: glipizide (Glucotrol), glyburide (DiaBeta, Micronase), and glimepiride (Amaryl), based on their pharmacokinetic profiles. Second-generation sulfonylureas tend to be prescribed more frequently because of their tolerability and dosing schedule.

How do they work?

The sulfonylureas act in three ways by (1) stimulating the release of insulin from the pancreas, (2) inhibiting the process of forming glucose from amino acids and fatty acids in the liver, and (3) increasing the number of insulin receptors to target cells.

How are they used?

The sulfonylureas are used for treatment of mild to moderately severe type 2 diabetes mellitus that cannot be controlled by diet alone, and in patients who do not have complications of diabetes.

What are the adverse effects?

The adverse effects of the sulfonylureas include hypoglycemia due to overdosage, allergic skin reactions, fainting, confusion, blurred vision, depression of bone marrow, and GI disturbances.

What are the contraindications and interactions?

The sulfonylureas are contraindicated in hypersensitivity to these agents. They should be avoided in patients with diabetes complicated by severe infection, acidosis, and severe renal, hepatic, or thyroid insufficiency. Safe use of the sulfonylurea drugs during pregnancy, in nursing mothers, and in children has not been established. These agents should be used cautiously in older adult patients and in those with Addison's disease or hepatic porphyria.

What are the important points patients should know?

Teach patients that oral hypoglycemic drugs are not the same as insulin. They enhance the effectiveness of insulin. Instruct patients taking sulfonylureas to avoid alcohol because a disulfiram-like reaction may occur. Symptoms of this reaction include fever, chills, diarrhea, abdominal pain, and severe nausea and vomiting.

Biguanides

Metformin (Fortamet, Glucophage) is a biguanide compound that keeps the blood sugar levels from rising too high or too fast after meals. This agent does not necessarily decrease blood glucose.

How do they work?

Biguanides act by promoting glucose uptake into cells through enhanced insulin-receptor binding and by decreasing the production of glucose in the liver. They slow glucose absorption and increase glucose removal from the blood without causing hypoglycemia. They may also reduce glucagon levels.

How are they used?

Biguanides are used for type 2 diabetes when no response occurs to sulfonylureas. They may be combined with sulfonylureas, in which case dose reduction of the biguanide agent would be needed.

What are the adverse effects?

Common adverse effects of biguanides include anorexia, GI upset (such as diarrhea, nausea, and vomiting), and lactic acidosis (rare).

What are the contraindications and interactions?

Biguanides are contraindicated in patients with renal disease, alcoholism, hepatic disease, or chronic cardiopulmonary dysfunction. Biguanides interact with amiloride, calcium channel blockers, cimetidine, digoxin, furosemide, morphine, procainamide, quinidine, quinine, ranitidine, trimethoprim, triamterene, and vancomycin.

What are the important points patients should know?

Instruct patients that biguanides should be taken with meals to minimize the effect of gastric irritation. Because these agents have a slow onset, glucose control may take up to 2 weeks to establish. Instruct patients to limit alcohol intake because the combination can increase the risk of lactic acidosis.

Thiazolidinediones

Two thiazolidinediones are currently available: pioglitazone (Actos) and rosiglitazone (Avandia). A third compound, troglitazone, was withdrawn from the market because of hepatic toxicity.

How do they work?

The thiazolidinediones improve cell sensitivity to insulin via the stimulation of a receptor in skeletal muscle, liver, and fat cells.

How are they used?

These agents are used as adjuncts to diet in the treatment of type 2 diabetes.

What are the adverse effects?

Common adverse effects include edema, anemia, headache, back pain, fatigue, weight gain, and hypoglycemia. Hepatic function needs to be closely monitored during therapy for signs of hepatic impairment.

What are the contraindications and interactions?

The thiazolidinediones are contraindicated in patients who have hypersensitivity to these agents. These drugs should be avoided in patients who have active liver impairment or during pregnancy and lactation. Safety and efficacy in children younger than 18 have not been established. Drug interactions between insulin and the thiazolidinediones may increase risk of heart failure or edema, or enhance hypoglycemia with oral antidiabetic agents. Ketoconazole and herbs such as garlic and ginseng may potentiate hypoglycemic effects.

What are the important points patients should know?

Advise patients to contact their physicians if any of the following symptoms develop during thiazolidinedione therapy because these symptoms may indicate hepatic dysfunction: dark urine, jaundice, abdominal pain, nausea, vomiting, anorexia, or fatigue.

Alpha-Glucosidase Inhibitors

Dietary carbohydrates require enzymatic degradation by α-glucosidase to monosaccharides within the GI tract to enable absorption. The α-glucosidase-inhibitors such as acarbose (Precose) and miglitol (Glyset) make up a unique class of drugs that act on this enzyme in the small intestine.

How do they work?

Alpha-glucosidase inhibitors inhibit or delay the absorption of sugar from the GI tract.

How are they used?

Alpha-glucosidase inhibitors are used as monotherapy or in combination with a sulfonylurea in patients with type 2 diabetes mellitus.

What are the adverse effects?

Prominent adverse effects include flatulence, diarrhea, and abdominal pain; they result from the appearance of undigested carbohydrate in the colon that is then fermented into short-chain fatty acids, releasing gas. Hypoglycemia may occur with concurrent sulfonylurea treatment.

What are the contraindications and interactions?
Alpha-glucosidase inhibitors are contraindicated in patients with inflammatory bowel disease or any intestinal condition that could be worsened by gas and distention. Because both miglitol (Glyset) and acarbose (Precose) are absorbed from the gut, these medications should not be prescribed in patients with renal impairment. Acarbose has been associated with reversible hepatic enzyme elevation and should be used with caution in the presence of hepatic disease.

What are the important points patients should know?
Instruct patients that insulin might be needed instead of, or to supplement, oral hypoglycemic drugs in times of infection, stress, or surgery.

✳ Apply Your Knowledge 22.3

The following questions focus on what you have just learned about the pancreatic hormones and hypoglycemic drugs. *See Appendix E for the correct answers.*

FILL IN THE BLANK
Select terms from your reading to fill in the blanks.

1. The alpha cells of the islets of Langerhans secrete _____.

2. Dysregulation of beta cell function of the pancreas may lead to a disorder known as _____.

3. An example of ultra-short-acting insulin is _____.

4. The most common adverse effect of insulin therapy is _____.

5. Long-acting insulins are used in the treatment of _____.

6. Combination of insulin 70/30 means _____ and _____.

7. There are now four chemical categories of orally used drugs that may lower blood sugar levels: the alpha-glucosidase inhibitors, biguanides, thiazolidinediones, and _____.

8. Sulfonylurea drugs are the mainstay of oral antidiabetic therapy and are classified as either _____ or _____.

LABELING
Answer the following drug-labeling questions using the label depicted.

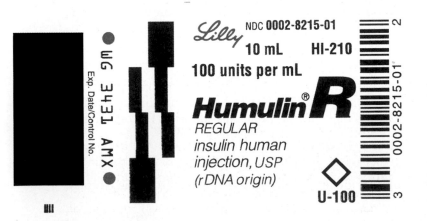

Copyright Eli Lilly and Company. Used with permission.

1. What is the generic name? _____

2. What is the dosage strength? _____

3. What is the name of the manufacturer of this drug? _____

4. What is the origin of this insulin? _____

5. What are the storage requirements for this drug? _____

Adrenal Glands

The adrenal glands sit on top of each kidney. The cortex, or outer portion of the adrenal gland, is one of the endocrine structures most vital for normal metabolic function. It is impossible for life to continue in the complete absence of adrenal cortical function.

ADRENOCORTICAL STEROIDS

The adrenal cortex secretes three types of steroid hormones: the glucocorticoids (also called adrenocortical hormones), mineralocorticoids, and gonadal corticoids. As a group, these hormones are called *corticosteroids*. In humans, *hydrocortisone* (cortisol) is the main glucocorticoid and *aldosterone* is the main mineralocorticoid. Gonadal corticoids are a group of androgens that mostly contain testosterone, estrogen, and progesterone. They will be discussed in detail in Chapter 23.

Adrenocorticotropic hormone (ACTH) is the primary stimulus to hydrocortisone secretion. ACTH is released in response to CRH. Adrenocortical hormones (glucocorticoids) and their effects on the human body are listed in Table 22-6 ■.

Table 22-6 ■ Adrenocortical Hormones and Their Effects

HORMONE	EFFECTS
Glucocorticoids	
Cortisone, hydrocortisone	Increase blood sugar levels, stimulate protein catabolism, mobilize fats, and decrease immunity and inflammatory responses
Mineralocorticoids	
Aldosterone	Cause sodium and water retention, increase blood pressure and blood volume
Gonadal Corticoids	
Androgens	Stimulate activity of the accessory male sex organs, promote development of male sex characteristics, or prevent changes in the latter following castration

Glucocorticoids

Glucocorticoids, such as cortisone (Cortistan, Cortone) and prednisone (Deltasone), have diverse effects including alterations in carbohydrate, protein, and lipid metabolism; maintenance of fluid and electrolyte balance; and preservation of normal function of the cardiovascular system, the immune system, the kidneys, skeletal muscle, endocrine system, and the nervous system. One of the major pharmacological uses of this class of drugs is based on their anti-inflammatory and immunosuppressive actions. A protective role for cortisol is apparent in the physiological response to severe stress that can increase daily production over tenfold.

The relative or complete absence of adrenocortical function, known as Addison's disease, is accompanied by loss of sodium chloride and water, retention of potassium, lowering of blood glucose and liver glycogen levels, increased sensitivity to insulin, nitrogen retention, and lymphocytosis. The disturbances in electrolyte metabolism are the cause of morbidity and mortality in most cases of severe adrenal insufficiency. Disorders caused by adrenal insufficiency can be corrected by administration of adrenal cortical extract or the pure adrenal cortical steroids now available. Overproduction of, or overtreatment with, glucocorticoids may cause Cushing's syndrome. Major adrenal corticosteroids (glucocorticoids) are listed in Table 22-7 ■.

How do they work?
The major actions of glucocorticoids are to suppress an acute inflammatory process and for immunosuppression.

How are they used?
Glucocorticoids are used for replacement therapy in adrenal insufficiency such as Addison's disease and congenital adrenal hyperplasia. Glucocorticoids are also used to

treat rheumatic, inflammatory, allergic, neoplastic, and other disorders. Glucocorticoids are of value in decreasing some cerebral edemas. Their value in the treatment of bacterial meningitis is probably due to the decreasing of edema. Topical or systemic glucocorticoids are used to treat certain skin diseases such as pruritus, psoriasis, and eczema.

What are the adverse effects?

When the glucocorticoids are used for short periods (less than 2 weeks), serious adverse effects, are unusual, even with moderately large doses. However, insomnia, behavioral changes, and acute peptic ulcers are occasionally observed even after only a few days of treatment.

Most patients who are given daily doses of 100 mg of hydrocortisone (Aeroseb-HC, Alphaderm) or more for longer than 2 weeks undergo a series of changes that have been termed **iatrogenic** (that is, produced inadvertently by medication or other treatment). Cushing's syndrome, acne, insomnia, and increased appetite are noted. In the treatment of dangerous or disabling disorders, these changes may not require cessation of therapy. However, the underlying metabolic changes accompanying them can be very serious by the time they become obvious, and eventually osteoporosis, diabetes, and aseptic necrosis of the hipbone may develop. Wound healing is also impaired under these circumstances.

What are the contraindications and interactions?

The corticosteroids are contraindicated in patients with peptic ulcer, heart disease, or hypertension with heart failure, certain infectious illnesses (such as varicella and tuberculosis), psychoses, diabetes, osteoporosis, and glaucoma.

Patients receiving these drugs must be monitored carefully for the development of hypoglycemia, glycosuria, sodium retention with edema or hypertension, hypokalemia, peptic ulcer, osteoporosis, and hidden infections. Glucocorticoids decrease the hypoglycemic activity of insulin and oral hypoglycemics, so that a change in dose of the antidiabetic drugs may be necessitated.

What are the important points patients should know?

Advise patients to take glucocorticoids as ordered. These drugs should not be stopped abruptly. Instead, the physician will organize the dose to be reduced over 1 to 2 weeks. Warn patients that they should not have any immunizations while taking these drugs, unless they have been approved by the physician. Advise patients to take oral drugs with food to prevent gastric irritation. Antacids or other anti-ulcer drugs may be prescribed to lessen the risk of ulceration.

Large doses of steroids may increase the patient's susceptibility to infection. Warn patients about this possibility and instruct them to notify their physicians of fever, cough, sore throat, or injuries that do not heal. They should inform other health-care professionals about their use of these drugs, especially prior to surgery.

Table 22-7 ■ Major Adrenal Corticosteroids (Glucocorticoids)

GENERIC NAME	TRADE NAME	AVERAGE ADULT DOSAGE	ROUTE OF ADMINISTRATION
betamethasone	Celestone, Betacort	0.6–7.2 mg/d	PO
cortisone	Cortistan, Cortone	20–300 mg/d in divided doses	PO
dexamethasone	Decadron	0.25–4 mg bid–qid	PO
hydrocortisone	Cetacort, Cortaid	0.5% cream applied daily qid	Topical
		10–320 mg tid–qid	PO
prednisolone	Delta-Cortef, Key-Pred, Prelone	5–60 mg/d qid	PO
prednisone	Deltasone	5–60 mg/d qid	PO
triamcinolone	Kenalog, Azmacort	4–48 mg/d qid	PO

Focus Point

Glucocorticoids

A patient who is taking glucocorticoids should understand the benefits and possible side effects of long-term use and be advised to report any new side effects. The patient should also be instructed to take oral doses with meals, avoid alcohol, limit sodium intake, and increase potassium intake.

Mineralocorticoids

Mineralocorticoids are a group of hormones secreted from the adrenal cortex. The most important mineralocorticoid in humans is aldosterone. Small amounts of desoxycorticosterone are also formed and released, although the amount is normally insignificant.

The rate of aldosterone secretion is subject to several influences. ACTH produces a moderate stimulation of its release, but this effect is not sustained for more than a few days in the normal individual.

How do they work?

Aldosterone and other steroids with mineralocorticoid properties regulate sodium and potassium balance in the blood by promoting the reabsorption of sodium from the distal convoluted and collecting ducts of the kidneys, which results in the excretion of potassium. Mineralocorticoids act by binding to the mineralocorticoid receptor in the cytoplasm of target cells, especially principal cells of the distal convoluted and collecting tubules.

How are they used?

Mineralocorticoids are used for replacement therapy for primary and secondary adrenocortical deficiency.

What are the adverse effects?

The adverse effects of mineralocorticoids can occur if the dosage is too high or prolonged, or if withdrawal is too rapid. They can cause edema, hypertension, congestive heart failure, increased sweating, or skin rashes. They can also cause hypokalemia, muscular weakness, and headache.

What are the contraindications and interactions?

Mineralocorticoids are contraindicated in patients with hypersensitivity to these agents and those with systemic fungal infections. They must be used cautiously in patients with Addison's disease or infection, and during pregnancy and lactation. Mineralocorticoids can decrease the effects of barbiturates, rifampin, and hydantoins.

What are the important points patients should know?

Advise patients to maintain a low-sodium and high-potassium diet if weight gain is an issue. Teach patients to recognize adverse effects of these drugs, which may include edema, hypertension, congestive heart failure, increased sweating, and skin rashes.

Focus Point

Addison's Disease

A ddison's disease is caused by adrenocortical insufficiency, which is characterized by an insidious onset of fatigue, weakness, lack of appetite, nausea and vomiting, weight loss, skin pigmentation, and hypotension.

✱ **Apply Your Knowledge 22.4** ▬▬▬▬▬

The following questions focus on what you have just learned about the adrenocortical steroids. *See Appendix E for the correct answers.*

MULTIPLE CHOICE

Select the correct answers from choices a–d.

1. The steroid hormones are produced by which of the following endocrine glands?

   a. Posterior pituitary

   b. Thymus

   c. Adrenal cortex

   d. Thyroid

2. In humans, the main glucocorticoid is:

   a. Testosterone

   b. Estrogen

   c. Aldosterone

   d. Hydrocortisone

3. The major actions of glucocorticoids are to suppress an acute inflammatory process and decrease the signs and symptoms of which of the following disorders or conditions?

   a. Allergic reactions

   b. Insomnia

   c. Acute peptic ulcer

   d. Osteoporosis

4. Which of the following glands releases aldosterone?

   a. Hypothalamus

   b. Anterior pituitary

   c. Pancreas

   d. Adrenal cortex

5. The most important mineralocorticoid in humans is:

   a. Cortisone

   b. Dexamethasone

   c. Aldosterone

   d. Prednisolone

6. Which of the following hormones is the primary stimulus to hydrocortisone secretion?

   a. Somatotropin hormone (GH)

   b. Adrenocorticotropin hormone (ACTH)

   c. Thyroid-stimulating hormone (TSH)

   d. Prolactin (PRL)

FILL IN THE BLANK

Select terms from your reading to fill in the blanks.

1. The adrenal cortex secretes three types of steroid hormones: the glucocorticoids (also called adrenocortical hormones), _____, and gonadocorticoids.

2. Gonadocorticoids are a group of _____ that mostly contain testosterone, estrogen, and progesterone.

3. Cortisone (Cortistan, Cortone) and prednisone (Deltatsone) are examples of _____.

4. The absence of adrenocortical function, known as _____ _____, is accompanied by loss of sodium chloride and water, retention of potassium, lowering of blood glucose and liver glycogen levels, increased sensitivity to insulin, nitrogen retention, and lymphocytosis.

5. Aldosterone regulates _____ and _____ balance in the blood.

Chapter Capsule

This section repeats the objectives from the beginning of the chapter and then provides a summary of the most important concepts for that objective. Use this section as a quick review and to check your knowledge.

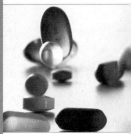

Objective 1: Describe the main functions of a hormone.

- ■ Regulate growth
- ■ Regulate blood glucose
- ■ Regulate intermediary metabolism
- ■ Maintain homeostasis

Objective 2: Explain the endocrine functions of the hypothalamus.

- ■ Sends directions via hormones to the pituitary gland
- ■ Controls the release of corticotropin-releasing hormone (CRH), growth-hormone–releasing hormone (GHRH), gonadotropin-releasing hormone (GnRH), and thyrotropin-releasing hormone (TRH)
- ■ Controls the release of anterior pituitary hormones

Objective 3: List six types of hormones that are secreted from the anterior pituitary gland.

- ■ Growth hormone
- ■ Adrenocorticotropin hormone
- ■ Thyroid-stimulating hormone
- ■ Follicle-stimulating hormone
- ■ Luteinizing hormone
- ■ Prolactin

Objective 4: Describe the role of the thyroid gland and its replacement and antithyroid drugs.

- ■ It secretes thyroxine (T4) and triiodothyronine (T3), which require iodized salt in the diet for synthesis, and calcitonin, which is involved with calcium homeostasis.

- Its absence or dysfunction can result in low to nonexistent levels of thyroid hormone (hypothyroidism), which lowers the basal metabolic rate, impairing growth and development.

- Its overactivity (hyperthyroidism) results in increased body metabolism, which can cause tachycardia, anxiety, weight loss, and other problems.

- Disorders of the thyroid gland are quite common; treatment indicates drug therapy.

- Levothyroxine is a commonly prescribed synthetic thyroid replacement hormone.

- Iodine or potassium iodide, radioactive iodine, and thioamide derivatives are the drugs of choice for antithyroid therapy.

Objective 5: Explain the pharmacotherapy of diabetes insipidus.

- Vasopressin is most often used to treat this disease, mainly for its antidiuretic effects.

Objective 6: Identify the role of hypoglycemic medications in treating diabetes mellitus.

- Insulin: lowers blood glucose levels by facilitating glucose uptake into body cells; controls the level of blood sugar but does not cure diabetes; insulin therapy required long-term; insulin used parenterally

- Oral antidiabetic drugs: sulfonylureas, biguanides, thiazolidinediones, and alpha-glucosidase inhibitors; these drugs are indicated for type 2 diabetes mellitus

- Sulfonylureas: stimulate the release of insulin; inhibit glucose formation; increase the number of insulin receptors to target cells

- Biguanides: promote glucose uptake into cells and decrease glucose production in the liver; slow glucose absorption and increase glucose removal from the blood without causing hypoglycemia; can also reduce glucagon levels

- Thiazolidinediones: improve body cell sensitivity to insulin via the stimulation of a receptor in skeletal muscle, liver, and fat cells

- Alpha-glucosidase inhibitors: delay or inhibit the absorption of sugar from the intestinal tract

Objective 7: Describe the adverse effects of insulin and corticosteroids.

- Insulin: lipodystrophy, allergic reactions, insulin resistance, hypokalemia, injection site reaction, pruritus, rash, hypoglycemic reactions (headache, hunger, weakness, sweating, tachycardia, confusion, emotional disturbances, coma, and death)

- Corticosteroids: insomnia, behavioral changes, acute peptic ulcers, Cushing's syndrome, acne, increased appetite, osteoporosis, diabetes, aseptic necrosis of the hipbone, impaired wound healing, edema, hypertension, congestive heart failure, increased sweating, skin rashes, hypokalemia, muscular weakness, and headache

Objective 8: Identify the two major classes of steroids.

- Glucocorticoids
- Mineralocorticoids

Internet Sites of Interest

- For an overview of diabetes, first click on "diabetes" in the right hand column, and then click-on images that provide illustrations of the endocrine glands, islets of Langerhans, pancreas, insulin production, glucose testing, insulin pump, and diabetes circulation in the foot, visit: **http://health.allrefer.com**

■   WebMD.com offers an in-depth look at diabetes prevention, treatment, and research at: **www.webmd.com**. Search for "diabetes."

■   To read an article about hypothyroidism diagnosis and treatment by a UCLA School of Medicine-Endocrinology Division professor, visit: **http://thyroid.about.com**. Search for "Hashimoto."

■   The Nemours Foundation sponsors a Web site that provides information about thyroid disease in children and adolescents: **www.kidshealth.org**. Enter the Parent Site and then search for "thyroid disease."

Chapter 23

Effects of Drugs on the Reproductive System

Chapter Objectives

After completing this chapter, you should be able to:

1. Describe the male and female reproductive structures.
2. Discuss the male and female sex hormones, and their effects on the reproductive system.
3. Explain the contraindications of estrogens.
4. Describe how oral contraceptives work to prevent pregnancy.
5. Discuss menopause and hormone therapy.
6. Provide information about androgens and anabolic steroids.
7. Explain the indications of androgens.
8. Discuss the major adverse effects of progestins.
9. Describe the contraindications of oral contraceptives.
10. Explain the mechanism of action of oxytocic drugs.

Key Terms

Androgens (page 501)

Estrogens (page 507)

Menorrhagia (men-no-RAH-jee-uh) (page 511)

Metrorrhagia (mee-tro-RAH-jee-uh) (page 511)

Oocytes (OO-oh-sites) (page 501)

Oxytocin (OK-see-TO-sin) (page 514)

Priapism (PRY-uh-pizm) (page 504)

Progesterones (page 507)

Ptosis (TOE-sis) (page 510)

Puberty (page 502)

Salpingitis (sal-pin-JY-tis) (page 509)

Sperm (page 501)

Testosterone (page 501)

PRACTICAL SCENARIO

A 34-year-old mother of three children has just been prescribed a combination oral contraceptive because she wants to avoid having any more children. She has never been on oral contraceptives before. Her physician told her about the possible side effects of the hormones, and what symptoms she should report immediately. She is now talking with you, and says that she works in a bar on the weekends, and her coworkers smoke. She says that her husband hates the smell of smoke on her clothes when she gets home from work. She also starts rummaging through her purse, looking for her car keys. She says that she can be very forgetful and loses everything, but she just attributes that to her crazy schedule and the kids.

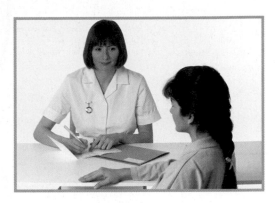

Antonia Deutsch ® Dorling Kindersley

Critical Thinking Questions

1. What are some key areas of concern that are raised in your discussion with Jane?
2. What teaching should you provide to Jane?

Introduction

The male and female reproductive systems are a connected series of organs and glands that produce and nurture sex cells, and transport them to sites of fertilization. Male sex cells are called **sperm**. Female sex cells are eggs, or **oocytes**. Some of the reproductive organs secrete hormones vital to the development and maintenance of secondary sex characteristics and regulation of reproductive physiology. These hormones are also the main drugs that affect the reproductive system. Some agents stimulate the secretions of hormones, whereas others block these same secretions. Drug therapy for disorders or conditions of the reproductive system can be very complicated, although the names of the drugs are familiar to many people.

Male Reproductive System

Organs of the male reproductive system produce and maintain male sex cells, or *sperm cells*; transport these cells and supporting fluids to the outside; and secrete male sex hormones. A male's *primary sex organs* (gonads) are the two testes, in which sperm cells and male sex hormones form. The accessory sex organs of the male reproductive system are the internal and external reproductive organs, including the epididymis, vas deferens, seminal vesicle, prostate gland, bulbourethral glands (Cowper's glands), scrotum, and penis (see Figure 23-1 ■). Table 23-1 ■ summarizes the function of the male reproductive organs.

MALE SEX HORMONES

Male sex hormones are called **androgens**. Testicular interstitial cells produce most of them, but the adrenal cortex synthesizes small amounts as well. **Testosterone** is the most abundant androgen. Its secretion begins during fetal development and continues for several weeks following birth; then, it nearly ceases during childhood. Between the

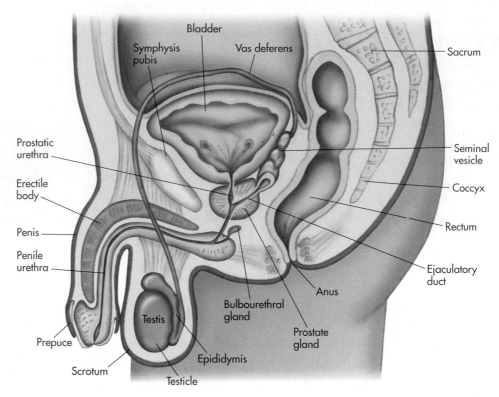

Figure 23-1 ■ The male reproductive system.

Table 23-1 ■ **Functions of the Male Reproductive System**

ORGAN	FUNCTION
Testes	
Interstitial cells	Produce and secrete testosterone
Seminiferous tubules	Produce sperm cells
Epididymis	Stores sperm cells
Vas deferens	Conveys sperm cells to ejaculatory duct
Seminal vesicles	Secrete an alkaline fluid containing nutrients and prostaglandins
Prostate gland	Secretes an alkaline fluid and enhances sperm cell motility
Bulbourethral glands	Secrete fluid that lubricates the end of the penis
Scrotum	Encloses, protects, and regulates the temperature of the testes
Penis	Conveys semen into the vagina during sexual intercourse

ages of 13 and 15, a young man's androgen production usually increases rapidly. This phase in development, when an individual becomes reproductively functional, is known as **puberty**. After puberty, testosterone secretion continues throughout the life of a male. The chief drugs that affect the male reproductive system are androgens and anabolic steroids (see Table 23-2 ■).

Table 23-2 ■ Male Hormones

GENERIC NAME	TRADE NAME	AVERAGE ADULT DOSAGE	ROUTE OF ADMINISTRATION
Androgens			
fluoxymesterone	Halotestin	5–20 mg/d	PO
methyltestosterone	Android, Virilon	10–50 mg/d in divided doses	PO (Buccal)
testosterone cypionate	Depo-Testosterone, Duratest	200–400 mg q2wk	IM
testosterone enanthate	Delatest, Delatestryl	50–400 mg q2–4wk	IM
testosterone (transdermal)	Androderm, Testoderm	Start with 6 mg/d; apply patch daily	Transdermal
Anabolic Steroids			
nandrolone	Durabolin	50–200 mg/wk	IM
oxandrolone	Oxandrin	1–5 mg/kg/d	PO
oxymetholone	Anadrol-50	2.5 mg bid–qid	PO
stanozolol	Winstrol	2 mg tid; then reduce to 2 mg/d or to 2 mg every other day	PO

Synthetic Androgens

Androgen therapy is often given to correct hypogonadism or to increase sperm production.

How do they work?

Synthetic steroids compound with both androgenic and anabolic activity to control the development and maintenance of secondary sexual characteristics. Androgenic activity is responsible for the growth spurt of the adolescent and for growth termination by epiphyseal closure. Anabolic activity increases protein metabolism and decreases its catabolism. Large doses suppress spermatogenesis, thereby causing testicular atrophy. Androgens antagonize the effects of estrogen excess in the female breasts and endometrium.

How are they used?

Testosterones are given to men and women for therapeutic purposes in various conditions. Their main indications in men are to supplement low levels of testosterone to correct hypogonadism (abnormally decreased gonadal function that results in retarded sexual development) or cryptorchidism (undescended testes). Androgens are also used to increase sperm production in cases of infertility. In females, they can be used in the palliative treatment of metastatic breast cancer. Androgens are also prescribed in women for treatment of postpartum breast engorgement, endometriosis, and fibrocystic breast disorder. These agents are able to stimulate increased production of red blood cells, protein synthesis, and muscle mass. Therefore, athletes may use androgens to improve athletic performance.

What are the adverse effects?

The common adverse effects of androgens include insomnia, excitation, skin flushing, nausea, vomiting, anorexia, diarrhea, and jaundice. Hypercalcemia, hypercholesterolemia, sodium retention, and water retention (especially in older adults) with edema are seen. The adverse effects of testosterone may also cause renal calculi, bladder irritability, and increased libido.

What are the secondary sexual characteristics?

What are the contraindications and interactions?

Androgens are contraindicated in patients with hypersensitivity or toxic reactions. These agents should be avoided in patients with serious cardiac, liver, or kidney disease. Androgens must not be prescribed in male patients with known or suspected prostatic or breast cancer. Testosterone (Androderm, Testopel) and other androgens cannot be used during pregnancy or lactation because of the possibility of virilization (the changes that occur as the male body develops, which are different from the development of the female body); that is, these substances would have undesired effects on a female. Androgens must be used cautiously in cardiac, liver, and kidney disease; prepubertal males; geriatric patients; and acute intermittent porphyria. Testosterone alters glucose tolerance tests and may increase creatinine and creatinine secretion. Androgens may suppress some clotting factors and may increase or decrease serum cholesterol.

What are the important points patients should know?

Advise patients about skin hygiene measures to reduce the severity of acne. Oral androgens should be taken with meals to reduce gastric upset. Instruct patients taking androgens to report **priapism** (painful and prolonged erection) because the dose would need to be reduced, and to also report decreased flow of urine because androgens can cause prostatic hypertrophy.

Focus on Geriatrics

Anabolic Steroids and Elderly Men

When anabolic steroids are given to elderly men, their risk of prostate cancer is increased.

✳ Apply Your Knowledge 23.1

The following questions focus on what you have just learned about the male reproductive system. *See Appendix E for the correct answers.*

MATCHING

Match the lettered definition to the numbered term.

TERM	DEFINITION
1. _____ Seminal vesicle	a. Produce sperm cells
2. _____ Seminiferous tubules	b. Secretes fluid that lubricates the end of the penis
3. _____ Scrotum	c. Secretes an alkaline fluid and contains prostaglandins
4. _____ Bulbourethral gland	d. Secrete testosterone
5. _____ Epididymis	e. Stores sperm cells
6. _____ Interstitial cells	f. Regulates temperature of the testes

MULTIPLE CHOICE

Choose the correct answers from choices a–e.

1. Testosterones are indicated for all of the following, except:

    a. Hypogonadism

    b. Cryptorchidism

    c. Endometriosis

    d. Increased sperm production

    e. Prostate cancer

2. Which of the following androgens or anabolic steroids is available by injection?

    a. Halotestin (fluoxymesterone)

    b. Depo-Testosterone (testosterone cypionate)

    c. Anadrol-50 (oxymetholone)

    d. Winstrol (stanozolol)

    e. Virilon (methyltestosterone)

3. If androgens are given to pregnant women, which of the following outcomes may be seen?

    a. Virilization

    b. Hypocalcemia

    c. Hypocholesterolemia

    d. Hypoglycemia

    e. Decreasing libido

4. The common adverse effects of androgens include all of the following, except:

    a. Jaundice

    b. Hypogonadism

    c. Insomnia

    d. Excitation

    e. Hypercalcemia

5. The development and maintenance of secondary sex characteristics in males depends on which of the following hormones?

    a. Estrogen

    b. Thyroxin

    c. Aldosterone

    d. Progesterone

    e. Testosterone

Female Reproductive System

The organs of the female reproductive system produce and maintain the female sex cells, the egg cells (or oocytes); transport these cells to the site of fertilization; provide a favorable environment for a developing fetus; propel the fetus outside the body during birth; and produce female sex hormones. A female's *primary* sex organs (gonads) are the two ovaries, which produce the female sex cells and sex hormones. The *accessory sex organs* of the female reproductive system are the internal and external reproductive organs. They include the ovaries, uterine tubes, uterus, vagina, labia majora, labia minora, clitoris, and vestibule (Figure 23-2 ■). Table 23-3 ■ summarizes the functions of the female reproductive organs.

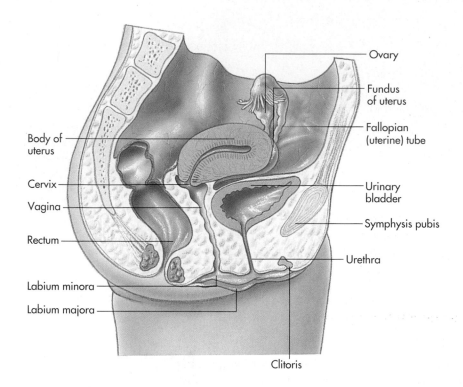

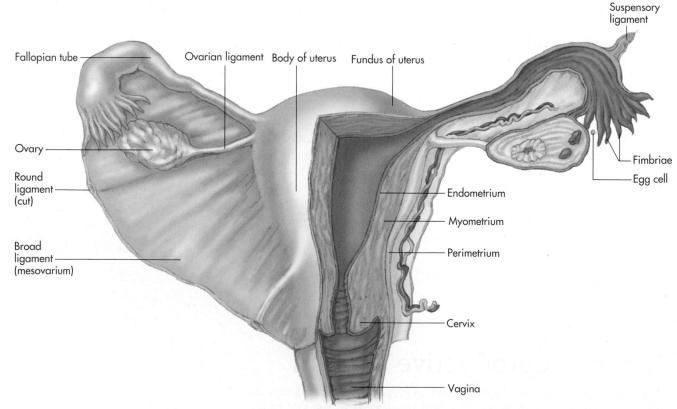

Figure 23-2 ■ The female reproductive system.

Table 23-3 ■ **Functions of the Female Reproductive System**

ORGAN	FUNCTION
Ovaries	Produce oocytes and female sex hormones
Uterine tubes	Convey oocytes toward the uterus and site of fertilization
Uterus	Protects and sustains embryo during pregnancy
Vagina	Conveys uterine secretions to outside of body; receives erect penis during sexual intercourse
Labia majora	Enclose and protect other external reproductive organs
Labia minora	Form margins of vestibule, protect openings of vagina and urethra
Clitoris	Produces feelings of pleasure and sexual stimulation
Vestibule	Space between labia minora that contains vaginal and urethral openings

FEMALE SEX HORMONES

The female body is reproductively immature until about age 10. Then, the hypothalamus begins to secrete increasing amounts of gonadotropin-releasing hormone (GnRH). GnRH, in turn, stimulates the anterior pituitary to release the gonadotropins FSH and LH. These hormones play primary roles in controlling female sex cell maturation, and in producing female sex hormones. Several tissues, including the tissues of the ovaries, adrenal cortices, and placenta (during pregnancy) secrete female sex hormones that belong to two major groups: **estrogens** and **progesterones.** Estradiol is the most abundant of the estrogens, which also include *estrone* and *estriol*.

The ovaries are the primary source of estrogens (in a nonpregnant female). At puberty, under the influence of the anterior pituitary, the ovaries secrete increasing amounts of estrogens. Estrogens stimulate enlargement of accessory organs, including the vagina, uterus, uterine tubes, ovaries, and external reproductive structures. Estrogens also develop and maintain the *female secondary sex characteristics*.

The ovaries are also the primary source of progesterone (in a nonpregnant female). This hormone promotes changes in the uterus during the female reproductive cycle, affects the mammary glands, and helps regulate the secretion of gonadotropins from the anterior pituitary. Androgen (male sex hormone) concentrations produce certain other changes in females at puberty. For example, increased hair growth in the pubic and axillary regions is due to androgens secreted by the adrenal cortices. Conversely, development of the female skeletal configuration, which includes narrow shoulders and broad hips, is a response to a low androgen concentration. Estrogens support the development and maintenance of reproductive organs and the secondary sex characteristics. Table 23-4 ■ summarizes the major synthetic estrogens.

Table 23-4 ■ **Major Synthetic Estrogens**

GENERIC NAME	TRADE NAME	AVERAGE ADULT DOSAGE	ROUTE OF ADMINISTRATION
conjugated estrogens	Premarin	0.3–2.5 mg/d in cycles; 25 mg by injection	PO, IM, IV
estradiol	Estrace	0.5–2 mg/d in cycles	PO
estradiol hemihydrate	Vagifem	25 mcg/d for 2 wk; then 25 mcg 2 times/wk	Vaginal
estradiol transdermal system	Alora, Estraderm	0.05–0.1 mg patch 2 times/wk	Transdermal
estradiol valerate	Delestrogen	5–20 mg q2–3wk	IM

(continued)

Table 23-4 ■ Major Synthetic Estrogens (*continued*)

GENERIC NAME	TRADE NAME	AVERAGE ADULT DOSAGE	ROUTE OF ADMINISTRATION
esterified estrogens	Estratab, Menest	0.3–1.25 mg/d	PO
estrone	Kestrone 5	0.1–0.5 mg 2–3 times/wk	IM
estropipate	Ogen, Ortho-Est	1–2 mg tid	PO

Synthetic Estrogens

(morning after pills)

The best known synthetic estrogen is diethylstilbestrol (Stilbestrol), which possesses most of the therapeutic and untoward actions of the natural estrogenic hormones. Since nonsteroidal estrogens lose little activity after oral administration, they have advantages over the natural estrogens, but the comparative toxicities are not clear.

How do they work?

Estrogens bind to intracellular receptors that stimulate DNA and RNA to synthesize proteins responsible for the effects of these hormones.

How are they used?

The estrogens are used in both genders, including replacement estrogen therapy in women who have had their ovaries removed during the reproductive years, in older women for the prevention and treatment of osteoporosis, and as palliative therapy for breast and prostatic carcinomas in men. Estrogens are also prescribed for abnormal bleeding (hormonal imbalance) and atrophic vaginitis.

What are the adverse effects?

The adverse effects of estrogen therapy include anorexia, nausea, vomiting, stomach cramping, flatulence, headaches, changes in libido (in females), edema of the lower extremities, and breast discomfort or enlargement. In males, feminization may occur, including changes in the fat deposit sites, atrophy of the sex organs, and loss of facial or body hair. Estrogens can cause retention of sodium and water, resulting in weight gain, edema, and hypertension.

What are the contraindications and interactions?

The estrogens are contraindicated in women with breast cancer, pregnancy, and lactation. Estrogens should be used with caution in patients with liver disease, gallbladder disease, endometriosis, pancreatitis, diabetes mellitus, heart failure, and kidney dysfunction.

Estrogens may interact with barbiturates, phenytoin, and rifampin, possibly causing decreased estrogen effects by increasing its metabolism. Estrogens may interfere with the effects of bromocriptine (Parlodel). They may also increase the levels and toxicity of cyclosporine (Restasis) and theophylline (Bronkodyl), and they may decrease the effectiveness of clofibrate (Atromid-S).

What are the important points patients should know?

Advise patients to take the drug exactly as prescribed and to not omit, increase, or decrease doses without the advice of their physician. Instruct patients about what to do when a dose is missed. Advise patients to review the package inserts to ensure understanding of estrogen therapy. Patients should not breastfeed while taking this drug.

Focus Point

Testosterone Use During Pregnancy

The use of testosterone during pregnancy can cause masculinization of the fetus, particularly if testosterone (androgen) therapy is provided during the first trimester of pregnancy.

Focus on Pediatrics

Estrogens During Pregnancy

Use of conjugated estrogens during the first trimester of pregnancy may increase the risk of fetal malformations, including cleft palate, heart defect, dislocated hips, absent tibiae, and polydactylia (presence of more than five digits on the hands or feet).

Focus on Geriatrics

Estrogen and Menopause

In women taking an estrogen preparation on a long-term basis after menopause, a progestin should be added to estrogen preparations to prevent endometrial hyperplasia and endometrial carcinoma. This practice is not necessary for women who have had a hysterectomy.

Progestins

Progesterone is the primary progestational substance that is naturally produced by ovarian cells of the corpus luteum. It has a physiological action that is unique and distinct from estrogen. Progestin derivatives are synthetic drugs. Table 23-5 ■ provides a summary of several progestins and combination products.

How do they work?

Progesterone transforms the endometrium from a proliferative to a secretory state; it suppresses pituitary gonadotropin secretion, thereby blocking follicular maturation and ovulation. Acting with estrogen, it promotes mammary gland development without causing lactation, and it increases body temperature 1 °F at the time of ovulation. The synthetic progestins are usually preferred for clinical use because of the decreased effectiveness of progesterone when administered orally.

How are they used?

The progestins are prescribed for secondary amenorrhea, functional uterine bleeding, endometriosis, and premenstrual syndrome. As an intrauterine agent (Progestasert), and in combination with estrogens, a progestin provides fertility control, largely supplanted by new progestins, which have longer action and may be taken orally.

What are the adverse effects?

Progestins may result in many adverse effects, and the incidence and intensity of these reactions may be varied. They may cause vaginal candidiasis, chloasma, cervical erosion, breakthrough bleeding, dysmenorrhea, amenorrhea, breast tenderness, edema, acne, pruritus, and mental depression. Thromboembolic disorder, pulmonary embolism, changes in vision, nausea, vomiting, and abdominal cramps are also seen.

What are the contraindications and interactions?

Progestins are contraindicated in patients who are hypersensitive to these agents. Progestins must be avoided in patients with known or suspected breast or genital malignancies. These agents are contraindicated in patients with impaired liver disease, undiagnosed vaginal bleeding, miscarriage, thrombophlebitis, and thromboembolic disorders. Progestins should be used cautiously in anemia, diabetes mellitus, history of psychic depression, previous ectopic pregnancy, presence or history of **salpingitis** (an inflammation or infection of a fallopian tube), and unresolved abnormal Pap smear. Barbiturates, carbamazepine (Tegretol), phenytoin (Dilantin), and rifampin (Rifadin) may alter contraceptive effectiveness. Ketoconazole (Nizoral) may inhibit progesterone metabolism.

What are the important points patients should know?

Advise patients to avoid exposure to UV light and prolonged periods of time in the sun. Tell patients to inform their physician promptly if any of the following occurs: sudden severe headache or vomiting, dizziness or fainting, numbness in an arm or leg, and acute chest pain. Advise patients to also report unexplained sudden or gradual, partial or complete loss of vision, **ptosis** (drooping eyelid), or diplopia. The physician should be notified if the patient becomes pregnant or suspects pregnancy. Patients should not breastfeed while taking these drugs.

Table 23-5 ■ Progestins

GENERIC NAME	TRADE NAME	AVERAGE ADULT DOSAGE	ROUTE OF ADMINISTRATION
hydroxyprogesterone caproate in oil	Hylutin	375 mg q4 weeks	IM
medroxyprogesterone	Amen, Provera	2–10 mg/d × 5–10 d	PO
	Depo-Provera	150 mg q3 mo or 400–1000 mg/wk	IM
megestrol	Megace	40–30 mg 1–4 times/d in divided doses	PO
norethindrone	Micronor, Norlutin	2.5–10 mg in cycles	PO
Combination Products			
estrogen and androgen	Estratest	Tablets of 1.25 mg estrogen/2.5 mg androgen	PO
estrogen and androgen	Depo-Testadiol	2 mg estrogen/50 mg/mL androgen	IM
estrogens and progestins combined	Activelle	Tablets of 1 mg estradiol/0.5 mg norethindrone acetate	PO

Focus Point

Estrogen–Progestin Combinations for Postmenopausal Women

The use of estrogen–progestin combinations for postmenopausal women is very controversial. There are benefits in protection against osteoporosis and colon cancer, but there is an increased relative risk of cardiovascular disease, breast cancer, and thromboembolism.

CONTRACEPTION

The contraceptive methods most commonly used in the United States are (in order of popularity): oral contraceptives (hormones), condoms, withdrawal (coitus interruptus), progestin injections, spermicides, diaphragms, progestin subdermal implants, and intrauterine devices (IUDs). Each method has advantages and disadvantages. In this chapter, only contraceptive hormones are discussed.

Contraceptive Hormones

Oral contraceptives usually consist of combinations of estrogen and progesterone derivatives to prevent pregnancy. Oral contraceptives are also available that contain only progesterone (progestin). Progestin-only contraceptives have a slightly higher failure rate (pregnancy) than do the combination agents. Table 23-6 ■ lists the various types of oral contraceptives.

estrogen, progesterone

4th week placebo

How do they work?

Oral contraceptives provide negative feedback to the hypothalamus and inhibit gonadotropin-releasing hormone. Therefore, the pituitary does not secrete FSH to stimulate ovulation. The endometrium of the uterus becomes thin, and the cervical mucus becomes thick and impervious to sperm. The mechanism of action is not fully understood.

How are they used?

Oral contraceptives are based on hormonal contraception. Combination tablets are taken every day for 3 weeks and then not taken during the fourth week to allow for withdrawal bleeding. Progestin alone is given in a small dose every day and is recommended only when estrogen is contraindicated, for example, during breastfeeding.

What are the adverse effects?

The adverse effects of oral contraceptives include nausea, abdominal pain, gallbladder disease, hepatic adenomas, breast tenderness or pain, weight gain, thromboembolism, stroke, headache, nervousness, dizziness, hypertension, myocardial infarction, and thrombophlebitis. Oral contraceptives may also cause amenorrhea, dysmenorrhea, **menorrhagia** (abnormally heavy or prolonged menstruation), and **metrorrhagia** (uterine bleeding that occurs independent of the normal menstrual period). Other adverse effects include decreased libido and vaginal candidiasis (fungal infection).

What are the contraindications and interactions?

Oral contraceptives are contraindicated in hypersensitivity of any component of the products. These agents should be avoided in pregnant women, in women who suspect pregnancy, and in women with genital bleeding of unknown etiology, thrombophlebitis, or history of thrombophlebitis. Oral contraceptives must be avoided in patients with coronary artery disease; liver dysfunction; carcinoma of the endometrium, breast, or other known estrogen-dependent neoplasia; severe hypertension; and diabetes with vascular involvement. Antibiotics, barbiturates, carbamazepine (Tegretol), fosphenytoin (Cerebyx), griseofulvin (Fulvicin), modafinil (Provigil), phenytoin (Dilantin), and rifampin (Rifadin) may decrease contraceptive effectiveness.

What are the important points patients should know?

Instruct women who are using oral contraceptives to follow the schedule for receiving these agents and to use alternative forms of barrier contraception while taking antibiotics. OTC drugs, including vitamin C or acetaminophen, should not be used without consulting the physician. Instruct patients to report episodes of calf pain or tenderness, shortness of breath, chest pain, visual disturbances, drooping eyelids, or double vision.

Table 23-6 ■ Types of Oral Contraceptives

GENERIC NAME	TRADE NAME	AVERAGE PRESCRIBED DOSAGE
Monophasic Combinations		
estinyl estradiol/desogestrel	Desogen, Mircette	1 active tablet/d for 21 d; then none for 7 d
estinyl estradiol/ethynodiol	Demulen	1 active tablet/d for 21 d; then none for 7 d
estinyl estradiol/levonorgestrel	Alesse, Levlen	30 mcg ethinyl estradiol/0.15 mg levonorgestrel in cycles
estinyl estradiol/norgestimate	Levora, Ortho-cyclin	1 active tablet/d for 21 d; then none for 7 d
estinyl estradiol/norgestrel	Lo-Ovral, Ovral	30 mcg estinyl estradiol/0.3 mg norgestrel in cycles
estrogen/progestin	Alesse-28, Necon 1/35	1 active tablet/d for 21 d; then none for 7 d
ethinyl estradiol/drospirenone	Yasmin	1 active tablet/d for 21 d; then none for 7 d
ethinyl estradiol/norethindrone	Brevicon, Genora	35 mcg ethinyl estradiol/0.5 mg norethindrone in cycles
mestranol/norethindrone	Genora 1/50, Nelova 1/50	50 mcg mestranol/1 mg norethindrone in cycles

(continued)

Table 23-6 ■ Types of Oral Contraceptives (*continued*)

GENERIC NAME	TRADE NAME	AVERAGE PRESCRIBED DOSAGE
Biphasic Combinations		
ethinyl estradiol/norethindrone	Nelova 10/11, Ortho-Novum 10/11	35 mcg ethinyl estradiol/0.5 mg norethindrone (×10 tablets) or 1 mg norethindrone (×11 tablets) in cycles
Triphasic Combinations		
ethinyl estradiol/levonorgestrel	Tri-Levlen, Triphasil	30 mcg ethinyl estradiol (×6 or 10 d) or 40 mcg ethinyl estradiol (×5 days)/0.05 mg levonorgestrel (×6 d) or 0.075 mg levonorgestrel (×5 d) or 0.125 mg levonorgestrel (×10 d) in cycles
ethinyl estradiol/norethindrone	Ortho-Novum 7/7/7, Tri/Norinyl	35 mcg ethinyl estradiol/0.5 mg norethindrone (×5 or 7 d) or 1 mg norethindrone (×9 d) in cycles
ethinyl estradiol/norgestimate	Ortho TriCyclen	1 active tablet/d for 21 d; then none for 7 d
Estrophasic Combinations		
ethinyl estradiol/norethindrone	Estrostep	1 active tablet/d for 21 d; then none for 7 d
Progestin-Only Medications		
norethindrone	Micronor, Nor-Q.D.	0.35 mg/d starting on Day 1 of menstrual flow, continuing indefinitely
norgestrel	Ovrette	0.075 mg/d starting on Day 1 of menstrual flow, continuing indefinitely

[handwritten annotation: (birthcontrol) side effect.]

Focus Point

Oral Contraceptives and Surgery

Oral contraceptives should be discontinued at least 4 weeks before a surgical procedure because of the risk for postoperative thromboembolic complications.

✳ Apply Your Knowledge 23.2

The following questions focus on what you have just learned about the female reproductive system and female sex hormones. *See Appendix E for the correct answers.*

MULTIPLE CHOICE

Choose the correct answers from choices a–e.

1. Estrogen therapy is contraindicated in women with which of the following disorders?

    a. Meningitis

    b. Cystitis

    c. Breast cancer

    d. Bone cancer

    e. Brain cancer

2. Which of the following is the most abundant of the estrogens?

   a. Estrone

   b. Estradiol

   c. Estriol

   d. Megestrol

   e. Conjugated estrogen

3. Which of the following hormones increases hair growth in the pubic and axillary regions?

   a. Growth hormone

   b. Progesterone

   c. Estrogen

   d. Androgen of the adrenal cortices

   e. Aldosterone

4. Which of the following hormones suppresses pituitary gonadotropin secretion to prevent ovulation?

   a. Progesterone

   b. Estrogen

   c. Insulin

   d. Corticosteroid

   e. Thyroxin

5. Progestins are contraindicated in patients with known or suspected:

   a. Functional uterine bleeding

   b. Premenstrual syndrome

   c. Endometriosis

   d. Genital malignancy

   e. Genital herpes

FILL IN THE BLANK

Select terms from your reading to fill in the blanks.

1. Estrogen therapy in men may cause _____.

2. Progesterone is the primary progestational substance produced by ovarian cells of the _____.

3. Estrogens stimulate enlargement of accessory organs of the female reproductive system, including the _____, _____, _____, _____, and _____.

4. The hypothalamus secretes gonadotropin-releasing hormone to stimulate the _____ to release the _____.

5. For the patient taking an estrogen preparation on a long-term basis, a progestin should be added to prevent _____ and _____.

MATCHING

Match the lettered term to the numbered definition.

DEFINITION	TERM
1. _____ Space between the labia minora	a. Clitoris
2. _____ Protect(s) openings of the vagina and urethra	b. Uterus
3. _____ Produce(s) oocytes	c. Labia minora
4. _____ Produce(s) feelings of pleasure	d. Ovaries
5. _____ Sustain(s) embryo during pregnancy	e. Vestibule

Focus on Natural Products

Kelp for Menorrhagia

Kelp is seaweed found in the Atlantic and Pacific Oceans that, in traditional herbal medicine, has been used to treat menorrhagia. It is available as a fluid or soft extract, tablets or gel tabs, and in dried whole plant form. Until more research is done, kelp should not be used during pregnancy and lactation, and should not be given to children, the elderly, or persons with cardiac disorders. It may decrease the effects of thyroid hormones.

Focus Point

Smoking and Oral Contraceptives

Women must avoid smoking while using oral contraceptives. Smoking greatly increases the risk of serious cardiovascular adverse effects.

LABOR AND DELIVERY

Pregnancy usually continues for 38 weeks after conception. Pregnancy ends with the *birth process*. A period of rapid changes and intense physical demands on the pregnant woman begins hours or days before the birth.

The declining progesterone concentration plays a major role in initiating birth. During pregnancy, progesterone suppresses uterine contractions. As the placenta ages, the progesterone concentration within the uterus declines, which stimulates synthesis of a prostaglandin that promotes uterine contractions. At the same time, the cervix begins to thin and then open. Changes in the cervix may begin a week or two weeks before other signs of labor occur.

Another stimulant of the birth process is the stretching of uterine and vaginal tissues late in the pregnancy. This initiates nerve impulses to the hypothalamus, which in turn signals the posterior pituitary gland to release the hormone **oxytocin**. Oxytocin stimulates powerful uterine contractions and aids labor in its later stages.

Uterine relaxants are useful in the process of preterm labor. These agents decrease uterine contraction and prolong the pregnancy to permit the fetus to develop more fully, therefore promoting neonatal survival. Oxytocic agents and uterine relaxants are listed in Table 23-7 ■.

Table 23-7 ■ Effects of Drugs on Labor and Delivery

GENERIC NAME	TRADE NAME	AVERAGE ADULT DOSAGE	ROUTE OF ADMINISTRATION
Oxytocics			
ergonovine	Ergotrate	0.2 mg q2–4h	IM, IV, IV
methylergonovine	Methergine	0.2–0.4 mg q6–12 h until danger of atony passes (2–7 d)	PO
		0.2 mg q2–4 h (max: 5 doses)	IM, IV

Table 23-7 ■ Effects of Drugs on Labor and Delivery

GENERIC NAME	TRADE NAME	AVERAGE ADULT DOSAGE	ROUTE OF ADMINISTRATION
oxytocin	Pitocin	Antepartum: 1 mU/min, increase by 1 mU/min q15min (max: 20 mU/min)	IV
		Postpartum: Infuse total of 10 U at rate of 20–40 mU/min after delivery	
Uterine Relaxants			
ritodrine	Yutopar	0.05–0.35 mg/min	IV
terbutaline	Brethaire	10 mcg/min q10min to 80 mcg/min	IV
		250 mg/h until contractions stop	SC
		2.5 mg q4–6h until delivery	PO

[handwritten annotation next to oxytocin: "excelerates delivery."]

Oxytocic Agents

Oxytocic drugs are able to induce uterine contractions before birth in normal labor. These agents are desirable in early vaginal delivery to stimulate the uterus.

How do they work?
Oxytocic drugs are identical pharmacologically to the oxytocic principle of the posterior pituitary gland. By direct action on uterine muscle, this produces phasic contractions characteristic of normal delivery. These agents also promote the milk ejection (letdown) reflex in nursing mothers, thereby increasing the flow of milk. Uterine sensitivity to oxytocin (Pitocin) increases during the gestation period and peaks sharply before birth.

How are they used?
Oxytocic drugs are used to initiate or improve uterine contraction at term only in carefully selected patients, only after the cervix is dilated, and after presentation of the fetus has occurred. These drugs are also used to stimulate letdown reflex in nursing mothers and to relieve pain from breast engorgement. Oxytocic drugs are prescribed for management of inevitable, incomplete, or missed abortion; control of postpartum hemorrhage; and promotion of postpartum uterine involution. Oxytocic drugs are also used to induce labor in cases of maternal diabetes and preeclampsia or eclampsia.

What are the adverse effects?
The adverse effects of oxytocic drugs are varied. Generally, they cause nausea, vomiting, maternal cardiac arrhythmias, hypertensive episodes, chest pain, dizziness, headache, and intracranial (within the cranium) hemorrhage. Allergic reactions may also occur.

What are the contraindications and interactions?
The oxytocic preparations are contraindicated in hypersensitive patients. Ergonovine (Ergotrate) and methylergonovine (Methergine) must be avoided in patients with hypertension and preeclampsia. They are not to be used to induce labor or prior to delivery of the placenta. Oxytocin injection is contraindicated in patients with significant cephalopelvic disproportion (the fetal head is too large to pass through the mother's pelvis), an unfavorable fetal position or presentation (undeliverable without conversion before delivery), obstetric emergencies in which the benefit-to-risk ratio for mother or fetus favors surgical intervention, and fetal distress in which delivery is not imminent. Oxytocin should be avoided in placenta previa or in those with previous cesarean section.

Oxytocic drugs may interact with vasoconstrictor drugs, causing severe hypertension. They may also interact with cyclopropane anesthesia, causing hypotension, maternal bradycardia, and arrhythmias. Some herbal supplements, such as ephedra and mahuang, may cause hypertension.

What are the important points patients should know?

Instruct patients to report severe cramping, increased bleeding, cold or numb fingers or toes, nausea, vomiting, chest pain, and sudden, severe headache immediately to health-care providers. Advise patients to avoid breastfeeding while taking ergonovine or methylergonovine.

Uterine Relaxants

Uterine relaxants are beta$_2$-adrenergic agonists that are prescribed as uterine relaxants in the management of preterm (premature) labor. Ritodrine (Yutopar) and terbutaline (Bricanyl) are two drugs currently used as uterine relaxants.

How do they work?

Beta$_2$-adrenergic agonists are clinically effective in preventing or delaying preterm labor because of their tocolytic effect. Uterine contractions decrease in frequency and intensity during treatment.

How are they used?

Beta$_2$-adrenergic agonists are used to manage premature labor in selected patients.

What are the adverse effects?

Ritodrine and terbutaline alter maternal and fetal heart rates and maternal blood pressure (dose-related). They can also cause chest pain, palpitations, arrhythmias, and pulmonary edema. Additional common adverse effects of beta$_2$-adrenergic agonists include headache, nausea, vomiting, nervousness, restlessness, sweating, and emotional upset.

What are the contraindications and interactions?

Ritodrine should be avoided in patients with antepartum hemorrhage, eclampsia, uncontrolled diabetes mellitus, bronchial asthma, and pulmonary hypertension. Terbutaline is contraindicated in patients with severe cardiac disorders, digital toxicity, and hypertension. Both ritodrine and terbutaline are given cautiously in patients with cardiac disease, hyperthyroidism, seizure disorders, and migraine headaches.

Corticosteroids may interact with ritodrine and may precipitate pulmonary edema. Epinephrine (Bronkaid Mist) and other sympathomimetic bronchodilators may increase the effects of terbutaline.

What are the important points patients should know?

Advise patients about the potential adverse effects and drug interactions of these agents. Instruct women to avoid breastfeeding while taking beta$_2$-adrenergic agonist drugs. Patients must be instructed to review instructions for use of inhalators and how to take their own pulses.

✳ Apply Your Knowledge 23.3

The following questions focus on what you have just learned about labor and delivery, and drugs that affect labor and delivery. *See Appendix E for the correct answers.*

MATCHING

Match the lettered drug trade name to the numbered generic name.

GENERIC NAME	TRADE NAME
1. _____ ritodrine	a. Ergotrate
2. _____ oxytocin	b. Methergine
3. _____ ergonovine	c. Brethaire
4. _____ terbutaline	d. Pitocin
5. _____ methylergonovine	e. Yutopar

MULTIPLE CHOICE

Choose the correct answer from choices a–e.

1. Which of the following hormones is released by the posterior pituitary gland?

    a. Prolactin

    b. Growth hormone

    c. Diuretic hormone

    d. Oxytocin

    e. Estrogen

2. Which of the following hormones promotes the milk ejection (letdown) reflex?

    a. Oxytocin

    b. Prolactin

    c. Estrogen

    d. Testosterone

    e. Growth hormone

3. Which of the following agents can be used to manage premature labor in selected patients?

    a. Epinephrine

    b. Testosterone

    c. Oxytocin

    d. Terbutaline

    e. Corticosteroid

4. The oxytocic preparations are contraindicated in all of the following conditions, except:

    a. to induce labor

    b. to promote milk ejection

    c. in hypertension

    d. in preeclampsia

    e. in placenta previa

5. Which of the following hormones plays a major role in initiating birth?

    a. Estrogen

    b. Oxytocin

    c. Prolactin

    d. Progesterone

    e. Prolactin

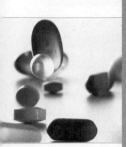

Chapter Capsule

This section repeats the objectives from the beginning of the chapter and then provides a summary of the most important concepts for that objective. Use this section as a quick review and to check your knowledge.

Objective 1: Describe the male and female reproductive structures.

- Male—testes, epididymis, vas deferens, seminal vesicle, prostate gland, bulbourethral (Cowper's) glands, scrotum, penis
- Female—ovaries, uterine tubes, uterus, vagina, labia majora, labia minora, clitoris, and vestibule

Objective 2: Discuss the male and female sex hormones, and their effects on the reproductive system.

- Male sex hormones—androgens
  - Testosterone—most abundant
  - Between 13 and 15 years of age, a young man's androgen production usually increases rapidly as he reaches puberty
  - After puberty, testosterone secretion continues throughout the life of a male
- Female sex hormones: estrogen and progesterone
  - Several tissues, including the tissues of the ovaries, adrenal cortices, and placenta (during pregnancy), secrete female sex hormones
  - Estradiol—most abundant estrogen
  - At puberty, under the influence of the anterior pituitary, the ovaries secrete increasing amounts of estrogens, which stimulate enlargement of accessory organs, including the vagina, uterus, uterine tubes, ovaries, and external reproductive structures
  - Estrogens—develop and maintain *female secondary sex characteristics*
  - Progesterone promotes changes in the uterus during the female reproductive cycle, affects the mammary glands, and helps regulate the secretion of gonadotropins from the anterior pituitary

Objective 3: Explain the contraindications of estrogens.

- Contraindicated in women with breast cancer, or who are pregnant or lactating
- Used with caution in liver disease, gallbladder disease, endometriosis, pancreatitis, diabetes mellitus, heart failure, and kidney dysfunction

Objective 4: Describe how oral contraceptives work to prevent pregnancy.

- Provide negative feedback to the hypothalamus and inhibit gonadotropin-releasing hormone
- Pituitary does not secrete FSH to stimulate ovulation; endometrium of the uterus becomes thin; and cervical mucus becomes thick and impervious to sperm

Objective 5: Discuss menopause and hormone therapy.

- Postmenopausal patients who are on long-term estrogen therapy should be given progestin, too, to prevent endometrial hyperplasia and endometrial carcinoma
- Progestin is not given to women who have had a hysterectomy

Objective 6: Provide information about androgens and anabolic steroids.

- Chief drugs that affect the male reproductive system

- Synthetic steroids that compound with both androgenic and anabolic activity to control the development and maintenance of secondary sexual characteristics

- Androgenic activity: responsible for growth spurt of adolescents and growth termination by epiphyseal closure

- Anabolic activity: increases protein metabolism and decreases its catabolism; large doses suppress spermatogenesis, thereby causing testicular atrophy

- Androgens: antagonize effects of estrogen excess in the female breasts and endometrium

Objective 7: Explain the indications of androgens.

- Main indications in men: to supplement low levels of testosterone to correct hypogonadism or cryptorchidism

- Also used to increase sperm production in cases of infertility

- Indications in women: palliative treatment of metastatic breast cancer; for treatment of postpartum breast engorgement, endometriosis, and fibrocystic breast disorder

- Able to stimulate increased production of red blood cells, protein synthesis, and muscle mass; athletes may use androgens to improve athletic performance

Objective 8: Discuss the major adverse effects of progestins.

- Vaginal candidiasis, chloasma, cervical erosion, breakthrough bleeding, dysmenorrhea, amenorrhea, breast tenderness, edema, acne, pruritus, and mental depression

- Thromboembolic disorder, pulmonary embolism, changes in vision, nausea, vomiting, and abdominal cramps also seen

Objective 9: Describe the contraindications of oral contraceptives.

- Hypersensitivity of any component of the products; should be avoided in pregnant women, women who suspect pregnancy, women with genital bleeding of unknown etiology, thrombophlebitis, or history of thrombophlebitis

- Must be avoided in patients with coronary artery disease, liver dysfunction, carcinoma of the endometrium, breast, or other known estrogen-dependent neoplasia, severe hypertension, and diabetes with vascular involvement

Objective 10: Explain the mechanism of action of oxytocic drugs.

- Identical pharmacologically to the oxytocic principle of posterior pituitary

- By direct action on uterine muscle, they produce phasic contractions characteristic of normal delivery

- They also promote milk ejection (letdown) reflex in nursing mothers, thereby increasing flow of milk

- Uterine sensitivity to oxytocin (Pitocin) increases during the gestation period and peaks sharply before birth

Internet Sites of Interest

- Further information about contraceptive options can be found at: **http://womenshealth.about.com**. Search for "prevent pregnancy."

- Personal stories of menopause and hormone therapy are available at: **www.4woman.gov/Menopause**

- Visit the National Institute on Drug Abuse at **http://www.nida.nih.gov/Infofacts/Steroids.html** for information on anabolic steroids.

- Information about the safety, availability, and efficacy of emergency contraception is available at: **www.contraceptiononline.org**. Click on "The Contraception Report."

Chapter Objectives

After completing this chapter, you should be able to:

1. Describe the major parts of the digestive system.
2. Explain how medications are absorbed from the gastrointestinal (GI) tract and metabolized.
3. Describe the use of histamine-2 (H_2)-receptor antagonists in the treatment of peptic ulcers.
4. Describe the use of antacids in the treatment of peptic ulcers.
5. Explain the effects of prostaglandins on the digestive tract.
6. List four generic names and trade names of proton pump inhibitors.
7. Explain the problems associated with laxative use.
8. Describe the drug treatment for diarrhea.
9. Describe the mechanism of action of bulk-forming laxatives, osmotic laxatives, and laxative stimulants.

Chapter 24

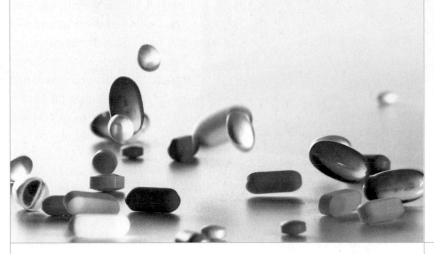

Effects of Drugs on Gastrointestinal Disorders

Key Terms

Alimentary canal (page 522)
Aluminum hydroxide (page 526)
Amylase (AM-mil-lace) (page 522)

Magnesium carbonate (page 526)
Melanosis (page 536)
Osmosis (oz-MOH-sis) (page 534)

Paralytic ileus (par-uh-LIT-tik ILL-ee-us) (page 533)
Ulcers (page 523)

PRACTICAL SCENARIO

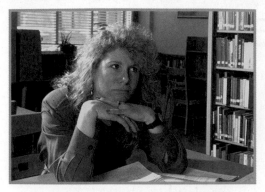

Source: Antonia Deutsch
© Dorling Kindersley.

A 26-year-old woman in graduate school visits the family physician because for the past 3 to 4 months, she has been experiencing gnawing pains in her upper-middle abdomen. When you ask her what seems to precipitate the pain, she is unable to say for sure. She says she feels the best in the early morning before eating. As the day progresses, she usually feels worse and worse and takes Mylanta or Milk of Magnesia to relieve the pain. Sometimes her pain is accompanied by severe diarrhea, and she has been tired, weak, and nauseous. In response to your question about stress, she tells you she is under extreme stress because she is preparing to defend her thesis for her Ph.D. She has been smoking more cigarettes than usual and drinking 6 to 8 cups of coffee each morning. In the evening, she often has a few glasses of wine to help her relax.

Critical Thinking Questions

1. Based on this patient's complaints, lifestyle, and use of OTC medications, what do you expect may be the cause of her initial complaint of upper middle of abdomen pain and her symptoms of fatigue, weakness, and nausea?

2. What diagnostic tests do you anticipate the physician ordering and for what possible diagnoses?

3. Instead of OTC antacids, what are the other choices for this patient to relieve her symptoms? Is there a class of medications that you think might be the better choice for her, and if so, why?

Introduction

Growth of the body depends on the consumption, absorption, and metabolism of food. The gastrointestinal (GI) tract is involved in the first essential components of these processes and is subject to many disease conditions, some of which are very common. It is not surprising that there are a number of drugs to treat these varying conditions. Because of the number of drugs available, it is helpful for discussion to divide the GI tract into two parts: the upper part (from the mouth to the stomach) and the lower part (from the duodenum to the anus). Some problems of the GI tract, specifically nausea and vomiting, are sometimes associated with the central nervous system (CNS).

The Digestive System

The digestive system consists of the alimentary canal, which extends about 8 meters from the mouth to the anus, and several accessory organs that secrete substances used in the process of digestion into the canal. The **alimentary canal** includes the mouth, pharynx, esophagus, stomach, small intestine, large intestine, rectum, and anus; the accessory organs include the salivary glands, liver, gallbladder, and pancreas (Figure 24-1 ■). Overall, the digestive system is a tube, open at both ends, that has a surface area of 186 square meters. It supplies nutrients for body cells. Therefore, digestion changes food into its simpler constituents prior to absorption.

Primary digestion occurs in the mouth. When food is ingested in the mouth, it is chewed and mixed with saliva that is excreted from the three major pairs of salivary glands: the parotid, submandibular, and sublingual glands. Saliva contains the digestive enzyme **amylase**. The three processes—digestion, absorption, and metabolism—begin here in the mouth.

Organ	Primary Functions
Salivary Glands	Provide lubrication, produce buffers and the enzymes that begin digestion
Pharynx	Passageway connected to esophagus
Esophagus	Delivers food to stomach
Stomach	Secretes acids and enzymes
Small Intestine	Secretes digestive enzymes, absorbs nutrients
Liver	Secretes bile, regulates blood chemistry
Gallbladder	Stores bile for release into small intestine
Pancreas	Secretes digestive enzymes and buffers; contains endocrine cells
Large Intestine	Removes water from fecal material, stores waste

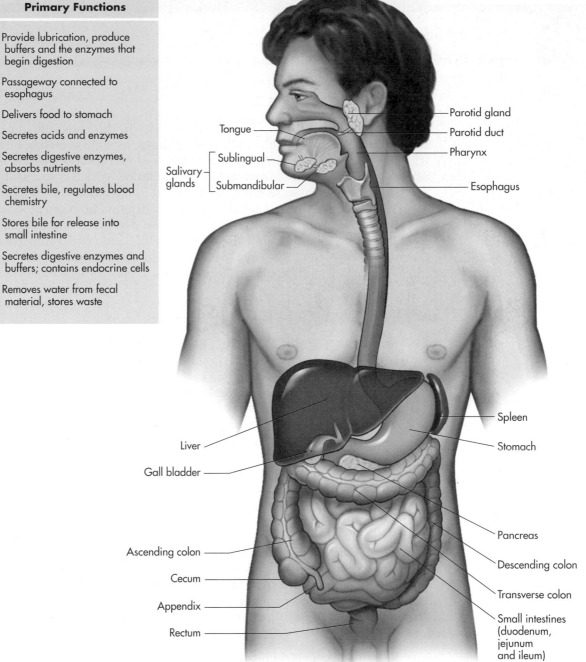

Figure 24-1 ■ The disgestive system.

The 25-cm-long esophagus is a straight tube through which food passes from the pharynx to the stomach. When food enters the stomach from the mouth and esophagus, it is mixed with stomach juices that include hydrochloric acid and some enzymes such as pepsin, which breaks it into much smaller, digestible pieces. The final stages of chemical digestion occur in the small intestine, where almost all nutrients from the ingested food are absorbed. Excessive secretions of hydrochloric acid, under certain conditions, may break down the gastric surface and cause sores or **ulcers** (breaks in mucuos membranes with loss of surface tissue, disintegration, and necrosis). The term *gastric ulcer* is used interchangeably with *peptic ulcer* for this condition. Peptic ulcer disease (PUD) is the most common disorder of the stomach.

Focus Point

Gastric Juice

The 40 million cells that line the stomach's interior can secrete 2 to 3 quarts (about 2 to 3 liters) of gastric juice per day—no wonder peptic ulcer disease is so common!

The liver is the center of metabolic activity in the body, playing a very important role in the digestion and absorption of nutrients, as well as metabolic activities. Detoxification (removal of toxins from the blood) and secretion of bile are the key functions of the liver. The pancreas secretes pancreatic juice, which contains digestive enzymes such as amylase, lipase, and nucleases, to aid in digestion.

The small intestine is a tubular organ that extends from the pyloric sphincter of the stomach to the beginning of the large intestine. The small intestine receives secretions from the pancreas and liver. It also completes digestion of the nutrients and absorbs the products of digestion. The small intestine transports residue to the large intestine. The large intestine absorbs water and electrolytes. It also forms and stores feces.

Peptic Ulcers

The problems associated with hyperacidity and excessive pepsin activity, some of which may be related to lifestyle choices, may eventually lead to the formation of a gastric or duodenal ulcer. Alcohol and caffeine have been linked to irritation of the mucosal lining of both the esophagus and stomach. Smoking has been linked to greater volume and concentration of gastric acid. Upper GI radiography is usually performed to diagnose PUD or gastroesophageal reflux disease (GERD).

Several groups of drugs have revolutionized the pharmacologic treatment of ulcers. There are three receptors in the stomach wall that need to be stimulated to cause the production of hydrochloric acid. These are the histamine-2 (H_2)-receptors, muscarinic cholinergic receptors, and gastrin receptors. Gastric ulcers are caused mainly by a defect in mucus production, whereas duodenal ulcers usually result from an increase in acid production. This makes the treatment of each somewhat different.

Many cases of gastric ulcer or gastritis (inflammation of the stomach) are due to the bacterium *Helicobacter pylori*. In bacteria-related peptic ulcers, successful treatment usually includes a combination of antibacterials such as metronidazole (Flagyl), amoxicillin (Amoxil), or tetracyclines, with agents such as colloidal bismuth or omeprazole (Prilosec). Colloidal bismuth in combination with two antibacterials is sometimes referred to as "triple therapy." Table 24-1 ■ summarizes drugs commonly used to treat peptic ulcers.

Table 24-1 ■ Drugs Commonly Used in Peptic Ulcer Disease

GENERIC NAME	TRADE NAME	AVERAGE ADULT DOSAGE	ROUTE OF ADMINISTRATION
Antacids			
aluminum hydroxide	Amphojel	600 mg tid–qid	PO
calcium carbonate	Titralac, Tums	1–2 g bid–tid	PO
calcium carbonate with magnesium hydroxide	Mylanta Gel-caps, Rolaids	2–4 capsules or tablets PRN (max: 12 tablets/d)	PO
magaldrate	Riopan	480–1,080 mg (5–10 mL suspension or 1–2 tablets) 4 times/d (max: 20 tablets or 100 mL/d)	PO

Table 24-1 ■ Drugs Commonly Used in Peptic Ulcer Disease

GENERIC NAME	TRADE NAME	AVERAGE ADULT DOSAGE	ROUTE OF ADMINISTRATION
magnesium hydroxide	Milk of Magnesia	2.4–4.8 g (30–60 mL)/d in 1 or more divided doses	PO
magnesium hydroxide / aluminum hydroxide with simethicone	Mylanta, Maalox Plus	10–20 mL PRN (max: 120 mL/d) or 2–4 tablets PRN (max: 24 tablets/d)	PO
sodium bicarbonate	Alka-Seltzer, baking soda	0.3–2 g 1–4 times/d or 1/2 tsp of powder in glass of water	PO
H₂-Receptor Antagonists			
cimetidine	Tagamet	800 mg/d in divided doses	PO
		300 mg q6–8h	IM, IV
famotidine	Pepcid	20–40 mg/d in divided doses	PO
		20 mg q12h	IV
nizatidine	Axid	300 mg at bedtime or in 2 divided doses	PO
ranitidine	Zantac	300 mg/d in 2 divided doses	PO
		50 mg q6–8h; 150–300 mg/24 h by continuous infusion	IV
Proton Pump Inhibitors			
esomeprazole	Nexium	20–40 mg/d	PO
lansoprazole	Prevacid	15–30 mg/d	PO
omeprazole	Prilosec	20–40 mg/d	PO
pantoprazole	Protonix	40 mg/d for 8–16 wk	PO
		40 mg/d for 7–10 d	IV
rabeprazole	AcipHex	20 mg/d	PO
Combination Medications			
bismuth-tetracycline-metronidazole	Helidac	1 blister pack/d for 14 d	PO
bismuth-ranitidine	Tritec	1 blister pack/d for 14 d	PO
Prostaglandins			
misoprostol	Cytotec	100–200 mcg qid with food	PO

Antacids

Antacids are alkaline compounds that may be used to neutralize hydrochloric acid in the stomach, thereby relieving the pain of hyperacidity, or even peptic ulcer.

How do they work?

The antacids are weak bases that readily combine with and neutralize hydrochloric acid. The combination of an antacid with digestive acid produces water and carbon dioxide gas.

How are they used?

The bases used in antacid preparations are usually basic compounds of aluminum, magnesium, sodium, calcium, and potassium. Of these, the most common are **aluminum hydroxide** (Amphojel) and **magnesium carbonate**, usually used in combination. Antacids counteract hyperacidity of the stomach, protect from peptic ulcers, and promote ulcer healing.

What are the adverse effects?

Depending on the type of antacid, the most common adverse effects may be diarrhea or constipation. For example, the magnesium and sodium-containing antacids may cause diarrhea. Calcium and aluminum-containing products can produce constipation. The other adverse effects that are less common, but more serious, include anorexia, weakness, bone pain, and tremors (aluminum-containing antacids). Hypermagnesemia may produce nausea, vomiting, confusion, renal calculi, metabolic alkalosis, and headache. Neurologic disorders sometimes occur with the use of calcium-containing antacids.

What are the contraindications and interactions?

The contraindications of antacids depend on their compounds: For example, calcium carbonate (Tums) should not be used in hypercalcemia and hyperparathyroidism, vitamin D overdosage, and decalcifying tumors. Calcium carbonate is also contraindicated in severe renal disease, renal calculi, ventricular fibrillation, and pregnancy. Magnesium-containing antacids are contraindicated in hypermagnesemia and pregnancy.

Antacids should be used cautiously in patients with impaired kidney function, lactation, and dialysis of the kidneys. Calcium carbonate should be used with caution in older adults and in lactating patients. Some antacids may interact with digoxin (Lanoxin). Calcium-containing antacids may decrease absorption of tetracyclines and ciprofloxacin (Cipro).

What are the important points patients should know?

Instruct patients to take antacids 1 to 3 hours after meals and at bedtime. Patients must avoid taking antacids within 1 to 2 hours of other oral medications. Advise them to increase fluid intake to about 3,000 mL per day to prevent kidney stones. Instruct those with heart disease, or those on sodium-restricted diets, to avoid antacids high in sodium content. Teach patients to alternate an aluminum- or calcium-salt antacid with a magnesium-salt antacid to prevent diarrhea or constipation. Remind patients that antacids should be used only for symptomatic relief and that they should notify their physician if relief does not occur in a day or two.

Focus on Geriatrics

Cautious Use of Tums in Older Adults

Calcium carbonate (Tums) should be used with caution in older adults because it is contraindicated in a wide variety of diseases and conditions that affect the elderly, including calcium loss due to immobilization, renal disease, renal calculi, ventricular fibrillation, and cardiac disease.

H$_2$-Receptor Antagonists

The H$_2$-receptor antagonists, of which cimetidine (Tagamet) is the prototype, were a huge discovery in the treatment of PUD and GERD.

How do they work?

Acid secretion is stimulated by H$_2$-receptor activation. H$_2$-receptor antagonists reduce the secretion of gastric acid from stomach cells by blocking these receptors.

How are they used?

H_2-receptor antagonists are used in short-term treatment of active duodenal ulcer and prevention of ulcer recurrence (at reduced dosage). They are also used for short-term treatment of active benign gastric ulcer, pathologic hypersecretory conditions such as Zollinger–Ellison syndrome, and heartburn.

What are the adverse effects?

The most common adverse effects are GI disturbances, headache, drowsiness, confusion, agitation, hallucinations, and reversible impotence. H_2-receptor antagonists may also cause cardiac arrhythmias and cardiac arrest after rapid IV bolus dose.

What are the contraindications and interactions?

These medications are contraindicated in patients with known hypersensitivity to cimetidine (Tagamet) or other H_2-receptor antagonists. They must not be used in lactating or pregnant patients, or in children younger than 16 years.

What are the important points patients should know?

Warn patients to avoid smoking and drinking alcohol while taking H_2-receptor antagonists because these substances can impede the effectiveness of the drug.

Proton Pump Inhibitors

Several compounds have been investigated because of their ability to block hydrochloric acid production.

How do they work?

The formation of hydrochloric acid depends on the production of hydrogen ions (protons) in the parietal cells, and proton pump inhibitors block this production.

How are they used?

Proton pump inhibitors are used to heal stomach and duodenal ulcers, and to relieve symptoms of GERD and esophagitis.

What are the adverse effects?

The common adverse effects of proton pump inhibitors include headache, dizziness, fatigue, diarrhea, abdominal pain, nausea, skin rash, and, rarely, hematuria.

What are the contraindications and interactions?

Long-term use of proton pump inhibitors for GERD or duodenal ulcers is contraindicated. These drugs should not be used in hypersensitive patients or in children younger than 18 years. Proton pump inhibitors should be avoided in pregnancy and in patients with GI bleeding.

What are the important points patients should know?

Advise patients that treatment with proton pump inhibitors is for a short course of therapy only. Treatment is usually limited to about 4–8 weeks.

Focus on Pediatrics

Use Care in Choosing OTC Medications for Children

OTC formulations of omeprazole, such as Prilosec and Zegerid, must not be used in children younger than 18. Omeprazole has not been significantly tested in children.

Prostaglandins

The prostaglandins are perhaps the most versatile and powerful substances used to treat GI disorders. They affect GI motility and gastric acid secretions.

How do they work?

Prostaglandins produce a variety of actions on the body. The effects of these substances (related to the stomach) include inhibition of gastric acid and gastrin production, stimulation of mucus, and secretion of bicarbonate. The prostaglandin analogue misoprostol (Cytotec) is most commonly used, and, though not as effective as the H_2-receptor antagonists, it has been effective in some cases when treatment with the latter has not been effective.

How are they used?

Prostaglandins tend to be antagonistic to ulcer formation in both the stomach and the duodenum. This avenue seems to offer a promising new approach to ulcer therapeutics in certain cases. Prostaglandins are used to prevent complications of gastric ulcers that result from nonsteroidal anti-inflammatory drugs (NSAIDs), especially in patients at high risk for complications from a gastric ulcer—for example, older adults and patients with a concomitant debilitating disease or a history of ulcers. These drugs are taken for the duration of NSAID therapy and do not interfere with the efficacy of the NSAID.

What are the adverse effects?

Prostaglandins, such as misoprostol (Cytotec), can cause diarrhea in some patients, which is usually mild and of short duration. The only other significant adverse effect is menorrhagia in women.

What are the contraindications and interactions?

Prostaglandins should not be used in pregnancy because they may induce premature labor by increasing uterine tone and contractility. Prostaglandins are contraindicated in lactation and in a history of allergies to prostaglandins.

What are the important points patients should know?

Ask female patients if they are, or might be, pregnant because prostaglandins are contraindicated. Tell female patients that these agents may cause women of childbearing age to experience spontaneous abortion, so they should use reliable contraception. Advise patients that diarrhea may occur with these drugs but will disappear after the first month of therapy.

❋ Apply Your Knowledge 24.1 ▬▬▬▬

The following questions focus on what you have just learned about the digestive system, peptic ulcers, and related medications. *See Appendix E for the correct answers.*

FILL IN THE BLANK

Select terms from your reading to fill in the blanks.

1. The accessory organs of the digestive system include the _____, _____, _____, and _____.

2. Three processes that occur in the alimentary canal include _____, _____, and _____.

3. Excessive secretions of hydrochloric acid in the stomach may cause _____.

4. The length of the digestive system extends about _____ from the mouth to the anus, and the surface of it is about _____ square meters.

5. The most common disorder of the stomach is _____.

6. A normal adult's stomach can secrete _____ of gastric juice per day.

7. The liver plays a key role in _____.

8. Completion of the digestion of food occurs in the _____.

MULTIPLE CHOICE

Choose the correct answer from choices a–d.

1. Cimetidine is the prototype of a histamine-receptor antagonist that:

   a. Causes sedation

   b. Is useful for motion sickness

   c. Enhances hepatic drug-metabolizing enzymes

   d. Reduces gastric acid secretion

2. All of the following are receptors in the stomach wall that need to be stimulated to cause the production of hydrochloric acid, except:

   a. H_1-receptors

   b. Muscarinic cholinergic receptors

   c. Gastrin receptors

   d. H_2-receptors

3. Which of the following antimicrobials is used for treatment of gastric ulcer due to the presence of Helicobacter pylori?

   a. Rifampin

   b. Metronidazole

   c. Sulfamethizole

   d. Vancomycin

4. The most common adverse effect of antacids containing calcium or aluminum is:

   a. Constipation

   b. Decreased respiration

   c. Bone pain

   d. Hypotension

5. Which of the following is an example of a prostaglandin that tends to be antagonistic to stomach ulcer formation?

   a. Clotrimazole

   b. Ketoconazole

   c. Misoprostol

   d. Tioconazole

Diarrhea

Diarrhea is defined as an increase in volume, fluidity, or frequency of bowel movements, relative to a particular individual's usual pattern. The causes of this condition are numerous, and consequently, the treatments are varied. In many instances, drug intervention is not required. For example, antidiarrheals are not used in the case of infective gastroenteritis, in which the diarrhea is a protective mechanism used by the body to flush out the offending pathogen. Clearly, the use of drugs to slow down GI motility in such circumstances would be inadvisable. Similarly, the use of antibiotics in diarrhea-causing bacterial infections of the GI tract may kill the offending pathogen, but also kill off some normal bacterial flora. Indeed, the World Health Organization (WHO) recommends that the first-line emergency treatment for diarrhea be rehydration and electrolyte replacement therapy. Diarrhea is usually self-limiting and resolves without further effects. The antidiarrheal drugs may be classified as opioids, synthetic opioid medications, and adsorbents (Table 24-2 ■).

Table 24-2 ■ **Classifications of Antidiarrheal Drugs**

GENERIC NAME	TRADE NAME	TYPE	COMMENTS
bismuth subsalicylate	Pepto-Bismol	Adsorbent	OTC
camphorated opium tincture (paregoric)	(generic)	Opioid	Schedule III
difenoxin hydrochloride with atropine sulfate	Motofen	Opioid	Schedule IV
diphenoxylate hydrochloride with atropine sulfate	Logen, Lomanate, Lomotil, Lonox	Opioid	Schedule V
kaolin and pectin	Kao-Span, Kaolin with Pectin, K-C	Adsorbent	OTC
loperamide	Immodium, Kaopectate III, Maalox Antidiarrheal	Opioid	OTC (Abuse is very low, and it is not classified as a controlled substance.)

Focus Point

Acute Diarrhea in Adults

Usually acute diarrhea in adults is self-limiting. Treatment with an antidiarrheal agent is usually unnecessary. However, symptomatic control may help some adults.

Opioid and Synthetic Opioid Drugs

These drugs require a prescription and are controlled substances. Opioid antidiarrheals are the most effective drugs for controlling diarrhea. Table 24-3 ■ lists the most common antidiarrheals.

How do they work?

Most of the narcotic analgesics can act on opioid receptors in the GI tract and are actually stimulants at these receptors. The stimulus increases the segmentation or mixing movements of the gut and simultaneously decreases the peristaltic movements. These effects, in turn, slow down forward movement and, at the same time, reabsorption.

How are they used?

The most commonly used opioid antidiarrheal drug is camphorated opium tincture (paregoric; generic only). This is a Schedule III drug and requires a prescription. When paregoric is combined with another drug, the medication becomes a Schedule V product—that is, if the combination contains less than 25 mL of paregoric per 100 mL of preparation.

What are the adverse effects?

The main adverse effect of these drugs is a reversal in the movement of the bowels that results in constipation. Other possible adverse effects include nausea, vomiting, agitation, drowsiness, tachycardia, and numbness of the hands and feet.

What are the contraindications and interactions?

Opioid preparations are contraindicated in intestinal obstruction and should be avoided in children younger than 6 years. In patients who have chronic diarrhea, treatment with opioids is not recommended.

What are the important points patients should know?
Encourage patients to keep a record of bowel movements while they are on the medication to determine its effectiveness and possible constipating effect. Advise patients to ingest a clear fluid diet for a few days, avoid fruit juices, and maintain fluid intake of about 3000 mL per day. Patients should avoid the use of alcohol because it promotes diuresis.

Table 24-3 ■ The Most Common Antidiarrheals

GENERIC NAME	TRADE NAME	AVERAGE ADULT DOSAGE	ROUTE OF ADMINISTRATION
bismuth subsalicylate	Pepto-Bismol	30 mL or 2 tablets q30–60 min PRN (max: 8 doses/d)	PO
camphorated opium tincture (paregoric)	(Schedule III generic)	5–10 mL after loose stool, q2h up to 4 times PRN	PO
difenoxin hydrochloride with atropine sulfate	Motofen	Initial dose: 2 tablets (1 mg each); then 1 tablet after each loose stool, or 1 tablet q3–4 h, PRN (max: 8 mg/d)	PO
diphenoxylate hydrochloride with atropine sulfate	Logen, Lomanate, Lomotil, Lonox	Initial dose: 2.5–5 mg tid–qid Maintenance: 2.5 mg bid–tid	PO (solution or tablets)
kaolin and pectin	Kao-Span, Kaolin w/Pectin, K-C	60–120 mL of regular suspension, or 45–90 mL of concentrated suspension after each loose stool	PO
loperamide	Imodium, Kaopectate III, Maalox Antidiarrheal	Initial dose: 4 mg; then 2 mg after each loose stool (max: 16 mg/d)	PO

Focus on Geriatrics

Elderly Patients and Opioid Antidiarrheals

Vital signs should be monitored regularly in older patients taking opioid antidiarrheals. These drugs may cause respiratory depression and decreased blood pressure in elderly individuals.

Adsorbents

The other class of antidiarrheals is adsorbents (see Table 24-3). These preparations are still used in some parts of the world because they are inexpensive and relatively effective.

How do they work?
Adsorbents act by coating the walls of the GI tract and adsorbing the toxins that might be implicated in causing diarrhea.

How are they used?
These medications are usually taken after each loose bowel movement until the diarrhea is controlled.

What are the adverse effects?
Adsorbents may cause constipation, which is usually mild and transient.

What are the contraindications and interactions?

The contraindications of adsorbents include a suspected obstructive bowel lesion, pseudomembranous colitis, diarrhea (associated with bacterial toxins), and the presence of fever. They should not be used for more than 48 hours without medical direction. Safety during pregnancy or lactation is not established. Adsorbents may interact with chloroquine (Aralen), digoxin (Lanoxin), penicillamine (Cuprimine), tetracycline (Achromycin), ciprofloxacin (Cipro), and many other drugs.

What are the important points patients should know?

Instruct patients not to exceed prescribed dosages and to notify their physician if diarrhea is not controlled within 48 hours or if fever develops. Women taking these drugs should not breastfeed without consulting their physician.

✳ Apply Your Knowledge 24.2

The following questions focus on what you have just learned about antidiarrheals. *See Appendix E for the correct answers.*

SOUND-ALIKE DRUG NAMES

Circle the correct answers.

1. Which of the following antidiarrheals is marketed under the trade name Motofen?

    difenoxin hydrochloride with atropine sulfate, or

    diphenoxylate hydrochloride with atropine sulfate

2. Which of the following antidiarrheal trade names corresponds to the generic drug kaolin and pectin?

    Kao-Span

    Kaopectate III

3. Which of the following is an antidiarrheal?

    paromomycin

    paregoric

4. Which of the following is sold under the trade name Immodium?

    loperamide

    lorazepam

5. Which of the following is the generic name for Pepto-Bismol?

    bisoprolol fumarate

    bismuth subsalicylate

MULTIPLE CHOICE

Choose the correct answers from choices a–d.

1. Diarrhea is defined as an increase in volume, fluidity, or frequency of:

    a. Emesis

    b. Digestion

    c. Alkaline components

    d. Bowel movements

2. The first-line emergency treatment for severe diarrhea should be electrolyte replacement therapy and:

   a. Emesis

   b. Antiemetics

   c. Rehydration

   d. Proton pump inhibitors

3. The most effective drugs for controlling diarrhea are:

   a. Opioids

   b. Prostaglandins

   c. Adsorbents

   d. Laxatives

4. Antidiarrheals that act by coating the walls of the GI tract, and are relatively inexpensive, are known as:

   a. Osmotics

   b. Opioids

   c. Adsorbents

   d. Absorbents

5. Because of their ability to cause respiratory depression in elderly patients, which of the following antidiarrheals require that vital signs be regularly monitored?

   a. Electrolytes

   b. Opiates and opiate-related drugs

   c. Osmotics

   d. Chloroquines

Constipation

Many people misunderstand the meaning of the word *constipation* and, therefore, resort to the use of laxatives in cases of what could be termed as "perceived" constipation, that is, slow gut transit time. A common cause of constipation is dehydration due to inadequate liquid ingestion, especially in hot weather and among elderly individuals. Nondietary constipation can be due to **paralytic ileus** (no peristaltic movements in the intestines), which can occur after abdominal surgery. Many drugs, particularly those with antimuscarinic activity, can slow down peristalsis and lead to constipation.

Laxatives, used to combat constipation, are among the most misused drugs because of misperceptions about constipation. Individuals tend to self-treat with easily available OTC drugs. Overuse of laxatives can, in turn, cause constipation. Laxatives are classified into several different categories, depending on their mechanism of action: osmotic (saline) laxatives, stool softeners, stimulants, and bulk-forming laxatives. Table 24-4 ■ presents the characteristics of different laxative categories.

Table 24-4 ■ Categories of Laxatives

GENERIC NAME	TRADE NAME	AVERAGE ADULT DOSAGE	ROUTE OF ADMINISTRATION
Osmotic Laxatives			
lactulose	Cephulac, Chronulac	30–60 mL/d PRN	PO
magnesium citrate	Citrate of Magnesia, Citroma	240 mL/d in 8 oz of water	PO
magnesium hydroxide	Magnesia Magma, Milk of Magnesia	2.4–4.8 g (30–60 mL)/d in 1 or more divided doses	PO
magnesium sulfate	Epsom Salt	10–15 g/d in 8 oz of water	PO
Stool Softeners			
docusate calcium	DCS, Surfak	50–500 mg/d	PO
docusate potassium	Dialose, Diocto-K	50–500 mg/d	PO
docusate sodium	Colace, Dio-Sul	50–500 mg/d	PO
		50–100 mg added to enema fluid	Rectal
glycerin	Glycerol, Osmoglyn	Insert 1 suppository of 5–15 mL of enema high into rectum and retain for 15 min	Rectal
Stimulant Laxatives			
bisacodyl	Apo-Bisacodyl, Dulcolax	5–15 mg PRN (max: 30 mg for special procedures)	PO
		10 mg PRN	Rectal
cascara sagrada	Cascara Sagrada Aromatic Fluidextract, Cascara Sagrada Fluidextract	Tablets: 325–1,000 mg/d; Aromatic Fluidextract: 2–6 mL/d; Fluidextract: 0.5–1.5 mL/d	PO
senna (sennosides)	Black-Draught, Senokot	Standard concentrate: 1–2 tablets or $\frac{1}{2}$–1 tsp at bedtime (max: 4 tablets or 2 tsp bid); Syrup: 10–15 mL at bedtime	PO
Bulk-Forming Laxatives			
polycarbophil	FiberCon, Mitrolan	1 g qid PRN (max: 6 g/d)	PO
psyllium hydrophilic mucilloid	Metamucil, Serutan	1–2 rounded tsp or 1 packet 1–3 times/d PRN	PO

Osmotic Laxatives

Osmotic (or saline) laxatives are a mixture of sodium and magnesium salts.

How do they work?

These drugs work via **osmosis**, in which sodium and magnesium ions attract water into the bowel, causing a more liquid stool to be formed. The contents are hypertonic, causing water to be retained, and if the osmotic pressure is great enough, it can pull water from the bowel's capillaries back into the bowel lumen. This results in a rise in pressure and volume in the colon and rectum, leading to stimulation of the defecation reflex.

How are they used?

Osmotic laxatives are used for short-term treatment of occasional constipation. They also have been used in treatment of poisoning by mineral acids and arsenic, or as mouthwash to neutralize acidity.

What are the adverse effects?

Common adverse effects include nausea, vomiting, abdominal cramps, diarrhea, weakness, lethargy, and electrolyte imbalance. In severe cases, they may cause hypotension, bradycardia, mental depression, and coma.

What are the contraindications and interactions?

The use of osmotic laxatives is contraindicated in patients with renal impairment and hypertension, because sodium ions can be absorbed and accumulate in the blood.

What are the important points patients should know?

Instruct patients that the action of osmotic laxatives does not occur until the drugs reach the colon; therefore, about 24 to 48 hours are needed before an effect results. Advise patients not to self-medicate with another laxative while waiting for the onset of action. Patients should notify their physician if diarrhea (more than two to three soft stools per day) persists more than 24 to 48 hours after taking a laxative. Diarrhea is a sign of overdosage. Dose adjustment may be indicated. Women should not breastfeed while taking these drugs without consulting their physician.

Focus Point

Laxative Abuse

The potential abuse of laxatives should be evaluated in patients suspected of having bulimia nervosa or anorexia nervosa. Elderly patients, whose diets and changing digestive systems may cause them to perceive constipation, may also overuse laxatives. Be alert for volume depletion, which causes serious electrolyte imbalances, especially among elderly patients.

Stool Softeners

Stool softeners are sometimes known as emollients or surfactants. Few of these compounds are in common use. One of them is docusate sodium (Colace).

How do they work?

Docusate sodium has detergent-like properties and seems to act mainly by holding water molecules in the fecal material, thus rendering them softer and easier to pass. Because the main mechanism of action is the softening process, these laxatives do not work quickly. Their effect usually takes several days to become apparent.

How are they used?

Stool softeners are used to ease bowel movements in constipated patients. They are used prophylactically in patients who should avoid straining during defecation, and for treatment of constipation associated with hard and dry stools.

What are the adverse effects?

Stool softeners may cause mild abdominal cramps, diarrhea, nausea, and bitter taste.

What are the contraindications and interactions?

Stool softeners are contraindicated in atonic constipation, nausea, vomiting, abdominal pain, and intestinal obstruction or perforation. These drugs should be used cautiously in patients with a history of congestive heart failure, edema, and diabetes mellitus. Docusate may interact and increase systemic absorption of mineral oil (Milkinol), which is also commonly used as a lubricant to treat constipation.

What are the important points patients should know?
Instruct patients to take sufficient liquids with each dose and increase fluid intake during the day. Advise them that docusate should not be taken for prolonged dietary management.

Focus Point

Diabetes and Laxatives

The blood glucose levels of patients with diabetes must be carefully monitored while taking laxatives that contain high amounts of lactose and galactose.

Laxative Stimulants

Laxative stimulants include cascara sagrada (Cascara Sagrada Fluidextract) and senna (Senokot).

How do they work?
Laxative stimulants are true purgatives in that they directly affect the walls of either the small or large intestine. They cause an increase in peristaltic movements, leading to defecation.

How are they used?
Laxative stimulants are used for temporary relief of constipation in various disease conditions and to prevent straining during defecation. Laxative stimulants are sometimes used with magnesium hydroxide (Milk of Magnesia).

What are the adverse effects?
Common adverse effects of laxative stimulants include anorexia, nausea, gripping, abnormally loose stools, constipation rebound, and **melanosis** (abnormal dark pigmentation) of the colon. They may cause discoloration of urine and hypokalemia.

What are the contraindications and interactions?
Laxative stimulants are contraindicated in patients with abdominal pain, fecal impaction, GI bleeding, ulcerations, appendicitis, and intestinal obstruction. They should not be used during pregnancy or in patients with congestive heart failure. Laxative stimulants should be used cautiously in lactating women and patients with renal impairment, diabetes, or rectal bleeding. They may interact with oral anticoagulants and decrease their effect.

What are the important points patients should know?
Instruct patients that frequent or prolonged use of irritant cathartics disrupts normal reflex activity of the colon and rectum, leading to drug dependence for evacuation.

Bulk-Forming Laxatives

The proper functioning of the bowel is dependent on the presence of adequate amounts of liquids as well as dietary fiber. Dietary fiber consists of plant products such as cellulose, hemicellulose, and lignin, which are all found in high quantities in the outer coating of seeds and grains. Many vegetables and fruits also contain high amounts of fiber. These substances are not digestible (to any great extent) in humans and, therefore, add bulk to the colonic contents, which stimulates forward propulsive movements and the defecation reflex. Examples of bulk-forming laxatives are psyllium hydrophilic mucilloid (Metamucil) and polycarbophil (FiberCon).

How do they work?

Bulk-forming laxatives absorb free water in the intestinal tract and oppose the dehydrating forces of the bowel by forming a gelatinous mass.

How are they used?

Bulk-forming laxatives are used in chronic atonic or spastic constipation and constipation associated with rectal disorders or anorectal surgery.

What are the adverse effects?

Common adverse effects include nausea and vomiting, diarrhea (with excessive use), and abdominal cramps.

What are the contraindications and interactions?

Bulk-forming laxatives are contraindicated in esophageal and intestinal obstruction, nausea, vomiting, fecal impaction, undiagnosed abdominal pain, appendicitis, and in children younger than age 2. They should be used cautiously in diabetes, pregnancy, and during lactation. Bulk-forming laxatives may decrease absorption and clinical effects of antibiotics, warfarin (Coumadin), digoxin (Lanoxin), nitrofurantoin (Nitrofan), and salicylates.

What are the important points patients should know?

Instruct patients who are on a low-sodium or low-calorie diet to note the sugar and sodium content of these preparations. Some of them contain natural sugars, whereas others contain artificial sweeteners. Be sure that patients understand that these drugs work to relieve both diarrhea and constipation by restoring a more normal moisture level to the stool. These drugs may reduce appetite if taken before meals. Women should not breast feed while taking these drugs without consulting their physician.

✱ Apply Your Knowledge 24.3 ▬▬▬

The following questions focus on what you have just learned about laxatives. *See Appendix E for the correct answers.*

MULTIPLE CHOICE

Choose the correct answer from choices a–d.

1. Which of the following is the trade name of bisacodyl?

    a. Dulcolax

    b. Milk of Magnesia

    c. Senokot

    d. Glycerol

2. Which of the following is not an adverse effect of laxative stimulants?

    a. Nausea

    b. Constipation rebound

    c. Hyperkalemia

    d. Melanosis of the colon

3. Which of the following is a trade name of lactulose (an osmotic laxative)?

    a. Epsom salt

    b. Osmoglyn

    c. Dulcolax

    d. Chronulac

(*continued*)

Apply Your Knowledge 24.3 (continued)

4. The proper function of the bowel is dependent on the presence of adequate amounts of liquids, as well as:

   a. Dietary lipid, which contains saturated fat

   b. Dietary protein, which contains low cholesterol

   c. Dietary fiber, which contains cellulose

   d. Nondietary fat

5. Bulk-forming laxatives are contraindicated in children younger than age:

   a. 16 years

   b. 12 years

   c. 6 years

   d. 2 years

FILL IN THE BLANK

Select terms from your reading to fill in the blanks.

1. Nondietary constipation can be due to _____, which can occur after abdominal surgery.

2. Many drugs, particularly those with _____ activity, can lead to constipation.

3. Osmotic laxatives are used for _____ of occasional constipation.

4. Stool softeners are sometimes known as _____ or _____.

5. Common adverse effects of bulk-forming laxatives include _____, _____, _____, and _____.

Vomiting

Vomiting is an act of disgorging the contents of the stomach through the mouth. It is also called *emesis*. Infectious diseases can directly irritate vomiting centers to inhibit impulses going to the stomach. Certain drugs, radiation, and chemotherapy may irritate the GI tract or stimulate the chemoreceptor trigger zone and vomiting center in the brain (medulla). After surgery, particularly abdominal surgery, nausea and vomiting are common. The main neurotransmitters that produce nausea and vomiting include dopamine, serotonin, and acetylcholine.

Emetics

Emetic drugs can induce vomiting. Vomiting is a reflex primarily controlled by the medulla oblongata of the brain (often affected by drugs such as morphine and digitalis).

How do they work?

Ipecac syrup has both central and peripheral emetic actions, but after oral administration, the peripheral action is predominant. Vomiting is triggered by intense irritation of the mucosal layer of the intestinal wall. Not surprisingly, the central action comprises stimulation of the vomiting center via the chemoreceptor trigger zone in the medulla.

How are they used?

Ipecac syrup is used as an emergency emetic to remove unabsorbed ingested poisons. The use of ipecac syrup as an emetic is controversial and in decline. In some regions, its use has been completely abandoned in the clinical setting, and it is not recommended for the treatment of poisoning in the home.

What are the adverse effects?

The adverse effects of ipecac syrup may include stiff muscles, severe myopathy, convulsions, and coma. Cardiac arrhythmias, chest pain, dyspnea, hypotension, and fatal myocarditis may also occur. Diarrhea and mild GI upset are seen in some cases.

What are the contraindications and interactions?

Ipecac syrup is contraindicated in comatose, semicomatose, or deeply sedated patients. It should not be used in patients who are in shock or having seizures, or in patients with impaired cardiac function. Ipecac syrup must be used cautiously during pregnancy, lactation, or in infants younger than 6 months old.

What are the important points patients should know?

Instruct patients or their families to call an emergency room, poison control center, or physician before using ipecac syrup. Patients should not breast feed after using this drug without consulting their physician.

Focus Point

Ipecac Toxicity

The misuse of ipecac has occurred in persons with eating disorders such as bulimia and may result in ipecac toxicity. Patients must immediately report to their physician if vomiting persists longer than 2 to 3 hours after ipecac syrup is given.

Antiemetics

Antiemetics are agents used to prevent or relieve nausea and vomiting that may be caused by many different disorders. Table 24-5 ■ shows the most commonly used antiemetics.

How do they work?

The mechanism of action of antiemetics is largely unknown, except that they help to relax the portion of the brain controlling the muscles that cause vomiting.

How are they used?

The antiemetics are used for prevention or treatment of nausea and vomiting, especially to treat motion sickness and radiation or postchemotherapy vomiting.

What are the adverse effects?

Drowsiness is a common adverse effect of antiemetics. Additional adverse effects include confusion, dry mouth, headache, hypotension, hypersensitivity reactions, and blurred vision.

What are the contraindications and interactions?

Antiemetic drugs should be avoided in patients with known hypersensitivity to these medications, coma, and severe central nervous system depression. Antiemetics are contraindicated during pregnancy or lactation, especially during the first trimester. Antiemetics are also contraindicated if there is nausea and vomiting with an undiagnosed condition. This is especially true in suspected appendicitis, intestinal obstruction, brain tumors, or drug toxicity. Different types of antiemetics may have different drug interactions. For example, serotonin antagonists usually have no drug interactions, whereas the effects of dopamine are altered by antiemetics.

What are the important points patients should know?

Advise patients who are taking antiemetics to avoid driving a car and operating heavy machinery. Instruct them to avoid alcohol because it intensifies the sedative effects of antiemetics. Pregnant women should avoid antiemetics during the first trimester. Non-pharmacological measures for nausea are safer and more appropriate. These measures include small, frequent meals, dry biscuits, and a quiet environment. Advise patients with travel sickness to take antiemetics 30 minutes prior to travel.

Focus on Natural Products

Ginger for Nausea

For thousands of years, the Chinese have used ginger medicinally to treat nausea, vomiting, morning sickness, and motion sickness. Studies have shown ginger to be about as effective as OTC medications sold for these purposes. It is also said to have anti-inflammatory properties and is given to patients who have arthritis. Ginger is also used to soothe coughing or for fever. Because ginger may affect blood clotting, it should be avoided by patients who are taking anticoagulants.

Table 24-5 ■ The Most Commonly Used Antiemetics

GENERIC NAME	TRADE NAME	AVERAGE ADULT DOSAGE	ROUTE OF ADMINISTRATION
Dopamine Antagonists			
haloperidol	Haldol	1–2 mg q12 h	PO
chlorpromazine	Thorazine	10–25 mg q4–6 h	PO, IM, IV
perphenazine	Trilafon	8–16 mg/d	PO, IM, IV
prochlorperazine	Compazine	5–10 mg tid–qid	PO, IM, IV, Rectal
promethazine	Phenergan	25 mg q4–6 h	PO, IM, IV, Rectal
thiethylperazine	Torecan	10 mg 1–3 times/d	PO, IM, Rectal
Other			
metoclopramide	Reglan	1–2 mg/kg 30 min prior to chemotherapy and q2–4 h PRN	IV
Serotonin Antagonists			
granisetron	Kytril	1 mg 1 h prior to chemotherapy	PO, IV
granisetron ondansetron	Zofran	4–8 mg tid	PO, IV
Antihistamines			
dimenhydrinate	Dramamine	50–100 mg q4–6 h PRN	PO, IM, IV
diphenhydramine	Benadryl	10–50 mg q4–6 h PRN	PO, IM, IV
hydroxyzine	Atarax, Vistaril	25–100 mg q6h PRN	PO, IM
meclizine	Antivert, Bonine	25–50 mg/d	PO
Anticholinergics			
scopolamine	Transderm-Scop	0.5 mg q72h	Transdermal
trimethobenzamide	Tigan	250 mg tid–qid	PO, Rectal

✸ Apply Your Knowledge 24.4

The following questions focus on what you have just learned about vomiting, emetics, and antiemetics. *See Appendix E for the correct answers.*

FILL IN THE BLANK

Select terms from your reading to fill in the blanks.

1. Ipecac syrup is used as an emergency emetic to remove _____.

2. Vomiting is a reflex primarily controlled by the _____.

3. Ipecac syrup is contraindicated in _____, _____, or _____ patients, and in patients experiencing _____ or _____.

4. Ipecac syrup must be used cautiously during pregnancy, lactation, and in infants younger than _____.

5. The use of ipecac syrup as an emetic is controversial, and is _____.

MATCHING

Match the lettered drug trade name to the numbered generic drug name.

GENERIC NAME	TRADE NAME
1. _____ meclizine	a. Trilafon
2. _____ promethazine	b. Atarax
3. _____ butyrophenones	c. Zofran
4. _____ granisetron	d. Thorazine
5. _____ chlorpromazine	e. Phenergan
6. _____ perphenazine	f. Kytril
7. _____ ondansetron	g. Haldol
8. _____ hydroxyzine	h. Bonine

Chapter Capsule

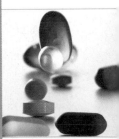

This section repeats the objectives from the beginning of the chapter and the provides a summary of the most important concepts for that objective. Use this section as a quick review and to check your knowledge.

Objective 1: Describe the major parts of the digestive system.

- Alimentary canal, including the mouth, pharynx, esophagus, stomach, small intestine, large intestine, rectum, and anus
- Accessory organs, including salivary glands, liver, gallbladder, and pancreas

Objective 2: Explain how medications are absorbed in the gastrointestinal (GI) tract, and metabolized.

- Stomach juices mix with a substance and break it down for absorption
- Chemical digestion occurs in the small intestine
- The liver is the center of metabolic activity and is very important in digestion, absorption, and metabolic activities

Objective 3: Describe the use of histamine-2 (H$_2$)-receptor antagonists in the treatment of peptic ulcers.

- Short-term treatment of active duodenal ulcer and prevention of ulcer recurrence (at reduced dosage) after it is healed
- Short-term treatment of active benign gastric ulcer, pathologic hypersecretory conditions such as Zollinger–Ellison syndrome, and heartburn

Objective 4: Describe the use of antacids in the treatment of peptic ulcers.

- For hyperacidity of the stomach, to protect from peptic ulcers, and to promote peptic ulcer healing

Objective 5: Explain the effects of prostaglandins on the digestive tract.

- Most versatile and powerful substances used to treat GI disorders
- Involved in GI motility and gastric acid secretions
- Inhibit gastric acid and gastrin production, mucus production, and bicarbonate secretion
- Prostaglandin analogue misoprostol (Cytotec) is most commonly used.

Objective 6: List four generic names and trade names of proton pump inhibitors.

- esomeprazole (Nexium)
- lansoprazole (Prevacid)
- omeprazole (Prilosec)
- pantoprazole (Protonix)

Objective 7: Explain the problems associated with laxative use.

- Nausea, vomiting, abdominal cramps, diarrhea, weakness, reduced appetite, lethargy, bitter taste, anorexia, gripping, constipation rebound, melanosis of the colon, discoloration of urine, hypokalemia, and electrolyte imbalance
- In severe cases, hypotension, bradycardia, mental depression, and coma
- Contraindicated in patients with renal impairment, atonic constipation, nausea, vomiting, abdominal pain, fecal impaction, esophageal obstruction, intestinal obstruction, intestinal perforation, GI bleeding, ulcerations, appendicitis, hypertension, and in patients younger than 2 years
- Cautious use in patients with history of congestive heart failure, edema, rectal bleeding, and diabetes mellitus

Objective 8: Describe the drug treatment for diarrhea.

- Opioid and synthetic opioid drugs: most effective
- Absorbents: inexpensive and, to a certain extent, effective

Objective 9: Describe the mechanism of action of bulk-forming laxatives, osmotic laxatives, and laxative stimulants.

- Bulk-forming laxatives: absorb free water in the intestinal tract and oppose the dehydrating forces of the bowel by forming a gelatinous mass
- Osmotic laxatives: use the ions of sodium and magnesium to attract water (osmosis), which causes a more liquid stool to be formed. Hypertonic contents cause water to be retained and to be pulled from the bowel's capillaries back into the bowel lumen, resulting in a rise in pressure and volume in the colon and rectum, leading to stimulation of the defecation reflex
- Laxative stimulants: true purgatives that cause an increase in peristaltic movements and lead to defecation

Internet Sites of Interest

- The National Institute of Diabetes and Digestive and Kidney Diseases (NIDDK) at: **http://digestive.niddk.nih.gov**, presents information on how the digestive system works. The information is appropriate for patient teaching. Search for "digestive system."

- The same NIDDK site provides information on peptic ulcer disease. Search for "peptic ulcer."

- The Family Doctor Web site offers information on the use of OTC laxatives at: **http://familydoctor.org**. Search for "laxatives."

- For information on the use of laxatives, see Medical News Today at: **www.medicalnewstoday.com**. Search for "laxative use."

Chapter 25

Effects of Drugs on Respiratory Disorders

Chapter Objectives

1. Describe the upper and lower respiratory tracts.
2. List the most commonly used medications for asthma.
3. Explain xanthine derivatives in the treatment of asthma.
4. Describe the mechanism of action of leukotriene inhibitors.
5. Explain the contraindications of mast cell stabilizers.
6. Describe the use of opioid cough suppressants.
7. Define expectorants and mucolytic agents.
8. Explain the mechanism of action of decongestants.

Key Terms

Alveolar duct (al-vee-OH-lar DUKT) (page 545)

Alveolar sacs (page 545)

Alveoli (al-VEE-oh-lie) (page 545)

Antitussives (an-tee-TUSS-ivz) (page 557)

Asthma (page 547)

Atelectasis (at-tuh-LEK-tuh-sis) (page 559)

Bronchioles (BRONG-kee-ols) (page 545)

Bronchitis (page 552)

Bronchodilators (page 550)

Bronchospasm (page 552)

Cystic fibrosis (SIS-tik fy-BRO-sis) (page 559)

Decongestants, (page 559)

Emphysema (em-fih-ZEE-muh) (page 553)

Expectorants (page 558)

Leukotriene inhibitors (loo-ko-TRY-een) (page 554)

Mast cells (page 555)

Mucolytics (myoo-ko-LIT-tiks) (page 558)

Nebulizer (NEH-byoo-ly-zer) (page 552)

Nonproductive cough (page 557)

Productive cough (page 557)

Xanthine derivatives (ZAN-theen) (page 553)

PRACTICAL SCENARIO

A 60-year-old man with a history of depression and hypertension visited his local pharmacy to buy a decongestant and cough suppressant for a bad chest cold. He asked the pharmacist to recommend a brand. The pharmacist recommended Sudafed (pseudoephedrine) for his congestion and Robitussin DM (dextromethorphan) for his cough. At home, the man took the recommended dose of each medicine. Within 1 hour, he began having palpitations, chest pains, and severe headache. He was sweating and his heart rate was 120 beats per minute. His wife called the emergency medical services (EMS). The EMS team obtained an ECG and asked the man's medical history. The man reported taking phenelzine (Nardil) for depression and atenolol (Tenormin) for hypertension. His wife stated that he had just taken Sudafed and Robitussin for his cold and cough. The EMS team stabilized his heart rate and transferred him to the hospital for observation.

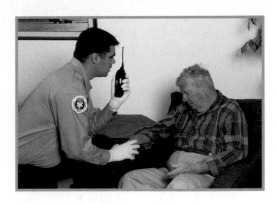

Critical Thinking Questions

1. What is the significance of the man's use of phenelzine, atenolol, and the OTC cold and cough medications?
2. What mistake did the pharmacist make in helping the man choose OTC cough and cold preparations?
3. What patient teaching would you provide this patient if he was seen in your office for a routine checkup and review of his prescriptions?

Introduction

All cells of the body require oxygen to break down nutrients and thereby release energy and produce energy (adenosine triphosphate [ATP]). The cells must also excrete the carbon dioxide that results from the process. Obtaining oxygen and removing carbon dioxide are the primary functions of the respiratory system, which includes tubes that filter incoming air and transport air into and out of the lungs, as well as microscopic air sacs where gases are exchanged. The respiratory organs also entrap particles from incoming air, help control the temperature and water content of the air, produce vocal sounds, and participate in the sense of smell and the regulation of blood pH.

Organs of the Respiratory System

The organs of the respiratory system can be divided into two groups, or tracts. Those in the *upper respiratory tract* include the nose, nasal cavity, paranasal sinuses, and pharynx. Those in the *lower respiratory tract* include the larynx, trachea, bronchial tree, and lungs (Figure 25-1 ■).

The lower respiratory tract is essential for the exchange of oxygen and carbon dioxide. As the bronchi enter the lungs, they subdivide into bronchial tubes and small **bronchioles** (which are 1 mm or less in diameter and have abundant smooth muscle and elastic fibers). At the end of each bronchiole is an **alveolar duct**. These ducts lead to thin-walled out-pouchings called **alveolar sacs**. Alveolar sacs lead to smaller microscopic air sacs called **alveoli**, which lie within capillary networks (Figure 25-2 ■).

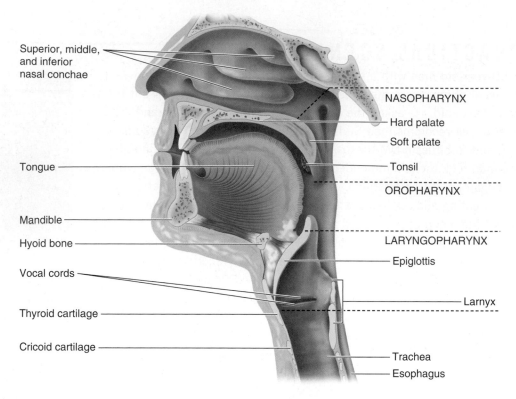

A

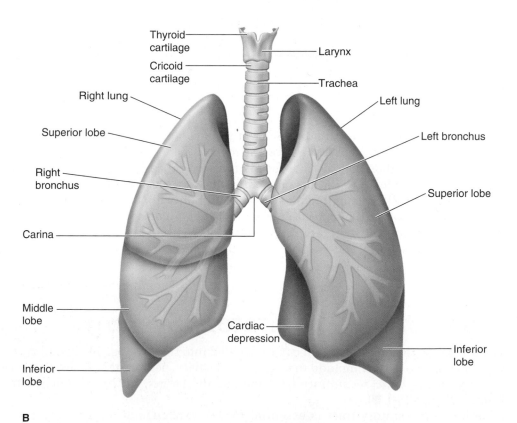

B

Figure 25-1 ■ (A) The upper and lower (B) respiratory tracts.

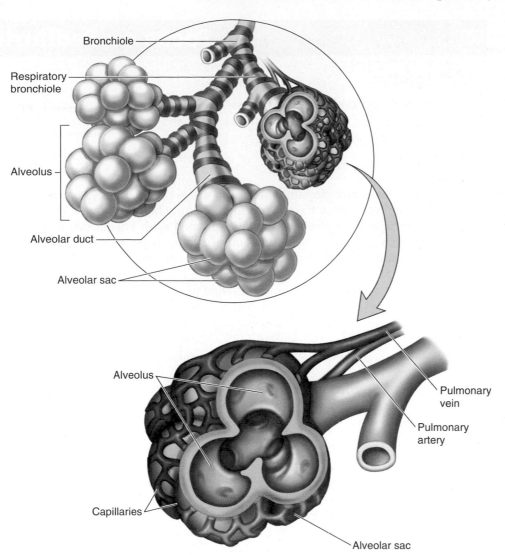

Figure 25-2 ■ Bronchioles and alveoli.

Drug Effects on Asthma

Asthma is a chronic disease caused by the increased reactivity of the tracheobronchial tree to various stimuli. It is a leading cause of chronic illness and school absenteeism in children (Figure 25-3 ■). Asthma is also one of the most common chronic conditions in the United States, affecting about 16 million Americans.

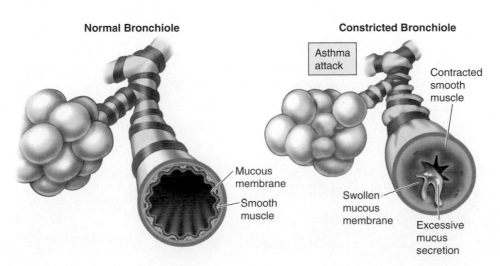

Figure 25-3 ■ The effects of asthma on the bronchioles.

Focus on Pediatrics

Isoproterenol for Asthma

Isoproterenol (Isuprel) is often used to treat status asthmaticus in children, even though such use is not a labeled indication. Parents should tell their children that saliva and sputum may appear pink after inhalation treatment, and that this is normal.

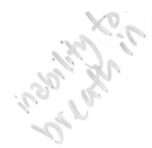

Asthma is frequently classified according to its cause: allergy, exercise-induced, or infections of the respiratory tract. Symptoms include breathlessness, cough, wheezing, and chest tightness. The airway becomes inflamed with edema (abnormal accumulation of fluid) and mucous plugs; hyperactivity of the bronchial tree adds to the symptoms. During asthmatic attacks, when bronchiole constriction and increased secretions are present, bronchodilators are used for relief. Classifications of the most common medications that are used for asthma are listed in Table 25-1 ■.

Table 25-1 ■ The Most Common Antiasthma Drugs

GENERIC NAME	TRADE NAME	AVERAGE ADULT DOSAGE	ROUTE OF ADMINISTRATION
Beta$_2$-Adrenergic Agonists			
albuterol	Proventil, Ventolin	2–4 mg tid	PO
		1–2 inhalations q4–6h; 2 inhalations before exercise	Inhalation
epinephrine	EpiPen	Individualized: solution 1:1,000, 0.3–0.5 mL	Inhalation, subcutaneous, IM
formoterol	Foradil	One 12-mg capsule q12h using aerolizer inhaler	Inhalation
ipratropium	Aerolizer Atrovent	2 inhalations qid at 4-h intervals (max: 12 inhalations in 24 h)	MDI
		500 mcg (1 unit-dose vial) q6–8h	Nebulizer
		Intranasal: 2 sprays of 0.06% in each nostril tid–qid up to 4 d	Nasal
isoetharine	Bronkosol	3–7 inhalations 1:3 dilution or 4 inhalations	Inhalation
isoproterenol	Isuprel	Inhalations 4–6 times/d (max: 6 inhalations in any hour during 24-h period)	Inhalation (MDI)
		Solution: 0.5 mL of 0.5% solution diluted to 2–2.5 mL with water or saline over 10–20 min up to 5 times/d	IPPB
levalbuterol	Xopenex	0.63 mg by nebulization tid q6–8 h, may increase to 1.25 mg tid if needed	Inhalation
metaproterenol	Alupent	20 mg q6–8h	PO
		2–3 inhalations q3–4h (max: 12 inhalations/d)	MDI
		5–10 inhalations of undiluted 5% solution	Nebulizer
		2.5 mL of 0.4–0.6% solution q4–6h	IPPB

Table 25-1 ■ The Most Common Antiasthma Drugs

GENERIC NAME	TRADE NAME	AVERAGE ADULT DOSAGE	ROUTE OF ADMINISTRATION
pirbuterol	Maxair	2 inhalations (0.4 mg) q6h (max: 12 inhalations/d)	Inhalation
salmeterol	Serevent	2 inhalations of aerosol (42 mcg) or 1 powder diskus (50 mcg) bid, 12h apart	Inhalation
terbutaline	Brethine	2.5–5 mg tid at 6-h intervals (max: 15 mg/d)	PO
		0.25 mg q15–30 min up to 0.5 mg in 4 h	Subcutaneous
		2 inhalations separated by 60 sec q4–6h	Inhalation
Xanthine Derivatives			
aminophylline	Somophyllin, Truphylline	Loading dose: 6 mg/kg over 30 min Maintenance dose: 0.25–0.75 mg/kg/h	IV
		0.6 mg/kg/h qid	PO
dyphylline	Dilor, Dyflex, Dyline-GG, Lufyllin, Neothylline, Thylline	200–800 mg q6h up to 15 mg/kg qid	PO
		250–500 mg q6h (max: 15 mg/kg qid)	IM
oxtriphylline	Choledyl	200–800 mg q6h up to 15 mg/kg	PO
theophylline	Somophyllin, Theo-Dur, Theolair, and others	Loading dose: 5 mg/kg	PO
		Maintenance dose: 0.5 mg/kg/h (IV) or q8–12h (sustained release)	PO/IV
Corticosteroids			
beclomethasone	Beclovent, Beconase*, QVAR, Vancenase, Vanceril	2 inhalations tid–qid up to 20 inhalations/d	Inhalation, Nasal
budesonide	Pulmicort, Rhinocort, Turbuhaler	Maintenance: 1–2 inhalations (200 mcg/inhalation 1–2 times/d)	Inhalation
dexamethasone	Aeroseb-Dex, Decadron, Decaspray	Up to 3 inhalations tid–qid (max: 800 mcg bid)	Inhalation
flunisolide	AeroBid, Nasalide, Nasarel	2 sprays orally, or intranasally in each nostril bid; may increase to tid if needed	PO, Nasal
fluticasone	Flonase, Flovent	100 mcg (1 inhalation in each nostril 1–2 times/d (max: 4 times/d)	Nasal
		1–2 inhalations bid	Inhalation
hydrocortisone	Cortaid, Dermacort	10–320 mg/d in 3–4 divided doses (max: 2 g/d)	PO

*Beconase AQ is a nasal spray; Beconase is also available as an inhalation aerosol.

(continued)

Table 25-1 ■ The Most Common Antiasthma Drugs (*continued*)

GENERIC NAME	TRADE NAME	AVERAGE ADULT DOSAGE	ROUTE OF ADMINISTRATION
mometasone furoate monohydrate	Nasonex	2 sprays (50 mcg each) in each nostril/d	Nasal
prednisolone	Delta-Cortef, Prelone	5–60 mg/d in single or divided doses	PO
prednisone	Deltasone, Meticorten	40 mg q12h for 3–5 d	PO
triamcinolone	Azmacort, Tri-Nasal	2 puffs 3–4 times/d or 4 puffs bid	Inhalation
		2 spray/nostril once daily (max: 8 sprays/d)	Nasal
Leukotriene Inhibitors			
montelukast	Singulair	10 mg at bedtime	PO
zafirlukast	Accolate	20 mg bid	PO
zileuton	Zyflo	600 mg qid	PO
Mast Cell Stabilizers			
cromolyn	Intal, NasalCrom	1 spray or 1 capsule inhaled qid	MDI
		1 spray in each nostril 3–6 time/d at regular intervals	Nasal
nedocromil	Alocril, Tilade	2 inhalations qid at regular intervals (NOT for acute asthma attacks!)	Inhalation
Combination Drugs			
fluticasone with salmeterol	Advair Diskus, Advair HFA	1 puff bid approx, 12h apart	Inhalation

IPPB = intermittent positive pressure breathing; MDI = metered-dose inhaler

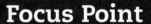

Focus Point

Severe Asthma

Severe forms of asthma are associated with frequent attacks of wheezing dyspnea, especially at night, and chronic limitation of activity. Asthma causes contraction of airway smooth muscle, mucosal thickening, and abnormally thick plugs of mucus.

BRONCHODILATORS

Bronchodilators are agents that widen the diameter of the bronchial tubes. They include beta$_2$-adrenergic agonists, such as salmeterol (Serevent) and xanthines, such as theophylline (Theo-Dur) and aminophylline (Truphylline, Somophyllin).

✳ Apply Your Knowledge 25.1

The following questions focus on what you have just learned about organs of the respiratory system and drug effects on asthma. *See Appendix E for the correct answers.*

MULTIPLE CHOICE

Choose the correct answer from choices a–d.

1. Bronchodilators are used for relief during asthmatic attacks when which of the following are present?

    a. Bronchiole dilation and decreased secretion

    b. Excretion of carbon dioxide

    c. Pink sputum

    d. Bronchiole contraction and increased secretion

2. Organs of the upper respiratory tract include the:

    a. Larynx

    b. Trachea

    c. Paranasal sinuses

    d. Lungs

3. Which of the following parts of the respiratory tract are attached to alveoli?

    a. Trachea

    b. Esophagus

    c. Bronchioles

    d. Paranasal sinuses

4. Microscopic air sacs that lie within capillary networks are known as:

    a. Bronchial tubes

    b. Alveoli

    c. Alveolar sacs

    d. Bronchodilators

5. Which of the following is one of the leading causes of absenteeism in school-aged children?

    a. Laryngitis

    b. Asthma

    c. Otitis media

    d. Bronchitis

FILL IN THE BLANK

Select terms from your reading to fill in the blanks.

1. Asthma is one of the most common chronic conditions in the United States, affecting about _____.

2. During asthmatic attacks, when bronchiole constriction is present, _____ are used for relief.

3. The primary functions of the respiratory system are obtaining _____.

4. The upper respiratory tract includes the _____.

5. The lower respiratory tract includes the _____.

Beta₂-Adrenergic Agonists

Beta₂-adrenergic agonists are drugs of choice in the treatment of *acute* bronchoconstriction, and they have replaced some of the older agents such as epinephrine because they cause fewer cardiac adverse effects. Some of these drugs (isoproterenol [Isuprel]) produce therapeutic effects immediately but last for 2 to 3 hours, whereas other drugs, like salmeterol (Serevent), provide 12 hours of therapy.

How do they work?

Beta₂-adrenergic agonists produce bronchodilation by relaxing smooth muscles of the bronchial tree. This effect decreases airway resistance, facilitates mucus drainage, and increases vital capacity.

How are they used?

Beta₂-adrenergic agonists are used to relieve **bronchospasm** (contraction of smooth muscle in the walls of the bronchi and bronchioles) associated with acute or chronic asthma, **bronchitis** (inflammation of the mucous membrane of the bronchial tubes), or other reversible obstructive airway diseases. Some of them are also used to prevent exercise-induced bronchospasm. Many of these types of agents are inhaled using a **nebulizer** (a device that disperses a fine-particle mist of medication into the deeper parts of the respiratory tract).

What are the adverse effects?

Adverse effects of beta₂-adrenergic drugs such as epinephrine (EpiPen) and isoproterenol (Isuprel) may cause restlessness, headache, dizziness, palpitations, tachycardia, insomnia, nausea, vomiting, and anorexia.

What are the contraindications and interactions?

Contraindications are hypersensitivity to sympathomimetic amines; narrow-angle glaucoma; and hemorrhagic and traumatic or cardiogenic shock. Safety during pregnancy or lactation is not established. Beta₂-adrenergic drugs should be used cautiously in older adults or debilitated patients and in those with prostatic hypertrophy, hypertension, diabetes mellitus, hyperthyroidism, Parkinson's disease, tuberculosis, and psychoneurosis. No significant drug interactions with beta₂-adrenergic agents have been reported.

What are the important points patients should know?

Instruct patients not to exceed the recommended dosage. They should use caution if driving or performing tasks that require alertness. Advise patients to eat small, frequent meals to avoid nausea, vomiting, or a change in taste. Instruct patients to immediately report chest pain, dizziness, insomnia, weakness, tremors, irregular heartbeat, difficulty breathing, productive cough, or lack of therapeutic effects to their physician.

Focus on Geriatrics

Cautious Use of Beta₂-Adrenergic Drugs in Elderly Patients

Care must be taken when using beta₂-adrenergic drugs such as epinephrine in older adults. These drugs are contraindicated in numerous conditions that affect elderly patients, including hypertension, Parkinson's disease, heart disease, glaucoma, and arteriosclerosis.

Xanthine Derivatives

Xanthine derivatives are a group of drugs chemically related to caffeine that dilate bronchioles in the lungs. Xanthines are most often used to treat asthma and are administered by the oral or IV route. Examples of xanthenes include aminophylline (Truphylline, Somophyllin) and theophylline (Theo-Dur).

How do they work?

Xanthine derivatives relax smooth muscle by direct action on the bronchi and pulmonary vessels. They stimulate the medullary respiratory center, resulting in an increase in the vital capacity of the lungs. Methylxanthines (such as caffeine) are bases of xanthine derivatives, which must be converted to theophylline. Theophylline (Theo-Dur) has a narrow therapeutic range and is not used as commonly today.

How are they used?

Xanthine derivatives are used for prophylaxis and the symptomatic relief of bronchial asthma, as well as bronchospasm associated with chronic bronchitis and **emphysema** (a condition in which the walls between the alveoli lose their elasticity. The alveoli become weakened and break. Air is trapped in the alveoli and exchange of oxygen and carbon dioxide is reduced.)

What are the adverse effects?

The common adverse effects of xanthine derivatives include palpitations, tachycardia, flushing, hypotension, insomnia, nervousness, nausea, vomiting, diarrhea, tachypnea, and respiratory arrest.

What are the contraindications and interactions?

Xanthine derivatives are contraindicated in hypersensitivity to these agents. Xanthine preparations should not be given to patients who have coronary artery disease, history of angina pectoris, or severe renal or liver impairment. Safety during pregnancy or lactation is not established. Xanthine derivatives should be used cautiously in children and older adults, and in those with hyperthyroidism, hypertension, peptic ulcer, prostatic hypertrophy, glaucoma, and diabetes mellitus.

The xanthine drugs may produce drug interactions with antibiotics, rifampin (Rifadin), phenobarbital (Bellatal), phenytoin (Dilantin), cimetidine (Tagamet), and caffeine.

What are the important point patients should know?

Advise patients to take these medications at the same time every day. They should avoid charbroiled food (or food cooked using charcoal), which may increase theophylline (Theo-Dur) elimination and reduce the half-life as much as 50%. Instruct patients to limit caffeine intake because it may increase the incidence of adverse effects. Instruct them to avoid cigarette smoking, which may significantly lower the plasma concentration of xanthine drugs. Women should not breast feed while taking these drugs without consulting a physician.

Focus on Geriatrics

Cautious Use of Xanthines

Xanthine derivatives must be used cautiously in older adults because their adverse effects include severe hypotension and cardiac arrest, which have higher fatality rates in this group of patients.

Corticosteroids

Corticosteroids, such as prednisone (Deltasone), are steroid hormones used to treat a wide variety of inflammatory diseases. Inhaled corticosteroids help prevent asthmatic attacks. Oral corticosteroids are used for the short-term management of acute severe asthma.

How do they work?

The precise mechanism of action of corticosteroids is not known. It is thought that they diminish the activation of inflammatory cells and increase the production of anti-inflammatory mediators, which in turn reduces mucus production and edema, and decreases airway obstruction.

How are they used?

Corticosteroids are used to treat respiratory conditions such as nasal congestion and allergic conditions such as rhinitis and asthma.

What are the adverse effects?

The adverse effects of corticosteroids include irritation of mucous membranes, headache, pharyngitis, epistaxis, nausea, vomiting, asthma-like symptoms, and coughing. Less common adverse effects include blood in the nasal mucous, runny nose, abdominal pain, diarrhea, fever, flu-like symptoms, body aches, dizziness, and bronchitis.

What are the contraindications and interactions?

Corticosteroids are contraindicated in patients with known hypersensitivity to these types of drugs. They should not be used if symptoms of hypercorticism (such as Cushing's syndrome) are present. They must be used with caution in patients with immune system infections, tuberculosis, herpes simplex, ulcers, nasal surgery, and nasal trauma, and in women who are pregnant or lactating. They should not be used in children younger than age 4. Corticosteroids may interact with ritonavir (Norvir), ketoconazole (Nizoral), other cytochrome P450 inhibitors, and other inhaled corticosteroids.

What are the important points patients should know?

Advise patients to avoid exposure to chickenpox or measles while taking corticosteroids and to contact their physician if exposure occurs. Women who are pregnant or lactating should not use corticosteroids without their physician's approval.

Focus on Pediatrics

Growth Retardation and Corticosteroids

Growth retardation is of particular concern when corticosteroids are used in children. Guidelines for use of corticosteroids with certain age groups of children must be followed closely.

Leukotriene Inhibitors

Leukotriene inhibitors, such as zafirlukast (Accolate), are bronchodilator and leukotriene-receptor antagonists. Leukotrienes are metabolized from arachidonic acid, which is also responsible for forming prostaglandins. Leukotrienes cause inflammation and allergic reactions. They increase edema, vascular permeability, and mucus in bronchioles.

How do they work?

A leukotriene inhibitor blocks either the synthesis of, or the body's inflammatory responses to, leukotrienes. Blocking the receptors also blocks the tissue's inflammatory response. Thus, leukotriene inhibitors control asthmatic attacks.

How are they used?
Leukotriene inhibitors are used in the prophylaxis and treatment of chronic asthma or allergic rhinitis.

What are the adverse effects?
Adverse effects of leukotriene inhibitors include arrhythmias, dizziness, light-headedness, anxiety, headache, and euphoria. Common adverse effects are nausea, diarrhea, dry mouth, and abdominal discomfort.

What are the contraindications and interactions?
Leukotriene inhibitors are contraindicated in hypersensitive patients and in those with severe asthma attacks, bronchoconstriction due to asthma or nonsteroidal anti-inflammatory drugs (NSAIDs), and status asthmaticus. They should not be used by lactating women and should be used cautiously in patients with severe liver disease, pregnant patients, and children younger than 12 months. No significant drug interactions with leukotriene inhibitor agents have been reported.

What are the important points patients should know?
Instruct patients not to use these drugs for reversal of an acute asthmatic attack, and instead to inform their physician if they need short-acting inhaled bronchodilators more often than leukotriene inhibitors.

Focus Point

Oral Administration Advantage

The principal advantage of leukotriene inhibitors is that they are taken orally. Some patients (especially children) do not comply well with inhaled medications.

Mast Cell Stabilizers

Mast cells are large cells found in connective tissue that contain a wide variety of biochemicals, including histamine. Mast cells are involved in inflammation secondary to injuries and infections, and they are sometimes implicated in allergic reactions. A mast cell stabilizer is able to stabilize mast cell membranes against rupture caused by antigenic substances. As a result, less histamine and other inflammatory substances are released in airway tissue. Examples of mast cell stabilizers include cromolyn (Intal) and nedocromil (Tilade).

How do they work?
Mast cell stabilizers are synthetic asthma-prophylactic agents with unique action. They inhibit the release of bronchoconstrictors such as histamine from sensitized pulmonary mast cells, thereby suppressing an allergic response.

How are they used?
Cromolyn sodium (Intal) is used primarily for prophylaxis of mild to moderate seasonal and perennial bronchial asthma and allergic rhinitis. It is also used for prevention of exercise-related bronchospasm, and prevention of acute bronchospasm induced by known pollutants or antigens. Nedocromil sodium (Tilade) is used as maintenance therapy for patients with mild to moderate asthma.

What are the adverse effects?
Common adverse effects include nausea, vomiting, dry mouth, throat irritation, cough, hoarseness, slightly bitter aftertaste, headache, dizziness, urticaria, and rash.

What are the contraindications and interactions?

Mast cell stabilizers are contraindicated in patients with coronary artery disease or history of arrhythmias, dyspnea, acute asthma, and status asthmaticus. These agents should not be used during pregnancy or in children younger than age 6. Cromolyn sodium (Intal) should be given cautiously in patients with renal or hepatic dysfunction. No clinically significant interactions with cromolyn sodium or nedocromil sodium have been established.

What are the important points patients should know?

Advise patients that throat irritation, cough, and hoarseness can be minimized by gargling with water, drinking a few swallows of water, or sucking on a lozenge after each treatment. Women should not breast feed while taking these drugs.

Focus on Geriatrics

Contraindications of Mast Cell Stabilizers

Mast cell stabilizers such as cromolyn are contraindicated in patients with coronary artery disease, history of arrhythmias, and renal or hepatic dysfunction—all conditions with higher rates of occurrence in elderly patients.

✳ Apply Your Knowledge 25.2

The following questions focus on what you have just learned about the various types of drugs used for respiratory disorders. *See Appendix E for the correct answers.*

FILL IN THE BLANK

Select terms from your reading to fill in the blanks.

1. Bronchodilators widen the diameter of the bronchial tubes by _____.

2. Beta$_2$-adrenergic agonists may be used to relieve _____ and _____.

3. Xanthine derivatives are used to treat respiratory disorders such as asthma and _____.

4. Leukotriene inhibitors are to be used for _____, and not _____ asthmatic attacks.

5. Mast cells are large cells found in _____.

MATCHING

Match the lettered drug trade name to the numbered generic drug name.

GENERIC NAME	TRADE NAME
1. _____ epinephrine	a. Intal
2. _____ aminophylline	b. Singulair
3. _____ theophylline	c. Truphylline
4. _____ cromolyn	d. EpiPen
5. _____ montelukast	e. Theo-Dur

Table 25-2 ■ Major Types of Cough Suppressants

GENERIC NAME	TRADE NAME	AVERAGE ADULT DOSAGE	ROUTE OF ADMINISTRATION
Opioids			
chlorpheniramine and hydrocodone	Tussionex	5 mL bid	PO
hydrocodone	Hycodan, Robidone A	5–10 mg q4–6h PRN (max: 15 mg/dose)	PO
codeine	(generic only)	10–20 mg q4–6h PRN (max: 120 mg/d)	PO
Nonopioids			
benzonatate	Tessalon Perles	100–200 mg tid (max: 600 mg/d)	PO
dextromethorphan	Robitussin DM, Romilar CF	10–20 mg q4h or 30 mg q6–8h (max: 120 mg/d) or 60 mg of sustained-action liquid bid	PO
diphenhydramine	Benadryl, Benahist	25 mg q4–6h (max: 100 mg/d)	PO

cause: respiratory depression. (handwritten annotation)

Antitussives

Antitussives are agents that reduce coughing. They are also called *cough suppressants.* The initial stimulus for a cough probably arises in the bronchial mucosa, where irritation results in bronchoconstriction. *Coughing* is a sudden expulsion of air from the lungs and through the mouth. A cough is often described as productive or nonproductive. A **productive cough** brings up fluid or mucus from the lungs. A **nonproductive cough** is a sudden ejection of air from the lungs and through the mouth that does not expel (produce) mucus or fluid from the throat or lungs. Antitussives are classified into two major groups: opioid and nonopioid. Various cough suppression agents are summarized in Table 25-2 ■.

How do they work?

The opioid cough suppressants cause respiratory depression similar to that of morphine. An antitussive action occurs at doses that are lower than those required for analgesia. Examples of opioid cough suppressants are codeine (many trade names), hydrocodone (Histussin), and chlorpheniramine/hydrocodone (Tussionex).

Nonopioid cough suppressants, such as dextromethorphan (Robitussin DM, Vicks Formula 44 Cough) do not suppress respiration. These drugs reduce the activity of peripheral cough receptors and appear to increase the threshold of the central cough center.

How are they used?

The opioid cough suppressants are used to suppress nonproductive cough, but they have limited use because of unwanted side effects. Codeine and hydrocodone (Histussin) are not generally effective but are used because they elevate the cough threshold.

Nonopioid cough suppressants are indicated for temporary relief of cough spasms in nonproductive coughs due to colds, pertussis, and influenza. The major nonopioid cough suppressants are over-the-counter (OTC) medications.

What are the adverse effects?

The adverse effects of antitussives may include difficulty breathing, drowsiness, skin rash, itching, dizziness, constipation, nausea, nervousness, and restlessness.

Respiratory Depletion (handwritten annotation)

What are the contraindications and interactions?

Antitussives are contraindicated in patients with known hypersensitivity, asthma, emphysema, diabetes, heart disease, seizure conditions, thyroid conditions, chronic bronchitis, and liver disease. They should be used only if directed by a physician in women who are pregnant or lactating.

Antitussives interact with monoamine oxidase (MAO) inhibitors, alcohol, sedatives and hypnotics, cold and allergy medications, muscle relaxants, and analgesics.

What are the important points patients should know?

Advise patients to call their physician if coughing does not improve, or if it lasts longer than 1 week, worsens, or produces yellow-colored mucus. They should also contact their physician if symptoms of fever, rash, sore throat, vomiting, or continuing headache occur.

Focus on Natural Products

Natural Expectorant

Wild cherry bark acts as an expectorant and also a mild sedative. It is available in syrup and tincture forms. It is good for coughs, colds, bronchitis, and asthma. However, wild cherry bark should not be used during pregnancy.

Focus Point

Opioids for Cough

Opioid analgesics are among the most effective drugs used as cough suppressants. Their effect is often achieved at doses below those required to produce analgesia. For example, 15 mg of codeine is usually sufficient to relieve coughing.

Expectorants and Mucolytics

Expectorants and **mucolytics** are medications that are capable of dissolving or promoting liquefaction of mucus in the lungs. They also facilitate the elimination of mucus through coughing. These medications (Table 25-3 ■) are available OTC and by prescription. Expectorants and mucolytics include acetylcysteine (Mucomyst), guaifenesin (Fenesin), and dornase alfa (Pulmozyme).

How do they work? common drug

Acetylcysteine (Mucomyst) lowers viscosity and facilitates the removal of secretions. Guaifenesin (Fenesin) enhances reflex outflow of respiratory tract fluids by irritation of gastric mucosa.

How are they used?

These agents are used as adjuvant therapy in patients with abnormal, sticky, or thickened mucous secretions in acute and chronic bronchopulmonary disease, and in pulmonary complications of **cystic fibrosis** (a disorder marked by abnormal secretions of the exocrine glands causing obstruction of bronchial pathways), tracheostomy, and **atelectasis** (absence of gas from the lungs).

What are the adverse effects?

The adverse effects of these expectorants and mucolytics are not significant. A low incidence of nausea and drowsiness is reported.

What are the contraindications and interactions?

Expectorants and mucolytics are contraindicated in patients with hypersensitivity to these agents. They should be avoided in pregnancy and lactation. Guaifenesin may interact with heparin therapy by inhibiting platelet function and increasing the risk of hemorrhage.

What are the important points patients should know?

Instruct patients to increase fluid intake to help loosen mucus and drink at least 8 glasses of fluids daily. They should contact their physician if cough persists beyond 1 week. Advise women to avoid breast feeding while taking these drugs without their physician's approval.

Table 25-3 ■ Expectorants and Mucolytics

GENERIC NAME	TRADE NAME	AVERAGE ADULT DOSAGE	ROUTE OF ADMINISTRATION
acetylcysteine	Mucomyst	10 mL of 20% solution, or 2–20 mL of 10% solution q2–6 h	Inhalation
dornase alfa	Pulmozyme	2.5 mg/d inhaled through nebulizer	Inhalation
guaifenesin	Fenesin, Humibid	100–400 mg q4h	PO
potassium iodide	Pima, SSKI	300–1,000 mg after meals bid–tid up to 1.5 g tid	PO

Decongestants

Decongestants are a class of drugs that reverse excessive blood flow (congestion) into an area. These agents are available in both oral and nasal preparations. Table 25-4 ■ shows the most commonly used decongestants, such as pseudoephedrine (Sudafed).

How do they work?

Decongestants are vasoconstricting agents that shrink the swollen mucous membranes of the nasal airway passage of the upper respiratory tract. Most oral agents are adrenergic medications, or medications that mimic the effects of the sympathetic nervous system.

How are they used?

The most common uses for decongestants are for the relief of nasal congestion due to the common cold, upper respiratory allergies, and sinusitis.

What are the adverse effects?

All patients may experience nervousness, insomnia, restlessness, dizziness, headaches, and irritability. Decongestants may also cause tachycardia, blurred vision, nausea, and vomiting.

What are the contraindications and interactions?

Decongestants should not be used by patients who are taking other sympathomimetic drugs. They also are contraindicated in patients with diabetes, heart disease, uncontrolled hypertension, hyperthyroidism, and prostatic hypertrophy.

Nasal decongestants may cause severe hypertension with certain MAO inhibitors. They may also decrease the vasopressor response with reserpine (Serpalan), methyldopa (Aldomet), and urine acidifiers. Nasal decongestants increase the duration of action of urine alkalinizers (sodium citrate, lactate, and sodium bicarbonate). They decrease the antihypertensive effects of methyldopa (Aldomet).

What are the important points patients should know?

Instruct patients to avoid taking oral decongestants within 2 hours of bedtime because pseudoephedrine (Sudafed) may act as a stimulant. Advise patients to discontinue the medication and consult their physician if extreme restlessness or signs of sensitivity occur. Women should not breast feed while taking decongestants without consulting their physician.

Table 25-4 ■ The Most Commonly Used Decongestants

GENERIC NAME	TRADE NAME	AVERAGE ADULT DOSAGE	ROUTE OF ADMINISTRATION
Oral Decongestants			
pseudoephedrine	Sudafed	60 mg q4–6h or 120 mg sustained release q12h	PO
Combination Decongestants/Antihistamines			
cetirizine-pseudoephedrine	Zyrtec-D	5–10 mg once daily	PO
clemastine fumarate	Tavist	1.34 mg bid, may increase to 8.04 mg/d	PO
fexofenadine-pseudoephedrine	Allegra D	60 mg tid	PO
loratadine-pseudoephedrine	Claritin-D and others	10 mg/d on empty stomach	PO
naproxen-pseudoephedrine	Aleve Cold & Sinus	275–1,100 mg/d	PO
Nasal Decongestants			
phenazoline 0.05%	Allerest	2 drops or sprays in each nostril q3–6h up to 3–5 d	Nasal
oxymetazoline 0.05%	Afrin	2–3 drops in each nostril bid up to 3–5 d	Nasal
phenylephrine 1%	Neo-Synephrine, Sinex	1–2 drops in each nostril q3–4h	Nasal
tetrahydrozoline 0.1%	Tyzine	2–4 drops in each nostril q3h PRN	Nasal drops

* Apply Your Knowledge 25.3

The following questions focus on what you have just learned about antitussives and decongestants. *See Appendix E for the correct answers.*

FILL IN THE BLANK

Select terms from your reading to fill in the blanks.

1. Antitussives are agents that _____.

2. Antitussives are classified into two major groups: _____ and _____.

3. Decongestants are agents that reverse _____ of nasal cavities.

4. Mucolytics and expectorants are used in pulmonary complications of cystic fibrosis and _____, or _____.

5. Decongestants are vasoconstricting agents that shrink the _____ of the nasal airway passages of the upper respiratory tract.

MATCHING

Match the lettered drug trade name to the numbered generic drug name.

GENERIC NAME	TRADE NAME
1. _____ clemastine fumarate	a. Zyrtec-D
2. _____ fexofenadine-pseudoephedrine	b. Neo-Synephrine
3. _____ phenylephrine 1%	c. Allegra-D
4. _____ cetirizine-pseudoephedrine	d. Aleve Cold & Sinus
5. _____ loratadine-pseudoephedrine	e. Claritan-D
6. _____ naproxen-pseudoephedrine	f. Tavist

Chapter Capsule

This section repeats the objectives from the beginning of the chapter and then provides a summary of the most important concepts for that objective. Use this section as a quick review and to check your knowledge.

Objective 1: Describe the upper and lower respiratory tracts.

- Upper respiratory tract—nose, nasal cavity, paranasal sinuses, and pharynx
- Lower respiratory tract—larynx, trachea, bronchial tree, and lungs

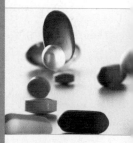

Objective 2: List the most commonly used medications for asthma.

- Asthma—most commonly treated by bronchodilators, xanthine derivatives, leukotriene inhibitors, corticosteroids, and mast cell stabilizers

Objective 3: Explain xanthine derivatives in the treatment of asthma.

- Xanthine derivatives—treat asthma by relaxing smooth muscle via direct action on the bronchi and pulmonary vessels

Objective 4: Describe the mechanism of action of leukotriene inhibitors.

- Leukotriene inhibitors—block either the synthesis of leukotrienes or the body's inflammatory responses to leukotrienes

Objective 5: Explain the contraindications of mast cell stabilizers.

- Mast cell stabilizers—contraindicated in patients with coronary artery disease, history of arrhythmias, dyspnea, acute asthma, status asthmaticus, during pregnancy, and in children under the age of 6 years; cromolyn sodium (Intal) should be used cautiously in renal or hepatic dysfunction

Objective 6: Describe the use of opioid cough suppressants.

- Opioid cough suppressants—used to suppress nonproductive cough, but limited use because of unwanted side effects; codeine and hydrocodone (Histussin) not as effective, but used to elevate the cough threshold

Objective 7: Define expectorants and mucolytic agents.

- Expectorants and mucolytics—medications capable of dissolving or promote liquefying of mucus in the lungs and facilitating elimination of mucus through coughing

Objective 8: Explain the mechanism of action of decongestants.

- Decongestants—vasoconstricting agents that shrink the swollen mucous membranes of the nasal airway passage of the upper respiratory tract; most oral agents—adrenergic medications or medications that mimic the effects of the sympathetic nervous system

 ## Internet Sites of Interest

- Information on various asthma topics and guidelines are available on the National Heart Lung and Blood Institute Web site at: **www.nhlbi.nih.gov**. Search for "asthma."

- The Family Doctor offers useful information on OTC decongestants at: **http://familydoctor.org/**. Search for "over the counter decongestants."

- Various lung disorders, including asthma and cough, are discussed in detail on the American Lung Association Web site at: **http://www.lungusa.org/**

- The Asthma and Allergy Foundation of America provides information, advocacy, and research on asthma at: **http://www.aafa.org/**

- A wealth of information about asthma and its treatments (including alternative therapies), screening tools, and prevention tips are found at MedlinePlus: **http://www.nlm.nih.gov/medlineplus/asthma.html**

Checkpoint Review 5

Select the best answer for the following questions.

1. Which of the following hormones is secreted by the kidneys?
   a. Vasopressin
   b. Oxytocin
   c. Luteinizing
   d. Erythropoietin

2. Following the proximal convoluted tubule is the:
   a. Distal convoluted tubule
   b. Loop of Henle
   c. Glomerular capsule
   d. Collecting duct

3. Which of the following is a major adverse effect of potassium-sparing diuretics?
   a. Hyperkalemia
   b. Hypercalcemia
   c. Hypokalemia
   d. Hypocalcemia

4. Antidiuretic hormone is also called:
   a. Oxytocin
   b. Adrenocorticotropic hormone
   c. Vasopressin
   d. Prolactin

5. Graves' disease is characterized by:
   a. Hypothyroidism
   b. Hyperthyroidism
   c. Myxedema
   d. Cretinism

6. Iodide is used alone for which of the following disorders or conditions?
   a. Hyperkalemia
   b. Hyperthyroidism
   c. Acute bronchitis
   d. Asthma

7. Propylthiouracil is classified as a (an):
   a. Diuretic drug
   b. Antihistamine
   c. Antithyroid agent
   d. Antihypertensive agent

8. Glucagon hormone is secreted by which of the following glands?

   a. Pancreas
   b. Thymus
   c. Thyroid
   d. Adrenal gland

9. The sulfonylureas are categorized as:
   a. Oral hypoglycemics
   b. Oral contraceptives
   c. Oral anticoagulants
   d. Loop diuretics

10. The alpha cells of the islets of the pancreas secrete:
    a. Insulin
    b. Thymosin
    c. Heparin
    d. Glucagon

11. Which of the following agents is used for nasal congestion and asthma?
    a. Furosemide
    b. Corticosteroids
    c. Potassium iodide
    d. Regular insulin

12. Loop diuretics are toxic to which of the following organs of the body?
    a. Ears
    b. Eyes
    c. Lungs
    d. Ovaries

13. Which of the following chronic conditions of the lungs is the most common in the United States?
    a. Nasal polyps
    b. Pneumonia
    c. Asthma
    d. Pulmonary edema

14. Bronchodilators that widen the diameter of the bronchial tubes include which of the following agents?
    a. Corticosteroids
    b. Narrow spectrum antibiotics
    c. Beta$_2$-adrenergic agonists
    d. Alpha$_2$-adrenergic agonists

15. Gestational diabetes develops during:
    a. Childhood
    b. The neonatal period
    c. Lactation
    d. Pregnancy

16. The antacids are all:

   a. Weak acids

   b. Weak alkalines

   c. Strong acids

   d. Strong alkalines

17. Which of the following are among the most misused drugs?

   a. Opioid analgesics

   b. Antidiarrheals

   c. Laxatives

   d. Antacids

18. All of the following are indications of androgens in women, except:

   a. Postpartum breast engorgement

   b. Fibrocystic breast disorders

   c. Breast cancer

   d. Endometriosis

19. Which of the following portions of the body secretes gonadotropin-releasing hormone?

   a. The hypothalamus

   b. The anterior pituitary

   c. The posterior pituitary

   d. The ovaries

20. The patient who is receiving insulin should be taught to be cautious about which of the following adverse effects?

   a. Malignant hyperthermia

   b. Severe hypotension

   c. Hypoglycemic reaction

   d. Malignant hypertension

21. Which of the following are the most effective drugs for controlling diarrhea?

   a. Osmotics

   b. Electrolytes

   c. Adsorbents

   d. Opioid antidiarrheals

22. A 70/30 combination of insulin means:

   a. NPH 70% and Regular insulin 30%

   b. NPH 30% and Regular insulin 70%

   c. NPH 30% and Novolin 70%

   d. NPH 70% and Novolin 30%

23. Stool softeners are sometimes called:

   a. Laxatives

   b. Osmotics

   c. Adsorbents

   d. Emollients

24. Which of the following is the best known synthetic estrogen?

   a. Norethindrone

   b. Diethylstilbestrol

   c. Megestrol

   d. Norgestrel

25. Which of the following is the trade name of insulin glargine (long-acting)?

   a. Novolin

   b. Lantus

   c. Humalog

   d. Humulin U

26. Which of the following chemical substances increases sodium ion reabsorption in the distal convoluted tubules and collecting ducts of the nephrons?

   a. Erythropoietin

   b. Insulin

   c. Glucagon

   d. Aldosterone

27. Water balance is regulated by the secretion of which of the following hormones?

   a. Vasopressin

   b. Thyroxin

   c. Erythropoietin

   d. Growth hormone

28. Exophthalmos (protrusion of the eyeball) is seen in which of the following conditions or disorders?

   a. Hyperparathyroidism

   b. Hyperthyroidism

   c. Hypertension

   d. Myxedema

29. Laxative stimulants are contraindicated in all of the following conditions, except:

   a. Fecal impaction

   b. Abdominal pain

   c. Pregnancy

   d. Constipation

30. Which of the following diuretics are used primarily for cerebral edema?

   a. Osmotic agents

   b. Carbonic anhydrase inhibitors

   c. Thiazide agents

   d. Loop diuretics

31. Which of the following portions of the male reproductive system stores sperm cells?

   a. Vas deferens

   b. Prostate gland

   c. Scrotum

   d. Epididymis

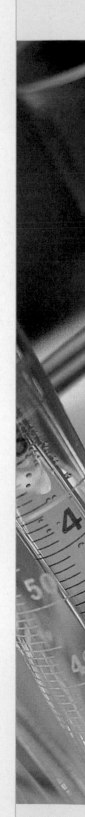

32. Which of the following agents stimulates powerful uterine contractions?

    a. Prolactin
    b. Progesterone
    c. Oxytocin
    d. Estrogen

33. Which of the following is the trade name of spironolactone?

    a. Dyrenium
    b. Aldactone
    c. Midamor
    d. Lasix

34. Which of the following drugs is an antiemetic?

    a. Ipecac
    b. Chlorpromazine
    c. Magnesium hydroxide
    d. Senna

35. Uterine relaxants include which of the following agents?

    a. Beta$_2$-adrenergic agonists
    b. Alpha$_2$-adrenergic agonists
    c. Cholinergic agonists
    d. Oxytocin hormone

36. Estrogen therapy in older women is used to prevent or treat which of the following disorders or conditions?

    a. Breast cancer
    b. Pregnancy
    c. Endometriosis
    d. Osteoporosis

37. Stoppage of blood flow is known as:

    a. Hemopoiesis
    b. Hemostasis
    c. Hemosiderosis
    d. Hemolysis

38. Which of the following chemical substances is released from the platelets?

    a. Serotonin
    b. Heparin
    c. Histamine
    d. Fibrinogen

39. Tagamet and Zantac are known as which of the following?

    a. Histamine agonists
    b. Histamine antagonists
    c. Antispasmodics
    d. Antacids

40. Which of the following is an example of an oral anticoagulant?

    a. Heparin
    b. Urokinase
    c. Streptokinase
    d. Coumadin

41. Allergic rhinitis is also known as:

    a. Rhinovirus
    b. Coryza
    c. Hives
    d. Hay fever

42. Which of the following anticoagulants should not be used during pregnancy?

    a. Warfarin
    b. Heparin
    c. Enoxaparin
    d. Ardeparin

43. The adrenal medulla synthesizes, stores, and secretes which of the following?

    a. Epinephrine and norepinephrine
    b. Androgen and glucocorticoids
    c. Parathormone
    d. Thyroxine

44. All of the following leafy green foods contain vitamin K, except:

    a. Parsley
    b. Swiss chard
    c. Spinach
    d. Sweet potatoes

45. Patients should be instructed to avoid exposure to UV light while taking which of the following drugs?

    a. Coumarin derivatives
    b. Thrombolytics
    c. Xanthine derivatives
    d. Progestins

46. Xanthine derivatives are used for prophylaxis and the symptomatic relief of which of the following conditions or disorders?

    a. Bronchial asthma
    b. Osteoporosis
    c. Dementia
    d. Pancreatitis

47. The process of blood clotting occurs in a series of sequential steps which are referred to as a:

    a. Prothrombin activator
    b. Cascade
    c. Thrombus
    d. Low-molecular-weight heparin

48. Most of the circulating clotting proteins are synthesized by which of the following organs in the human body?

    a. Lungs
    b. Liver
    c. Bones
    d. Brain

49. Conjugated estrogens (during the first trimester) may increase the risk for which of the following?

    a. Dysrhythmia in the fetus
    b. Heart failure in the fetus and infant
    c. Malabsorption in the infant
    d. Malformations in the fetus and infant

50. Which of the following is an example of antiplatelet agents?

    a. Heparin
    b. Abciximab
    c. Abbokinase
    d. Warfarin

For questions 51–55, match the lettered drug class to the numbered description.

DESCRIPTION

51. _____ Converted to theophylline

52. _____ Causes masculinization of the fetus

53. _____ Used to treat gastrointestinal disorders

54. _____ Metabolized from arachidonic acid

55. _____ Produces phasic contractions characteristic of normal delivery

DRUG CLASS

a. Leukotriene inhibitors
b. Oxytocic agents
c. Prostaglandins
d. Androgen derivatives
e. Xanthine derivatives

For questions 56–60, match the lettered drug trade name to the numbered drug generic name.

GENERIC NAME	TRADE NAME
56. _____ dalteparin	a. Lovenox
57. _____ danaparoid	b. Innohep
58. _____ ardeparin	c. Orgaran
59. _____ enoxaparin	d. Fragmin
60. _____ tinzaparin	e. Normiflo

Select terms from your reading to fill in the blanks.

61. Oral androgens should be taken with meals to reduce _____.

62. The testes secrete _____.

63. The best known synthetic _____ is diethyl-stilbestrol (Stilbestrol).

64. The ovaries are the primary source of progesterones and _____.

65. Primary digestion occurs in the _____.

66. H_2-receptor antagonists are used in short-term treatment of active _____.

67. The prostaglandins are involved in gastrointestinal _____ and gastric acid secretions.

68. Bronchodilators include _____ adrenergic agonists and _____.

69. Leukotriene inhibitors are bronchodilators and leukotriene receptor _____.

70. The pancreas is an accessory organ of the _____.

Chapter 26

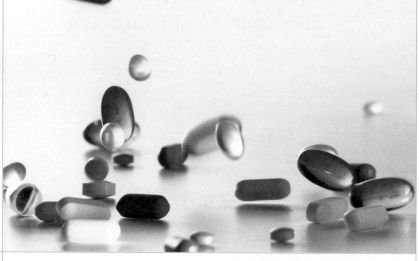

Effects of Drugs on Musculoskeletal Disorders

Chapter Objectives

After completing this chapter, you should be able to:

1. Describe the major functions of the skeletal system.
2. Identify the most common bisphosphonate agents used for osteoporosis.
3. Define rheumatoid arthritis.
4. List the major drugs used for rheumatoid arthritis.
5. Describe the major indications of methotrexate.
6. Explain gouty arthritis and the cause of gout.
7. Describe the mechanism of action of colchicine.
8. Explain the indications of allopurinol.
9. Name three disorders that may cause spasticity.
10. List commonly used central skeletal muscle relaxants.

Key Terms

Dysphagia (dis-FAY-jee-uh)
(page 572)

Flatulence (FLAT-yoo-lentz)
(page 572)

Hyperuricemia (hy-per-yoo-rih-SEE-mee-uh) (page 580)

Nephrotic syndrome (neh-FROT-ik)
(page 582)

Oligospermia (ol-lih-go-SPER-mee-uh)
(page 578)

Osteopenia (os-tee-oh-PEE-nee-uh)
(page 570)

Osteoporosis (os-tee-oh-por-OH-sis)
(page 570)

Spasticity (spas-TIH-sih-tee)
(page 583)

PRACTICAL SCENARIO

Leonora, a slightly built, 73-year-old woman, visits her long-time family physician complaining of low-grade but constant back pain. The nurse's exam finds that her weight has remained consistent over time, but she has lost almost 2 inches in height in the last 10 years. Reviewing her chart, the doctor notes that Leonora has been postmenopausal for more than 25 years, declined to take hormone replacement therapy, and 2 years ago broke her ankle stepping off a curb into the street. Physical examination shows kyphosis (humpback). The physician orders a DEXA scan to measure bone density, but tells Leonora that even without the results of the scan, she is quite sure that the osteopenia most people experience as they get older has, in this case, degenerated into osteoporosis.

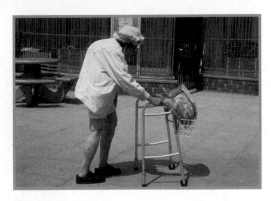

Bill Aron/PhotoEdit Inc.

Critical Thinking Questions

1. What is the significance of the fact that Leonora has been postmenopausal for many years?

2. What is the difference between osteopenia and osteoporosis, and why does one lead to a reduction in height in patients?

3. Would drug therapy or lifestyle changes work best for Leonora in managing her osteoporosis?

Introduction

Disorders of the musculoskeletal system are very common in people of all ages. Musculoskeletal conditions include osteoarthritis, muscle spasms, gout, bursitis, tendonitis, and rheumatoid arthritis. Medications used to treat these conditions include skeletal muscle relaxants, nonsteroidal anti-inflammatory drugs (NSAIDs), aspirin, and gold salts.

Musculoskeletal System

The musculoskeletal system consists of two body systems: (1) the muscular system and (2) the skeletal system. The muscular system includes three types of muscle tissues: (1) skeletal muscle, (2) cardiac muscle, and (3) smooth muscle. Skeletal muscle, which is discussed in this chapter, contains connective tissues, nerves, and blood vessels. Skeletal muscles produce movement, maintain posture and body position, support soft tissue, and maintain body temperature.

The skeletal system includes the bones of the skeleton, and the cartilages, ligaments, and other connective tissues that stabilize or connect the bones. The five primary functions of the skeletal system are: (1) support, (2) storage of minerals and lipids, (3) blood cell production, (4) protection, and (5) leverage (Figure 26-1 ■).

Calcium is the most abundant mineral in the human body. Its proper balance and interaction with other minerals and hormones is essential to optimal functioning of several body systems, particularly the musculoskeletal system. A typical human body contains 1 to 2 kg of calcium, with roughly 99% of it deposited in the skeleton. Calcium ion homeostasis is maintained by a negative feedback system involving a pair of hormones with opposing effects. These hormones—parathyroid hormone and calcitonin—coordinate the storage, absorption, and excretion of calcium ions. Three target sites are involved: (1) bones (storage), (2) digestive tract (absorption), and (3) kidneys (excretion).

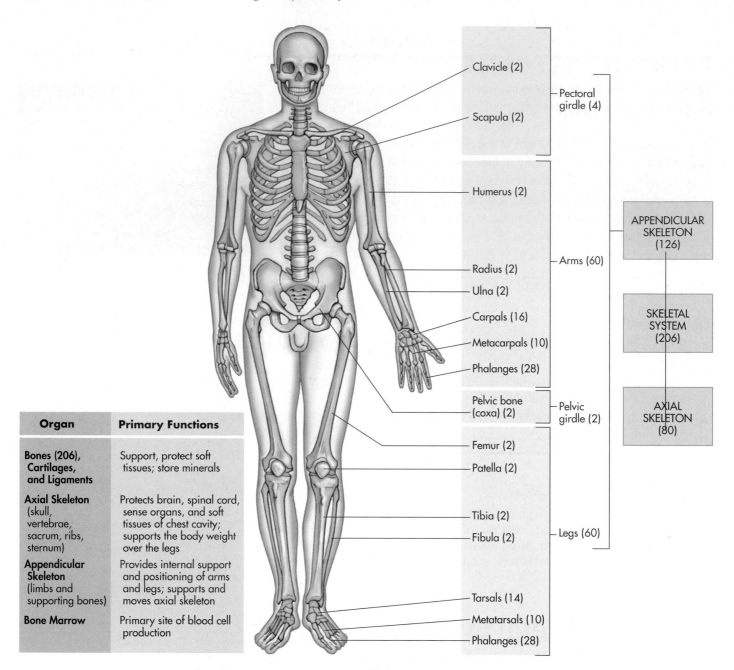

Organ	Primary Functions
Bones (206), Cartilages, and Ligaments	Support, protect soft tissues; store minerals
Axial Skeleton (skull, vertebrae, sacrum, ribs, sternum)	Protects brain, spinal cord, sense organs, and soft tissues of chest cavity; supports the body weight over the legs
Appendicular Skeleton (limbs and supporting bones)	Provides internal support and positioning of arms and legs; supports and moves axial skeleton
Bone Marrow	Primary site of blood cell production

Figure 26-1 ■ The skeletal system and its functions.

Osteoporosis

The bones of the skeleton become thinner and weaker as a normal part of the aging process. Inadequate ossification (the process of bone formation) is called **osteopenia**, and most people become slightly osteopenic as they age. This reduction in bone mass begins between the ages of 30 and 40.

When the reduction in bone mass is sufficient to compromise normal function, the condition is known as **osteoporosis**. The fragile bones that result are likely to break when exposed to stresses that younger individuals could easily tolerate. For example, a hip fracture can occur when a woman in her 90s simply tries to stand. Any fractures that do occur lead to loss of independence and immobility that further weakens the skeleton.

With its loss of normal bone density, osteoporosis leads literally to porous bone that can be described as being compressible like a sponge, rather than dense like a brick. It occurs more often in women than in men, especially in postmenopausal women, whose levels of the hormone estrogen are greatly decreased. Osteoporosis can cause permanent disability if not arrested, and treatment varies depending on the cause.

AGENTS AFFECTING POSTMENOPAUSAL OSTEOPOROSIS

Treatment of postmenopausal osteoporosis is an important area of new drug development because estrogen replacement therapy (ERT) and hormone replacement therapy (HRT), once popular forms of treatment for several postmenopausal conditions, including osteoporosis, have been associated with increased cardiovascular problems as well as the potential increased risk of endometrial and breast cancer in some patients (Table 26-1 ■). New drug developments include the selective estrogen-receptor modulators (SERMs) such as raloxifene (Evista), plus new-generation bisphosphonates.

prevent occurance of osteoporosis

Table 26-1 ■ Drugs Used to Treat Osteoporosis

GENERIC NAME	TRADE NAME	AVERAGE ADULT DOSAGE	ROUTE OF ADMINISTRATION
Bisphosphonates			
alendronate sodium	Fosamax, Fosamax-70	5–10 mg/d 70 mg once a wk	PO
risedronate sodium	Actonel	5 mg/d	PO
Hormonal Agents			
calcitonin salmon	Calcimar, Miacalcin	1 spray/d	Intranasal spray
raloxifene	Evista	60 mg/d	PO
sodium fluoride	Slow Fluoride	In cycles	PO

Bisphosphonates

The first bisphosphonate available for clinical use was etidronate (Didronel), but several new analogues are now available, including pamidronate (Aredia), alendronate (Fosamax), tiludronate (Skelid), and risedronate (Actonel). For treatment of osteoporosis, only alendronate (Fosamax) and risedronate (Actonel) are used. Alendronate (Fosamax) was the first oral bisphosphonate to be approved for the treatment and prevention of osteoporosis in postmenopausal women.

How do they work?
Alendronate is a highly selective inhibitor of bone demineralization and resorption (breakdown). It appears to increase bone mineral density. The mechanism of action of risedronate is not fully understood.

How are they used?
Only alendronate and risedronate have been approved for the treatment of osteoporosis, but other bisphosphonates are used for other purposes. For example, etidronate, pamidronate, and tiludronate are used for Paget's disease, a disorder similar to osteoporosis in that bones become very weak and brittle, but are characterized by constant bone resorption and formation, resulting in enlarged and abnormal bones. Pamidronate is also indicated for hypercalcemia of malignancy. Ibandronate sodium (Boniva) is a once-monthly medication for postmenopausal osteoarthritis used to build bone mass and maintain bone density.

What are the adverse effects?

Several gastrointestinal (GI) adverse effects may occur that include **flatulence** (presence of excess gas in the stomach and intestines), acid regurgitation, **dysphagia** (difficulty in swallowing), and gastritis. Other effects include headache, musculoskeletal pain, and rash.

What are the contraindications and interactions?

Alendronate and risedronate are contraindicated in hypersensitivity to these agents, severe renal impairment, hypocalcemia, lactation, and pregnancy. These agents should be used cautiously in patients with renal impairment, congestive heart failure, hyperphosphatemia, liver disease, fever or infection, and peptic ulcer. Calcium and food (especially dairy products) reduce alendronate absorption.

What are the important points patients should know?

Review with patients the correct administration of these medications, and advise patients to report fever, especially when accompanied by arthralgia and myalgia. Instruct patients to take the drugs at least 30 minutes before food, beverages, or other medications. Women should not breast feed while taking these drugs.

Hormonal Agents

For patients who are unable to take ERT or bisphosphonates, hormonal agents such as calcitonin (Calcimar, Miacalcin) or raloxifene (Evista) are often prescribed.

Calcitonin

Calcitonin is secreted by the parafollicular cells of the thyroid glands of mammals. Calcitonin is a natural product obtained from salmon. Human calcitonin is also available (Cibacalcin) but is not as potent or long lasting.

How does it work?

The principal effects of calcitonin are to lower serum calcium and phosphate by action on the bones and kidneys. Calcitonin inhibits bone resorption and lowers serum calcium. Thus, calcitonin increases bone density and reduces the risk of vertebral fractures.

How is it used?

Calcitonin is approved for the treatment of osteoporosis in postmenopausal women, hypercalcemia, and symptomatic Paget's disease.

What are the adverse effects?

The adverse effects of calcitonin include headache, eye pain, hypersensitivity reactions, and anaphylaxis (reported for human calcitonin [Cibacalcin] only). Urinary frequency, chills, chest pressure, weakness, dizziness, nasal congestion, and shortness of breath are other adverse effects of calcitonin.

What are the contraindications and interactions?

Calcitonin is contraindicated in patients with hypersensitivity to fish proteins or to synthetic calcitonin. It should be avoided in patients with a history of allergy. Safe use in children, pregnancy, and lactation is not established. Calcitonin should be used cautiously in patients with renal impairment and pernicious anemia. Calcitonin may interact with, and may decrease serum lithium (Eskalith) levels.

What are the important points patients should know?

Advise patients to watch for redness, warmth, or swelling at the injection site, and report any of these effects to their physicians, because it may indicate an inflammatory reaction. Instruct patients to consult their physicians before using OTC preparations such as some supervitamins, hematinics (which improve the condition of the blood), and antacids containing calcium and vitamin D.

Focus on Natural Products

DMSO

Dimethyl sulfoxide, also known as DMSO, has a long history as a topical agent that can help reduce pain and inflammation in various musculoskeletal disorders, such as tendonitis. DMSO should only be used under the guidance of a qualified health-care professional.

RALOXIFENE HYDROCHLORIDE

Raloxifene (Evista) is one of the selective estrogen-receptor modulators (SERMs) and is considered to be an estrogen antagonist.

How does it work?

Raloxifene acts by combining with estrogen receptors. It decreases bone resorption and increases bone mass and density by acting through the estrogen receptor. Raloxifene has not been associated with endometrial proliferation or the increased risk of uterine or breast cancers.

How is it used?

Raloxifene is used primarily to prevent and treat osteoporosis in postmenopausal women. It is also used to reduce the risk of breast cancer in postmenopausal women. This agent is able to reduce total serum cholesterol and low-density lipoprotein (LDL).

What are the adverse effects?

The adverse effects of raloxifene include hot flashes, migraines, headache, flu-like symptoms, uterine disorders, vaginal bleeding, urinary tract disorders, and breast pain. Other adverse effects are depression, insomnia, and dizziness.

What are the contraindications and interactions?

Raloxifene is contraindicated in women who are, or who might become pregnant, and in those with active (or history of) venous thromboembolic events (for example, pulmonary embolism or retinal vein thrombosis). It is also contraindicated with concurrent use of systemic ERT. Raloxifene should be used cautiously with diazepam (Valium), lidocaine (Anestacon), and diazoxide (Proglycem). It can interact with cholestyramine (Questran) and warfarin (Coumadin).

What are the important points patients should know?

Advise patients to contact their physician immediately if unexplained calf pain or tenderness occurs. They should avoid prolonged restriction of movement during travel. Be sure patients are aware that raloxifene (Evista) can induce hot flashes. Patients should not breast feed while taking this drug.

Focus Point

Raloxifene

Raloxifene is the first of the selective estrogen-receptor modulators to be approved for the prevention of osteoporosis.

✳ Apply Your Knowledge 26.1

The following questions focus on what you have just learned about the musculoskeletal system, osteoporosis, and related medications. *See Appendix E for the correct answers.*

FILL IN THE BLANK
Select terms from your reading to fill in the blanks.

1. The primary functions of the skeletal system include _____, _____, _____, _____, and _____.

2. Three types of muscle tissues are _____, _____, and _____ muscle.

3. Inadequate ossification is known as _____.

4. Calcium ion homeostasis involves a pair of hormones known as _____ and _____.

5. Raloxifene is considered an estrogen antagonist and is a selective _____ (SERM).

MATCHING
Match the lettered drug trade name to the numbered generic drug name.

GENERIC NAME	TRADE NAME
1. _____ salmon calcitonin	a. Vivactil
2. _____ raloxifene	b. Actonel
3. _____ risedronate sodium	c. Fosamax
4. _____ alendronate sodium	d. Evista
5. _____ calcium carbonate	e. Miacalcin

Rheumatoid Arthritis

Rheumatoid arthritis (RA) is a systemic autoimmune disease that involves inflammation of the membranes lining the joints and often affects internal organs. Most patients exhibit a chronic fluctuating course of disease that can result in progressive joint destruction, deformity, and disability. It occurs two to three times more often in women, and the peak onset occurs between the fourth and sixth decades of life.

Most commonly, the joints first affected by RA include the metacarpophalangeal joints of the hands, metatarsophalangeal joints of the feet, and the wrists. Other areas affected by this disease include the spine, shoulders, ankles, and hips. Rheumatoid arthritis involves not only joint capsules, but also tendons, ligaments, and skeletal muscles. The goals in the management of RA are to:

✳ Prevent or control joint damage

✳ Prevent loss of function

✳ Decrease pain

✳ Maintain the patient's quality of life

✳ Avoid or minimize adverse effects of treatment

Antirheumatic Drugs

Drug therapy for RA involves the treatment of symptoms and use of disease-modifying agents. Drugs with anti-inflammatory activity are the agents of choice for the symptomatic relief of RA. Salicylates, NSAIDs, and COX-2 inhibitors (as discussed in Chapter 12) reduce joint pain and swelling, but they do not alter the course of the disease or prevent joint destruction. Corticosteroids have excellent anti-inflammatory activity and are immunosuppressants. Disease-modifying antirheumatic drugs (DMARDs) reduce or prevent joint damage and preserve joint function. DMARDs are listed in Table 26-2 ■.

Table 26-2 ■ Disease-Modifying Drugs for Rheumatoid Arthritis

GENERIC NAME	TRADE NAME	AVERAGE ADULT DOSAGE	ROUTE OF ADMINISTRATION
Gold Compounds			
auranofin	Ridaura	3–6 mg/d; may increase up to 3 mg tid after 6 mo	PO
aurothioglucose	Solganal	10–50 mg; initially: 10 mg; then increased weekly until 1 g is reached	IM
gold sodium thiomalate	Myochrysine	Dose may be continued at 25–50 mg every other wk for 2–20 wk	IM
Miscellaneous Agents			
adalimumab	Humira	40 mg every other week (may use 40 mg/wk if not on concomitant methotrexate)	Subcutaneous
etanercept	Enbrel	25 mg twice weekly or 0.08 mg/kg (or 50 mg) once weekly	Subcutaneous
hydroxychloroquine sulfate	Plaquenil	200–600 mg/d	PO
methotrexate	Folex, Mexate	2.5–5 mg bid for 3 doses/wk	PO
sulfasalazine	Azulfidine	250–500 mg/d (max: 8 g/d)	PO

GOLD COMPOUNDS

Gold compounds, such as auranofin (Ridaura), aurothioglucose (Solganal), and gold sodium thiomalate (Myochrysine), were first proved to be effective in a large group of patients in 1960. Because of their toxicity, they are used infrequently today.

How do they work?

The mechanism of anti-inflammatory action of gold compounds is not clearly understood. Gold uptake by macrophages with subsequent inhibition of migration and phagocytic action occurs, thereby suppressing immune responsiveness, which may be the principal mechanism of action.

How are they used?

Gold compounds are effective for active RA. They are generally used when adequate trials with salicylates or other NSAIDs have not been satisfactory.

What are the adverse effects?

The adverse effects of gold compounds include hypersensitivity, syncope, bradycardia, thickening of the tongue, and a metallic taste in the mouth. Hematologic abnormalities are thrombocytopenia, leukopenia, and aplastic anemia.

What are the contraindications and interactions?

These agents are contraindicated in patients with gold allergy or history of severe toxicity from previous therapy with gold or other heavy metals. Gold compounds should not be used in patients with uncontrolled diabetes mellitus, renal or hepatic insufficiency, or history of hepatitis. Gold compounds may increase the risk of blood dyscrasias if they are used with antimalarials, immunosuppressants, and penicillamine (Cuprimine), another DMARD.

What are the important points patients should know?

Be sure that patients are aware of possible adverse effects and know to report them to their physicians. If therapy is interrupted at the onset of gold toxicity, serious reactions can be avoided. Advise patients to report any unusual color or odor of their urine, and to avoid contact with anyone who has a cold, has had a recent vaccination, or has been recently exposed to a communicable disease.

Focus Point

Gold Compounds

Adverse reactions to gold compounds are most likely to occur during the second and third months of therapy. However, reactions may appear at any time during therapy, or even several months after treatment has been discontinued.

HYDROXYCHLOROQUINE

Hydroxychloroquine sulfate (Plaquenil) is classified as an anti-infective and an antimalarial. This agent is used mainly to treat malaria.

How does it work?

The mechanism of the anti-inflammatory action of this drug in rheumatic diseases is unclear.

How is it used?

Hydroxychloroquine is approved for RA but is not considered one of the most efficacious DMARDs. Hydroxychloroquine is often used for the treatment of lupus erythematosus.

What are the adverse effects?

The adverse effects of hydroxychloroquine are fatigue, headache, mood or mental changes, anxiety, retinopathy, blurred vision, and difficulty focusing. Other adverse effects include anorexia, nausea, vomiting, diarrhea, and abdominal cramps.

What are the contraindications and interactions?

Hydroxychloroquine is contraindicated in patients with known hypersensitivity to this agent. Safe use in pregnancy or lactation is not established. Hydroxychloroquine must be used cautiously in patients with hepatic disease, alcoholism, and impaired renal function.

   Aluminum- and magnesium-containing antacids and laxatives decrease hydroxychloroquine absorption. This agent may interfere with the response to rabies vaccine.

What are the important points patients should know?

Teach patients about the adverse effects and symptoms of prolonged therapy with this drug. Advise them to follow the drug regimen exactly as prescribed by their physicians, and make sure to keep this drug out of reach of children. Because this drug may cause damage to the eyes, advise patients to get regular eye exams. Instruct patients to avoid breastfeeding while taking this drug without consulting their physicians.

Focus on Pediatrics

Hydroxychloroquine

Hydroxychloroquine has not been established for safe use in juvenile arthritis. It should not be used during pregnancy, because it crosses the placental barrier, nor during lactation.

METHOTREXATE

Formerly called amethopterin, methotrexate (Folex, Mexate) was once considered the DMARD of first choice in the treatment of RA. However, newer DMARDs, such as adalimumab (Humira) and etanercept (Enbrel), are becoming first-choice agents (see Table 26-2).

1st agent nonsteroidal

2nd. methotroxide

How does it work?

Methotrexate is a folic-acid blocker and immunosuppressant that affects lymphocyte and macrophage function.

How is it used?

Methotrexate is principally used in combination regimens to maintain induced remissions in neoplastic diseases. Methotrexate is also used to treat severe psoriasis, psoriatic arthritis, and rheumatoid arthritis.

What are the adverse effects?

The most common toxicity of methotrexate is dose-related bone marrow suppression. Infertility with azoospermia (absence of living spermatozoa in the semen) and amenorrhea also occur. GI upset and mouth sores are less serious common adverse effects.

What are the contraindications and interactions?

Methotrexate is contraindicated in pregnancy and lactation; in men and women of childbearing age; hepatic and renal insufficiency; or preexisting blood dyscrasias. Methotrexate should be used cautiously in patients with infections, peptic ulcer, ulcerative colitis, cancer patients with preexisting bone marrow impairment, and poor nutritional status.

   Alcohol, azathioprine (Azasan), and sulfasalazine (Azulfidine) increase the risk of hepatotoxicity if used with methotrexate. Chloramphenicol (Chlorofair), sulfonamides, salicylates, NSAIDs, phenytoin (Dilantin), tetracyclines, and probenecid (Benemid) may increase methotrexate levels with increased toxicity.

What are the important points patients should know?

Be sure patients are aware of the dangers of this drug and know to promptly report any abnormal symptoms to their physicians. They should know that the most common adverse affects are stomach upset, mouth sores, headache, and drowsiness. Alcohol ingestion increases the incidence and severity of methotrexate hepatotoxicity. Instruct patients that they should not self-medicate with vitamins or over-the-counter (OTC) compounds that include folic acid, which alters methotrexate response. They should avoid exposure to sunlight and ultraviolet light, and wear sunglasses and sunscreen.

Focus Point

Methotrexate

Prolonged treatment with small frequent doses of methotrexate may lead to hepatotoxicity, which is best diagnosed by liver biopsy.

PENICILLAMINE

Penicillamine (Cuprimine) is a metabolite of penicillin and is rarely used today because of toxicity. Therefore, it will not be discussed here for the treatment of RA.

SULFASALAZINE

Sulfasalazine (Azulfidine) is a GI and anti-inflammatory agent.

How does it work?

Sulfasalazine is a locally acting sulfonamide that is believed to be converted by intestinal microflora to sulfapyridine, providing antibacterial action, and to 5-aminosalicylic acid or mesalamine, which may exert an anti-inflammatory effect. It may also inhibit prostaglandins that are known to cause diarrhea and affect mucosal transport, as well as interfere with absorption of fluids and electrolytes from the colon.

How is it used?

Sulfasalazine is effective in RA and reduces the rate of appearance of new joint damage. It has been used in juvenile chronic arthritis and ankylosing spondylitis.

What are the adverse effects?

Approximately 30% of patients using sulfasalazine discontinue the drug because of toxicity. Common adverse effects include nausea, vomiting, headache, and rash. Other adverse effects include anemia, **oligospermia** (a subnormal concentration of spermatozoa in the ejaculate), blood dyscrasias, liver injury, and allergic reactions.

What are the contraindications and interactions?

Sulfasalazine is contraindicated in patients with sensitivity to this agent or other sulfonamides and salicylates. It should not be used in patients with agranulocytosis, intestinal and urinary tract obstruction, or porphyria. Sulfasalazine is contraindicated in pregnancy and in children younger than 2 years of age. It should be used cautiously in patients with severe allergy or bronchial asthma, hepatic or renal impairment, and in children under the age of 6 years. Antibiotics may alter absorption of sulfasalazine.

What are the important points patients should know?

Instruct patients that this drug may color the urine and skin orange-yellow. Women should not breastfeed while taking sulfasalazine without consulting their physicians.

✸ Apply Your Knowledge 26.2

The following questions focus on what you have just learned about rheumatoid arthritis and antirheumatic drugs. *See Appendix E for the correct answers.*

MULTIPLE CHOICE

Select the correct answers from choices a–d.

1. Which of the following agents used to treat active rheumatoid arthritis can cause thickening of the tongue and metallic taste?

    a. Penicillamine

    b. Sulfasalazine

    c. Methotrexate

    d. Gold compounds

2. Aluminum-containing antacids may decrease absorption of which of the following anti-rheumatic drugs?

   a. Sulfasalazine

   b. Hydroxychloroquine

   c. Auranofin

   d. Penicillamine

3. Which of the following disease-modifying drugs for rheumatoid arthritis must be administered by intramuscular (IM) injection?

   a. Hydroxychloroquine

   b. Methotrexate

   c. Aurothioglucose

   d. Sulfasalazine

4. Which of the following is the oldest drug used to treat rheumatoid arthritis and is used infrequently today?

   a. Methotrexate

   b. Penicillamine

   c. Sulfasalazine

   d. Gold sodium thiomalate

5. Which of the following is a systemic autoimmune disorder?

   a. Gout

   b. Paget's disease

   c. Rheumatoid arthritis

   d. Osteoporosis

MATCHING

Match the lettered drug trade name to the numbered drug generic name.

GENERIC NAME	TRADE NAME
1. _____ methotrexate	a. Plaquenil
2. _____ sulfasalazine	b. Ridaura
3. _____ aurothioglucose	c. Azulfidine
4. _____ penicillamine	d. Myochrysine
5. _____ auranofin	e. Solganal
6. _____ gold sodium thiomalate	f. Cuprimine
7. _____ hydroxychloroquine sulfate	g. Folex

Gout and Gouty Arthritis

Several distinct diseases are characterized by crystal deposition in and around joint spaces. This deposition can lead to acute inflammation of the joint. Gout is a metabolic disorder of sodium urate deposition (which involves uric acid crystals), in which uric acid accumulates in the bloodstream or joint cavities, causing inflammation and pain. Gout is classified as primary, secondary, or gouty arthritis. Primary gout is a disease primarily of the adult male with a peak incidence in the fifth decade of life.

The cause of gout is either the overproduction or underexcretion of uric acid. Primary gout generally is caused by overproduction of uric acid and may be due to enzyme deficiencies in the metabolic pathway for purines or genetic dysfunction. Secondary gout, characterized by underexcretion of uric acid, may be caused by diminished renal function, interaction with various medications, or unknown causes.

Primary gout has three manifestations: (1) asymptomatic **hyperuricemia** (elevated uric-acid blood level), (2) acute gouty arthritis, and (3) chronic gouty arthritis. In *acute gouty arthritis*, the onset of the attack is abrupt and typically occurs at night or early in the morning as synovial fluid is reabsorbed. In acute gouty arthritis, immobilization of the affected joints, most often the big toes, heels, ankles, wrists, fingers, elbows, or knees, is very important.

DRUGS FOR GOUTY ARTHRITIS

Anti-inflammatory drug therapy should begin immediately, and urate-lowering drugs should not be given until the acute attack has been controlled. Specific drugs include colchicine, allopurinol, NSAIDs, and corticosteroids (Table 26-3 ■).

Table 26-3 ■ Anti-Gout Medications

GENERIC NAME	TRADE NAME	AVERAGE ADULT DOSAGE	ROUTE OF ADMINISTRATION
allopurinol	Aloprim, Zyloprim	200–800 mg/d	PO, IV
colchicine	colchicine (generic only)	0.5–0.6 mg/d prophylactically; 0.5–1.2 mg q1–2 h for acute attack	PO
probenecid	Benemid	250–500 mg bid	PO
sulfinpyrazone	Anturane	100–400 mg/d	PO

COLCHICINE

Colchicine is an anti-inflammatory agent specifically used for gout and is ineffective for any other disease. Colchicine is not an analgesic, so it does not relieve the symptoms of any condition but gout.

How does it work?

Colchicine acts by inhibiting the formation of white blood cells, which decreases joint inflammation.

How is it used?

Colchicine may be used to treat acute gouty attacks or to reduce the incidence of attacks in chronic gout.

What are the adverse effects?

The most common adverse effects are GI disturbances, such as nausea, vomiting, diarrhea, and abdominal pain. Colchicine may decrease intestinal absorption of vitamin B_{12}.

What are the contraindications and interactions?

Colchicine is contraindicated in blood dyscrasias, severe GI conditions, severe renal conditions, severe hepatic conditions, and severe cardiac disease. Use of IV colchicine is contraindicated in patients with both renal and hepatic dysfunction. Severe local irritation can result from subcutaneous or intramuscular (IM) use. It is also contraindicated during pregnancy, and its safe use in children has not been established.

What are the important points patients should know?

Instruct patients taking colchicine at home to withhold the drug and report to their physicians any onset of GI symptoms or signs of bone marrow depression (nausea, sore throat, bleeding gums, sore mouth, fever, fatigue, malaise, and unusual bleeding or bruising). Advise patients to keep colchicine on hand at all times to start therapy or to increase dosage, if a physician directs, at the first suggestion of an acute attack. Advise patients to avoid beer, ale, and wine because they may precipitate gouty attack. Women taking colchicine should not breast feed without consulting their physicians.

Focus on Geriatrics

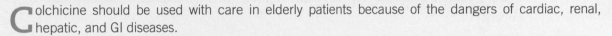

Colchicine Use in Elderly Patients

Colchicine should be used with care in elderly patients because of the dangers of cardiac, renal, hepatic, and GI diseases.

ALLOPURINOL

Allopurinol (Aloprim, Zyloprim) is known as an anti-gout agent because it improves the solubility of uric acid. It is used for chronic gout and will not relieve an attack already started. The drug must be taken regularly for a few months to be effective.

How does it work?

Allopurinol reduces endogenous uric acid by selectively inhibiting action of xanthine oxidase, the enzyme responsible for converting xanthine derivatives to uric acid (the end product of purine catabolism). Allopurinol has no analgesic, anti-inflammatory, or uricosuric (increasing excretion of uric acid) actions.

How is it used?

Allopurinol is used to control primary hyperuricemia that accompanies severe gout and to prevent possibilities of acute gouty attack.

What are the adverse effects?

Allopurinol may cause drowsiness, headache, dizziness, nausea, vomiting, diarrhea, and abdominal pain. In some cases, this agent may cause hepatotoxicity and renal insufficiency. Allopurinol can produce pruritus and skin rash.

What are the contraindications and interactions?

Allopurinol is contraindicated in patients with hypersensitivity to this agent. Allopurinol is also contraindicated as initial treatment for acute gouty attacks. This medication should be avoided in children (except in those with hyperuricemia secondary to cancer and chemotherapy). Safety during pregnancy or lactation is not established. Allopurinol should be used cautiously in patients with impaired hepatic or renal function, history of peptic ulcer, lower GI tract disease, and bone marrow depression.

Drug interaction of allopurinol with alcohol, caffeine, and thiazide diuretics may increase the uric-acid level; it may increase the risk of skin rash if used with ampicillin (Amcill) and amoxicillin (Amoxil). Allopurinol enhances the anticoagulant effect of warfarin (Coumadin).

What are the important points patients should know?

Advise patients to drink enough fluid (at least 3,000 mL, or 3 quarts, per day) to produce urine output of at least 2,000 mL, or 2 quarts, per day. Instruct patients to report diminishing urine output, cloudy urine, unusual color or odor to urine, pain or discomfort on urination, and onset of itching or rash. Tell patients to stop taking allopurinol if a skin rash appears even after 5 or more weeks of therapy. Patients should minimize exposure to ultraviolet light or sunlight and not drive or engage in potentially hazardous activities until their response to this drug is known. This drug should only be taken under constant medical supervision, and women taking allopurinol should not breast feed without consulting their physicians.

Uricosuric Agents

Probenecid (Benemid) and sulfinpyrazone (Anturane) are uricosuric drugs that are employed to decrease the amount of urate in patients with increasingly frequent gouty attacks.

How do they work?

These agents work by competitively inhibiting renal tubular reabsorption of uric acid, thereby promoting its excretion and reducing serum urate levels.

How are they used?

Uricosuric therapy should be initiated if several acute attacks of gouty arthritis have occurred or when plasma levels of uric acid in patients with gout are so high that tissue damage is almost inevitable.

What are the adverse effects?

Adverse effects of uricosuric agents do not provide a basis for preferring one or the other. Both of these organic acids cause gastrointestinal irritation, but sulfinpyrazone is more active in this regard. Probenecid is more likely to cause allergic dermatitis, but a rash may appear after the use of either compound. Another adverse effect of using probenecid is **nephrotic syndrome** (a clinical state characterized by edema, various abnormal substances present in the urine, decreased plasma albumin, and usually, increased blood cholesterol).

What are the contraindications and interactions?

Uricosuric therapy is contraindicated in patients with blood dyscrasias and uric-acid kidney stones. Safety during pregnancy, lactation, or in children younger than 2 years of age is not established. These agents should be used cautiously in patients with history of peptic ulcer.

Salicylates may decrease uricosuric activity and methotrexate (Folex, Mexate, Rheumatrex) elimination. There is an increased risk of nitrofurantoin (Furadantin) toxicity if used with probenecid or sulfinpyrazone.

What are the important points patients should know?

Advise patients to drink fluids liberally (approximately 3,000 mL per day) to maintain daily urine output of at least 2,000 mL or more. Physicians may advise restriction of high-purine foods during early therapy until uric-acid levels stabilize. Foods high in purine include organ meats (sweetbreads, liver, kidneys), meat extracts, meat soups, and gravy. Instruct patients to avoid alcohol because it may increase serum urate levels. They should be instructed not to stop taking these drugs, or to take aspirin or other OTC medications, without first consulting their physicians.

Focus Point

Uricosuric Therapy

Urate-lowering drugs should not be started until after the acute attack has completely resolved, a process that takes 2 to 3 weeks.

✳ Apply Your Knowledge 26.3

The following questions focus on what you have just learned about gouty arthritis and its drug therapy. *See Appendix E for the correct answers.*

FILL IN THE BLANK
Select terms from your reading to fill in the blanks.

1. Gout is a disorder of sodium _____.

2. The cause of gout is either the _____ or _____ of uric acid.

3. Colchicine is an anti-inflammatory agent specifically used for _____.

4. Allopurinol reduces endogenous uric acid by selectively inhibiting the action of _____.

5. Allopurinol is contraindicated as the initial treatment for _____.

6. Colchicine is not an analgesic and does not relieve the symptoms of any condition except _____.

7. Allopurinol is used to control primary _____.

8. For the treatment of gout, _____ should begin immediately, and urate-lowering drugs should not be given until the _____ has been controlled.

9. Uricosuric drugs include _____ and _____.

10. Uricosuric therapy should be initiated if several _____ attacks of _____ have occurred.

MATCHING
Match the lettered drug trade name to the numbered drug generic name.

GENERIC NAME	TRADE NAME
1. _____ allopurinol	a. Indocin
2. _____ indomethacin	b. Anturane
3. _____ probenecid	c. Benemid
4. _____ sulfinpyrazone	d. Alloprin (Alloprin is a trade name in Canada only.)

Muscle Spasms and Pain

Muscular spasms and pain are often associated with traumatic injuries and **spasticity** (inability of opposing muscle groups to move in a coordinated manner) from chronic debilitating disorders such as cerebral palsy, strokes, or head and spinal cord injuries. Muscle spasms can also be caused by overmedication with antipsychotic drugs, epilepsy, and hypocalcemia. Transmission of impulses from motor nerves to muscle cells occurs across spaces known as *neuromuscular junctions.* These spaces are sensitive to chemical changes in their immediate environment. Therefore, somatic motor nerve impulses cannot be generated, which may also decrease the availability of calcium ions to the myofibrillar contractile system.

There are two types of muscle spasms: *tonic* and *clonic* spasms. A single, prolonged contraction is called a tonic spasm, whereas multiple, rapidly repeated contractions are known as clonic spasms. Most muscle spasms and strains are self-limited and respond to rest, physical therapy, and short-term use of aspirin and other analgesics.

SKELETAL MUSCLE RELAXANTS

Treatment of muscle spasms may be both nonpharmacologic and pharmacologic (muscle relaxants). Nonpharmacologic treatments include immobilization of the affected muscle, application of heat or cold, ultrasound, hydrotherapy, and massage. Local anesthesia may also effect relaxation of limited muscle groups, and local anesthetic block of efferent somatic motor outflow is sometimes used to relieve localized skeletal muscle spasms.

Spasticity results from increased muscle tone due to hyperexcitable neurons, or the lack of inhibition in the spinal cord (or at the skeletal muscles). Many neurologic disorders that cause spasticity require the long-term use of muscle relaxants. The skeletal muscles are voluntary muscles under control of the central nervous system (CNS). Skeletal muscle relaxants work by blocking somatic motor nerve impulses through depression of specific neurons within the CNS.

Centrally Acting Muscle Relaxants

These agents, such as baclofen (Lioresal), cyclobenzaprine (Flexeril), and lorazepam (Ativan), relieve symptoms of muscular stiffness and rigidity. Centrally acting muscle relaxants improve mobility of the part of the body that is affected. Pharmacotherapy for muscle spasms can be a combination of analgesics, anti-inflammatory medications, and centrally acting skeletal muscle relaxants. The centrally acting muscle relaxants are listed in Table 26-4 ■.

How do they work?
The exact mechanism of action of these agents is unknown, but they may affect the brain or spinal cord to inhibit upper motor neuron activity.

How are they used?
Skeletal muscle relaxants are used to treat local spasms to reduce pain and increase range of motion. Baclofen (Lioresal) is often a drug of first choice because of its wide safety margin.

What are the adverse effects?
All of the centrally acting agents can cause sedation. Common adverse effects include drowsiness, dizziness, weakness, and fatigue. Tizanidine (Zanaflex) and other centrally acting agents may cause hallucinations or *ataxia* (loss of coordination, such as that caused by benzodiazepines).

What are the contraindications and interactions?
Baclofen (Lioresal) is contraindicated in bacteremia (the presence of viable bacteria in circulating blood) and clotting disorders. Carisoprodol (Soma) should be avoided in patients with acute intermittent porphyria and in children younger than age 5. Clonazepam (Klonopin) is contraindicated in liver disease and glaucoma. None of the centrally acting muscle relaxants should be used during pregnancy and lactation.

Centrally acting muscle relaxants such as baclofen should not be used with alcohol and other CNS depressants, monamine oxidase (MAO) inhibitors, and antihistamines. Baclofen may increase blood glucose levels, making it necessary to increase dosage of sulfonylureas and insulin.

What are the important points patients should know?

Instruct patients to avoid consuming alcoholic beverages and other CNS depressants because this combination will potentiate CNS depression. Incidence of CNS symptoms are reportedly high in patients older than 40 years. Advise patients with diabetes to closely monitor blood glucose for loss of glycemic control. Patients should avoid driving and using heavy machinery until the effect is stabilized because these drugs are prone to cause drowsiness and dizziness. Tell patients to report all adverse reactions to their physician. Instruct patients not to self-dose with OTC drugs without their physician's approval. These drugs should not be stopped abruptly, and the stopping of these drugs should be directed by a physician. Instruct female patients that these drugs should not be taken during pregnancy or while breastfeeding.

Table 26-4 ■ Centrally Acting Muscle Relaxants

GENERIC NAME	TRADE NAME	AVERAGE ADULT DOSAGE	ROUTE OF ADMINISTRATION
baclofen	Lioresal	15–80 mg/d in divided doses	PO
carisoprodol	Soma	350 mg tid–qid	PO
chlorphenesin carbamate	Maolate	400–800 mg/d in divided doses	PO
chlorzoxazone	Paraflex, Parafon	250–750 mg tid–qid	PO
clonazepam	Klonopin	0.5–20 mg tid	PO
cyclobenzaprine	Flexeril	10–60 mg/d in divided doses	PO
dantrolene	Dantrium	Initially: 25 mg/d; then 50–400 mg/d in divided doses	PO
diazepam	Valium	2–10 mg bid–qid	PO
		2–10 mg	IM, IV
lorazepam	Ativan	1–10 mg bid–tid	PO
methocarbamol	Robaxin	1.5 g qid for 2–3 d; then 4–4.5 g/d in 3–6 divided doses	PO
		0.5–1 g q8h	IM
		1–3 g/d in div. doses (max: rate of 300 mg/min)	IV
orphenadrine citrate	Banflex, Norflex	100 mg bid	PO
		60 mg bid	IM, IV

Focus Point

Baclofen

Baclofen (Lioresal) is at least as effective as diazepam (Valium) in reducing spasticity and produces much less sedation.

✳ Apply Your Knowledge 26.4

The following questions focus on what you have just learned about skeletal muscle relaxants and centrally acting muscle relaxants. *See Appendix E for the correct answers.*

MATCHING
Match the lettered drug trade name to the numbered drug generic name.

GENERIC NAME	TRADE NAME
1. _____ lorazepam	a. Dantrium
2. _____ metaxalone	b. Flexeril
3. _____ baclofen	c. Lioresal
4. _____ orphenadrine	d. Skelaxin
5. _____ cyclobenzaprine	e. Norflex
6. _____ dantrolene	f. Ativan

MULTIPLE CHOICE
Select the correct answers from choices a–d.

1. Rapidly repeated contractions of skeletal muscles are called:
   a. Clonic spasms
   b. Colic spasms
   c. Tonic spasms
   d. Cardiac spasms

2. All of the following are nonpharmacological therapies for skeletal muscle spasms, except:
   a. Ultrasound
   b. Hydrotherapy
   c. Electroshock
   d. Immobilization

3. Which of the following is often a drug of first choice for local spasms?
   a. cyclobenzaprine (Flexeril)
   b. diazepam (Valium)
   c. methocarbamol (Robaxin)
   d. baclofen (Lioresal)

4. Baclofen is contraindicated in which of the following conditions?
   a. Peptic ulcer
   b. Clotting disorders
   c. Acute intermittent porphyria
   d. Asthma

5. Muscle spasms may be caused by all of the following, except:
   a. Hypocalcemia
   b. Epilepsy
   c. Hypertension
   d. Hypercalcemia

Chapter Capsule

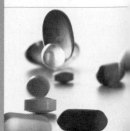

This section repeats the objectives from the beginning of the chapter and then provides the most important concept for that objective. Use this section as a quick review and to check your knowledge.

Objective 1: Describe the major functions of the skeletal system.

- Support, storage of minerals and lipids, blood cell production, protection, and leverage

Objective 2: Identify the most common bisphosphonate agents used for osteoporosis.

- Alendronate (Fosamax)—first oral bisphosphonate approved for treatment and prevention of osteoporosis in postmenopausal women
- Risedronate (Actonel)

Objective 3: Define rheumatoid arthritis.

- Systemic autoimmune disease; involves inflammation of the membranes lining the joints; often affects internal organs
- A chronic fluctuating course of disease that can result in progressive joint destruction, deformity, and disability
- Occurs two to three times more often in women; peak onset between the fourth and sixth decades of life

Objective 4: List the major drugs used for rheumatoid arthritis.

- Treatment of symptoms—drugs with anti-inflammatory activity, such as salicylates, NSAIDs, and COX-2 inhibitors; corticosteroids have excellent anti-inflammatory activity and are immunosuppressants
- Treatment to prevent joint damage and preserve joint function—disease-modifying antirheumatic drugs (DMARDs), such as methotrexate (Folex, Mexate), sulfasalazine (Azulfidine), etanercept (Enbrel) and adalimumab (Humira)

Objective 5: Describe the major indications of methotrexate.

- Principally used in combination regimens to maintain induced remissions in neoplastic diseases; also used to treat severe psoriasis, psoriatic arthritis, and rheumatoid arthritis

Objective 6: Explain gouty arthritis and the cause of gout.

- Disorder of sodium urate deposition (which involves uric-acid crystals) characterized by crystal deposition in and about joint spaces, which can lead to acute inflammation of the joint
- Primarily a disease of the adult male, with peak incidence in the fifth decade of life
- Caused by either the overproduction or the underexcretion of uric acid
- Primary gout has three manifestations—asymptomatic hyperuricemia, acute gouty arthritis, and chronic gouty arthritis
- Onset of *acute gouty arthritis* is abrupt, typically occurring at night or early in the morning as synovial fluid is reabsorbed

Objective 7: Describe the mechanism of action of colchicine.

- Inhibits the formation of white blood cells to decrease joint inflammation

Objective 8: Explain the indications of allopurinol.

- Used to control primary hyperuricemia (high levels of uric acid in the blood circulation) that accompanies severe gout and to prevent acute gouty attack

Objective 9: Name three disorders that may cause spasticity.

- Cerebral palsy
- Stroke
- Head or spinal cord injuries

Objective 10: List commonly used central skeletal muscle relaxants.

- baclofen (Lioresal)
- carisoprodol (Soma)
- chlorphenesin carbamate (Maolate)
- chlorzoxazone (Paraflex, Parafon)
- clonazepam (Klonopin)
- cyclobenzaprine (Flexeril)
- dantrolene (Dantrium)
- diazepam (Valium)
- lorazepam (Ativan)
- methocarbamol (Robaxin)
- orphenadrine citrate (Banflex, Norflex)

Internet Sites of Interest

- The National Institute of Neurological Disorders and Stroke, a division of the NIH, provides information about spasticity and its treatments at: **www.ninds.nih.gov**. Search for "spasticity."

- MedicineNet.com provides an in-depth look at rheumatoid arthritis at: **www.medicinenet.com**. Search for "rheumatoid arthritis."

- Johns Hopkins University, Division of Rheumatology, offers a comprehensive discussion about treatments for rheumatoid arthritis at: **www.hopkins-arthritis.som.jhmi.edu**. Click on "rheumatoid arthritis" in left-hand column.

- For more information about the rheumatoid arthritis drug methotrexate (Folex, Mexate, Rheumatrex) visit: **www.rxlist.com**. Click on "methotrexate."

Chapter Objectives

After completing this chapter, you should be able to:

1. Describe the structure and function of the eye.

2. Explain glaucoma and types of glaucoma.

3. State the rationale for use and the mechanism of action of carbonic anhydrase inhibitors in the treatment of glaucoma.

4. Identify direct-acting miotics (cholinergic drugs) and list two generic and trade names.

5. Explain mydriatic agents and their indications.

6. State the mechanism of action of antimuscarinics.

Chapter 27

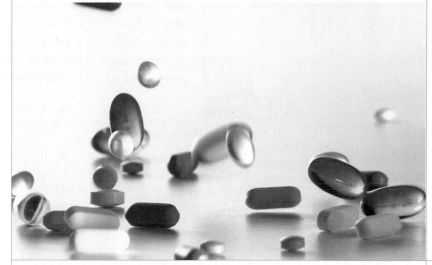

Effects of Drugs on Eye Disorders

Key Terms

Accommodation (page 590)

Aqueous humor (AY–kwee–us) (page 591)

Blepharitis (blef-fah-RY-tis) (page 599)

Cataract (page 592)

Choroid layer (KO-royd) (page 590)

Ciliary body (SIL-ee-ayr-ee) (page 590)

Ciliary muscle (page 590)

Cornea (page 590)

Glaucoma (glauw-KO-ma) (page 592)

Iris (page 591)

Lens (page 590)

Optic nerve (page 590)

Photoreceptors (page 591)

Pupil (page 591)

Retina (page 591)

Retinal detachment (page 596)

Retinopathy (ret-tin-NOP-pa-thee) (page 592)

Sclera (page 590)

Vitreous humor (VIT-ree-us) (page 592)

PRACTICAL SCENARIO

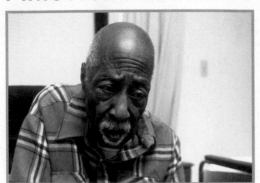

A 72-year-old African-American man with a history of hypertension, coronary artery disease, and diabetes mellitus presents with the inability to clearly see objects at a distance and visual field loss. He also states that 2 days ago, he missed some stairs as he was walking up to the second floor of his home. The physician conducts an eye examination and determines that the patient's intraocular pressure is 25 mm Hg, there is no hemorrhage in the retina, and his right eye has a mild cataract. The physician diagnoses this patient as having glaucoma.

Critical Thinking Questions

1. After the physician leaves the room, the patient asks the medical assistant about this condition. How should the medical assistant explain the diagnosis to this patient, including its complications and possible relationship to his other disorders?

2. What treatment options would you tell the patient are available?

3. What would you tell the patient about his lifestyle that may be helpful with regard to this diagnosis?

Introduction

A number of the key drug groups mentioned elsewhere in the text are used in ophthalmology. Drug groups such as the antimicrobials, corticosteroids, adrenergic drugs, muscarinic drugs, and nonsteroidal anti-inflammatory drugs (NSAIDs) have ophthalmic indications. In this chapter, the effects of these drugs on the eye will be emphasized.

Structure and Function of the Eye

The eye is a hollow, spherical structure about 2.5 cm in diameter. Its wall has three distinct layers. These layers consist of an outer layer (**sclera**), a middle layer (**choroid layer** or "coat"), and an inner layer (retina). The spaces within the eye are filled with fluids that support its wall and internal parts.

The anterior of the sclera bulges forward as the transparent **cornea**, the window of the eye, and helps to focus entering light rays. Along the circumference, the cornea is continuous with the sclera (the white portion of the eye). In the back of the eye, the **optic nerve** and certain blood vessels pierce the sclera.

The middle layer includes the choroid layer, ciliary body, and iris (Figure 27-1 ■). The choroid layer contains many pigment-producing melanocytes. The melanin that these cells produce absorbs excess light and helps to keep the inside of the eye dark.

The **ciliary body**, which is the thickest part of the middle layer, extends forward from the choroid layer and forms an internal ring around the front of the eye, which constitutes the **ciliary muscle**. Many strong but delicate fibers, called *suspensory ligaments,* extend inward from the ciliary processes and hold the transparent **lens** in position. The distal ends of these fibers attach along the margin of a thin capsule that surrounds the lens. The ciliary muscles and suspensory ligaments, along with the structure of the lens itself, enable the lens to adjust shape to facilitate focusing, a phenomenon called **accommodation**. The functions of the ciliary body are controlled by the parasympathetic nervous system. The uveal tract of the eye consists of the iris, ciliary body, and choroid.

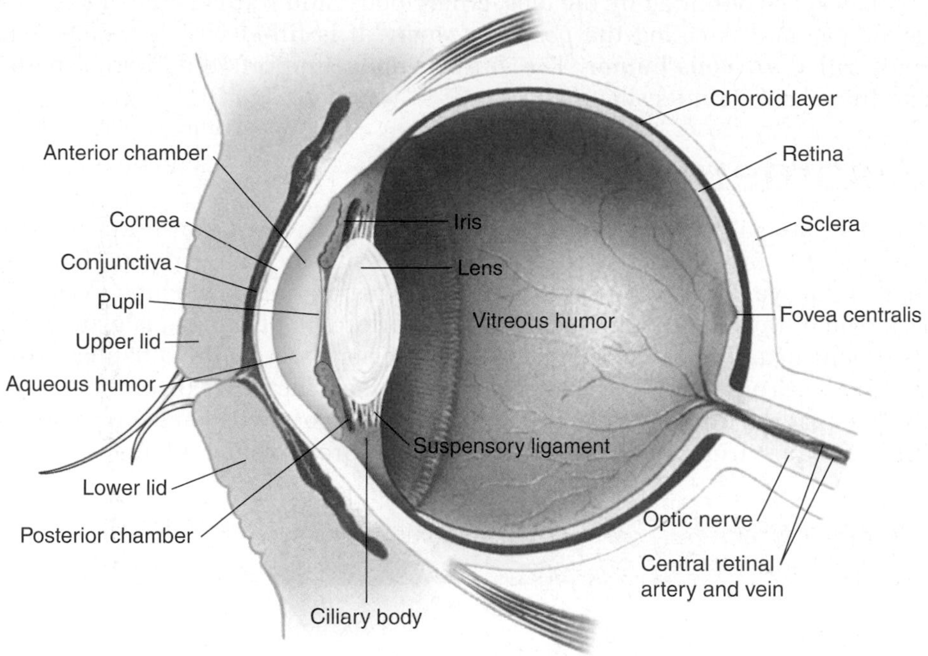

Figure 27-1 ■ Anatomy of the eye.

The **iris** is a thin diaphragm composed mostly of connective tissue and smooth muscle fibers. From the outside, the iris is the colored portion of the eye. The ciliary body secretes a watery fluid called **aqueous humor** into the posterior chamber. The iris extends forward from the periphery of the ciliary body and lies between the cornea and lens (see Figure 27–1). The fluid circulates from this chamber through the **pupil**, a circular opening in the center of the iris, and into the anterior chamber. Aqueous humor fills the space between the cornea and lens, helps nourish these parts, and aids in maintaining the shape of the front of the eye. It subsequently leaves the anterior chamber through veins and a special drainage canal, the scleral venous sinus (Schlemm canal), located in its wall at the junction of the cornea and the sclera. The iris consists of circular and radially arranged bands of smooth muscle, innervated by the autonomic nervous system, that control the size of the pupil. The autonomic nervous system plays an important part in the regulation of the eye functions. Structures such as the iris, ciliary body, lens, lacrimal glands, and ocular vasculature receive autonomic innervation. The effects of this stimulation are summarized in Table 27-1 ■.

The inner layer consists of the **retina**, which contains the visual receptor cells (**photoreceptors**). This layer is continuous with the optic nerve in the back of the eye and extends forward on the inner layer of the eyeball.

Table 27-1 ■ Effect of Autonomic Nervous System on the Eye

PARTS OF THE EYE	EFFECTS OF SYMPATHETIC STIMULATION	EFFECTS OF PARASYMPATHETIC STIMULATION
Ciliary muscle	Relaxation (for far vision)	Accommodation
Ciliary processes	Vasoconstriction of ciliary processes increases aqueous humor production	Increased outflow of aqueous humor and vasodilation
Iris	Contraction of the radial muscle: pupil dilation (mydriasis)	Contraction of the circular muscle: pupil constriction (miosis)
Conjunctival vasculature	Vasoconstriction	Vasodilation
Conjunctival vasculature	Vasoconstriction	Vasodilation
Lacrimal apparatus	Vasoconstriction	Increased secretion and vasodilation

The space bounded by the lens, ciliary body, and retina is the largest compartment of the eye and is called the *posterior cavity*. It is filled with a transparent, jelly-like fluid called **vitreous humor**. The vitreous body supports the internal parts of the eye and helps maintain its shape.

Disorders of the Eye

The eyes are subject to various disorders, some of which are serious. These disorders may include inflammation, infections, injuries, glaucoma, **cataract** (an opacity of the lens of the eye), and diabetic **retinopathy** (degeneration of the blood vessels of the retina). One of the most common and serious disorders of the eye is glaucoma, for which treatment usually begins with medication. Therefore, in this chapter, most emphasis will be on drugs used in treatment of glaucoma. The other disorders or conditions of the eye that are initially treated with lasers or surgery will not be discussed here. Anti-inflammatory drugs and antibiotics have been previously explained in other chapters.

Focus on Pediatrics

Congenital Cataracts

Congenital cataracts may result from chromosomal abnormalities and maternal diseases during pregnancy. If the cataracts are dense and obscure the view of the optic disk, an ophthalmologist must determine the possible long-term effects on the infant's vision, and surgery may be recommended.

Glaucoma

Glaucoma damages the optic nerve and is often caused by elevated intraocular pressure. This elevation of the intraocular pressure (IOP) results from excessive production of aqueous humor or diminished ocular fluid outflow. When the pressure is persistently high, blindness may occur secondary to optic nerve damage. Glaucoma is the second most common cause of blindness in the United States (cataract is number one). Normal IOP ranges from 11 to 21 mm Hg; however, this level may not necessarily be healthy for all people. Some people with normal pressure develop optic nerve injury. In contrast, many patients have IOP of more than 21 mm Hg without any optic nerve injury (ocular hypertension). The two types of glaucoma include acute angle-closure and chronic open-angle glaucoma. Figure 27-2 ■ shows the normal condition of the eye, as well as open-angle and angle-closure glaucoma.

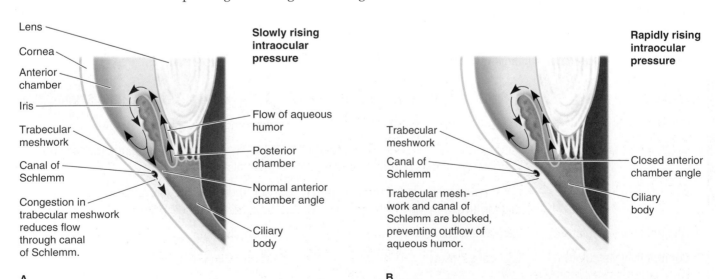

Figure 27-2 ■ The pathophysiology of glaucoma: (A) slowly rising IOP; (B) rapidly rising IOP.

Open-angle glaucoma is by far the more common form, accounting for about 90 percent of cases. Risk factors for primary open-angle glaucoma are listed in Table 27-2 ■. This type of glaucoma is generally responsive to drug therapy. Other treatments for open-angle glaucoma may include lasers or surgery. Most of the drugs used in the treatment of open-angle glaucoma are also used in the acute management of narrow-angle glaucoma prior to operation.

Table 27-2 ■ Risk Factors for Primary Open-angle Glaucoma

Elevated intraocular pressure	Diabetes
Older age	Hypertension
Family history	Myopia
Black race	Use of corticosteroids

Angle-closure glaucoma accounts for 10% of all glaucomas in the United States. Angle-closure glaucoma can be primary due to pupillary block. It is most common among Eskimos and Asians. Primary angle closure is more common in women, elderly patients, and patients with a family history of angle-closure glaucoma.

Focus on Geriatrics

Glaucoma in Elderly Adult

Although glaucoma can occur in any age group, it is six times more common in persons older than 60 years.

✳ Apply Your Knowledge 27.1

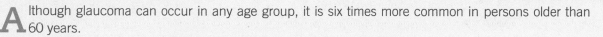

The following questions focus on what you have just learned about the structure and functions of the eye, and the most common eye disorders. *See Appendix E for the correct answers.*

FILL IN THE BLANK
Select terms from your reading to fill in the blanks.

1. The iris is a thin diaphragm composed of connective tissue and _____.

2. The space bounded by the lens, ciliary body, and retina is a compartment of the eye that is known as the _____.

3. The ocular disease that most commonly causes blindness is _____.

4. The anterior of the sclera that bulges forward is called the _____.

5. The choroid layer (or coat) contains many melanocytes that produce _____.

6. The most inner layer of the eye is the _____.

7. The iris consists of smooth muscle that is innervated by the _____ nervous system.

8. The suspensory ligaments hold the _____.

9. The risk factors for glaucoma include age older than 60 years and use of _____.

10. Open-angle glaucoma is by far the _____ form.

OPHTHALMIC PREPARATIONS TO TREAT GLAUCOMA

Drug therapy is directed toward reducing the raised IOP. In general, the medications used either reduce the formation of aqueous humor or enhance the drainage of aqueous humor from the eye. Some drugs, such as adrenaline, possess both of these actions. The drugs used for treatment of glaucoma include beta-adrenergic blockers, cholinergic direct-acting agents (miotics), cholinesterase inhibitors, sympathomimetics, carbonic anhydrase inhibitors, and prostaglandin inhibitors (Table 27-3 ■).

Table 27-3 ■ Drug Therapies in Glaucoma that Decrease Formation of Aqueous Humor

GENERIC NAME	TRADE NAME	AVERAGE ADULT DOSAGE	ROUTE OF ADMINISTRATION
Beta-Adrenergic Blocking Agents			
betaxolol	Betoptic, Kerlone	1 drop 0.5% solution bid	Topical
carteolol	Ocupress	1 drop 1% solution bid	Topical
levobunolol	Betagan	1–2 drops 0.25–0.5% solution 1–2 times/d	Topical
metipranolol	OptiPranolol	1 drop 0.3% solution bid	Topical
timolol	Betimol, Timoptic	1–2 drops of 0.25–0.5% solution 1–2 times/d	Topical
Alpha$_2$–Adrenergic Blocking Agents			
apraclonidine	Lopidine	1 drop 0.5% solution bid	Topical
brimonidine tartrate	Alphagan P	1 drop 0.2% solution bid	Topical
Carbonic Anhydrase Inhibitors			
acetazolamide	Diamox	250 mg 1–4 times/d	PO
dichlorphenamide	Daranide, Oratrol	100–200 mg followed by 100 mg bid	PO
dorzolamide hydrochloride	Trusopt	1 drop 2% solution tid	PO
methazolamide	Neptazane	50–100 mg bid–tid	PO
Osmotic Diuretics			
glycerine anhydrous	Ophthalgan	1–1.8 g/kg 1–1.5 h before ocular surgery; may repeat q5h	PO
isosorbide	Ismotic	1–3 g/kg bid–qid	PO
mannitol	Osmitrol	1.5–2 mg/kg as a 15–25% solution over 30–60 min	IV

Beta-Adrenergic Blockers

Beta-blocker agents are relatively safe, highly efficacious, act longer than the cholinergic agonists, and have no effects on pupil size or accommodation.

How do they work?

Beta-blockers lower the cyclic adenosine monophosphate (cAMP) levels within the ciliary body necessary for aqueous humor production. This reduces elevated IOP in chronic open-angle glaucoma by reducing the formation of aqueous humor.

How are they used?

The beta-blockers are considered the drugs of first choice in the treatment of intraocular hypertension and chronic open-angle glaucoma.

What are the adverse effects?

The most common adverse effects are local, mild ocular stinging, dry eyes, tearing, blurred vision, and eye irritation. Beta-adrenergic blockers may also have the adverse effects of systemic beta blockers. These agents may mask symptoms of acute hypoglycemia in diabetic patients (tachycardia and tremor, but not sweating). Beta-adrenergic blockers may precipitate thyrotoxic crisis in patients with hyperthyroidism.

What are the contraindications and interactions?

Beta-adrenergic blockers are contraindicated in patients with angle-closure glaucoma (unless used with a miotic), sinus bradycardia, and cardiogenic shock. Safety during pregnancy and in children younger than 18 years is not established. These drugs should be used cautiously in patients with heart failure or diabetes mellitus, in those who have evidence of airflow obstruction, and during lactation.

Reserpine (Serpalan) may interact with beta-blockers and cause addictive hypotensive effects or bradycardia. Verapamil (Calan) may cause addictive heart block.

What are the important points patients should know?

Advise patients to report unusual or significant changes in pulse rate to their physician according to the parameters provided. Instruct patients to follow their dosing regimen exactly as prescribed. They should not stop these drugs abruptly. Instruct patients to report difficulty in breathing promptly to their physician because the drug may need to be withdrawn.

Carbonic Anhydrase Inhibitors

Carbonic anhydrase inhibitors are diuretic agents, but they are also available as eye preparations.

How do they work?

Carbonic anhydrase inhibitors act on the enzyme responsible for the conversion of carbon dioxide to bicarbonate and hydrogen ions. The mechanism of action of this group (in glaucoma) is different from that described for the kidneys in Chapter 21. In the eye, carbonic anhydrase plays a significant role in aqueous humor formation by the ciliary body cells. In the ciliary bodies, carbonic anhydrase facilitates the secretion of bicarbonate ions in the aqueous humour. Carbonic anhydrase inhibitors therefore decrease the formation of aqueous humour.

How are they used?

Glaucoma has become the main clinical indication for the carbonic anhydrase inhibitors. Most of these drugs must be administered systemically. Dorzolamide (Trusopt) is available in a topical preparation.

What are the adverse effects?

The carbonic anhydrase inhibitors are closely related to the sulfanilamide antibacterial agents. As such, they produce a similar profile of adverse effects, including skin rashes, kidney stones, and aplastic anemia. Other adverse effects associated with this group are depression, anorexia, and electrolyte imbalances (especially potassium).

What are the contraindications and interactions?

Carbonic anhydrase inhibitors are contraindicated in patients with chronic noncongestive angle-closure glaucoma. These drugs should be avoided in patients with hypersensitivity and marked renal or hepatic dysfunction. Safety during pregnancy or lactation is not established. Carbonic anhydrase inhibitors should be used cautiously in patients with a history of hypercalciuria, diabetes mellitus, gout, and asthma. These drugs may interact with amphetamines, ephedrine (Efedron), and procainamide (Procan) to decrease renal excretion.

What are the important points patients should know?

Instruct patients to avoid touching the eye with the tip of the drug dispenser. Tell them to discontinue the drug and report to their physician if ocular irritations, infection, or systemic hypersensitivity occurs. Be sure to advise patients that some of these drugs may cause drowsiness and that they should avoid hazardous activities until the response to drugs is known. If patients are using oral medications (acetazolamide), they should report numbness, tingling, burning, drowsiness, visual problems, sore throat, fever, and renal problems. Advise them to eat potassium-rich foods and take potassium supplements while taking acetazolamide in high doses or for prolonged periods.

Focus on Natural Products

Bilberry for Eye Health

The berries, roots, and leaves of the bilberry plant have been used to improve night vision, to prevent cataracts, macular degeneration, and glaucoma, and to prevent and treat diabetic retinopathy and myopia. However, it should be avoided during pregnancy and lactation, and may cause constipation if large amounts of the dried fruit are consumed. Higher-than-recommended doses of this herb for extended periods will result in toxicity and may even result in death.

Osmotic Diuretics

Osmotic diuretic drugs are commonly used in patients needing eye surgery or for acute closed-angle glaucoma. These agents include glycerin anhydrous (Ophthalgan), isosorbide (Ismo), and mannitol (Osmitrol). Osmotic diuretics were discussed in Chapter 21.

Direct-Acting Miotics (Cholinergic Agents)

Miotic muscarine agonists (Table 27-4 ■) are agents that constrict the pupils. Miotics are often used to treat glaucoma.

How do they work?

Miotic agents act primarily to increase the drainage of aqueous humour out of the anterior cavity through the canal of Schlemm. They achieve this effect through miosis (pupil constriction) and contraction of the ciliary muscles responsible for accommodation. These effects are mediated by the parasympathetic nervous system.

How are they used?

The muscarinic agonists are used in open-angle and angle-closure glaucoma. Examples of muscarinics include acetylcholine chloride, pilocarpine (Adsorbocarpine), and carbachol (Miostat).

What are the adverse effects?

Systemic adverse effects of topical muscarinic agonists are few, with headache being the most common. The most common adverse effect of the muscarinic agonists on the eye is pupil constriction.

What are the contraindications and interactions?

Cholinergic agents (miotics) are contraindicated in patients with hypersensitivity, contact allergy, cataract, **retinal detachment** (separation of the retina from the corneal layer), and depression. Cholinergic drugs may interact with monamine oxidase (MAO) inhibitors and cause increased risk of hypertensive emergency. They may increase the effects of beta blockers and other antihypertensives on blood pressure and heart rate.

What are the important points patients should know?

Advise patients to use caution during nighttime driving and in performing hazardous activities in poor light. Instruct them to report to their physician if any sensitivity or severe adverse drug reactions occur.

Table 27-4 ■ Drug Therapy in Glaucoma that Increases the Outflow of Aqueous Humor

GENERIC NAME	TRADE NAME	AVERAGE ADULT DOSAGE	ROUTE OF ADMINISTRATION
Direct-Acting Miotics (Cholinergic Agents)			
carbachol	Isopto Carboptic, Miostat	1–2 drops 0.75%–3% solution q4h–tid	Topical
pilocarpine hydrochloride	Isopto Carpine Miocarpine	1 drop of 1% solution in affected eye	Topical
Indirect-Acting Miotics (Cholinesterase Inhibitors)			
demecarium bromide	Humorsol	1–2 drops of 0.125%–0.25% solution 2 times/wk	Topical
physostigmine salicylate	Antilirium	1 drop of 0.25%–0.5% solution 1–4 times/d	Topical
Sympathomimetics			
dipivefrin hydrochloride	Propine	1 drop in eye q12h	Topical
epinephrine borate	Epinal	1–2 drops as needed	Topical
phenylephrine hydrochloride	Neo-Synephrine	1 drop of 2.5% or 10% solution before examination	Topical
Prostaglandins and Prostamides			
bimatoprost	Lumigan	1 drop of 0.03% solution daily in the evening	Topical
latanoprost	Xalatan	1 drop of 1.5 mg solution daily in the evening	Topical
travoprost	Travatan	1 drop in affected eye(s) once daily in the evening	Topical
unoprostone	Rescula	1 drop of 0.15% solution bid	Topical

Indirect-Acting Miotics (Cholinesterase Inhibitors)

The cholinesterase inhibitors are more potent and longer acting than the direct-acting miotic agents.

How do they work?
Cholinesterase inhibitors produce severe miosis and muscle contractions. These actions cause a decreased resistance to aqueous outflow.

How are they used?
Cholinesterase inhibitors are used to treat open-angle glaucoma. Examples of this group include demecarium (Humorsol) and physostigmine (Antilirium).

What are the adverse effects?
Ophthalmic-related adverse effects of cholinesterase inhibitors include lacrimation, burning conjunctivitis, retinal detachment, and conjunctival thickening. Systematic adverse effects are nausea, vomiting, diarrhea, abdominal cramps, difficulty breathing, urinary incontinence, salivation, and fainting.

What are the contraindications and interactions?
Cholinesterase inhibitors are contraindicated in patients with hypersensitivity to these agents. The drugs are also contraindicated in patients with any acute inflammatory

disorders of the eye, and during pregnancy or lactation. The cholinesterase inhibitors should be used cautiously in patients with chronic angle-closure glaucoma, or in patients with myasthenia gravis. Drug interactions occur with carbachol (Miostat), beta blockers, atropine (Atropisol), ipratropium (Atrovent), and echothiophate (Phospholine Iodide).

What are the important points patients should know?
Instruct patients that aching around the eyebrows or temporary burning or stinging may occur initially but usually disappears as the body adjusts to the medication. Vision may be temporarily blurred or unstable after applying eye drops. Advise patients to use caution if driving or performing duties requiring clear vision. Because the medication may cause sensitivity to bright light, instruct patients to wear sunglasses. Advise patients to inform the doctor about changes in vision, eye pain, sweating, nausea, vomiting, diarrhea, difficulty breathing, increased urination or salivation, or irregular heartbeat.

Focus Point

Eye Protection and Insecticides/Pesticides

Individuals working with insecticides or pesticides that contain organophosphate or carbonate, and using cholinesterase inhibitors, must wear respiratory masks, change their clothes frequently, and wash exposed clothes thoroughly.

Sympathomimetic Agents

Sympathomimetics have both alpha- and beta-adrenergic activity (see Chapter 15). Apraclonidine (Iopidine) and brimonidine (Alphagan P) are relatively selective alpha$_2$ agonists. Dipivefrin (Propine) and phenylephrine (AK-Dilate Ophthalmic) are beta-adrenergic agonists.

How do they act?
The sympathomimetics can decrease the formation of aqueous humor and increase its outflow by activating adrenoreceptors associated with the ciliary body.

How are they used?
The sympathomimetic drugs we have listed can be used in the management of glaucoma.

What are the adverse effects?
Common adverse effects of dipivefrine and phenylephrine include headache, blurred vision, a stinging sensation during instillation, and increased sensitivity to light. *Rebound nasal congestion* (hyperemia and edema of mucosa), nasal burning, and sneezing may also occur. Other adverse effects of sympathomimetics include palpitation, tachycardia, bradycardia (overdosage), extrasytoles, hypertension, sweating, sleeplessness, anxiety, and dizziness.

What are the contraindications and interactions?
Sympathomimetic agents are contraindicated in patients with hypersensitivity to these drugs, or in patients with severe coronary disease, severe hypertension, angle-closure glaucoma (ophthalmic preparations), pregnancy, and lactation. Ophthalmic solution (10%) of dipivefrin (Propine) and phenylephrine (AK-Dilate Ophthalmic) should be used cautiously in cardiovascular disease, diabetes mellitus, hyperthyroidism, hypertension, pregnancy, elderly patients, and in infants. Epinephrine (Bronkaid Mist) should not be used while wearing soft lenses because discoloration of lenses may occur. There are no known drug interactions with ophthalmic preparations. Dobutamine (Dobutrex) may increase risk of hypertension when it is given along with beta-adrenergic blockers. The effects of dopamine (Dopastat) may be increased

when given with a tricyclic antidepressant or monoamine oxidase inhibitor. Epinephrine may interact with a tricyclic antidepressant and cause increased risk of sympathomimetic effects. Excessive hypertension may occur when epinephrine is used with propranolol (Inderal).

What are the important points patients should know?

Patients should be aware that the instillation of 2.5 to 10% strength ophthalmic solution can cause burning and stinging. Instruct them to not exceed recommended dosage regardless of formulation. Tell patients that systemic absorption from nasal and conjunctival membranes could occur. Instruct patients to discontinue the drug and report to their physician if adverse effects occur, and to wear sunglasses in bright light because the pupils will be large and the eyes may be more sensitive to light than usual. Advise patients that some ophthalmic solutions may stain contact lenses.

Focus Point

Eyedrops and Contact Lenses

Patients with contact lenses must remove them and leave them out for at least 15 minutes after administration of eyedrop preparations.

Prostaglandin Agonists

Research has shown that prostaglandins also have a role in the movement of aqueous humor through the eye.

How do they work?

Prostaglandin agonist agents increase aqueous humor outflow by reducing congestion in the *trabecular meshwork*, resulting in lowered intraocular pressure

How are they used?

Prostaglandin agonists are used in the treatment of open-angle glaucoma and intraocular hypertension to lower IOP. Travoprost (Travatan) can be used as first-line monotherapy or in combination with timolol.

What are the adverse effects?

The ocular adverse effects of prostaglandin agonists include ocular dryness, visual disturbance, ocular burning, foreign body sensation, eye pain, pigmentation of the periocular skin, **blepharitis** (inflammation of one or both eyes), cataract, ocular irritation, eye discharge, tearing, increase pigmentation of the iris, and photophobia.

What are the contraindications and interactions?

Prostaglandin agonists should be avoided in patients with hypersensitivity and during pregnancy. These agents are to be used cautiously in patients with active intraocular inflammation, those wearing contact lenses, and in lactating women. These agents may interact with thimerosal (Mersol) and other topical ophthalmic drugs.

What are the important points patients should know?

Instruct patients, especially those with green eyes, of a possible change in iris pigmentation, which is an irreversible condition.

Focus Point

Allergic Blepharoconjunctivitis

Apraclonidine (Iopidine) should be used only for the short-term for lowering intraocular pressure, because with chronic use it is associated with allergic blepharoconjunctivitis.

✳ Apply Your Knowledge 27.2

The following questions focus on what you have just learned about the treatment of glaucoma. *See Appendix E for the correct answers.*

MATCHING

Match the lettered drug trade name to the numbered generic drug name.

GENERIC NAME	TRADE NAME
1. _____ carteolol	a. Ismotic
2. _____ metipranolol	b. Miostat
3. _____ acetazolamide	c. Antilirium
4. _____ dorzolamide	d. Epinal
5. _____ isosorbide	e. Diamox
6. _____ epinephryl borate	f. Neo-Synephrine
7. _____ latanoprost	g. Xalatan
8. _____ phenylephrine	h. Ocupress
9. _____ physostigmine	i. Trusopt
10. _____ carbachol	j. OptiPranolol

MULTIPLE CHOICE

Choose the correct answers from choices a–d.

1. Which of the following drugs is used in the treatment of glaucoma and requires a high-potassium diet?
   a. Dichlorphenamide
   b. Glycerin anhydrous
   c. Betaxolol
   d. Acetazolamide

2. Miotic agents achieve increased drainage of aqueous humor by which of the following mechanisms?
   a. Miosis and contraction of the ciliary muscles
   b. Miosis and relaxation of the ciliary muscles
   c. Mydriasis and relaxation of the ciliary muscles
   d. Only mydriasis

3. The most common adverse effect of the muscarinic agonists on the eye is:
   a. Conjunctivitis
   b. Cataract
   c. Pupil constriction
   d. Pupil relaxation

4. Cholinesterase inhibitors are used to treat:
   a. Chronic angle-closure glaucoma
   b. Open-angle glaucoma
   c. Acute abdominal cramps
   d. Salivation

5. The trade name of bimatoprost is which of the following?
   a. Lumigan
   b. Diamox
   c. Alphagan P
   d. Neo-Synephrine

DRUG THERAPY FOR MINOR EYE CONDITIONS

There is a broad range of agents indicated for eye examinations, minor irritations, and injury. These drugs include antimicrobials, local anesthetics, and anti-inflammatories. Antimicrobials and anti-inflammatory drugs were discussed in Chapters 8, 9, and 12. Some drugs, including mydriatic drugs and cycloplegic agents, are used for ophthalmic examinations.

Mydriatic Agents

Mydriatic drugs are agents that dilate the pupil of the eye. These drugs are commonly used during eye examinations to permit examination of the retina. Examples of mydriatics or sympathomimetics include hydroxyamphetamine (Paredrine) and phenylephrine hydrochloride (Mydfrin), which are used to dilate pupils in angle-closure glaucoma. These drugs were discussed previously in this chapter.

Cycloplegics (Anticholinergic) Agents

Cycloplegic drugs (Table 27-5 ■) cause paralysis of ciliary muscles resulting in pupillary dilation.

How do they work?

Antimuscarinic agents such as atropine (Atropisol), homatropine (AK-Homatropine), and cyclopentolate (Ak-Pentolate) act by blocking all muscarinic responses to acetylcholine. The mechanism of action of anticholinergic agents includes mydriasis (pupillary dilation) and cycloplegia (paralysis of ciliary muscles).

How are they used?

Anticholinergic drugs are used locally by inserting drops in the eyes for eye exams, and preoperatively for eye surgery; however, they can also aggravate glaucoma-producing mydriasis and cycloplegia.

What are the adverse effects?

Antimuscarinic drugs may cause mydriasis, blurred vision, photophobia, increased IOP, cyclopegia, eye dryness, and local redness.

What are the contraindications and interactions?

Contraindications include hypersensitivity to antimuscarinic drugs, angle-closure glaucoma, urinary bladder neck obstruction caused by prostatic hypertrophy, intestinal atony, severe ulcerative colitis, tachycardia secondary to cardiac insufficiency, acute bleeding, and myasthenia gravis. Safety during pregnancy or lactation is not established.

Antimuscarinic agents should be used cautiously in elderly patients and in patients with brain damage (in children), hyperthyroidism, asthma, and hepatic or renal disease. Antimuscarinic drugs may interact with the ocular antihypertensive effects of carbachol (Miostat), pilocarpine (Adsorbocarpine), and physostigmine (Antilirium).

What are the important points patients should know?

Instruct patients to use caution when driving or engaging in other potentially hazardous activities because these drugs may cause blurred vision. Patients should be advised to avoid touching the dropper to any skin or eye surface. Advise patients to not wear soft contact lenses when eyedrops are being inserted and to immediately report difficulty breathing; swelling of the lips, tongue, or face; hives; palpitations; and unusual behavior.

Table 27-5 ■ Cycloplegics (Anticholinergic Drugs)

GENERIC NAME	TRADE NAME	AVERAGE ADULT DOSAGE	ROUTE OF ADMINISTRATION
atropine sulfate	Isopto Atropine Atropisol	1 drop of 0.5% solution daily	Topical
cyclopentolate	Cyclogyl, Pentolair	1 drop of 0.5%–2% solution 40–50 min before surgery	Topical
homatropine	Isopto Homatropine Isopto Hyoscine	1–2 drops of 2% or 5% solution before eye exam	Topical
scopolamine hydrobromide	Mydriacyl	1–2 drops of 0.25% solution 1 h before eye exam	Topical
tropicamide	Tropicacyl	1–2 drops of 0.5%–1% solution before eye exam	Topical

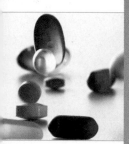

Chapter Capsule

This section repeats the objectives from the beginning of the chapter and then provides a summary of the most important concepts for that objective. Use this section as a quick review and to check your knowledge.

Objective 1: Describe the structure and function of the eye.

- A hollow, spherical structure about 2.5 cm in diameter with three distinct layers in its walls: an outer layer (sclera), a middle layer (choroid layer or "coat"), and an inner layer (retina)
- Spaces within the eye—filled with fluids that support its wall and internal parts
- Structures—the iris, ciliary body, lens, lacrimal glands, and ocular vasculature receive autonomic innervation

Objective 2: Explain glaucoma and types of glaucoma.

- Damage to the optic nerve, often caused by elevated IOP
- Results from excessive production of aqueous humor or diminished ocular fluid outflow
- Can cause blindness secondary to optic nerve damage
- Two types of glaucoma—acute angle-closure and chronic open-angle

Objective 3: State the rationale for use and the mechanism of action of carbonic anhydrase inhibitors in the treatment of glaucoma.

- Plays a significant role in aqueous humor formation by the ciliary body cells of the eye
- Facilitates the secretion of bicarbonate ions in the aqueous humor, decreasing formation of aqueous humor
- Main clinical indication—glaucoma
- Most administered systemically

Objective 4: Identify direct-acting miotics (cholinergic drugs) and list two generic and trade names.

- Agents that constrict the pupil; often used to treat glaucoma
- Carbachol (Miostat, Isopto Carboptic)
- Pilocarpine hydrochloride (Miocarpine, Isopto Carpine)

Objective 5: Explain mydriatic agents and their indications.

- Agents that dilate the pupil of the eye; commonly used during eye examinations to permit examination of the retina

- Used locally by inserting drops in the eyes for eye exams, and preoperatively for eye surgery; however, can aggravate glaucoma-producing mydriasis and cycloplegia

Objective 6: State the mechanism of action of antimuscarinics.

- Act by blocking all muscarinic responses to acetylcholine

- Mechanism of action of antimuscarinic agents—mydriasis (pupillary dilation) and cycloplegia (paralysis of ciliary muscles)

 Internet Sites of Interest

- Learn more about glaucoma at the Glaucoma Research Foundation Web site: **www.glaucoma.org**.

- More information about carbonic anhydrase inhibitors can be found on the Mayo Clinic Web site at **www.mayoclinic.com**. Select "Drugs & Supplements" at the top of the page. Then search for "carbonic anhydrase inhibitors."

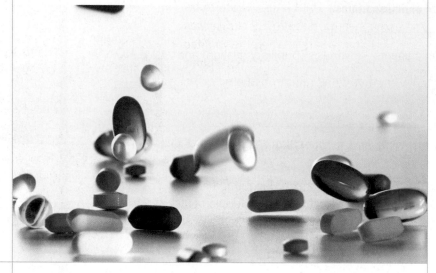

Chapter 28

Toxicology

Chapter Objectives

After completing this chapter, you should be able to:

1. Predict some symptoms that signify specific types of poisonings.

2. Explain steps that can be taken to prevent poisonings from occurring.

3. Differentiate several types of poisonings for which activated charcoal is used to absorb the toxic agent.

4. Explain the six major services offered by the poison control center network.

5. Identify the most common types of poisonings in the United States.

6. Discuss the type of alcohol that has the greatest toxic effects on the human body.

7. Recognize two types of poisonings listed as true "medical emergencies."

8. Discuss a leading cause of death in opiate poisoning.

9. Name the type of salicylate found in 30 million American households.

10. Contrast the treatments for scorpion stings and snake bites.

Key Terms

Activated charcoal (page 608)

Antivenom (page 622)

Chelating agents (kee-LAY-ting) (page 619)

Child-resistant packaging (page 605)

Emesis (EH-meh-sis) (page 607)

Ethanol (EH-the-nol) (page 611)

Gastric lavage (luh-VAAZH) (page 607)

Hemodialysis (hee-mo-dy-AL-uh-sis) (page 611)

Hemoperfusion (hee-mo-per-FU-zhun) (page 607)

Hyperkalemia (hy-per-kah-LEE-mee-uh) (page 618)

Hyperthermia (hy-per-THER-mee-uh) (page 614)

Hypoxia (hy-POK-see-uh) (page 615)

Intoxication (in-tok-sih-KAY-shun) (page 612)

Medical emergency (page 616)

Pneumonitis (new-moh-NY-tis) (page 611)

Toxic agent (page 606)

Toxicologists (tok-sih-KAW-loh-jistz) (page 610)

Universal antidote (AN-tih-doht) (page 609)

Urticaria (er-tih-KEH-ree-uh) (page 613)

Whole bowel irrigation (page 619)

PRACTICAL SCENARIO

A pregnant mother checked on her 2-year-old son who had been napping in his crib for nearly 4 hours. She found vomitus in the crib next to her son and couldn't arouse the child. She called the emergency medical service (EMS). They arrived and found the child's breathing to be rapid (27 breaths/minute) and his heart rate to be 139 beats per minute. The child was cyanotic and appeared to be in shock. He was transported to the nearby emergency department (ED) immediately, where he vomited again. The ED staff noted pill fragments in the vomitus. Further investigation found these fragments to be *radiopaque* (relative impenetrability by radiation such as X-rays).

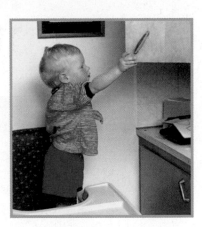

Critical Thinking Questions

1. What do you think the child ingested, and what are the clues that lead you to this suspicion?

2. What other signs or symptoms might you expect to find in this child and what tests might confirm what the child ingested?

Source: Ball, Jane W., Binder Ruth C., *Child Health Nursing: Partnering with Children and Families*, 1st e, p. 451, ©2006. Reprinted by permission of Prentice Hall, Inc., Upper Saddle River, NJ.

Introduction

Toxicology is the basic science that deals with poisoning, particularly the effects of drugs or other chemicals that cause injury, illness, or death to a living organism. Humans are surrounded by a chemical environment wherein substances may be inhaled, ingested, or absorbed through the skin. Poisons produce toxic effects at concentrations that change the normal state of the organism.

Approximately 10 million people are poisoned annually in the United States, and 4,000 of these poisonings are fatal (see the Centers of Disease Control and Prevention Web site at: http://www.cdc.gov/ncipc/factsheets/poisoning.htm for statistics). Depressed persons may use poisons to attempt suicide. Other high-risk groups for poisoning include elderly adults (medication mix-ups), hospitalized patients (medication errors), workers exposed to occupational chemicals, and children younger than 6 years of age (accidents). Accidental poisonings may occur with nontherapeutic chemicals such as heavy metals, pesticides, and domestic agents (for example, household cleaners and disinfectants). Overdosing with abused drugs is another form of poisoning. In some cases of poisoning, there are specific antidotes available, and they will be discussed in this chapter.

Prevention

Child-resistant packaging (for example, blister packs or special lids requiring the user to press downward and turn simultaneously) was introduced in 1972. Since then, accidental deaths from lethal poisonings, via medicines and household chemicals, have been reduced, especially for children younger than age 5. This and other poison-prevention programs have made an impact on reducing accidental poisoning cases in the United States.

If poisoning is suspected, you should call the poison control center immediately (1-800-222-1222). Teach your patients prevention tips as follows:

✳ Keep chemicals and medicines locked up and out of sight.

✳ Keep these substances in their original containers.

✳ Read all labels before using.

✳ Leave original labels intact on all products.

✳ Check dosages every time medication is administered.

✳ Make sure there is plenty of light when reading medication labels.

✳ Clean out medicine cabinets regularly.

✳ Always dispose of unneeded medications safely, and rinse containers before discarding.

Focus on Pediatrics

Preventing Poisonings in Children

■ Close child-resistant packaging properly after use.

■ Never let young children out of sight while potential poisons are in use.

■ Don't take medicines in front of children.

■ Refer to medicine as *medicine*, and make sure that children understand that it is not candy.

Another method of prevention is the use of *aversive agents,* which are nontoxic substances added to poisonous substances to cause an offensive smell or taste. The use of aversive agents is controversial: Some scientists think they are best used when added to relatively palatable toxic substances. Most experts, however, think that this method of prevention should only be used in products that are highly toxic.

Poison Detection

Careful evaluation of a person who has been affected by a toxic substance is essential to determine which of the treatment steps take priority and by which route the poison should be removed, if removal is possible. Patients who may have been poisoned must be correctly diagnosed. Most poisoning syndromes can simulate other diseases, although some chemical substances cause uniquely characteristic toxic effects. Poisoning usually is included in differential diagnoses of acute hepatic or renal insufficiency, bone-marrow depression, acute psychosis, convulsions, and coma. Poisoning may not be considered (but should be) when the major manifestation is a mild psychiatric disturbance or neurological disorder, skin eruptions, pulmonary congestion, hypotension, fever, bleeding, or abdominal pain. Patients may be unaware of exposure to a poison, such as with chronic insidious intoxications, or after attempted abortion or suicide. They may also be unwilling to admit exposure to a poison. Identification of the **toxic agent** (poisonous or harmful substance) should always be attempted because specific antidotal therapy is obviously impossible without first identifying the toxic agent in question.

Specific poisons have some clinical features that lead to accurate diagnosis, including:

(handwritten note: (lack of) blue color of skin.)

✳ Cyanide: unmistakable odor of bitter almonds on patient's breath

✳ Insecticides: gastrointestinal (GI) hyperactivity, salivation, and pupillary constriction

✳ Carbon monoxide: cherry-colored flush of the skin and mucous membranes

Body fluids should be chemically analyzed to definitively identify the intoxicating agent. Relatively simple lab procedures can identify common poisons such as aspirin and barbiturates, although others require more complex toxicology studies. Chronic intoxications may be diagnosed and evaluated through chemical analyses of body tissues or fluids.

✳ Apply Your Knowledge 28.1

The following questions focus on what you just learned about poison prevention and detection. *See Appendix E for the correct answer.*

FILL IN THE BLANK

Select terms from your reading to fill in the blanks.

1. _____ packaging and other poison prevention programs have reduced accidental poisonings in the United States.

2. If poisoning is suspected, you should call the _____ immediately.

3. Poisoning by _____ causes an unmistakable odor.

4. Specific antidotal therapy is impossible without identifying the _____.

5. Poisoning by _____ causes a cherry-colored flush of the skin and mucous membranes.

6. The addition of _____ to toxic substances helps prevent ingestion because of unpleasant odors and tastes.

7. Gastrointestinal hyperactivity, salivation, and pupillary constriction are clinical symptoms of poisoning with _____.

Treatment of Poisoning

Supporting vital signs, preventing further poison absorption, enhancing poison elimination, administering specific antidotes, and preventing reexposure are the major treatment goals for poisoned patients. Specific treatment depends on the severity of poisoning, the time of presentation as compared to the time of exposure, the route and amount of exposure, and the identity of the poison. Removal of ingested substances can be attempted in several ways:

✳ By directly removing poisons from the stomach (if the poisoning is detected early)

✳ By increasing the rate of transit of poisons through the large intestine (even though little or no absorption occurs there, and this step may therefore not be effective)

✳ By removing or filtering it from the blood circulation (if the substance has probably already been absorbed into the system, or was injected)

Various methods exist for eliminating poisons from the gastrointestinal tract, including :

✳ **Emesis** (vomiting)

✳ **Gastric lavage** (washing out the stomach with sterile water or a salt-water solution)

✳ Cathartics

✳ Diuretics

✳ Dialysis

✳ Blood exchange transfusions or **hemoperfusion** (removing poisons from blood by passing it through a tube containing treated charcoal or ion-exchange resins).

EMETICS

The most popularly used emetic is ipecac syrup, which is an extract from the roots of the *Caephalis ipecacuanha* plant. One of its active principal ingredients, emetine, triggers vomiting by intensely irritating the intestinal wall's mucosal layers. Its central action stimulates the vomiting center in the medulla, via the chemoreceptor trigger zone. For most patients, 30 mL of ipecac syrup is given, followed by a second dose

induction of vomit is for swallen tablets

after 30 minutes if vomiting has not begun. Younger children are given between 15 and 25 mL depending on age. After ipecac is administered, patients are asked to drink 100 to 200 mL of water to stretch the stomach muscles and produce a more complete emptying of the stomach during emesis.

In the case of ingestion of corrosives, emesis is contraindicated because these poisons can cause further damage to the esophagus, pharynx, and mouth if they are ejected from the stomach. The practice of giving a glass of milk to a fully conscious person who has ingested poison to cause emesis has been abandoned for the same reason. Other contraindications for emesis include altered consciousness, ingestion of volatile petroleum products, and impaired gag reflex.

Some areas of the world have stopped using ipecac syrup as an emetic because it does not cause complete stomach emptying, it acts as a sedative in children, and it could be used to cause emesis in a patient who has ingested a poison that has not been identified as corrosive. Also, until the effects of emetics have subsided (usually up to 2 hours), absorbents cannot be used to treat the toxic agent.

Focus on Pediatrics

Use of Ipecac

The American Academy of Pediatrics (AAP) recommends that syrup of ipecac no longer be used routinely as a home treatment strategy. Until now, the AAP advised that parents keep a 1-ounce bottle of syrup of ipecac in the home to induce vomiting if it was feared that a child had swallowed a poisonous substance. Use of ipecac is now recommended only on the advice of a physician or the poison control center.

ADSORBENTS

Particles of **activated charcoal** (charcoal that has been treated with oxygen) is used to bind to molecules of ingested poisons and reduce absorption into the blood through the stomach walls. A dose ratio of at least 10 parts charcoal to 1 part estimated dose of poison is recommended, although it is often difficult to correctly estimate how much poison has been ingested. Activated charcoal is very effective in treating poisonings from cardiac glycosides (plant-derived agents used to stimulate the heart) and methylxanthines (commonly used as stimulants and bronchodilators). It is effective in treating heavy metal or corrosive chemical poisonings.

Often, activated charcoal is administered after emesis, although some medical professionals believe that a sufficient dose of charcoal without emesis is adequate in certain poisoning cases. Activated charcoal should not be administered along with ipecac syrup, until after the vomiting induced by ipecac has subsided. Also, the charcoal should be discarded if it becomes moist, because it will have decreased ability to bind to the molecules of the poison.

CATHARTIC AGENTS

Osmotic cathartics are often used to reduce absorption of toxic substances because they shorten the transit time of chemicals through the GI tract. Commonly used cathartic agents include sorbitol (a slowly absorbed sugar alcohol) and soluble salts of either magnesium or sodium. These agents raise the osmotic pressure of the intestinal contents, thereby retaining water. This increase in intestinal bulk stimulates peristalsis in the bowel. Care must be taken to avoid dehydration due to poor water absorption.

Because sodium sulphate, Milk of Magnesia, and Epsom salt are inorganic salts that are poorly absorbed, they are ideal cathartic agents. Sorbitol is still preferred because the inorganic salts increase sodium load and can cause certain problems in patients who have cardiovascular or renal disease. Magnesium sulfate products should be avoided in patients with impaired renal function because excessive magnesium plasma levels can occur, leading to unconsciousness because of CNS depressive effects.

Poison Antidotes

Activated charcoal is an effective, nonspecific absorbent of many materials and was once considered to be a **universal antidote** (that is, one agent that will counteract all poisons). For a long period, a combination of activated charcoal, tannic acid, and magnesium oxide was considered to be the universal antidote. It has now been established that tannic acid and magnesium oxide have no significant efficacy and may actually impede the one active ingredient, activated charcoal. A long-advocated home remedy of burned toast and strong tea was also considered a universal antidote, but this concoction has no merit. In fact, there is no true universal antidote but rather just a few specific antidotes available for use in situations of clinical overdosage.

Few specific antidotes are available for use in situations of clinical overdosage. Antidotes neutralize, antagonize the effects of, or facilitate the elimination of the chemical substance. They are available against poisoning with the following substances: anticholinesterase (neostigmine and physostigmine), atropine, iron, narcotics, benzodiazepines, heparin, warfarin, and digoxin (see Table 28-1 ■). The advantage of specific antidotes is that other interventions (for example, gastric lavage, artificial ventilation, and so on) become unnecessary.

Table 28-1 ■ Poisons and Antidotes

POISONS	ANTIDOTES
Acetaminophen overdose	N-acetylcysteine
Anticholinesterase overdose	pralidoxime iodide
Atropine overdose	physostigmine
Benzodiazepine overdose	flumazenil
Carbon monoxide poisoning	oxygen
Cyanide poisoning	amyl nitrate
Digoxin overdose	atropine or phenytoin
Heparin overdose	protamine sulphate
Iron poisoning	deferoxamine
Methanol poisoning	ethanol
Opiate overdose	naloxone
Organophosphate poisoning	atropine or pralidoxime
Warfarin overdose	vitamin K_1

✳ Apply Your Knowledge 28.2

The following exercises focus on what you just learned about treatments for poisoning. *See Appendix E for the correct answers.*

MATCHING

Match the lettered antidote to its the numbered poison or overdose.

POISON/OVERDOSE	ANTIDOTE
1. _____ Opiate overdose	a. Protamine sulfate
2. _____ Atropine overdose	b. Amyl nitrate
3. _____ Heparin overdose	c. Physostigmine
4. _____ Cyanide poisoning	d. Atropine
5. _____ Organophosphate poisoning	e. Naloxone

(*continued*)

Apply Your Knowledge 28.2 (continued)

FILL IN THE BLANK

Select terms from your reading to fill in the blanks.

1. Specific treatment, for poisoning depends on the time of _____ as compared to the time of _____.

2. Besides cathartics, diuretics, and diuresis, another three methods for removing poisons from the GI tract include _____, _____, and _____.

3. One of the principal active ingredients of ipecac syrup is _____, which triggers vomiting by intensely irritating the intestinal wall's mucosal layers.

4. Ipecac's central action is to stimulate the vomiting center in the _____, via the _____ trigger zone.

5. Activated charcoal should be _____ if it becomes moist.

6. A slowly absorbed sugar alcohol, _____, is used as a cathartic to stimulate peristalsis in the bowel.

7. Cathartic agents act by raising the _____ of the intestinal contents, thereby _____ water.

8. Inorganic _____, such as sodium sulphate, are good cathartic agents because they are _____ absorbed.

9. A contraindication for using magnesium sulfate products as cathartics is impaired _____ function, which can lead to unconsciousness because of CNS depressive effects.

Poison Control Centers

More than 600 poison control centers exist in the United States (see the Web site for the American Association of Poison Control Centers at http://www.aapcc.org/). Through this network, poison treatment information is available at no charge, 24 hours a day. The Illinois chapter of the American Academy of Pediatrics in Chicago established the first poison control center, followed soon after by the Duke University Poison Control Center in North Carolina. These two centers promoted the idea of countrywide poison control centers. The FDA established the National Clearinghouse for Poison Control Centers in 1957 to collect and standardize product toxicology data. This agency reproduced their data on large file cards, distributing them to the nationwide poison control centers.

Since 1953, public health has been positively affected by U.S. poison control centers, with reductions in morbidity and mortality and decreased costs of health care brought about by the efforts of poison specialists, clinical **toxicologists** (those who study poisons and toxic agents and their treatments), and medical toxicologists.

The poison control centers offer six major services:

1. Community education about poison prevention

2. Health-care provider education in the recognition and management of poisonings

3. Emergency telephone treatment recommendations for all types of poisonings, drug overdoses, and chemical exposures provided to nonmedical and medical callers. Most callers (about 80%) are not in the health-care profession, but may be family members, childcare providers, or actual poisoning victims.

4. Research and surveillance of human poison exposures, including occupational and environmental exposures, as well as those related to chemicals and drugs

5. Telephone follow-up for all patients (hospitalized or not) to assess progress and recommend additional poison treatment that may be required

6. Training of future toxicologists

Specific Poisons

Nonprescription drugs, household products, solvents, pesticides, and poisonous plants are among the most common sources of poisons affecting the general population. Some household products contain potential health risks if they are ingested or inhaled, or if they come into contact with skin or eyes. The National Library of Medicine's Household Products Database provides consumer-friendly information on many of these products and their potential effects. The following discussion of specific poisons stresses their action and the recognition or treatment of clinical poisoning.

ACETAMINOPHEN

Acetaminophen (Tylenol and others) is one of the drugs most commonly involved in accidental poisonings and suicide attempts. Acute ingestion of more than 150 to 200 mg/kg in children, or a total of 8 g in adults, is considered potentially toxic.

In early stages of toxicity, the patient is asymptomatic or has nausea and vomiting. After 2 or 3 days, there is evidence of liver injury. In severe cases, liver failure occurs, resulting in hepatic encephalopathy and death. Renal failure may also occur.

The antidote is acetylcysteine, which is most effective when given early and should be started within 8 to 10 hours if possible. A liver transplant may be required for patients with severe hepatic failure.

ALCOHOLS

Although there are many different kinds of alcohol, the term *alcohol* usually refers to ethyl alcohol, or **ethanol** (a flammable, colorless chemical compound produced by fermentation of grain). Methyl, propyl, butyl, and amyl alcohols are examples of other alcohols that are very toxic when taken orally. Alcohols are commonly used today, including as sterilizing agents and as rubbing alcohol, in solvents, aftershave, antifreeze, all sorts of cleaning solutions, and nail polish removers. Alcohols are central nervous system depressants. Isopropyl alcohol is absorbed rapidly from the stomach and lungs and is distributed in body water. It is metabolized to acetone in the liver by the enzyme alcohol dehydrogenase. As much as 20% is excreted unchanged in urine. Ingestion produces gastric irritation, and aspiration raises the danger of vomiting. The systemic effects of isopropyl alcohol are similar to those of ethyl alcohol, but isopropyl alcohol is twice as potent. Emesis should be induced, or gastric lavage performed. **Hemodialysis** (a method in which the patient's blood is passed through a tube to a semipermeable membrane [dialyzer] that filters out waste products, and the cleansed blood is then returned back to the body) effectively removes it and should be considered for patients with high serum levels who do not respond to conservative therapy. Activated charcoal is ineffective in treating this type of poisoning.

ETHYLENE GLYCOL

Ethylene glycol is commonly used in antifreeze and windshield de-icing solutions. This form is sometimes colorless and has a sweet taste. Ethylene glycol is metabolized in the liver and may cause severe damage to this organ. Between 1 and 12 hours after ingestion, the patient may suffer from nausea and vomiting, ataxia, seizures, cerebral edema, coma, and death. Between 12 and 14 hours, the signs and symptoms include tachypnea, cyanosis, tachycardia, pulmonary edema, and **pneumonitis** (inflammation of the lungs).

Gastric lavage should be performed within 30 minutes of ingestion of ethylene glycol. The intravenous administration of a 10% solution of ethanol is used, as well as hemodialysis.

METHANOL

Methanol, or methyl alcohol (wood alcohol), has a number of industrial and domestic uses such as in gas-line antifreeze, windshield-washer fluid, and as a solvent in photocopier solutions. Methanol is far more toxic to the human body than ethanol because it is metabolized into formaldehyde. **Intoxication** (an abnormal state induced by a chemical agent such as a drug, serum, or toxin; essentially, a poisoning) with methanol can lead to permanent disability and sometimes death.

Like ethanol, methanol is a CNS depressant and can cause euphoria and muscle weakness, depending on the rate of formation of formic acid. Clinical manifestation of intoxication includes visual disturbances, bradycardia, seizures, metabolic acidosis, respiratory depression, and coma. Methanol can also cause blindness and permanent damage to the retina.

The treatment for methanol poisoning is gastric lavage and the intravenous administration of a 10% solution of ethanol. Hemodialysis is also effective in helping clear methanol from the body.

✳ Apply Your Knowledge 28.3

The following exercises focus on what you have just learned about poison control centers and some specific types of poisonings. *See Appendix E for the correct answers.*

MULTIPLE CHOICE

Choose the correct answer for each question from among choices a–d.

1. The six services offered by the poison control centers include all of the following EXCEPT:

   a. Community education about poison prevention

   b. Emergency telephone treatment recommendations

   c. Research and surveillance of human poison exposures

   d. Telephone follow-up for hospitalized patients only

2. One of the drugs most commonly involved in accidental poisonings and suicide attempts is:

   a. Acetaminophen

   b. Acetylcysteine

   c. Codeine

   d. Epinephrine

3. Alcohols are:

   a. Nitrates

   b. Polishes

   c. CNS depressants

   d. CNS stimulants

4. Acetylcysteine is the antidote for:

   a. Methanol

   b. Acetaminophen

   c. Ethanol

   d. Ethylene glycol

5. Ethylene glycol is commonly used in:

   a. Brake fluid

   b. Sweetened foods

   c. Gasoline

   d. Antifreeze

6. Methanol is far more toxic to the human body than ethanol because it is metabolized into:

a. Formaldehyde

b. Formalin

c. Carbon monoxide

d. Carbon dioxide

FILL IN THE BLANK

Select terms from your reading to fill in the blanks.

1. Nonprescription drugs, household products, solvents, pesticides, and poisonous plants are among the most _____ sources of poisons affecting the general population.

2. A toxic dose of acetaminophen in adults is _____ or more grams.

3. Liver injury begins in 2 or 3 days in patients poisoned with _____ .

4. Acetylcysteine is most effective as an antidote for acetaminophen when given within _____ hours of poisoning.

5. Isopropyl alcohol is metabolized to _____ in the liver by the enzyme alcohol dehydrogenase.

6. Symptoms of _____ poisoning that occur within 1 to 12 hours include nausea and vomiting, ataxia, seizures, cerebral edema, coma, and death.

ANTICOAGULANTS

Anticoagulants are agents that prevent formation of blood clots (*thrombi*). Risk factors for clot formation include age of the patient (older than 40 years), immobility (bed rest for more than 4 days), pregnancy, obesity, high-dose estrogen therapy, surgery (lower limbs), malignancy, and varicose veins. Anticoagulant agents are not effective for an existing clot, but they decrease the ability of the blood to clot, and prevent formation of other clots. Heparin and warfarin are commonly used anticoagulants in the United States.

HEPARIN

Heparin is one of the potent anticoagulants naturally obtained from the liver and lungs of domestic animals. In humans, it is usually found in mast cells (large tissue cells in blood vessels of the skin and bone marrow that contain histamine and heparin). Heparin is available in only parenteral dosage forms for intravenous and subcutaneous administration. It is primarily metabolized in the liver.

Bleeding is the most common complication of heparin administration. This usually presents as epistaxis (nose bleed), ecchymoses (effusion of blood beneath the skin), hematuria (blood in the urine), or melena (passage of blood in the stool). Bleeding may be due to an excess or overdose of heparin administration. Heparin also may produce allergies and osteoporosis. Heparin allergy can manifest as fever or **urticaria** (vascular reaction of the skin characterized by a rash and severe itching). Life-threatening bleeding should be treated with immediate reversal of the heparin effect via a slow intravenous infusion of protamine sulfate. Protamine strongly neutralizes the heparin molecule.

WARFARIN

Warfarin is a synthetic derivative of dicoumarol. It is one of the most commonly used oral anticoagulants. Warfarin is absorbed from the small intestine, bound to albumin, and carried to the liver. The major complication of warfarin therapy is bleeding. As with heparin therapy, warfarin should be withheld from patients with known severe hypertension, recent surgery, and bleeding disorders. Pregnant patients should not receive warfarin because it crosses the placenta and can produce hemorrhage in the neonate. Birth defects due to warfarin can occur throughout gestation. Administration of phytonadione (vitamin K) is recommended. Patients who are bleeding may require the administration of blood products that contain clotting factors.

AMPHETAMINES

Stimulant agents can cause toxicity when abused. In the United States, the most commonly abused stimulants include methamphetamine ("crank," "crystal meth") and cocaine ("crack") as well as legal drugs such as pseudoephedrine (Sudafed) and ephedrine. Caffeine is also found combined with pseudoephedrine or ephedrine in pills sold as amphetamine substitutes. At the doses usually used by stimulant abusers, euphoria and fatigue are accompanied by a sense of power and well-being. At higher doses, agitation, restlessness, and acute psychosis may occur, accompanied by hypertension and tachycardia. Very high fever can cause brain damage and hypotension, as well as renal failure. There is no specific antidote. Seizures and **hyperthermia** (a condition of increased body heat; body temperatures above 104 °F [40 °C] are life-threatening; brain death begins at 106 °F [41 °C]).

Focus Point

Caffeine in Supplements

Caffeine is often added to dietary supplements sold as "metabolic enhancers" or "fat-burners."

ANTIHISTAMINES

Manifestations of antihistamine poisoning include CNS excitement or depression. Drowsiness, stupor, and coma may occur in adults, and there is a wide variation in patient tolerance to antihistamines. Treatment is supportive and focused on removing any unabsorbed drug while maintaining vital functions. Phenobarbital or diazepam may be used to control convulsions.

Focus on Pediatrics

Antihistamines in Young Children

Use of antihistamines in infants and young children may cause serious side effects such as convulsions (seizures). Children are generally more sensitive to the effects of antihistamines, which can include nightmares or unusual excitement, nervousness, restlessness, or irritability.

BENZODIAZEPINES

Benzodiazepines are weak, lipid-soluble acids that are readily absorbed. They exhibit 85 to 99% protein binding in the plasma and are mainly eliminated by hepatic metabolism. Their CNS depressant effects begin less than 30 minutes after acute overdose. When benzodiazepines are combined with other CNS depressants, coma and respiratory depression can occur, which can also happen with ultra-short-acting benzodiazepines. Early in the course of poisoning, excitation may occur. The method of choice for GI decontamination from benzodiazepines is activated charcoal, and respiratory support should be provided as necessary.

✳ Apply Your Knowledge 28.4

The following exercises focus on what you have just learned about poisoning with anticoagulants, amphetamines, antihistamines, and benzodiazepines. *See Appendix E for the correct answers.*

FILL IN THE BLANK

Select terms from your reading to fill in the blanks.

1. The major complication from use or overuse of the anticoagulants heparin and warfarin is _____.

2. In the United States, two commonly abused amphetamines are _____, also known as _____, and _____, also known as _____.

3. Convulsions caused by antihistamine poisoning may be treated with either _____ or _____.

4. When benzodiazepines are combined with other CNS depressants, _____ and _____ can occur.

5. The method of choice for GI decontamination from benzodiazepines is _____.

MATCHING

Match the lettered agent to the numbered overdose sign or symptom. Some lettered terms may be used more than once.

OVERDOSE SIGN OR SYMPTOM	AGENT
1. _____ Epistaxis, ecchymoses, hematuria	a. Antihistamines
2. _____ Acute psychosis, hypertension, tachycardia	b. Benzodiazepines
3. _____ Drowsiness, stupor, coma	c. Heparin and warfarin
4. _____ Seizures and hyperthermia	d. Amphetamines
5. _____ Coma and respiratory depression	

BLEACHES

Bleaches cause corrosive action in the mouth, pharynx, and esophagus that is similar to that caused by sodium hydroxide. The solution used for chlorinating swimming pools contains 20% sodium hypochlorite, whereas industrial strength bleaches contain 10% or more. (Household bleaches, including Clorox®, contain 3 to 6%.) Treatment consists of dilution of ingested bleach with water or milk.

CARBON MONOXIDE

Colorless, odorless, tasteless, and nonirritating, carbon monoxide (CO) is a gas that is present in the exhaust of internal combustion engines, improperly maintained heating systems, improperly ventilated charcoal cookers or fireplaces, and industrial furnaces such as those in steel mills. Automobile exhaust contains between 3 and 7%, but CO is responsible for about 3,500 accidental deaths and suicides in the United States every year. Its toxic effects are the result of tissue **hypoxia** (lack of oxygen). Severe CO poisoning causes a characteristic cherry color in the skin and mucous membranes. Treatment requires effective ventilation with pure oxygen (O_2). Ventilation should be artificially supported if necessary. Diuretics and steroids are used to treat resultant cerebral edema. Tips for preventing CO poisoning are found in Table 28-2 ■.

Table 28-2 ■ **Tips for Avoiding CO Poisoning**

- Install a CO detector in the house and check its battery whenever smoke detector batteries are checked.
- Avoid burning anything in an unproperly vented stove or fireplace.
- Never heat a house with a gas oven.
- Never run a generator in an enclosed space or outside a window where the exhaust could blow indoors.
- Never warm up a car in an enclosed garage.
- Clean snow out of car tailpipes.

COCAINE

Cocaine abuse occurs in nearly all economic and social levels of society (see Chapter 16). This agent is highly addictive—perhaps not as a physical addiction, but instead as a strongly psychological addiction. The danger of snorting cocaine is nasal congestion, which can lead to necrosis of the nasal mucosa and septum. Overdose can lead to cardiac dysrhythmias and death.

CORROSIVES

Corrosive acids (including hydrofluoric, sulfuric, and phosphoric acids) are used in toilet bowl cleaners, automobile battery fluid, laboratories, and industry. Sulfuric acid is used along with hydrofluoric acids as a stone cleaner. Toxic effects are due to direct chemical action. Ingestion of corrosives is almost always with suicidal intent. If ingested, these acids produce irritation, severe pain, bleeding, and severe burns in the mouth, esophagus, and stomach. Profound shock may develop, which may be fatal. Ingestion of corrosives is treated by immediate dilution with large amounts of water or milk. The use of emesis or gastric lavage is contraindicated because of the danger of perforation. If emesis or gastric lavage is required, diagnostic esophagoscopy should be performed in the first 24 hours after ingestion.

CYANIDE

An exceedingly potent and rapid-acting poison, cyanide is a true **medical emergency** (an injury or illness that poses an immediate threat to a person's health or life and requires help from a doctor or hospital). However, specific and effective antidotal therapy is available. This type of poisoning may result from inhalation of hydrocyanic acid (for instance, in a house fire when rubber, plastic, or silk burns; or in industries such as photography, chemical research, plastics or metal industries) or from ingestion of soluble inorganic cyanide salts (usually intentional). Also, some plants (for example, apricot pits and cassava potatoes) contain amygdaline and other substances that release cyanide when digested. Treatment is highly effective if given quickly. The chemical antidotes to cyanide should be immediately available wherever emergency medical care is offered. Diagnosis may be made by a characteristic odor of bitter almonds on the patient's breath. The preferred treatment is to administer nitrite to produce methemoglobin. Supportive measures should be instituted as soon as possible (especially, artificial respiration with 100% oxygen).

DIGOXIN

One of the most common cardiac glycosides is digoxin. Its major active ingredients come from the digitalis plant. The margin between effective therapy and dangerous toxicity is very narrow. Heart rate, rhythm, and function, assessed via ECG, are used to maintain therapeutic levels. Side effects and blood digitalis levels must also be monitored.

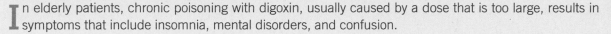

Focus on Geriatrics

Chronic Digoxin Poisoning

In elderly patients, chronic poisoning with digoxin, usually caused by a dose that is too large, results in symptoms that include insomnia, mental disorders, and confusion.

Early signs of poisoning by digoxin include anorexia, nausea, and vomiting. There are also other adverse effects such as headache, abdominal cramping, lethargy, diarrhea, vertigo, fatigue, irritability, muscle weakness, blurred vision, seizures, bradycardia, diplopia, and electrolyte imbalance.

Digoxin is contraindicated in patients with severe pulmonary disease, hypothyroidism, acute myocardial infarction, impaired renal function, and in pregnant or lactating women. To treat digoxin poisoning, activated charcoal is preferred. Lavage or ipecac may be used, but these are less often used.

 ## Apply Your Knowledge 28.5

The following exercises focus on what you just learned about poisoning with bleaches, carbon monoxide, cocaine, corrosives, cyanide, and digoxin. *See Appendix E for the correct answers.*

MULTIPLE CHOICE

Choose the correct answers from choices a–d.

1. Treatment for poisoning with bleach includes:
   a. Dilution with water or alcohol
   b. Dilution with water or milk
   c. Administration of ipecac
   d. Administration of activated charcoal

2. A sign of severe CO poisoning is:
   a. Blue-colored skin and mucous membranes
   b. Cherry-colored skin and mucous membranes
   c. Hyperventilation
   d. Hypoventilation

3. Overdose of cocaine may lead to:
   a. Cardiac dysrhythmias
   b. Hypoxia
   c. Addiction
   d. Drowsiness

4. Ingestion of corrosives is almost always:
   a. Related to the workplace
   b. Accidental
   c. Suicidal
   d. Related to housekeeping

(continued)

Apply Your Knowledge 28.5 (continued)

5. Cyanide poisoning causes an unmistakable breath odor of:

   a. Cherries

   b. Apricots

   c. Rubber

   d. Bitter almonds

6. Chronic poisoning with digoxin in the elderly usually results from too small of a dose.

   a. Carelessness

   b. Hyperthyroidism

   c. Doses that are too high

   d. Liver disease

MATCHING

Match the lettered treatment for overdose/poisoning to its numbered agent. Some lettered treatments may be used more than once.

AGENT	TREATMENT
1. _____ Digoxin	a. Activated charcoal
2. _____ CO	b. Nitrites
3. _____ Cocaine	c. Dilution with milk or water
4. _____ Cyanide	d. 100% oxygen
5. _____ Bleach	e. There is no specific antidote
6. _____ Corrosives	

ELECTROLYTES

Electrolytes are compounds that dissociate into ions when dissolved in water and include magnesium, potassium, sodium, and chloride. Their concentrations differ in blood plasma and other tissues. Serious imbalances of these compounds can be toxic (see Chapter 21).

Magnesium

The magnesium ion is a profound depressant of the CNS. Magnesium sulfate is used intravenously as a hypotensive agent and orally as a cathartic. In a patient with normal renal function, poisoning after oral or rectal administration is unlikely. However, in the presence of impaired renal function, an oral dose of 30 grams may be fatal. Magnesium causes GI irritation when ingested, and systemic poisoning can cause hypotension, hypothermia, coma, paralysis, and respiratory failure. Treatment includes the IV administration of 10 mL of a 10% solution of calcium gluconate.

Potassium

Potassium in the body helps to regulate neuromuscular excitability and muscle contraction. However, lethal or near-lethal overdose of potassium via the IV route is a frequent error associated with IV fluid therapy. The chief sign of potassium poisoning is the development of **hyperkalemia** (higher than normal levels of potassium in the bloodstream), which is easily verified by conducting a serum potassium level test.

Treatment is usually effective if the condition is discovered quickly; it consists of administration of calcium to combat cardiac toxicity, or sodium bicarbonate or glucose/insulin, which sends potassium into the cells.

Iron

Iron is essential for the synthesis of hemoglobin. When iron levels are deficient, replacement iron may be supplied by ferrous sulfate or iron dextran. However, iron overdose is the leading cause of fatal poisonings in children, and causes hemorrhagic necrosis, as well as possible bowel perforation. Signs and symptoms include vomiting, diarrhea, and abdominal pain. For severe overdose, **whole bowel irrigation** (WBI) is indicated. WBI is the rapid administration of large volumes of an osmotically balanced polyethylene glycol solution given orally or via a nasogastric tube, to flush out the entire GI tract. Serious iron intoxication requires the use of deferoxamine, which turns the urine a reddish color. The patient is sufficiently detoxified when the urine returns to normal color.

ISONIAZID (INH)

The mainstay of antitubercular therapy is isoniazid, which is usually combined with similar agents such as rifampin and pyrazinamide. The most common adverse effects are fever, peripheral neuritis, jaundice, and skin rash. Hepatitis can be severe and fatal. Also, aplastic or hemolytic anemia and thrombocytopenia may occur. The treatment of isoniazid poisoning consists of administration of pyridoxine and, within 2 hours, gastric lavage; once the airway is secured, activated charcoal is administered at 10 times the amount of isoniazid ingested. Severe cases may benefit from the administration of sodium bicarbonate. Hemodialysis may be indicated if the patient does not respond to these standard treatments. The occurrence of hepatitis may require liver transplantation.

LEAD

Lead poisoning is one of the oldest occupational and environmental hazards in the world. Despite its recognized health threat, lead continues to have widespread commercial application. Distribution of lead into air, food, and water has declined considerably in the past two decades because of diminished use of lead in gasoline, paint, and other applications. Extensive evidence indicates that lead may have subtle subclinical adverse effects on nervous system function and on blood pressure, at blood lead concentrations once considered "normal" or "safe."

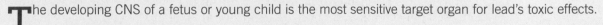

Focus on Pediatrics

Lead Toxicity in Children

The developing CNS of a fetus or young child is the most sensitive target organ for lead's toxic effects.

Adults are less sensitive than children to lead's CNS effects. Symptoms of acute poisoning include a metallic taste in the mouth, abdominal pain, vomiting, CNS depression, and respiratory failure. Treatment includes the administration of **chelating agents** (organic compounds capable of forming coordinate bonds with metals) to help the body rid itself of lead. For mild poisoning, the chelating agent penicillamine may be used alone; for severe poisoning, it may be used in combination with IV ethylenediaminetetraacetic acid (EDTA) and dimercaprol. For acute poisoning, gastric lavage is indicated.

LITHIUM

Lithium carbonate is the primary drug used to treat patients in manic states, such as those seen in bipolar disorder. Adverse effects include tremor, diarrhea, polydipsia, anorexia, polyuria, vomiting, blurred vision, albuminuria, hypothyroidism, hyperglycemia, and weight gain. Overdose may produce vomiting, diarrhea, muscle weakness, ataxia, and drowsiness.

After assessing airway condition, treatment of lithium overdose should consist of gastric lavage (if within 1 hour after ingestion), followed by administration of activated charcoal, whole bowel irrigation, and administration of sodium polystyrene sulfonate. Volume resuscitation with normal saline or one-half isotonic sodium chloride solution may be effective to enhance renal elimination in patients with mild to moderate toxicity. For severe intoxication, hemodialysis is indicated.

MERCURY

The only metal that is a liquid under ordinary conditions is metallic mercury. Acute mercury poisoning usually occurs through ingestion of inorganic mercuric salts or inhalation of metallic mercury vapor. Intoxication from mercuric salts causes a burning sensation in the throat, a metallic taste, discoloration and edema of the mouth, vomiting, bloody diarrhea, and shock. Side effects include renal failure and acute chemical pneumonia. Gastric lavage and activated charcoal should be administered in mercuric salt poisoning. Intramuscular dimercaprol can also be used.

✳ Apply Your Knowledge 28.6

The following exercises focus on what you have just learned about poisoning by electrolytes, lead, isoniazid, lithium, and mercury. *See Appendix E for the correct answer.*

MATCHING
Match the lettered therapy that may be part of the treatment of poisoning/overdose by the numbered agents.

AGENT	THERAPY
1. _____ Magnesium	a. Sodium bicarbonate
2. _____ Potassium	b. Sodium polystyrene sulfonate
3. _____ Iron	c. Calcium gluconate
4. _____ Isoniazid	d. Pyridoxine
5. _____ Lead	e. Deferoxamine
6. _____ Lithium	f. Chelating agents
7. _____ Mercury	g. Dimercaprol

FILL IN THE BLANK
Select terms from your reading to fill in the blanks.

1. Side effects of mercury poisoning include _____ failure and acute chemical _____.

2. Severe intoxication with _____ may require _____.

3. _____ are organic compounds capable of forming coordinate bonds with metals to rid the body of the poison.

4. Adults are _____ sensitive than children to the CNS effects of lead.

5. _____ is indicated for severe iron poisoning.

6. The chief sign of potassium poisoning is the development of _____.

7. The magnesium ion is a CNS _____.

8. Systemic poisoning with _____ can cause hypotension, hypothermia, coma, paralysis, and respiratory failure.

9. Lethal or near-lethal overdose of _____ via the IV route is a frequent error associated with IV fluid therapy.

10. _____ poisoning is one of the oldest occupational and environmental hazards in the world.

OPIOIDS

Morphine, heroin, and codeine decrease central and sympathetic nervous system activity. Intoxication is characterized by euphoria, drowsiness, and constricted pupils (in mild cases); and hypotension, bradycardia, hypothermia, coma, and respiratory arrest (in more severe cases). Death is usually caused by apnea or pulmonary aspiration of gastric contents. When patients arrive for care shortly after ingestion, the stomach should be emptied by gastric lavage or emesis, and activated charcoal should be administered. Narcotic intoxication can be reversed by the opioid antagonist naloxone.

ORGANOPHOSPHATES

Organophosphates include insecticides and chemical "nerve gases" such as sarin. They are absorbed through the skin, lungs, and GI tract. Widely distributed in tissues, organophosphates are slowly eliminated by hepatic metabolism. The time from exposure to onset of toxicity is usually 30 minutes to 2 hours. These agents may cause nausea, vomiting, urinary and fecal incontinence, abdominal cramps, increased bronchial secretions, wheezing, coughing, salivation, sweating, urinary frequency, and blurred vision. In severe poisoning, pulmonary edema, hypotension, and bradycardia may occur.

Treatment of organophosphate poisoning includes removing clothing that may have become contaminated and washing the skin with soap and water. GI decontamination should include use of activated charcoal. Supportive measures include treatment of seizures, ventilatory assistance, and oxygen administration.

PETROLEUM DISTILLATES

Petroleum distillates include gasoline, kerosene, diesel oil, and paint thinner. They are CNS depressants that damage cells by dissolving cellular lipids. Pulmonary damage occurs with pulmonary edema or pneumonitis and is a common, serious complication. A state that resembles alcohol intoxication may be induced by inhaling gasoline or kerosene vapors. Symptoms include nausea, headache, and a burning sensation in the chest. Oral ingestion causes irritation of upper mucous membranes in the GI tract. For treatment, extreme care must be used to prevent aspiration. Gastric emptying is indicated when large amounts have been ingested. For patients who are still alert, emesis may be induced. Oxygen therapy should also be given.

SALICYLATES

Aspirin is the most common salicylate—found in more than 30 million American households. The ingestion of 10 to 30 grams of aspirin or sodium salicylates may be fatal to adults. Intoxication may result from a cumulative effect of therapeutic administration of high doses. Toxic symptoms may begin at dosages of 3 grams per day. Therapeutic salicylate intoxication is usually mild and is called *salicylism*. Vertigo and hearing impairment are the earliest symptoms, and further overdosage causes nausea, vomiting, diarrhea, sweating, drowsiness, fever, and headache. CNS effects may progress to convulsions, hallucinations, cardiovascular collapse, coma, hyperthermia, pulmonary edema, and death. Treatment consists initially of inducing emesis, or of gastric lavage, after which activated charcoal, and then an osmotic cathartic, are administered. Artificial ventilation with oxygen may be used to treat respiratory depression, and convulsions may be treated with phenobarbital or diazepam. Hemodialysis and peritoneal dialysis are highly effective in cases of serious poisoning from salicylates.

THEOPHYLLINE

Theophylline is used to treat asthma and chronic obstructive pulmonary disease (COPD). It affects the cardiovascular, neurologic, GI, and metabolic systems. After an acute overdose, hypokalemia, hyperglycemia, hypercalcemia, hypophosphatemia, and acidosis commonly occur. Common symptoms of toxicity include nausea, vomiting, abdominal pain, hypomagnesemia, and tachycardia. Serious overdose results in seizures, hypotension, and significant dysrhythmias, which may result in cardiac arrest.

After airway, breathing, and circulation have been established, treatment of theophylline overdose consists of endotracheal intubation and gastric lavage. Activated charcoal with the possibility of sorbitol as a cathartic should be administered. Benzodiazepines and phenobarbital are indicated to treat seizures. Short-acting beta blockers may be used with caution, especially if hypotension is present. Serious toxicity may require hemoperfusion or hemodialysis.

✳ Apply Your Knowledge 28.7

The following exercises focus on what you have just learned about poisoning with opioids, organophosphates, petroleum distillates, salicylates, and theophylline. *See Appendix E for the correct answers.*

FILL IN THE BLANK
Select terms from your reading to fill in the blanks.

1. Opioids depress _____ and _____ nervous system activity.

2. Treatment of organophosphate poisoning includes removing _____.

3. Petroleum distillates are CNS depressants that damage cells by dissolving _____.

4. Poisoning with petroleum distillates produces a state similar to _____.

5. Salicylates are found in most American households and include _____.

6. _____ and _____ are the earliest symptoms of salicylate toxicity.

7. Serious overdose of theophylline results in _____, _____, and _____, which may result in _____.

8. Treatment of theophylline overdose consists of _____ and _____.

Bites and Stings

Bites and stings from various animals, including insects and reptiles, are among the most common traumatic complaints that involve poisons. This section discusses bites and/or stings from scorpions, spiders, and snakes.

SCORPIONS

Scorpions are common in the United States, but of the 30 different species, only two are deadly, and these are found in the southwestern states. Most stings occur in warmer months. The **antivenom** (purified antibodies against venoms or venom components) is derived from cat serum, and is used along with calcium gluconate and phenobarbital to treat scorpion stings. Opioids (such as codeine and morphine) are contraindicated because they enhance the scorpion venom's effects.

SPIDERS Bites

There are many types of spiders in the United States with poison harmful to human beings. Perhaps the most dangerous of these spiders is the black widow, which is common in warmer climates throughout the country. Female black widows can deliver a very painful bite and venom that affects the CNS. It can be fatal especially in infants, allergic persons, and elderly people, or in others, if left untreated. The venom must be neutralized with antivenom administered intravenously. For controlling muscle spasms caused by the spider's venom, IV calcium gluconate is given. Other appropriate treatments include antibiotics, tetanus immunization, oxygen, antihistamines, adrenaline, and muscle relaxants.

SNAKE BITES

Poisonous snakes bite about 7,000 people each year in the United States, and out of this number, 20 people die. These snakebites are medical emergencies and occur most often during summer afternoons in rocky or grassy areas. They are usually not fatal if prompt, correct treatment is given. The only poisonous snakes found in the United States are coral snakes and pit vipers (which include rattlesnakes and water moccasins). Most snakebites occur on the arms and legs. Bites to the head or trunk are most dangerous.

Correct first aid that is administered promptly can reduce venom absorption and prevent severe symptoms. The patient should not be given any beverages, food, or oral medications. Incision and suction may be successfully used only for pit viper bites that occurred less than 1 hour prior to treatment. Suction is also indicated if transport time to a medical facility would exceed 30 minutes. Mouth suction should not be used if the rescuer has oral ulcers, if the patient is close to a medical facility, or if the antivenom can be promptly given. Alcoholic drinks or stimulants speed venom absorption, so they should be avoided. Ice should not be applied to the bite because it will increase damage to the patient's tissues.

 Apply Your Knowledge 28.8

The following exercises focus on what you just learned about poisoning via bites and stings. *See Appendix E for the correct answers.*

MULTIPLE CHOICE
Choose the correct answers from choices a–d.

1. Most scorpion stings occur in:
   a. Warm temperatures
   b. Cold temperatures
   c. Northern states
   d. Mexico

2. These drugs enhance the effects of scorpion venom:
   a. Benzodiazepines
   b. Opioids
   c. Cardiac glycosides
   d. Barbiturates

3. The venom of female black widow spiders affects the:
   a. Heart
   b. GI tract
   c. CNS
   d. Liver

(continued)

Apply Your Knowledge 28.8 (continued)

4. The most dangerous snakebites are on the:
   a. Arms and legs
   b. Mouth
   c. Trunk and head
   d. Ankles

5. The following should not be applied to a snakebite because it will increase damage to the patient's tissues.
   a. Heat
   b. Lidocaine
   c. Bandages
   d. Ice

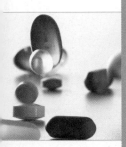

Chapter Capsule

This section repeats the objectives from the beginning of the chapter and then provides a summary of the most important concepts for that objective. Use this section as a quick review and to check your knowledge.

Objective 1: Predict some symptoms that signify specific types of poisonings.

- Unmistakable odor of bitter almonds on patient's breath—cyanide
- Gastrointestinal (GI) hyperactivity, salivation, and papillary constriction—insecticides
- Cherry-colored flush of the skin and mucous membranes—carbon monoxide (CO)

Objective 2: Explain steps that can be taken to prevent poisonings from occurring.

- Keep chemicals and medicines locked up and out of sight
- Keep these substances in their original containers
- Read all labels before using
- Leave original labels intact on all products
- Check dosages every time medication is administered
- Make sure there is plenty of light when reading medication labels
- Clean out medicine cabinets regularly
- Always dispose of unneeded medications safely, and rinse containers before discarding

Objective 3: Differentiate several types of poisonings for which activated charcoal is used to absorb the toxic agent.

- Cardiac glycosides (used to stimulate the heart)
- Methylxanthines (commonly used as stimulants and bronchodilators)
- Heavy metal or corrosive chemical poisonings

Objective 4: Explain the six major services offered by the poison control center network.

- Community education about poison prevention
- Health-care provider education in the recognition and management of poisonings
- Emergency telephone treatment recommendations for all types of poisonings, drug overdoses, and chemical exposures provided to nonmedical and medical callers

- Research and surveillance of human poison exposures, including occupational and environmental exposures, as well as those related to chemicals and drugs
- Telephone follow-up for all patients (hospitalized or not) to assess progress and recommend additional poison treatment that may be required
- Training of future toxicologists

Objective 5: Identify the most common types of poisonings in the United States

- Nonprescription drugs
- Household products
- Solvents
- Pesticides
- Poisonous plants

Objective 6: Discuss the type of alcohol that has the greatest toxic effects on the human body.

- Methanol—metabolizes into formaldehyde

Objective 7: Recognize two types of poisonings listed as true "medical emergencies."

- Cyanide—potent and rapid-acting poison
- Snake bites

Objective 8: Discuss a leading cause of death in opiate poisoning.

- Apnea or pulmonary aspiration of gastric contents

Objective 9: Name the type of salicylate found in 30 million American households.

- Aspirin

Objective 10: Contrast the treatments for scorpion stings and snake bites.

- Scorpion stings—antivenom derived from cat serum used with calcium gluconate and phenobarbital
- Snake bites—incision and suction for pit viper bites that occurred less than 1 hour prior to treatment; avoidance of beverages, food, or oral medications; transport to nearest medical facility

Internet Sites of Interest

- The National Institutes of Health provides an important Web site with information on the toxicity of common household products at: **http://householdproducts.nlm.nih.gov**
- The American Association of Poison Control Centers (AAPCC) Web site is at: **www.aapcc.org**. Be sure to keep the number of the Poison Control Center posted in your facility and provide patients with this information, especially parents of young children.
- On the Web site of the National Institute of Occupational Safety and Health at: **www.cdc.gov/niosh**, click on "Chemicals" for information concerning chemical toxicity.
- Provide parents of young children with information from Web sites such as: **http://www.epa.gov** and **http://www.niehs.nih.gov**. Search for "lead."

Chapter 29

Geriatrics

Chapter Objectives

After completing this chapter, you should be able to:

1. Discuss the process of aging.
2. Explain the leading causes of diseases and death in elderly patients older than age 65.
3. Identify the factors that influence drug absorption in older adults.
4. Discuss creatinine clearance in elderly patients and use the measurement formula.
5. Identify polypharmacy and its effects on elderly patients.
6. List common cardiovascular disorders in elderly individuals.
7. Discuss the effects of sedatives and hypnotics on elderly patients.
8. List six principles that are important in treating elderly patients.

Key Terms

Alzheimer's disease (AL-zhy-merz) (page 635)

Cognitive (page 627)

Creatinine clearance (kree-AT-tih-neen) (page 630)

Glycoprotein (page 629)

Polypharmacy (page 631)

Stroke (page 628)

Thiazides (page 633)

PRACTICAL SCENARIO

An 82-year-old man arrives at the hospital complaining of chest pains. An ECG test reveals congestive heart failure, and he is treated with various drugs including a diuretic and an ACE inhibitor. His condition stabilizes, and he is discharged. Seven days later, he experiences nausea and confusion. His doctor treats the nausea but does not treat the confusion, assuming it is related to senility. The patient develops a tremor in his hands, which is an adverse effect of the drug prescribed for his nausea. He is given benztropine, which then causes constipation. The doctor gives him docusate tablets for the constipation, but the patient's confusion increases until he is extremely anxious. Next, the doctor prescribes an antipsychotic, which calms the patient down, but results in depression. The doctor prescribes an antidepressant, but the patient soon dies from ventricular tachycardia.

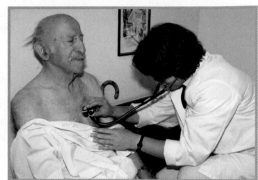

Critical Thinking Questions

1. What action by the physician may have led to this patient's death?
2. What are the principles that might have helped the physician make different drug therapy decisions for the patient?
3. What assumptions did the physician make early in the course of therapy that may have been unwarranted or incorrect?

Introduction

The process of aging is complex and includes biological, psychological, sociological, and behavioral changes. *Biologically*, the body gradually loses the ability to renew itself. Various body functions begin to slow down, and the vital senses become less acute. *Psychologically*, aging persons experience changing sensory processes; perception, motor skills, problem-solving ability, and emotions are frequently altered. *Sociologically*, they must cope with the changing roles and definitions of self that society imposes on elderly people. *Behaviorally*, aging individuals may move more slowly and have less dexterity.

Major changes that are not physiological also occur during the aging process and impact health, including **cognitive** (intellectual processes, such as thinking, reasoning, and remembering) changes, such as forgetting to take daily medications; economic changes due to decreased income, increased health expenses, and other factors; and unforeseen changes including the death of a spouse.

Geriatric Drug Therapy

The elderly population requires increased health-care attention. In the United States, the elderly population grew more than tenfold during the twentieth century. In 1900, there were just over 3 million Americans age 65 or older. In 2000, the same group numbered nearly 35 million. Drug therapy for geriatric patients requires specific knowledge of their physiology, pathology, and other age-related factors. Drug dosages must be adjusted according to an elderly patient's weight, amount of body fat, laboratory results (e.g., blood urea nitrogen [BUN], creatinine, serum protein, liver enzymes, electrolytes), and current health conditions.

Significant changes in common responses to certain drugs can occur in older people. Other drugs may affect elderly patients in only slightly differing ways. As people age, their drug usage patterns change—generally increasing—because the incidence of disease or multiple diseases increases with age. In addition, many older adults experience problems with nutrition and finances that may decrease dosing compliance in prescribed drugs. Health-care practitioners who deal with the elderly must be aware of these issues and understand how to deal with them. Equally important, it is essential for health-care personnel to be aware of the leading causes of death in the elderly.

Disease and Death in Elderly People

Heart disease and cancer have been the two leading causes of death among people 65 years of age and older for the past two decades. Over one-third (35%) of all deaths are due to heart disease, including heart attacks and chronic ischemic heart disease. Cancer accounts for about one-fifth (22%) of all deaths.

Other important chronic diseases among persons 65 years of age and older include **stroke** (cerebrovascular disease), chronic obstructive pulmonary disease, diabetes, pneumonia, and influenza. Alzheimer's disease and several important renal diseases (such as chronic nephritis and nephrotic syndrome) have gained significance as causes of death among the elderly population during the past two decades. Alzheimer's disease is now among the 10 leading causes of death for older white people, but not for other racial groups.

Physiologic Changes in Elderly Individuals

Most organ systems show a decline that begins during young adulthood and continues as people age. Individuals age differently, and the elderly accumulate physiologic deficiencies with the passage of time in varying amounts. The most important decline appears to be in the renal function. The physiologic changes in older adults are shown in Table 29-1 ■.

Table 29-1 ■ Physiologic Changes in Geriatric Patients

ORGANS	PHYSIOLOGIC CHANGES
Heart	Cardiac output and blood flow decrease.
Liver	Function of enzymes and blood flow decrease.
Kidneys	Blood flow, glomerular filtration, and nephron function decrease.
Stomach	Gastric secretions decrease.
Intestines	Peristalsis and motility decrease; first-pass effect decrease.

CHANGES IN PHARMACOKINETICS

Pharmacokinetics deal with the absorption, distribution, metabolism, and elimination of drugs as well as the amount of time each of these processes requires. In many cases, pharmacokinetics can explain why different people react differently to a drug.

Absorption

Although drug absorption is not altered in any major way with age, the rate at which some drugs are absorbed does change. Conditions that influence drug absorption in older adults include slower gastric emptying, altered nutritional habits, and greater use of over-the-counter (OTC) medications.

Distribution

Elderly people tend to have increased body fat, but reduced lean body mass, and reduced total body water (Table 29-2 ■).

Table 29-2 ■ Pharmacokinetic Changes Due to Aging

TYPE OF CHANGE	YOUNG ADULTS (BEGINNING AT AGE 20)	OLDER ADULTS (BEGINNING AT AGE 60)
Body fat	18–20% of body weight (men)	36–38% of body weight (men)
	26–33% of body weight (women)	38–45% of body weight (women)
Body water	61% of body weight	53% of body weight
Hepatic blood flow	100% in a young adult	55–60% in an older adult
Kidney weight	100% in a young adult	80% in an older adult
Lean body mass	19% of body weight	12% of body weight
Serum albumin	4.7 g/dL	3.8 g/dL

Serum albumin, which binds to many drugs, especially weak acids, is usually decreased. There may be a concurrent increase in **glycoprotein**, a specific serum protein that binds to many basic drugs. Changes such as these may alter a drug's appropriate loading dose. Because of decreased volume of distribution, the loading dose of a drug, such as digoxin (Lanoxin), should be reduced (if it is used at all) in an older person with heart failure. Because of reduced drug clearance, maintenance doses also may have to be reduced.

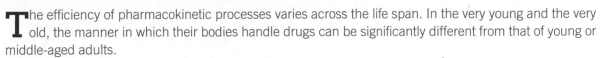

Focus Point

Age Affects Pharmacokinetic Process

The efficiency of pharmacokinetic processes varies across the life span. In the very young and the very old, the manner in which their bodies handle drugs can be significantly different from that of young or middle-aged adults.

Metabolism

The liver's capacity to metabolize drugs does not appear to consistently decline as age increases. This is true for all drugs. However, as we age the liver's ability to heal from an injury (such as from viral hepatitis or alcohol use) declines. The health-care professional should realize that a history of recent liver disease in an elderly patient should lead to caution when administering drugs that are mostly cleared by the liver. This is true even after the patient has apparently completely recovered from hepatic damage. Also in elderly people, heart failure and other diseases that affect liver function (such as malnutrition) are more common. Heart failure may alter liver metabolism and reduce hepatic blood flow. Impaired hepatic function also may result from severe nutritional deficiencies.

Elimination

Because of decreased cardiac output and blood flow in the circulatory system, the liver and kidneys are affected. By age 65, nephron function may decline by 35%, and after 70 years of age, blood flow to the kidneys may be decreased 40%.

Creatinine clearance is an indicator of the glomerular filtration rate. Evaluating renal function based on serum creatinine alone may not be accurate for older adults because of the decrease in muscle mass. Creatinine is a by product of the muscle breakdown of stored proteins. However, creatinine is primarily excreted by the kidneys. A decrease in muscle mass can cause a decrease in serum creatinine. In elderly patients, serum creatinine may be within normal values because of a lack of muscle mass, but there still could be a decrease in renal function. In young or middle-aged adults, serum creatinine would be increased with a decrease in renal function.

The serum creatinine level may be measured by the 24-hour creatinine clearance test to evaluate renal function. Creatinine clearance can also be calculated by the following formula:

$$\text{Creatine clearance in mL/min} = \frac{(140 - \text{age}) \times (\text{weight in kg})}{72 \times \text{serum creatinine in mg/dL}}$$

The normal creatinine clearance value for an adult is 80 to 130 mL/min.

With liver and kidney dysfunction, the efficacy of a drug dose is usually decreased. If several drugs are being taken, drug effects may be intensified in elderly patients. If the efficiency of the hepatic and renal systems is decreased, the half-life of the drug is prolonged, resulting in drug toxicity. Special medications must be administered in reduced dosages in elderly patients (Table 29-3 ■).

Table 29-3 ■ Medications Administered in Elderly Patients that Require Reduced Dosages

DRUG OR CLASS OF DRUG	ADVERSE EFFECTS
Aminoglycosides	Ototoxicity, nephrotoxicity
Carbamazepine (Carbatrol)	Ataxia, drowsiness
Cimetidine (Tagamet)	Confusion
Digoxin (Lanoxin)	Overdose toxicity
Levodopa (Dopar)	Hypotension
Morphine (Avinza)	Respiratory depression
Thioridazine (Mellaril)	Confusion
Thyroxine	Myocardial infarction
Vitamin D (Calcijex)	Renal toxicity
Warfarin (Coumadin)	Bleeding

CHANGES IN PHARMACODYNAMICS

The term *pharmacodynamics* refers to how drugs interact at target organs or receptor sites. Pharmacodynamics examines the way drugs bind with receptors, the concentration required to elicit a response, and the time required for each of these events. Because there is a lack of affinity to receptor sites throughout an elderly person's body, the pharmacodynamic response may be changed.

Many changes in pharmacodynamics in elderly individuals result from altered pharmacokinetics or diminished homeostatic responses. There may be changes with age in the characteristics or numbers of some receptors. The elderly patient may be more or less sensitive to drug action because of age-related changes in the central nervous system, changes in the number of drug receptors, and changes in the affinity of receptors to drugs. If the patient is more sensitive to the drug's action, the dose may need to be lowered, and vice versa. Changes in organ functions are important to consider in drug dosing. Most studies show that the elderly experience a decrease in responsiveness to β-adrenoceptor stimulants.

In the cardiovascular system of older adults who do not have obvious cardiac disease, the increment of cardiac output required by mild-to-moderate exercise is successfully provided until at least age 75. However, the increased output results mostly from increased stroke volume in the elderly (while in young adults, it results from tachycardia). Average blood pressure and symptomatic orthostatic hypotension both increase with age. An elderly patient should be checked for orthostatic hypotension during every physician visit. Other physiologic changes in older adults include increased blood sugar, impaired temperature regulation, and poor tolerance to hypothermia.

Focus on Natural Products

Yohimbe

Yohimbe is a natural supplement widely taken to treat erectile dysfunction. However, in the absence of standardization in dietary supplement labeling in the United States, there is no reliable way to determine the amount of the drug *yohimbine* that is contained in the supplement. Yohimbe is not recommended for patients with hypertension or hepatic, renal, or peptic ulcer disease—all common conditions affecting elderly individuals.

Polypharmacy

The practice of prescribing multiple medicines to a single patient simultaneously is called **polypharmacy**. In general, it is better to use as few medicines as possible. Polypharmacy increases the patient's costs for treatment, as well as increases the chances for multiple adverse effects and drug interactions. Administration of many drugs together is more common in the elderly population because of their need for different medical specialists and the use of OTC drugs and herbal therapies.

Polypharmacy may cause liver dysfunction, malnutrition, confusion, and falls. Liver dysfunction contributes to delirium or acute confusional state. Confusion and disturbances of perception (including misinterpretations of information) are commonly seen. Herbal preparations must be considered drugs as well, and use with prescribed medications contributes to polypharmacy.

Focus on Geriatrics

Polypharmacy

Multiple drug therapies may cause confusion in elderly patients and lead to medication errors and further drug interactions.

✳ Apply Your Knowledge 29.1

The following questions focus on what you have just learned about disease, death, and physiologic changes in elderly people. *See Appendix E for the correct answers.*

MULTIPLE CHOICE
Select the correct answers from choices a–d.

1. All of the following may result from polypharmacy, except:

   a. Increases in the patient's costs of treatment

   b. Increases in the chances for side effects

   c. Increases in liver functions

   d. Increases in the chances for drug interactions

2. The elderly patient may be more or less sensitive to drug action because of age-related changes in which of the following factors?

   a. Central nervous system

   b. Changes in the number of drug receptors

   c. Changes in the affinity of receptors to drugs

   d. All of the above

3. Creatinine clearance is an indicator of which of the following?

   a. Gastrointestinal tract absorption

   b. Glomerular filtration rate

   c. Gastrointestinal hormone secretion

   d. Glomerular inflammatory diseases

4. Serum albumin binds to many drugs, especially in which of the following conditions?

   a. Weak acids

   b. Weak bases

   c. Strong acids

   d. Strong bases

5. Which of the following types of diseases are the most common in elderly persons?

   a. Lung diseases

   b. Kidney diseases

   c. Liver diseases

   d. Heart diseases

FILL IN THE BLANK
Select terms from your reading to fill in the blanks.

1. Alzheimer's disease is now among the _____ leading causes of death among older white people.

2. The most important decline appears to be in the _____ function of older adults.

3. Drug dosages must be adjusted according to an elderly patient's weight, _____, _____ results, _____, and liver enzymes, or current health conditions.

4. Conditions that influence drug absorption among persons 65 years of age include slower gastric emptying, altered nutritional habits, and greater use of _____.

5. By age 65, a person's nephron function may decline by _____%.

Changes in the Effects of Drugs on Elderly Patients

Antihypertensives, cardiac glycosides, antiarrhythmics, central nervous system drugs (sedative–hypnotics, opioid analgesics, antidepressants, and antipsychotics, as well as medications used for Alzheimer's disease), anti-inflammatory drugs, antimicrobial drugs, and GI drugs (antiulcer drugs and laxatives) all have different effects on elderly patients. Drug selection for this group of patients is extremely important. Drugs with longer half-lives may accumulate and cause toxicity.

CARDIOVASCULAR DRUGS

Cardiovascular disorders such as hypertension, congestive heart failure, myocardial infarction, and stroke are very common in older adults. Almost one-third of all deaths in Western countries are attributed to heart disease. Many drugs can be used for these disorders, and some of them must be used cautiously in the elderly.

Antihypertensive Drugs

In the United States, blood pressure increases with age, especially in elderly women. It is clear that uncontrolled hypertension leads to serious health problems and, especially in the elderly, should be treated very seriously.

Weight reduction and salt restriction are indicated prior to drug therapy, which usually begins with **thiazides**, the most commonly prescribed class of diuretics. These agents often cause hyperglycemia, hyperuricemia, and hypokalemia in elderly patients, due to their higher incidence of arrhythmias, type II diabetes, and gout. It is important that antihypertensives be used in lowered doses. If the patient also has atherosclerotic angina, calcium channel blockers are effective and safe when their use is controlled. Beta blockers are prescribed less owing to their effects on patients with obstructive airway disease, though they are important if heart failure is present. ACE inhibitors are less useful unless diabetes or heart failure is present.

Alpha$_1$ blockers, such as prazosin (Minipress) and terazosin (Hytrin) and centrally acting alpha$_2$ agonists, such as methyldopa (Aldomet), clonidine (Catapres), guanabenz (Wytensin), and guanfacine (Tenex), are infrequently used for elderly patients because of their adverse effects.

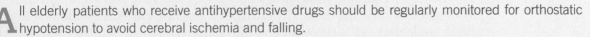

Focus on Geriatrics

Antihypertensives and Elderly Patients

All elderly patients who receive antihypertensive drugs should be regularly monitored for orthostatic hypotension to avoid cerebral ischemia and falling.

Cardiac Glycosides

Physicians often overuse cardiac glycosides, partially because of their fear of heart failure in elderly patients. Because older patients are more susceptible to arrhythmias, the toxic effects of cardiac glycosides are particularly dangerous, and long-term use of these drugs should be carefully monitored because of their narrow therapeutic range. The half-life of digoxin (Lanoxin) may be increased by 50% or more in elderly patients, and renal function must be considered when a dosing regimen is being contemplated. In geriatric patients, coronary atherosclerosis, hypokalemia, hypomagnesemia, and hypoxemia all contribute to a high incidence of digitalis-induced arrhythmias. Other less common digitalis toxicities, including delirium, endocrine abnormalities, and visual changes, are also seen in the elderly. With close monitoring of serum digoxin levels, creatinine clearance tests, and vital signs (the pulse should not be less than 60 beats per minute), digoxin is considered safe for older adults.

Antiarrhythmic Drugs

Treating elderly patients who have dysrhythmias (also called *arrhythmias*) is challenging. Clearances of quinidine and procainamide decrease, while their half-lives increase in aging patients. Older people exhibit changes in hemodynamic reserve, incidence of severe coronary disease, and different frequencies of electrolyte disturbances—all of which contribute to arrhythmias. Disopyramide (Norpace) should be avoided due to its major toxicities. The half-life of lidocaine (Anestacon) is increased in the elderly, and its loading dose should be reduced in geriatric patients to avoid toxicity.

Patients with atrial fibrillation, however, do as well with simple control of their ventricular rate as they do with conversion to normal sinus rhythm. For safety, measures should still be taken to reduce possible thromboembolism in chronic atrial fibrillation (such as with anticoagulant drugs or aspirin therapy).

Anticoagulants

Bleeding may occur with chronic use of anticoagulants in elderly patients. Warfarin (Coumadin) is 99% protein-bound, and with a decrease in serum albumin, which is common among older adults, there is an increase in free, unbound circulating warfarin. There is a significant risk for bleeding as a result. Regular testing to determine the level of warfarin in the blood and regulate anticoagulant drug therapy is essential for everyone taking the drug, particularly the elderly.

Focus Point

Prothrombin Time

Elderly patients who are taking anticoagulants must have periodic monitoring of prothrombin time (PT) or international normalized ratio (INR) to determine the level of anticoagulant in the blood and to regulate anticoagulant drug therapy.

CENTRAL NERVOUS SYSTEM DRUGS

Numerous drugs influence the action of chemical mediators and affect neurotransmitter release and reception. These drugs may act by blocking receptors and prevent the transmitters from binding them. CNS drugs for geriatric patients—sedative–hypnotics, narcotic analgesics, antidepressants, antipsychotics, and drugs used for Alzheimer's disease—are discussed in this section.

Sedatives and Hypnotics

Insomnia is a common problem for the elderly. Sedatives and hypnotics are the second most common group of drugs prescribed for or taken OTC by the elderly. In those who are 60 to 70 years old, the half-lives of many barbiturates and benzodiazepines show their greatest age-related increase. These agents are eliminated more slowly if the patient has reduced renal function or a liver disease. It is generally believed that elderly patients have more variances in their sensitivity to sedative and hypnotic drugs on a pharmacodynamic basis. In order to avoid injuries and accidents, ataxia and other motor impairments should be especially watched for in older individuals taking these drugs.

Narcotic Analgesics

Narcotics may cause dose-related adverse effects when taken by the elderly. Geriatric patients are often more sensitive to the respiratory effects of narcotic analgesics because of the way respiratory function changes with increased age. Patients should be evaluated regarding their sensitivity to these agents before administration, and caution should be continually used. Hypotension may also result from narcotic use. However, for conditions requiring strong analgesia (such as cancer), opioids are frequently underutilized for this group of patients. Good pain management plans are easily obtained, and underutilization of narcotic analgesics is generally unjustified.

Antidepressants and Antipsychotics

Phenothiazines, such as promazine (Prozine-50) and perphenazine (Phenazine), and phenothiazine-like drugs, such as haloperidol (Haldol), have sometimes been overused in managing psychiatric diseases in the elderly. These agents are effective in treating schizophrenia, delirium, dementia, aggressiveness, and paranoia, but are not fully satisfactory for geriatric patients. These drugs do not appear to be effective in dementia caused by Alzheimer's disease. When an antipsychotic drug that has sedative effects is required in the elderly, a phenothiazine such as thioridazine (Mellaril) is adequate, except in patients with preexisting extrapyramidal disease. Older drugs such as chlorpromazine (Thorazine) should be avoided in the elderly due to their orthostatic hypotension-inducing effects. Drug doses should be gradually increased according to the patient's tolerance and the desired therapeutic effect. There should be close monitoring for possible adverse effects.

The half-lives of some phenothiazines are increased in the geriatric population, and dosages should be started at just a fraction of the amounts used for young adults. Lithium (Eskalith) must be dosage-adjusted due to its clearance by the kidneys, and thiazide diuretics should not be used with lithium because it further reduces renal clearance.

Older adults are more likely to experience toxic effects of antidepressants, but they are just as responsive to them as other adults. Senile dementia and major depression must be carefully diagnosed, as they may resemble each other. If a tricyclic antidepressant is to be used, nortriptyline (Aventyl) and desipramine (Norpramin) are good choices because of their reduced antimuscarinic effects.

Focus Point

Depression and Suicide

The suicide rate among people older than age 65 is more than twice the national average, and psychiatric depression, a leading cause of suicide, is often undertreated in elderly patients.

Medications Used for Alzheimer's Disease

Alzheimer's disease is characterized by progressive memory and cognitive function impairment, which may lead to a completely vegetative state and, ultimately, death. The biochemical defects responsible for Alzheimer's disease have not been identified. It is believed that abnormal neuronal lipoprotein processing, together with changes in choline acetyltransferase, brain glutamate, dopamine, norepinephrine, serotonin, and somatostatin, are causative factors.

Cholinomimetic drugs are usually the focus of treatment for Alzheimer's patients. Cerebral vasodilators have been deemed ineffective. A cholinesterase inhibitor called tacrine (Cognex) enters the CNS quickly and has a duration of 6 to 8 hours. This drug apparently increases the release of acetylcholine from cholinergic nerve endings and may inhibit MAO, decrease the release of gamma-aminobutyric acid (GABA), and increase the release of norepinephrine, dopamine, and serotonin from nerve endings. However, it has significant toxic effects including nausea, vomiting, and liver toxicity.

CNS Drug Toxicities

Alzheimer's patients are often very sensitive to CNS toxicities of drugs that have antimuscarinic effects.

Donepezil (Aricept), rivastigmine (Exelon), and galantamine (Reminyl) have been shown to improve cognitive activity in some Alzheimer's patients. They may even reduce morbidity from other diseases and slightly prolong the life of the patient. These agents should be used with caution in patients receiving other cytochrome P450 enzyme inhibitors such as ketoconazole (Nizoral) and quinidine (Quinora).

ANTI-INFLAMMATORY DRUGS

For osteoarthritis and rheumatoid arthritis, nonsteroidal anti-inflammatory drugs (NSAIDs), such as naproxen (Naprosyn) and ibuprofen (Advil, Motrin), must be used with special care because of toxicity. Although aspirin causes GI irritation and bleeding, newer NSAIDs may cause irreversible kidney damage. They accumulate more rapidly in geriatric patients, especially in those with renal disease. Elderly patients receiving large doses of NSAIDs must be carefully monitored for changes in renal function.

For those who cannot tolerate full NSAID doses, corticosteroids, such as hydrocortisone (Cortef, Hydrocortone) and prednisone (Deltasone, Meticorten), are very useful. However, these agents can cause osteoporosis that is related to the dose and duration of corticosteroid therapy. Increased calcium and vitamin D intake may reduce these effects. Frequent exercise should also be encouraged during corticosteroid therapy.

GASTROINTESTINAL AGENTS

Histamine-2 (H_2)-receptor blockers are safer drugs than other antiulcer agents for the treatment of peptic ulcers. Ranitidine (Zantac), famotidine (Pepcid), and nizatidine (Axid) may be used for elderly patients. Cimetidine (Tagamet) is not suggested for the older adult because of its side effects and multiple potential drug interactions.

Laxatives are commonly taken by elderly patients. In long-term facilities such as nursing homes, 75% of older adult patients use laxatives on a daily basis. Fluid and electrolyte imbalances may occur with excessive use. Increased GI motility with laxative use may decrease the absorption of other drugs.

ANTIMICROBIAL DRUGS

Elderly patients appear to have reduced host defenses due to alterations in their T-lymphocyte function. As a result, they are more susceptible to serious infections and diseases such as cancer. Antimicrobial drugs have been used since 1940 to compensate for this deterioration of natural body defenses. Important changes in the half-lives of antimicrobial drugs may be expected due to decreased renal function. This is very important in the case of aminoglycosides owing to their toxicities to the kidneys and other organs. For example, the half-lives of gentamicin (Garamycin), kanamycin (Kantrex), and netilmicin (Netromycin) are more than doubled in elderly patients.

Penicillins, such as amoxicillin (Amoxil), cephalosporins, such as cefotaxime (Claforan), sulfonamides, such as sulfadiazine (Gantanol[3]) and tetracyclines, such as tetracycline HCI (Achromycin), are considered safe for the elderly. If the patient has a decrease in renal drug clearance and the drug has a prolonged half-life, the drug dose should be reduced.

✳ Apply Your Knowledge 29.2

The following questions focus on what you have just learned about changes in the effects of drugs on the elderly population. *See Appendix E for the correct answers.*

MATCHING
Match the lettered percentages of pharmacokinetic changes among the elderly population to the numbered types of pharmacokinetic change.

PHARMACOKINETIC CHANGES	PERCENTAGES OF CHANGES AMONG ELDERLY PEOPLE
1. _____ Body water	a. 55% to 60% in older adults
2. _____ Body fat	b. 12% of body weight
3. _____ Lean body mass	c. 53% of body weight
4. _____ Hepatic blood flow	d. 36% of body weight

FILL IN THE BLANK
Select terms from your reading to fill in the blanks.

1. Donepezil and galantamine should be used with caution in patients receiving other cytochrome _____ enzyme inhibitors, such as ketoconazole and quinidine.

2. H_2-receptor blockers include ranitidine, cimetidine, _____, and _____.

3. Thiazides are often the beginning treatment for hypertension in elderly patients, and these agents often cause hyperglycemia, hyperuricemia, and _____.

4. Morphine may cause dose-related adverse effects when taken by the elderly, because these patients are often more sensitive to _____ effects of narcotic analgesics.

5. Warfarin (Coumadin), an anticoagulant, is commonly prescribed for older adults, but causes a significant risk of _____.

Special Considerations

Inadequate health-care and prescription coverage often forces older patients to avoid taking required medications that are important for their quality of life. Newer NSAID therapies for arthritis treatment, for example, may cost more than $100 a month.

Focus Point

More Drugs Prescribed for the Elderly Population

People older than 65 account for more than 32% of the drugs prescribed in the United States, even though they represent only about 12% of the total population.

Noncompliance due to forgetfulness may result in patients not staying on a regular drug regimen, thereby greatly reducing effectiveness. Deliberate noncompliance may also occur, based on prior poor experience with a drug. Other noncompliance in taking drugs may be caused by physical disabilities or difficulty in using spoons, syringes, and other equipment. Enlisting the elderly patient as an educated, willing participant in drug therapies is vital. Labels should be large enough for patients to read, and any other impediments to sticking to a drug regimen should be noted and efforts made to overcome them.

Health-care practitioners should adhere to the following principles when treating elderly patients:

❋ Take drug histories carefully.

❋ Prescribe drugs only for specific, rational indications.

❋ Define the goal of drug therapy.

❋ Start with small doses, adjust slowly, and check blood levels when necessary.

❋ Maintain suspicion regarding drug reactions and interactions by knowing what other drugs the patient is taking.

❋ Keep the drug regimen as simple as possible. Try to use drugs that may be taken at the same time every day, and use the smallest number of drugs that is possible.

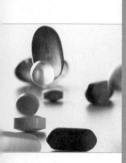

Chapter Capsule

This section repeats the objectives from the beginning of the chapter and then provides a summary of the most important concepts for that objective. Use this section as a quick review and to check your knowledge.

Objective 1: Discuss the process of aging.

■ Physiologic changes—decreased cardiac output and blood flow, function of liver enzymes and blood flow, kidney blood flow, glomerular filtration, nephron function, gastric secretions, peristalsis and motility, first-pass effect, body water, hepatic blood flow, kidney weight, lean body mass, and serum albumin, increased body fat

■ Biological, psychological, sociological, and behavioral changes; changes in sensory processes, and in roles and self-definitions; slowdown of physical movement; decreased dexterity

Objective 2: Explain the leading causes of diseases and death in elderly patients older than age 65.

■ Heart disease, including heart attacks and chronic ischemic heart disease: 35% of deaths among elderly individuals

■ Cancer—about 22% percent of deaths in the elderly population

■ Chronic diseases—stroke, chronic obstructive pulmonary disease, diabetes, pneumonia, and influenza

■ Alzheimer's disease and several serious renal diseases: increases over the past two decades as causes of death in elderly individuals

Objective 3: Identify the factors that influence drug absorption in older adults.

■ Slower gastric emptying

■ Altered nutritional habits

■ Greater use of OTC medications

Objective 4: Discuss creatinine clearance in elderly patients and use the measurement formula.

■ Creatinine clearance is an indicator of the glomerular filtration rate; creatinine is a by-product of the muscle breakdown of stored proteins, but is excreted primarily by the kidneys; serum creatinine level can be measured by the 24-hour creatinine clearance test to evaluate renal function

■ Creatinine clearance can also be calculated by the following formula:

$$\text{Creatinine clearance in mL/min} = \frac{(140 - \text{age}) \times (\text{weight in kg})}{72 \times \text{serum creatinine in mg/dL}}$$

Objective 5: Identify polypharmacy and its effects on elderly patients.

- Polypharmacy—prescribing multiple medicines to a single patient simultaneously by one or more physicians; taking herbal drugs in addition to prescribed drugs
- Effects—increased costs of treatment; increased chances for side effects and drug interactions; possible liver dysfunction, malnutrition, confusion, and falls

Objective 6: List common cardiovascular disorders in elderly individuals.

- Hypertension
- Congestive heart failure
- Myocardial infarction
- Stroke

Objective 7: Discuss the effects of sedatives and hypnotics on elderly patients.

- The half-lives of many sedatives and hypnotics increase in patients ages 60 to 70
- Reduced elimination of the drugs occurs if the patient has impaired renal function or a liver disease
- Elderly patients often have more variances in their sensitivity to these drugs
- Ataxia and other motor impairments can occur

Objective 8: List six principles that are important in treating elderly patients.

- Take drug histories carefully
- Prescribe drugs only for specific, rational indications
- Define the goal of drug therapy
- Start with small doses, adjust slowly, check blood levels
- Know what other drugs the patient is taking
- Keep the drug regimen as simple as possible

Internet Sites of Interest

- For a review of renally excreted drug dosing, visit:
  www.rxkinetics.com/renal.html
- WebMD presents an article on the prescribing of sedatives for elderly people with insomnia, based on material from the *British Medical Journal* at:
  www.webmd.com. Search for "sedatives elderly."
- PharmacyTimes.com offers "Understanding and Managing Polypharmacy in the Elderly" at: **www.pharmacytimes.com**. Search for "polypharmacy in the elderly."

Chapter 30

Pediatrics

PRACTICAL SCENARIO

Alice Wood, age 32, is breastfeeding her newborn. Alice has developed a cold and says she is not sleeping at night because of her symptoms. She wants to take an over-the-counter (OTC) decongestant and cough suppressant. But Alice's health-care provider instructed her that she cannot take any medication while breastfeeding without first checking with her physician. Alice is confused and questions you about this.

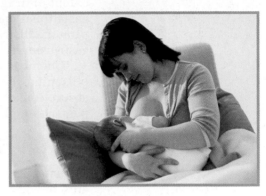

Ruth Jenkinson
© Dorling Kindersley.

Critical Thinking Questions

1. How would you address Alice's concerns?
2. Is it safe for Alice to take an OTC product for her cold symptoms while she is breastfeeding?
3. How can Alice help to minimize any effect on her infant from taking a medication?

Introduction

Lack of knowledge and understanding of the clinical pharmacology of specific drugs in pediatric patients, particularly in newborns, can result in many problems in drug therapy. The problem of establishing efficacy and dosing guidelines for infants is further complicated by the fact that the pharmacokinetics of many drugs changes greatly as an infant ages from birth to several months after birth. The dose-response relationships of some drugs may change markedly during the first few weeks after birth. Then, during the first few months of life, physiologic processes and their resulting pharmacokinetic variables change significantly. This is why it is vital to pay special attention to the pharmacokinetics of pediatric patients. The differences between younger patients and other groups have not been greatly researched.

The term **neonates** refers to newborns from birth to 28 days old, the **infant** is from 29 days old to walking age (typically 1 year), and the **toddler** is a child from approximately 1 year to 3 year of age.

Pharmacokinetics

The basic pharmacologic principles that apply to adults (see Chapter 1) also apply to neonates, infants, and younger children. Only the ways in which they differ in neonates and infants are discussed in this section.

DRUG ABSORPTION

In infants and children, the drug absorption process is similar to that of adults. Factors such as blood flow at the site of administration and gastrointestinal function influence drug absorption. These factors change rapidly soon after birth.

Physiologic conditions that can reduce the rate of blood flow to the site of administration include heart failure, cardiovascular shock, and vasoconstriction. For example, there is very little muscle mass in a preterm infant who is sick. Drugs may remain in the muscles and be absorbed more slowly than anticipated. If **peripheral blood circulation** (the circulation in the body's extremities) improves, a sudden increase of circulating drugs may result in potentially toxic drug concentrations. Drugs that can be especially dangerous in these situations include aminoglycoside antibiotics, anticonvulsants, and cardiac glycosides.

Due to rapidly changing biochemical and physiologic changes that occur in the gastrointestinal tract of infants, drugs that are inactivated by the low pH of gastric contents should not be given orally. **Peristalsis** (the rhythmic movement of the intestines) in neonates is irregular and may be slower than anticipated. Great care must be taken in administering drugs to neonates due to the unpredictability of their rates of absorption.

The rate of gastric emptying is an important determinant of the overall rate and extent of drug absorption. It is variable during the neonatal period and is affected by gestational maturity, postnatal age, and type of feeding. Gastroesophageal reflux, respiratory distress syndrome, and congenital heart disease in the neonate can delay gastric emptying.

Chemical agents applied to the skin of a premature infant may result in inadvertent poisoning. For example, drug toxicities in neonates are reported for percutaneous absorption of such agents as hexachlorophene (Phisohex), laundry detergents with pentachlorophenol, hydrocortisone (Alphaderm), and disinfectant solutions with aniline.

DRUG DISTRIBUTION

Neonates have higher percentages of water than adults. Extracellular water makes up 40% of body weight in neonates, as compared to 20% in adults. Most neonates experience diuresis in the first 2 days of life. It is important, especially for water-soluble drugs, to determine the concentration of a drug at receptor sites.

The amount of body fat in full-term neonates is about 15%. Organs that accumulate high concentrations of lipid-soluble drugs in older children may accumulate smaller amounts of these types of agents in younger infants. Another important factor is drug binding to plasma proteins. Albumin's affinity for acidic drugs and the total plasma protein concentration increase during the time from birth into early infancy. These do not reach normal adult values until 10 to 12 months of age. Usually, protein binding of drugs is lowered in neonates. This has been seen with local anesthetic drugs, diazepam (Valium), phenobarbital (Barbital), ampicillin (Amcill), and phenytoin (Dilantin). Therefore, the concentration of free (unbound) drug in plasma is increased. This results in greater drug effect or toxicity.

Focus on Pediatrics

Physiologic Impacts on Pharmacokinetics

The physiologic processes that influence pharmacokinetics in children include gastrointestinal function, tissue blood flow, body fluid levels, plasma protein concentrations, liver function, and renal function.

Certain drugs compete with serum bilirubin in binding to albumin. Drugs given to a neonate with jaundice can displace bilirubin from albumin, and because of the greater permeability of a neonate's blood–brain barrier, large amounts of bilirubin may enter the brain and cause **kernicterus**, which is a serious form of jaundice in newborns.

DRUG METABOLISM

Most drugs are metabolized in the liver. Drug-metabolizing oxidases and conjugating enzymes exhibit substantially lower activity in neonates. Because of these lower metabolic activities, many drugs have slow clearance rates and longer half-life elimination times. Drug doses and dosing schedules must be altered appropriately. If not, the neonate may experience adverse effects from drugs that are metabolized in the liver.

The limited knowledge and understanding of the clinical pharmacology of specific drugs in pediatric patients predispose this population to problems in the course of drug treatment, particularly in newborns and infants. There are no FDA requirements for pediatric studies, which means that determining appropriate efficacy and dosage guidelines for the therapeutic use of drugs in children must rely extensively on pharmacologic data derived primarily from adults. The problem of establishing efficacy and dosage guidelines for infants is further complicated by the fact that the pharmacokinetics of many drugs changes appreciably as an infant ages from birth (which is sometimes premature) to several months after birth. The dose-response relationships of some drugs may change markedly during the first few weeks after birth.

Pharmacokinetics and organ responsiveness also change dramatically during development from the embryonic and fetal periods to adulthood. Prematurely born neonates at gestations as short as 24 weeks are now surviving (a full-term **gestation**, or the period of fetal development from conception until birth, is 40 weeks).

DRUG EXCRETION

The glomerular filtration rate is much lower in newborns than in older children or adults. Based on body surface area, a neonate's glomerular filtration rate is only 30 to 40% that of an adult. Premature babies show an even lower glomerular filtration rate. However, glomerular filtration rates do improve greatly during the first week after birth. By the end of the third week, glomerular filtration is 50 to 60% of an adult's. Adult values are reached by the time an infant is 6 to 12 months old. Drugs that require renal function for elimination are removed from the body very slowly during the first weeks of life.

Toddlers may have shorter elimination half-lives of drugs than older children and adults, probably as a result of higher renal elimination and metabolism. One example concerns the drug digoxin. The dose per kilogram of this drug is much higher for toddlers than for adults, which is a fact that is still not fully understood.

✳ Apply Your Knowledge 30.1

The following questions focus on what you have just learned about pediatric pharmacokinetics. *See Appendix E for the correct answers.*

FILL IN THE BLANK
Select terms from your reading to fill in the blanks.

1. The dose-response relationships of some drugs may change markedly during the first _____.

2. Neonates have higher percentages of _____ than do adults.

3. Because of the greater permeability of a neonate's blood–brain barrier, large amounts of bilirubin may enter the brain and cause _____.

4. Toddlers may have shorter elimination half-lives of drugs than _____.

5. Due to lower metabolizing activities in neonates, many drugs have slow _____.

MULTIPLE CHOICE
Choose the correct answers from choices a–d.

1. Which of the following factors change rapidly soon after birth and influence drug absorption?
   a. Lesser permeability of the blood–brain barrier
   b. Greater organ responsiveness to a drug
   c. Blood flow at the site of administration
   d. Blood flow at the site of the kidneys

2. A sudden increase of circulating drug may result in potentially toxic drug concentrations in all of the following examples except:
   a. Cardiac glycosides
   b. Aminoglycoside antibiotics
   c. Amoxicillin antibiotics
   d. Anticonvulsants

(continued)

Apply Your Knowledge 30.1 (continued)

3. Neonates have higher percentages of water than do adults. Which of the following ratios is correct?

    a. 60/30

    b. 40/20

    c. 30/5

    d. 20/5

4. The amount of body fat in full-term neonates is about:

    a. 2%

    b. 7%

    c. 12%

    d. 15%

5. The affinity of albumin for acidic drug concentrations during the time from birth into early infancy may:

    a. Decrease

    b. Increase

    c. Stay the same

    d. Vary

Pediatric Dosage Forms and Compliance

Actual pediatric dosages are determined by taking into account the form of the drug and how a parent or caregiver will dispense it to the child. Elixirs and suspensions are popular forms for pediatric administration. **Elixirs** are alcoholic solutions that offer consistent dissolution and distribution of the drugs they contain. **Suspensions** are dosage forms that contain undissolved drug particles and must be shaken to evenly distribute them. This is essential because if a suspension drug form is not adequately shaken, it will cause dangerous variations in dosages. For example, an uneven distribution of drug is a potential cause of inefficacy or toxicity in children taking phenytoin (Dilantin) suspensions. The prescriber must provide proper instructions to the pharmacist and the child's parents or caregivers.

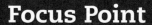

Focus Point

Pediatric Doses

Pediatric doses can be based on body surface area, age, and body weight.

Major dosing errors may result from incorrect calculations because many pediatric doses are calculated by using body weight. A common, but potentially fatal, mistake is that ten times the amount of medication is administered because a decimal point was placed incorrectly. A good rule to use in avoiding "decimal point errors" is to always use a zero to the left of a decimal point for doses that are less than "1" (Figure 30-1 ■). Also, zeros should not be used after decimal points if they are not needed.

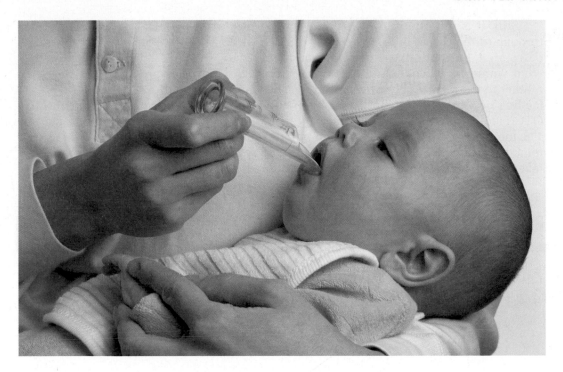

Figure 30-1 ■ Using the measuring device provided by the pharmacy or physician is important for giving the correct dose to children.
© Dorling Kindersley.

Pharmacodynamics

The mechanisms of action of drugs in newborns, infants, and children involve a complex sequence of events. An inadequate response to an effective concentration of a drug may result from the presence or absence of receptors, inadequate drug-receptor binding, or the inability of the organ or tissue to respond to the postreceptor signal. One particular drug may have a specific affinity for a special cell. Some drugs may act by affecting the enzyme functions of the body. Each of these events progresses at different rates during development, beginning with growth to biochemical maturation and eventually to structural maturation, at which point the organ can respond fully to the events initiated by a drug.

Certain drugs pose particular difficulties when used in neonates because of the unique character of their distribution or elimination in patients in this age group, or because of the unusual side effects they may cause. These drugs include the antibiotics, digoxin (Lanoxin), indomethacin (Indameth), and methylxanthines.

Focus Point

Pediatric Pharmacokinetic Differences

The differences in pharmacokinetics can lead to stronger or weaker drug effects in children compared with those in young adults.

Drug Administration During Lactation

Many women avoid breastfeeding because they incorrectly believe that drugs they may be taking are in sufficient quantities to cause great risk to their infants. In actuality, more babies die because of problems from baby formula than from the milk of their mothers.

Still, it is important to realize that most drugs taken by lactating women do pass through to the breast milk. Drug concentration in breast milk is usually low. In a one-day period, the amount of a drug that an infant receives from nursing is much less than what would be considered a "therapeutic dose." If a drug is prescribed as safe for a mother to take while she is breastfeeding, she should take it 1 to 2 hours before breast-feeding or 3 to 4 hours after breastfeeding to minimize the effect on the infant. Most OTC medications provide information on the label about its safety during lactation. The mother should avoid OTC products that contain multiple ingredients, such as cold remedies, as well as those containing more than 20% alcohol. The mother should not take more than the dosage listed on the product label.

Focus on Pediatrics

Drug Safety during Lactation

If data are not available about a certain drug and its effects on breastfeeding, the mother should not take it.

Many antibiotics are highly detectable in breast milk. Tetracyclines appear at about 70% of maternal serum concentrations and can stain the developing teeth of an infant. Isoniazid (Laniazid) can quickly reach equilibrium between maternal blood and breast milk. Its concentrations in breast milk can cause signs of pyridoxine deficiency in the infant if the mother does not take pyridoxine supplements (Beesix).

Sedatives and hypnotics can produce pharmacologic effects in nursing infants. Barbiturates can produce sedation and poor sucking reflexes; sedation can also be caused by chloral hydrate. Diazepam (Valium) can also sedate a nursing infant, but more importantly, can result in significant drug accumulation.

Heroin, methadone (Dolophine), and morphine (Avinza) can cause narcotic dependence in infants, and these infants may have to be tapered off, as would their mother. Excessive amounts of alcohol can produce alcoholic effects in infants. Lithium (Eskalith) enters breast milk in concentrations equal to those in maternal serum, and the baby may be exposed to relatively large amounts of this drug as a result. Radioactive substances can increase the risk of thyroid cancer in infants, and chemotherapeutic, cytotoxic, or immune-modulating agents are also potentially dangerous to the pediatric population. No matter what medication the breastfeeding mother is taking, she should monitor her infant for any signs of drug effect and report this to the infant's health-care provider.

Focus on Natural Products

Lobelia Dangers

Lobelia is found in dietary supplements that are marketed for use by children and infants, as well as pregnant women. Lobelia may be very dangerous to use because it contains alkaloids with pharmacologic actions that are similar to nicotine. It can cause either autonomic nervous system depression or stimulation, bronchial dilation, increased respiratory rate, respiratory depression, sweating, rapid heart rate, hypotension, and even coma or death.

Pediatric Drug Dosages *+ Formula (child)*

It is not always safe to proportionally reduce adult doses to determine safe pediatric doses. Patients should always follow their physician's instructions about pediatric dosages and double-check them with the drug manufacturer's product inserts and labels. The FDA is moving toward more stringent demands on the testing and thorough labeling of new drug products for children. The recommended pediatric dose, usually stated as milligrams per kilogram or milligrams per pound, should always be followed.

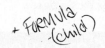 ## Apply Your Knowledge 30.2

The following questions focus on what you have just learned about pediatric dosage forms, doses, and compliance, pharmacodynamics, and drug administration during lactation. *See Appendix E for the correct answers.*

FILL IN THE BLANK
Select terms from your reading to fill in the blanks.

1. Tetracyclines show up as about 70% of maternal serum concentrations and can _____.

2. The use of isoniazid in breastfeeding infants can cause them to develop signs of _____.

3. Radioactive substances can increase the risk of _____ in infants while they are being breastfed by their mothers.

4. An inadequate response to an effective concentration of a drug may result from absence of _____ or _____.

5. Major dosing errors may result from incorrect calculations because many pediatric doses are calculated by using _____.

MATCHING
Match the lettered term to the numbered description.

DESCRIPTION	TERM
1. _____ Alcoholic solution that offers consistent dissolution and distribution of the drugs they contain	a. Suspension
2. _____ Drug that can result in significant drug accumulation in breastfed infants if present in mother's breast milk	b. Barbiturates
	c. Morphine
3. _____ Dosage form that contains undissolved drug particles	d. Elixir
4. _____ Drug class that can produce sedation and poor sucking reflex in breastfed infants if present in mother's breast milk	e. Diazepam
5. _____ A drug that can cause narcotic dependence in breastfed infants if present in mother's breast milk	

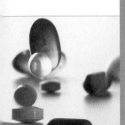

Chapter Capsule

This section repeats the objectives from the beginning of the chapter and then provides a summary of the most important concepts for that objective. Use this section as a quick review and to check your knowledge.

Objective 1: List drugs that may result in toxicity in newborns or infants.

- Drugs that can be especially dangerous to newborns or infants include aminoglycoside antibiotics, anticonvulsants, and cardiac glycosides

Objective 2: Describe drug toxicities in neonates from percutaneous absorption.

- Agents that may result in inadvertent poisoning in neonates include hexachlorophene, pentachlorophenol-containing laundry detergents, hydrocortisone, and aniline-containing disinfectant solutions

Objective 3: List three example drugs that should not be used in neonates because of their lowered protein binding.

- Local anesthetic drugs
- Diazepam
- Phenobarbital

Objective 4: Explain the factors affecting pharmacokinetics in children.

- Drug absorption—physiologic conditions that can reduce the rate of blood flow to the site of administration include heart failure, cardiovascular shock, and vasoconstriction; if peripheral blood circulation improves, a sudden increase of circulating drugs may result in potentially toxic drug concentrations; rate of gastric emptying
- Drug distribution—neonates have higher percentages of water than do adults; their amount of body fat is about 15%; another important factor is drug binding to plasma proteins; protein binding of drugs is lowered in neonates
- Drug metabolism—neonates exhibit substantially lower drug-metabolizing activities of oxidases and conjugating enzymes; the dose-response relationships of some drugs may change markedly during the first few weeks after birth
- Drug excretion—in newborns, the glomerular filtration rate is much lower than in older children or adults; drugs that require renal function for elimination are removed from the body very slowly during the first weeks of life

Objective 5: Describe the means by which adult doses must be adjusted for pediatric drug administration.

- Pediatric drug dosages are based on proportionally reduced adult doses
- They can be based on body surface area, age, and body weight

Objective 6: Discuss pharmacodynamics in newborns, infants, and children.

- An inadequate response to an effective concentration of a drug may result from the presence or absence of receptors, or inadequate drug-receptor binding
- A particular drug has a specific affinity for a special cell
- Some drugs may act by affecting the enzyme functions of the body
- Certain drugs pose particular difficulties when used in neonates because of the unique character of their distribution or elimination in patients in this age group, or because of the unusual side effects they may cause

Objective 7: List five drugs that produce pharmacologic effects in nursing infants.

■ Antibiotics

■ Sedatives and hypnotics

■ Heroin

■ Alcohol

■ Lithium

Objective 8: Explain the effects of radioactive substances in breast milk.

■ These substances can increase the risk of thyroid cancer in infants, and chemotherapeutic, cytotoxic, or immune-modulating agents are also potentially dangerous to babies

Internet Sites of Interest

■ Search this site for "pediatric pharmacotherapy": **www.medscape.com**.

■ This site provides information about medical assisting pharmacology, with calculation examples: **www.mapharm.com/med_calc_pedi.htm**

■ Search for "drugs and other substances in breast milk" at: **www.kidsgrowth.com**.

Checkpoint Review 6

Select the best answer for the following questions.

1. When the reduction in bone mass is sufficient to compromise normal function, this condition is known as which of the following?
   a. Osteocystoma
   b. Osteomalacia
   c. Osteopenia
   d. Osteoporosis

2. An opacity of the eye's lens is called:
   a. Glaucoma
   b. Cataract
   c. Retinopathy
   d. Choroiditis

3. An unmistakable odor of bitter almonds on a patient's breath suggests an accurate diagnosis of the presence of which of these toxic agents?
   a. Carbon monoxide
   b. Cocaine
   c. Bleach
   d. Cyanide

4. Which of the following antidotes is indicated to treat digoxin overdose?
   a. Phenytoin or atropine
   b. Naloxone
   c. Amyl nitrate
   d. Flumazenil

5. Elderly patients appear to have reduced host defenses due to alterations in the function of which of the following leukocytes?
   a. B-lymphocytes
   b. T-lymphocytes
   c. Macrophages
   d. Monocytes

6. Which of the following experiences the most age-related pharmacokinetic changes?
   a. Lean body mass
   b. Heart weight
   c. Kidney weight
   d. Body water

7. Which of the following age groups have higher percentages of water?
   a. Neonates
   b. Infants
   c. Teenagers
   d. Elderly

8. Gold sodium thiomalate (Myochrysine) is effective in which of the following disorders?
   a. Bronchitis
   b. Hepatitis
   c. Acute glomerulonephritis
   d. Active rheumatoid arthritis

9. All of the following are adverse effects of estrogen replacement therapy in the treatment of postmenopausal osteoporosis, except:
   a. Breast cancer
   b. Lung cancer
   c. Endometrial cancer
   d. Cardiovascular problems

10. Carbonic anhydrase inhibitors act on the enzyme responsible for the conversion of carbon dioxide to which of the following?
    a. Bicarbonate and calcium ions
    b. Bicarbonate and sodium ions
    c. Bicarbonate and hydrogen ions
    d. None of the above

11. Colchicine is used for which of the following conditions or diseases?
    a. Peptic ulcer
    b. Gout
    c. Severe hepatic conditions
    d. Severe cardiac disease

12. The drug of choice for opiate overdose is which of the following agents?
    a. Cyanide
    b. Amyl nitrate
    c. Naloxone
    d. Atropine

13. Which of the following drugs can lead to necrosis of the nasal septum?
    a. Cocaine
    b. Corrosive acid
    c. Cyanide
    d. Carbon monoxide

14. Prescribing multiple medications to a single patient simultaneously is called:
    a. Polydactylism
    b. Polypharmacy
    c. Pharmacology
    d. Polypharmacology

15. Which of the following is an example of a new drug that is a selective estrogen-receptor modulator for the treatment of postmenopausal osteoporosis?
    a. carisoprodol (Soma)
    b. lorazepam (Ativan)
    c. acetazolamide (Diamox)
    d. raloxifene (Evista)

16. Baclofen is at least as effective as which of the following drugs?
    a. lorazepam (Dantrium)
    b. dorzolamide (Trusopt)
    c. diazepam (Valium)
    d. levobunolol (Betagan)

17. Several drugs, even when applied directly to the eye, may have systemic effects. This is due to the drug entering via which of the following routes?
    a. The lungs
    b. The nasolacrimal ducts
    c. The mouth and nasopharyngeal ducts
    d. All of the above

18. The antivenom for scorpion venom is derived from the serum of which of the following animals?
    a. Cats
    b. Horses
    c. Pigs
    d. Chickens

19. Which of the following drug forms must be shaken to be evenly distributed before being given to a patient?
    a. Elixirs
    b. Syrups
    c. Suspensions
    d. Spirits

20. The anterior of the sclera of the eye that bulges forward is called the:
    a. Retina
    b. Pupil
    c. Iris
    d. Cornea

21. All of the following are primary functions of the skeletal system, except:
    a. Blood cell production
    b. Storage of minerals
    c. Production of heat and energy
    d. Protection of other organs

22. Which of the following is the generic name of Fosamax?
    a. risedronate sodium
    b. alendronate sodium
    c. raloxifene
    d. calcitonin salmon

23. Pharmacokinetics deal with all of the following, except:
    a. Distribution
    b. Elimination
    c. Metabolism
    d. Mechanisms of action

24. Most of the common disorders seen in elderly people concern which of the following systems?
    a. Respiratory
    b. Cardiovascular
    c. Urinary
    d. Integumentary

25. All elderly patients who receive antihypertensive drugs should be regularly monitored for:
    a. Orthostatic hypotension
    b. Hyperglycemia
    c. Hypouricemia
    d. Hypernatremia

26. Suicides are more than twice as common in which of the following age groups?
    a. Young children
    b. Teenagers
    c. Middle age adults
    d. Elderly adults

27. Which of the following is present in higher percentages in neonates as compared to adults?
    a. Water
    b. Fat
    c. Plasma protein
    d. Lean mass

28. Which of the following drug forms is most popular for pediatric administration?
    a. Powders and pills
    b. Intramuscular injections
    c. Elixirs and suspensions
    d. Suppositories

29. The most poisonous spider found in the United States is the:
    a. Brown recluse spider
    b. Tarantula
    c. Black widow spider
    d. Funnel-web spider

30. Tetracyclines show up as about 70% of maternal serum concentrations, and breastfeeding may cause which of the following adverse effects in infants?
    a. Staining of incoming teeth
    b. Staining of urine and tears
    c. Staining of skin and hair
    d. Renal failure

31. Organophosphates may be absorbed through which of the following parts of the body?

    a. Lungs
    b. Skin
    c. GI tract
    d. All of the above

32. Which of the following is used for controlling muscle spasms caused by a spider's venom?

    a. IV saline
    b. IV calcium gluconate
    c. IV potassium chloride
    d. None of the above

33. The most dangerous site on the body to be bitten by a snake is which of the following?

    a. Leg
    b. Arm
    c. Finger
    d. Head

34. Which of the following is a common and serious complication of diesel oil inhalation?

    a. Encephalitis
    b. Pneumonitis
    c. Hepatitis
    d. Renal failure

35. Exposure to radioactivity during pregnancy may increase the risk of cancer in infants. Which of the following organs is at most risk?

    a. Pancreas
    b. Thyroid
    c. Spleen
    d. Liver

36. Which of the following metals is a liquid under ordinary conditions?

    a. Iron
    b. Copper
    c. Mercury
    d. Lead

37. The ciliary body is the thickest part of which layer of the eye?

    a. Inner
    b. Middle
    c. Outer
    d. Inner and middle

38. Pigment-producing melanocytes are located in which of the following organs?

    a. Mouth
    b. Liver
    c. Spleen
    d. Eye

39. Cherry-colored flushing of the skin and mucus membranes is characteristic of poisoning by which of the following?

    a. Cyanide
    b. Carbon monoxide
    c. Atropine
    d. Acetaminophen

40. All of the following drugs may produce pharmacologic effects in nursing infants, except:

    a. Lithium and alcohol
    b. Antacids and vitamins
    c. Sedatives and hypnotics
    d. Heroin and antibiotics

41. Which of the following is the oldest occupational and environmental hazard in the world?

    a. Mercury poisoning
    b. Lithium poisoning
    c. Lead poisoning
    d. Heroin poisoning

42. Photoreceptors are located in which of the following portions of the eyes?

    a. Pupils
    b. Retina
    c. Aqueous humor
    d. Choroid

43. Which of the following is a systemic autoimmune disease?

    a. Osteoporosis
    b. Osteomyelitis
    c. Rheumatoid arthritis
    d. Rheumatoid fever

44. When the lenses of the eyes adjust shape and facilitate focusing, it is known as:

    a. Presbyopia
    b. Diplopia
    c. Amblyopia
    d. Accommodation

45. All of the following are risk factors for primary open-angle glaucoma, except:

    a. Myopia
    b. Diabetes
    c. Peptic ulcer
    d. Black race

46. When benzodiazepines are combined with other CNS depressants, which of the following adverse effects can occur?

    a. Coma and renal failure
    b. Coma and respiratory depression
    c. Hypertension
    d. Hyperthermia

47. Which of the following chemical substances is used in antifreeze and windshield de-icing solutions?

a. Methyl alcohol
b. Ethylene glycol
c. Ethanol
d. Methanol

48. Which of the following is one of the most common and serious disorders of the eye?

a. Retinal detachment
b. Conjunctivitis
c. Glaucoma
d. Cataract

49. Adverse effects of acetazolamide (Diamox) include:

a. Blurred vision, urinary retention
b. Dry mouth, thirst
c. Paresthesias, drowsiness, nausea
d. Congestive heart failure

50. Auranofin (Ridaura) is employed in the treatment of:

a. Rheumatoid arthritis
b. Multiple sclerosis
c. Ear infections
d. Ulcerative colitis

For questions 51-55, please match the lettered drug to the numbered description.

DESCRIPTION

51. _____ Also called "wood alcohol"
52. _____ Treats warfarin overdose
53. _____ No specific antidote
54. _____ Leads to cardiac dysrhythmias and death
55. _____ Treated with 100% oxygen

DRUG

a. Cocaine
b. Amphetamine
c. Vitamin K₁
d. Carbon monoxide
e. Methanol

For questions 56-60, match the lettered trade name to the numbered generic name.

GENERIC NAME

56. _____ mannitol
57. _____ timolol
58. _____ methocarbamol
59. _____ dantrolene
60. _____ acetazolamide

TRADE NAME

a. Diamox
b. Dantrium
c. Robaxin
d. Betimol
e. Osmitrol

Select terms from your reading to fill in the blanks.

61. Calcitonin is secreted by the parafollicular cells of the _____ gland.

62. Calcium is the most abundant mineral in the _____.

63. The three layers of the eye include the sclera, choroid, and _____.

64. The drugs of first choice in the treatment of intraocular hypertension are the _____.

65. In newborns, the glomerular filtration rate is much _____ than in older children or adults.

66. Creatinine clearance is an indicator of glomerular _____.

67. Administration of many drugs together is more common in the _____ because of the use of different physicians and specialties.

68. The only poisonous snakes found in the United States are _____ snakes and various types of pit vipers.

69. The treatment for methanol poisoning is gastric lavage and the intravenous administration of a 10% solution of _____.

70. The method of choice for GI decontamination from benzodiazepines is _____.

Glossary

Absence seizures Brief seizures characterized by arrest of activity and occasional muscle contractions and relaxations

Absorption The process of drug movement into the systemic circulation

Abuse potential The potential for a drug to cause dependence, abuse, or both

Accommodation Focusing of the lens of the eye

Acromegaly (ak-roh-MEHG-uh-lee) A disorder in which the extremities, such as the hands, feet, and head, are greatly enlarged

Activated charcoal Charcoal that has been treated with oxygen; used to reduce absorption of poisons in the body

Active immunity (ih-MYOO-nih-tee) A form of acquired immunity that develops in an individual in response to an immunogen

Acute (a) Characterized by sharpness or severity (acute pain, an acute infection); (b) having a sudden onset, sharp rise, and short course (an acute disease, an acute inflammation)

Addison's disease (ADD-iss-uns) Adrenocortical insufficiency caused by an autoimmune response to the adrenal gland

Additives Chemicals that are added to foods to facilitate their processing and preservation, to enhance their restorative or stimulating properties, and to control natural contaminants

Adenocarcinoma (ah-deh-no-kar-sih-NO-muh) A malignant tumor arising from a glandular origin

Adenohypophysis (add-eh-no-hy-PO-fih-sis) Anterior lobe of pituitary gland

Adjuvant (AJ-eh-vant) Aiding or contributing to

Adrenergic (add-ruh-NUR-jik) Referring to neurons that release norepinephrine, epinephrine, or dopamine

Adverse effects Harmful effects

Affinity Attractive force

Agonist (AH-go-nist) A drug that binds to a receptor and produces an appropriate physiologic response that is similar to what an endogenous substance would do

Akathisia (ak-kuh-THIS-zee-uh) Difficulty in initiating muscle movement

Alimentary canal Part of digestive system that includes the mouth, pharynx, esophagus, stomach, small intestine, large intestine, rectum, and anus

Alkaloids (AL-kuh-loyds) Organic nitrogen-containing compounds that are alkaline and usually bitter tasting; combine with acids to make a salt

Alkylating agents (AL-kih-lay-ting) Cause replacement of hydrogen by an alkyl group, specifically one that inhibits cell division and growth

Alopecia (al-o-PEE-shuh) Hair loss

Alpha tocopherol (AL-fa toh-KAW-fer-rol) Vitamin E; a substance that protects fragile red blood cell walls (mainly in premature infants) from breaking down

Alpha-adrenergic receptors (AL-fuh add-ruh-NUR-jik ree-SEP-ters) Parts of cells that respond to adrenaline

Aluminum hydroxide Base element used as an antacid

Alveolar duct (al-vee-OH-lar dukt) End of each bronchiole

Alveolar sacs Thin-walled air sacs in the bronchioles

Alveoli (al-VEE-oh-lie) Microscopic air sacs in the capillary networks of bronchioles

Alzheimer's disease (AL-zhymerz) A disease characterized by progressive memory and cognitive function impairment, which may lead to a completely vegetative state and, ultimately, death

Amylase (AM-mil-lace) Digestive enzyme

Anabolic steroids (AN-uh-bol-lik STER-oidz) Hormonal substances related to estrogen, progestins, testosterone, and corticosteroids, which promote muscle growth

Analgesia (ah-nul-JEE-zee-ah) Insensibility to pain without loss of consciousness

Analgesic (ah-nul-JEE-zik) Relating to, characterized by, or producing pain relief with or without antipyretic or anti-inflammatory action

Anaphylactic shock (an-nuh-fih-LAK-tik) A sudden and severe allergic reaction that may be life threatening

Androgens Male sex hormones

Anemia (uh-NEE-mee-uh) A deficiency of hemoglobin, red blood cell number, or red blood cell volume

Anesthesia (an-ess-THEE-zee-ah) Loss of sensation or consciousness

Anesthetics (an-ess-THET-iks) Substances that produce anesthesia

Angina pectoris (an-JY-nuh pek-TOR-iss) A common form of ischemic heart disease that often precedes and accompanies myocardial infarction; described as chest pain and squeezing pressure that can radiate to the jaw and arm

Anions (AN-eye-ons) Negatively charged ions

Antagonist (an-TAH-go-nist) An agent that acts in physiologic opposition; in pharmacology, it is an agent that prevents an agonist from binding to a receptor, thereby blocking its effects

Antibacterial spectrum (an-tie-BAK-tee-ree-ul SPEK-trum) The range of bacteria against which an agent is effective

Antibiotics (an-tie-by-AW-tik) Substances produced by microorganisms that, in low concentrations, are able to inhibit or kill other microorganisms

Antibodies (an-tih-BAH-deez) Special proteins manufactured by the lymphocytes when a foreign substance invades the body

Anticholinergics (AN-tee-kol-in-UR-jiks) Drugs that inhibit the actions of acetylcholine by occupying the acetylcholine receptors

Antidiuretic hormone (ADH) A hormone (also called *vasopressin*) that is released from the posterior lobe of the pituitary gland; exerts an antidiuretic effect; its absence can cause diabetes insipidus

Antigens (AN-tih-jenz) Specific chemical targets, usually pathogens, parts, or products of pathogens, or other foreign compounds, against which antibodies react

Antimetabolites (an-tee-meh-TAH-bo-lytz) Substances that prevent cancer cell growth by affecting DNA production; effective only against cells that are actively participating in cell metabolism

Antimicrobial (an-tie-my-KRO-bee-ul) Referring to an agent that destroys or inhibits the growth of microorganisms, especially pathogenic microorganisms

Antioxidant An agent that prevents cellular structure from being broken down by oxygen

Antipsychotics Any of the powerful tranquilizers (for example, phenothiazines or butyrophenones) used especially to treat psychosis and believed to act by blocking dopamine nervous receptors; also *neuroleptics*

Antipyretics (an-tih-pye-REH-tiks) Drugs that reduce elevated body temperature (fever) to normal levels

Antitumor antibiotics Agents made from natural products produced by species of the soil fungus *Streptomyces;* very effective in the treatment of certain tumors

Antitussives (an-tee-TUSS-ivz) Agents that reduce coughing

Antivenom Purified antibody against venoms or venom components

Apothecary system (ah-PAW-thuh-keh-ree) A very old English system of measurement that has been replaced by the metric system

Approved name A drug's nonproprietary (or generic) name

Aqueous humor (AY-kwee-us) Watery fluid that fills the space between the cornea and lens, helps nourish these parts, and aids in maintaining the shape of the front of the eye; secreted from the ciliary body

Arabic number A number commonly used in expressing quantity and value, such as 0, 1, 2, 3, 4, 5, 6, 7, 8, and 9

Ascorbic acid (as-SCOR-bik) Vitamin C; a substance required for building and maintaining strong tissues for wound healing, resistance to infection, and enhanced iron absorption

Aseptic (ay-SEP-tik) Hand washing and other precautions to reduce risk of infection

Asplenia (as-PLEN-ee-yuh) Loss of the spleen

Asthma A chronic disease caused by increased reactivity of the tracheobronchial tree to various stimuli

Ataxia An inability to coordinate muscle activity

Atelectasis (at-tuh-LEK-tuh-sis) Absence of gas in the lungs, causing collapse

Atrioventricular node (AY-tree-oh-ven-TRI-kyoo-ler) Node that provides the only normal conduction pathway between the atrial and ventricular syncytia; its fibers delay impulse transmission; located in the inferior portion of the septum, which separates the atria, and just beneath the endocardium

Atrium (AY-tree-um) Smaller upper receiving chamber of heart

Attenuated (ah-TEN-yoo-ay-ted) Reduced severity of (a disease) or virulence or vitality of a pathogenic agent

Automaticity (aw-toe-muh-TIH-sih-tee) The heart impulse's automatic, spontaneous initiation

Bacteria Single-celled organisms with a cell wall and cellular organelles that allow them to live independently in the environment

Bactericidal (bak-tee-ree-uh-SY-dul) Capable of killing microbes

Bacteriostatic (bak-tee-ree-oh-STAH-tik) Capable of inhibiting microbial growth

Basal ganglia A group of cell bodies in the medulla involved in the regulation of motor activity

Benign (be-NYN) Of a mild type or character that does not threaten health or life; related to cancer, slow growing

Beri-beri (BEH-ree BEH-ree) A disease caused by a deficiency of thiamine and characterized by edema, cardiovascular abnormalities, and neurologic symptoms

Beta-adrenergic receptors (BAY-tuh add-ruh-NUR-jik) Receptors that respond to norepinephrine or epinephrine

Bevel The slanted part at the needle's tip

Bioavailability The degree and rate at which a substance (as a drug) is absorbed into a living system or is made available at the site of physiologic activity

Biotransformation The process of conversion of drugs within the body

Blepharitis (blef-fah-RY-tis) Inflammation of one or both eyes

Blood pressure Commonly means *arterial pressure;* pressure created in the vessels by the pumping action of the heart; varies from one vessel to another within the systemic circuit

Blood volume Total amount of blood in vascular system

Booster A substance that increases the effectiveness of a medication

Bradycardia (bray-dee-KAR-dee-uh) An abnormally slow heartbeat

Bradykinesia (bray-dee-kuh-NEE-shuh) Extremely slow movement

Bradykinin (brah-dee-KYE-nin) A polypeptide that mediates inflammation, increases vasodilation, and contracts smooth muscle

Broad-spectrum Referring to agents that are effective against a wide range of organisms

Bronchioles (BRONG-kee-ols) The portion of the bronchial tubes that are less than 1 mm in diameter and have abundant smooth muscle and elastic fibers

Bronchitis Inflammation of the mucous membrane of the bronchial tubes

Bronchodilators Agents that widen the diameter of the bronchial tubes

Bronchospasm Contraction of smooth muscle in the walls of the bronchi and bronchioles

Bundle of His A large group of fibers that enter the upper part of the intraventricular septum and are divided into right and left bundle branches lying just beneath the endocardium, between the AV node and the Purkinje fibers; also known as the *atrioventricular bundle*

Calciferol (kal-SIH-fuh-rol) Vitamin D_3

Calcitonin (kal-sih-TOE-nin) A thyroid hormone that lowers blood levels of calcium and phosphate and promotes bone formation

Calcitriol (kal-SIH-tree-ol) The active vitamin D hormone

Calibrated Marked with graduated measurements

Candidiasis (kan-dih-dy-AY-sis) An infection or disease caused by *Candida,* especially *Candida albicans,* usually resulting from debilitation, physiologic change, prolonged administration of antibiotics, and barrier breakage

Cannula (KAN-yoo-luh) The actual metal length that makes up the majority of the needle; it is attached to the hub

Carcinogenic (kars-ih-no-JEN-ik) Cancer causing

Cardiac output Volume of blood pumped per minute

Carotene (KAH-roh-teen) Substance found in dark green and yellow vegetables and fruits and converted to vitamin A in the human body

Cataract A clouding of the lens of the eye or its surrounding transparent membrane that obstructs the passage of light

Catecholamines (kah-teh-KOH-luh-meenz) Any of various amines (epinephrine, norepinephrine, and dopamine) that contain a dihydroxybenzene ring, are derived from tyrosine, and function as hormones, neurotransmitters, or both

Cations (KAT-eye-ons) Positively charged ions

Cell-mediated immunity Immunity obtained when cells attack the antigens directly, rather than producing antibodies; lymphocytes are the primary cells that provide this immunity

Central nervous system Brain and spinal cord

Cerebrum (seh-REE-brum) Largest part of the brain that includes nerve centers associated with sensory and motor functions; provides higher mental functions, including memory and reasoning

Chelating (kee-LAY-ting) agents Organic compounds capable of forming coordinate bonds with metals

Chemical name The name describing the chemical makeup of a drug

Child-resistant packaging Blister packs, special lids requiring the user to press downward and turn simultaneously

Cholecalciferol (koh-luh-kal-SIH-feh-rol) Vitamin D_3; a substance that controls calcium metabolism in bone building

Cholesterol (koh-LES-teh-rol) A natural lipid found in cell membranes, particularly in animal muscle and organ cells

Cholinergic (kol-i-NUR-jik) Referring to neurons that release acetylcholine

Cholinergic blockers Drugs that inhibit the actions of acetylcholine by occupying the acetylcholine receptors

Choroid layer (KO-royd) Middle layer of the eye

Chronic lasting a long time or marked by frequent recurrence

Ciliary body (SIL-ee-ayr-ee) Thickest part of the middle layer of the eye; extends forward from the choroid layer and forms an internal ring around the front of the eye

Ciliary muscle Muscle in the eye that enables the lens to adjust shape to facilitate focusing

Coagulation (koh-ag-yew-LAY-shun) Blood clotting

Cobalamin (koh-BAL-luh-min) Vitamin B_{12}; a substance that promotes the normal function of all cells, especially normal blood formation, and is necessary for proper nervous system function

Cognitive Relating to intellectual processes, such as thinking, reasoning, and remembering

Common fraction A fraction that represents equal parts of a whole; subclassified as proper, improper, mixed, and complex

Congestive heart failure A condition in which the heart pumps blood at an insufficient rate, the kidneys retain salt and water, and fluid accumulates in interstitial spaces

Connective tissue Tissue that consists of fibroblasts, macrophages, and interlacing protein fibers (collagen) that supports, ensheathes, and binds together other tissues and includes adipose tissue, tendons, ligaments, aponeuroses, cartilage, and bone

Controlled substances Those drugs whose possession and use are controlled by the comprehensive Drug Abuse Prevention and Control Act

Conversion The changing of units

Convulsion An abnormal violent and involuntary contraction or series of contractions of the muscles; violent spasms

Cornea The window of the eye that helps to focus entering light rays

Creatinine (kree-AT-tih-neen) A chemical waste molecule produced in skeletal muscle tissue by the breakdown of creatine phosphate

Creatinine clearance An indicator of the glomerular filtration rate; creatinine, a byproduct of the muscle breakdown of stored proteins, is excreted by kidneys

Cretinism (KREE-ten-izm) A disorder of deficiency of thyroid hormones (hypothyroidism) during infancy that results in dwarfism and severe mental retardation

Cryoanesthesia (KRY-o-an-ess-THEE-zee-ah) Reduction of nerve conduction by localized cooling

Cushing's disease (KUSH-ings) A disease in which Cushing's syndrome is caused by a tumor in the pituitary gland

Cushing's syndrome A condition that affects the trunk of the body, in which a pad of fat develops between the shoulders, producing a buffalo hump, and the face becomes round and moon shaped

Cutaneous flush, (kew-TAY-nee-us) Skin reddening

Cyclooxygenase (SYE-klo-OKS-ih-jeh-nase) The name for a group of enzymes required to produce prostaglandins from arachidonic acid

Cystic fibrosis (SIS-tik fy-BRO-sis) A disorder marked by abnormal secretions of the exocrine glands causing obstruction of bronchial pathways

Decimals Any real numbers expressed as a fraction of 10

Decongestants A class of drugs that reverse excessive blood flow (congestion) into an area

Dehydration (dee-hy-DRAY-shun) Excessive loss of body water

Denominator (dee-NAW-mih-nay-ter) The part of a fraction that is below the line and that functions as the divisor of the numerator (number above the line)

Dermatitis (dur-mah-TY-tiss) Inflammation of the skin

Designer drugs drugs produced by a minor modification in the chemical structure of an existing drug, resulting in a new substance with similar pharmacologic effects

Desired dose The amount of drug to be administered at one time (must be in the same unit of measurement as the dosage unit)

Diabetes insipidus (dy-uh-BEE-tees in-SIP-uh-dus) A disorder that is caused by insufficient secretion of vasopressin by the pituitary gland or by a failure of the kidneys to respond to circulating vasopressin; characterized by intense thirst and excretion of large amounts of urine

Diabetes mellitus (dy-uh-BEE-tees MEL-uh-tiss) A serious endocrine disorder characterized by hyperglycemia (high blood glucose levels); resulting from deficient insulin secretion or decreased sensitivity of insulin receptors on target cells

Diastole Ventricles contract and eject blood

Dilutions (dye-LOO-shuns) Less concentrated mixtures

Dissolution (dis-oh-LOO-shun) The process of dissolving

Distribution The passage of an agent through blood or lymph to various body sites

Diuretics (dy-yoo-REH-tiks) Drugs that promote water loss from the body into the urine

Dose-effect relationship The relationship between the dose of a drug (or other agent) that produces harmful effects and the severity of the effects on the patient

Drams Fluidrams; apothecary unit of weight (equivalent to 1/8 ounce)

Dwarfism (DWARF-izm) A condition in which the body is abnormally undersized

Dysphagia (dis-FAY-jee-uh) Difficulty swallowing

Dysrhythmia (dis-RITH-mee-uh) Disturbance of the heart rhythm; also called *arrhythmia*

Eczema (ECK-zih-mah) The most common inflammatory skin condition, caused by endogenous and exogenous agents

Edema (eh-DEE-muh) An abnormal fluid accumulation in the body

Efflux (EE-flucks) The process of flowing out; something that is given off

Electrocardiogram (ECG/EKG) (ee-lek-tro-KAR-dee-oh-gram) A test that records the electrical activity of the heart; electrograph is the tracing made on paper

Elixirs (ee-LICKS-ers) Alcoholic solutions that offer consistent dissolution and distribution of the drugs they contain

Embolus (EM-bo-lus) An abnormal particle circulating in blood, such as an air bubble or blood clot

Emesis (EH-meh-sis) Vomiting

Emollients (ee-MOLE-ee-ents) Skin-softening agents

Emphysema (em-fih-ZEE-muh) Condition of the lung that is marked by distension and eventual rupture of the alveoli with progressive loss of pulmonary elasticity, that is accompanied by shortness of breath with or without cough, and that may lead to impaired heart action

Endocardium (en-do-kar-dee-um) The thin membrane lining the inside of the cardiac muscle

Endogenous (en-dah-jeh-nus) Caused by factors within the body or mind or arising from internal structural or functional causes (*endogenous* malnutrition or *endogenous* psychic depression); relating to or produced by metabolic synthesis in the body

Endorphins (en-DOR-finz) Any of a group of endogenous peptides (such as enkephalin and dynorphin) found especially in the brain that bind chiefly to opiate receptors and produce some of the same pharmacologic effects (such as pain relief) as do opiates

Enkephalins (en-KEH-fuh-linz) Peptides with opiate and analgesic activity that occur naturally in the brain and have a marked affinity for opiate receptors

Epicardium (ep-ih-Kar-dee-um) Membrane lining the outside of the myocardium

Epidural anesthesia (ep-eh-DUR-al) Anesthesia produced by injection of a local anesthetic into the epidural (lumbar or caudal) space via a catheter that allows repeated infusions

Epilepsy (EH-pih-lep-see) Various disorders marked by abnormal electrical discharges in the brain and typically manifested by sudden brief episodes of altered or diminished consciousness, involuntary movements, or convulsions

Erythema (ear-ih-thee-mah) Skin redness caused by capillary dilation

Estrogens One of two major groups of female sex hormones; stimulate enlargement of the vagina, uterus, uterine tubes, ovaries, and external reproductive structures

Ethanol (EH-the-nol) A flammable, colorless chemical compound produced by fermentation of grain

Ethics Standards of behavior, including concepts of right and wrong beyond what legal considerations are in any given situation

Excretion The last stage of pharmacokinetics that removes drugs from the system via the kidneys

Expectorants Medications capable of dissolving or promoting liquefaction of mucus in the lungs

Extremes The two outside terms in a proportion

Fiber A type of complex carbohydrate that does not supply energy or heat to the body

Fibrillation (fib-rih-LAY-shun) Very rapid, irregular contractions or twitching of the individual muscular fibers of the atria or ventricles

Fight-or-flight response Reaction in the body when faced by a sudden threat or source of stress

First-pass effect Immediate exposure of orally administered drugs to metabolism by liver enzymes before they reach the systemic circulation

Flatulence (FLAT-yoo-lentz) Presence of excess gas in the stomach and intestines

Flutter Rapid, regular atrial contractions that often produce sawtooth waves in an ECG; or rapid ventricular tachycardia that appears as a regular, undulating pattern in an ECG, without QRS and T waves as would normally be found

Fraction A number usually expressed in the form a/b; expresses one or more equal parts of a whole

Fungi (fung-guy) Nonphotosynthetic, eukaryotic single or multicellular organisms that are found throughout the environment; fungi have a cell wall containing *sterol*

Fungicidal (fun-jih-sy-dul) Having a killing action on fungi

Gastric lavage (luh-VAAZH) Washing out the stomach with sterile water or a salt-water solution

Gastrostomy tube (gah-straw-sto-mee) A surgically placed tube into the stomach; provides a route for feeding and administering medication

Gauge Diameter of the needle shaft that varies from #18 to #28; the larger the gauge, the smaller the shaft's diameter

Generic name A drug's approved, nonproprietary or official name

Gestation (jes-STAY-shun) The period of fetal development from conception until birth; about 40 weeks

Gestational diabetes mellitus (jeh-STAY-shuh-nul) May develop during pregnancy, and symptoms may be similar to type 2 diabetes

Gigantism (jy-GANT-izm) A condition in which the entire body or any of its parts is abnormally large

Gingival hyperplasia (JIN-jih-vul hi-per-PLAY-zhuh) An increase in the number of cells in the gums of the mouth, causing them to have a swollen appearance

Glaucoma (glauw-KO-muh) A disorder that damages the optic nerve and is often caused by elevated intraocular pressure

Globulins (GLOB-yoo-linz) Proteins present in blood that contain antibodies

Glomerular capsule (gloh-MAYR-yoo-lar KAP-sool) A thin-walled, sac-like structure of the renal corpuscle that surrounds the glomerulus

Glomerular filtration Separation of wastes from body water to produce urine; occurs in the glomerulus

Glomerulus (gloh-MAYR-yoo-lus) A filtering unit of the nephron composed of a cluster of blood capillaries

Glucagon (GLOO-kuh-gon) Hormone secreted when blood glucose levels are low

Glycoprotein A specific serum protein that binds to many basic drugs

Glycoside (GLY-ko-side) An organic compound that yields sugar and nonsugar substances when hydrolyzed; an important cardiac glycoside is digoxin

Goiter (GOY-ter) A swelling of the thyroid gland resulting from a shortage of iodine in the diet

Grain Basic unit of weight of the apothecary system

Gram The unit of weight of the metric system (equivalent to 15.432358 grains)

Gram-negative Refers to bacteria that cannot resist decolorization with alcohol after being treated with Gram's crystal violet; among these bacteria are *Escherichia coli*, *Salmonella*, and other *Enterobacteriaceae*, *Pseudomonas*, *Moraxella*, *Helicobacter*, and *Legionella*

Gram-positive Refers to bacteria that have the ability to resist decolorization with alcohol after being treated with Gram's crystal violet stain, imparting a violet color to the bacterium when viewed by microscope; includes *Bacillus*, *Listeria*, *Staphylococcus*, *Streptococcus*, *Enterococcus*, and *Clostridium*

Graves' disease A disorder in which the thyroid gland is overactive; characterized by numerous eye problems

Half-life ($t1/2$) The time taken for the blood or plasma concentration of the drug to decrease from full to one-half

Hemodialysis (hee-mo-dy-AL-uh-sis) A method in which the patient's blood is passed through a tube to a semipermeable membrane (dialyzer) that filters out waste products

Hemoperfusion (hee-mo-per-FU-zhun) The removal of poisons from blood by passing it through a tube containing treated charcoal or ion-exchange resins

Hemostasis (hee-mo-STAY-sis) A physiologic progression of several steps that stops bleeding

Heparin (HEH-puh-rin) An anticoagulant commonly administered subcutaneously

Household system System of measurement used in most American homes that is not precisely accurate

Hub Part of the needle that fits onto the syringe

Humoral (HYOO-moh-rul) immunity Immunity based on the antigen–antibody response; obtained when B cells produce circulating antibodies to act against an antigen

Hybridomas (hy-brih-DO-muhz) Fusion of a single immune cell to tumor cells that are grown in cultures

Hypercholesterolemia (hi-per-koh-les-ter-raw-LEE-mee-uh) Higher-than-normal levels of cholesterol in the blood

Hyperkalemia (hy-per-kah-LEE-mee-uh) An abnormally high amount of potassium ions in blood

Hyperplasia (hy-per-PLAY-shuh) Abnormal cell growth

Hypertension (hy-per-ten-shun) Blood pressure that is elevated above the normal limits

Hypertensive crisis Severely elevated blood pressure

Hyperthermia (hy-per-THER-mee-uh) A condition of increased body heat; body temperatures above 104°F (40°C) are life-threatening; brain death begins at 106°F (41°C)

Hyperthyroidism (hy-per-THY-royd-izm) Overactivity of the thyroid gland

Hyperuricemia (hy-per-yoo-rih-SEE-mee-uh) Elevated blood level of uric acid

Hypervitaminosis (hy-per-vy-tuh-mih-NOH-sis) Excess intake of vitamins

Hypodermic (hy-po-DUR-mik) Refers to administration of drugs under the skin; of or relating to the needles used

Hypoglycemia (hy-po-gly-SEE-mee-uh) An abnormally low blood glucose level

Hypokalemia (hy-po-kah-LEE-mee-uh) An abnormally low concentration of potassium ions in blood

Hyponatremia (hy-po-nuh-TREE-mee-uh) An abnormally low concentration of sodium ions in blood

Hypoparathyroidism (hy-po-par-uh-THY-royd-izm) A rare disorder in which the body produces little or no parathyroid hormone, resulting in an abnormally low level of blood calcium (hypocalcemia)

Hypopituitarism (hy-po-pih-TOO-ih-tayr-izm) Underactivity of the pituitary gland

Hypotension (hy-po-TEN-shun) An abnormal condition in which blood pressure is not adequate for full oxygenation of the tissues

Hypothyroidism (hy-po-THY-royd-izm) Underactivity of the thyroid gland

Hypoxia (hy-POK-see-uh) Lack of oxygen

Iatrogenic (eye-ah-troh-JEH-nik) Produced inadvertently by medication or other treatment

Immune response A specific defense of the body in response to a foreign substance

Immunity The ability to resist infection and disease through the activation of specific defenses

Immunocompromised (im-myoo-no-KOM-pro-miezd) A weakened immune system

Immunogen (ih-MYOO-no-jen) Antigen

Immunoglobulins (ih-myoon-o-GLOB-yoo-linz) Antibodies, derived from human plasma, that have been formed by the body to specific antigens

Improper fraction A fraction with a numerator that is greater than or the same as the denominator

Infant A child aged 29 days old to walking age (typically 1 year)

Injectable Medication that can be administered by intradermal (within the skin), subcutaneous (into fatty tissue under the skin), intramuscular (IM, into the muscle), and intravenous (IV, into the vein) injection

Insomnia (in-SOM-nee-uh) Inability to sleep normally

Insulin (IN-suh-lin) A pancreatic hormone that stimulates glucose metabolism

International units Units standardized by an international agreement; used to show the amount of drug required to produce a certain effect

Interstate commerce The commerce, traffic, transportation, and exchange between states of the United States

Intoxication (in-tok-sih-KAY-shun) An abnormal state induced by a chemical agent such as a drug, serum, or toxin; essentially, a poisoning

Invasive Pertaining to a route of medication administration that requires insertion of an instrument or device through the skin or a body orifice

Iris Thin diaphragm in the eye that is composed mostly of connective tissue and smooth muscle fibers; colored portion of eye

Ischemia (is-KEE-mee-uh) Insufficient blood flow to the myocardium

Islets of Langerhans (EYE-lits of LANG-ur-hans) Small clusters of cells within the pancreas

Isotypes (EYE-so-typz) Species of atoms of a chemical element with the same atomic number and position in the periodic table and nearly identical chemical behavior but with differing atomic mass or mass number and different physical properties

Keratinization (keh-rat-in-eh-ZAY-shun) Formation of keratin (a horny layer of skin)

Keratinocytes (keh-RAH-tin-oh-syts) Epidermal cells that produce keratin

Keratolytic (keh-rat-oh-LIH-tik) Referring to agents that separate or loosen the horny layer of the epidermis

Kernicterus (ker-NIK-ter-rus) A serious form of jaundice in the newborn

Legend drugs Prescription drugs

Lens Transparent part of eye; adjusts to facilitate focusing

Leukotriene inhibitors (loo-ko-TRY-een) Drugs that inhibit the production of leukotrienes, which are the cause of the inflammatory response in asthma

Lipophilic (lie-poh-FIL-lik) Related to the ability to dissolve more easily in lipids than in water

Liter (LEE-ter) The unit of volume of the metric system (equivalent to 1.056688 quarts)

Lithium (LITH-ee-um) A drug that reduces the activity of certain neurotransmitters and is used in the treatment of bipolar disorder

Loop of Henle (HEN-lee) A long, U-shaped part of the renal tubule extending through the medulla from the end of the proximal convoluted tubule to the beginning of the distal convoluted tubule

Lymph (limf) The fluid that flows through the lymphatic vessels

Lymphatic (lim-FAH-tik) vessels Network of vessels of the lymphatic system that begin in peripheral tissues and end at connections to the venous system

Lymphocytes (LIM-foh-sites) White blood cells that manufacture antibodies to overcome infection and disease

Lymphoid (LIM-foyd) organs Organs connected to the lymphatic vessels that contain large numbers of lymphocytes

Macrominerals (mak-ro-MIH-neh-ruls) Dietary minerals needed by the human body in high quantities

Macrophages (MAK-ro-fah-jez) Immune cells derived from monocytes

Magnesium carbonate Base element used as an antacid

Major minerals Elements that occur in large amounts in the body (i.e., calcium) and have a daily requirement of more that 100 mg/d

Malignant (mah-LIG-nent) In terms of cells, rapidly proliferating with an atypical appearance

Mast cells Large white blood cells found in connective tissue that contain a wide variety of biochemicals, including histamine; involved in inflammation secondary to injuries and infections and are sometimes implicated in allergic reactions

Means The two inside terms in a proportion

Medical emergency An injury or illness that poses an immediate threat to a person's health or life and requires help from a doctor or hospital

Melanosis Abnormal dark pigmentation

Menorrhagia (men-no-RAH-jee-uh) Abnormally heavy or prolonged menstruation

Metabolism The sum of chemical and physical changes in the tissues, consisting of anabolism and catabolism

Metastasis (meh-TAS-tuh-sis) The spreading of cancer cells from the primary site to secondary sites

Meter the unit of length of the metric system (equivalent to 39.37007874 inches)

Metric system Most common, most accurate, and safest system of measurement based on the decimal system

Metrorrhagia (mee-tro-RAH-jee-uh) Uterine bleeding that occurs independent of the normal menstrual period

Milliequivalents (mil-lee-ee-KWIH-vuh-lentz) Measurements used to indicate the strength of certain drugs; more specifically, an expression of the number of grams of equivalent weight of a drug contained in 1 mL of a normal solution

Minim (MIH-num) The basic unit of volume of the apothecary system

Minuend (min-YOO-end) In subtraction, the number from which another number (subtrahend) is subtracted

Mitosis (my-TOH-sis) The splitting of one cell into two new cells

Mixed fraction A fraction that has a whole number and a proper fraction combined and whose value is always greater than one

Monoclonal antibodies (maw-noh-KLO-nul) Types of human proteins that are produced by fusing a single immune cell to tumor cells that are grown in cultures

Mucolytics (myoo-ko-LIT-tiks) Medications capable of dissolving or promoting liquefaction of mucus in the lungs

Multiplicand (mul-tih-plih-KAND) The number that is to be multiplied by another number

Multiplier (MUL-tih-ply-er) The number that multiplies another number (multiplicand)

Muscarinic receptors (mus-kah-RIN-ik) Receptors that innervate smooth muscle and slow the heart rate

Mycoses (my-KOH-seez) Fungal infections

Myocardial infarction (my-oh-KAR-dee-ull in-FARK-shun) MI; heart attack; occurs when a portion of the heart is deprived of blood supply, causing cells to die

Myocardium (my-oh-KAR-dee-um) The middle layer and most important structure of the heart; contains the heart muscles that regulate cardiac output

Myxedema (mix-uh-DEE-muh) The most severe form of hypothyroidism; often develops in the older child or adult and is characterized by swelling of the hands, feet, and face (especially around the eyes); can lead to coma and death

Narcotic a medication that induces sleep or stupor and alters mood and behavior

Nasogastric (NG) tube (nay-zo-GAS-trik) Tube that is inserted through the nose for feeding or removing gastric secretions

Nebulizer (NEH-byoo-ly-zer) A device that disperses a fine-particle mist of medication into the deeper parts of the respiratory tract

Neonates (NEE-oh-nayts) Newborns from birth to 28 days old

Nephrons (NEH-fronz) Functional units of kidneys

Nephrotic syndrome (neh-FROT-ik) a clinical state characterized by edema, various abnormal substances present in the urine, decreased plasma albumin, and increased blood cholesterol

Neurohypophysis (noor-oh-hy-PO-fih-sis) Posterior lobe of pituitary gland

Neuroleptic Referring to psychotropic drugs used to treat psychosis

Neurons Nerve cells

Neurotransmitters (noo-roh-TRANZ-mih-ters) Certain chemical substances, concentrated in various parts of the central nervous system, that are released by neurons and allow communication from one nerve cell to another

Nicotinic receptors (nik-oh-TIN-ik) Receptors that respond to acetylcholine and nicotine and affect skeletal muscles

Nomogram (NAW-mo-gram) A numerical chart that shows relationships between two values

Nonproductive cough A sudden ejection of air from the lungs and through the mouth that does not expel (produce) mucus or fluid from the throat or lungs

Nuclear pharmacy A specialty area of pharmacy practice dedicated to the compounding and dispensing of radioactive materials for use in nuclear medicine procedures

Nucleoside (NOO-klee-oh-sied) Derived from a nucleic acid

Nucleotides (NOO-klee-oh-tiedz) The basic structural subunits of DNA

Numerator (NOO-meh-ray-ter) The top number in a fraction

Nystagmus (nis-TAG-mus) A constant, involuntary movement of the eye

Oligospermia (ol-lih-go-SPER-mee-uh) A subnormal concentration of spermatozoa in ejaculate

Oncogenes (ON-koh-jeenz) Cancer genes that develop from normal genes

Oocytes (OO-oh-sites) Female sex cells

Opiate (OH-pee-ut) A drug (as morphine, heroin, and codeine) containing or derived from opium and tending to induce sleep and to alleviate pain

Opioid (OH-pee-oyd) Possessing some properties characteristic of opiate narcotics but not derived from opium

Optic nerve Nerve that runs through back of the eye; transmits electrical pulses from the retina to the brain, providing vision

Orphan drugs Drugs developed under the Orphan Drug Act, which provides federal financial incentives to nonprofit and commercial organizations for development and marketing of drugs used to treat rare diseases (those that affect fewer than 200,000 people in the United States)

Osmolality (oz-moh-LAL-ih-tee) The concentration of particles in plasma

Osmosis (oz-MOH-sis) The process in which sodium and magnesium ions attract water into the bowel, causing a more liquid stool to be formed

Osteopenia (os-tee-oh-PEE-nee-uh) Reduced bone mass

Osteoporosis (os-tee-oh-por-OH-sis) Reduced bone mass that compromises normal function and often leads to fractures

Ounces Household unit of measurement of weight equivalent to 480 grains or 31.10349 g

Overdose A toxic dose of a drug or other substance

Oxytocin (awk-see-TOH-sin) A hormone that stimulates powerful uterine contractions; aids labor in its later stages

Palliative (PAH-lee-uh-tiv) Able to ease a disease's effects but not able to cure

Parasites (PAH-rah-syts) Protozoans, roundworms, flatworms, and arthropods

Parafollicular cells (par-uh-fo-LIK-u-lur) Cells in the thyroid gland that release calcitonin

Paralytic ileus (par-uh-LIT-ik ILL-ee-us) Absence of peristaltic movements in the intestines

Parasympathetic nervous system (pahr-ah-sim-pah-THET-ik) The part of the nervous system that slows the heart rate, increases intestinal and glandular activity, and relaxes muscles

Parasympatholytics (pahr-ah-sim-pah-tho-LIT-iks) Drugs that inhibit the actions of acetylcholine by occupying the acetylcholine receptors

Parenteral (puh-REN-teh-rul) Introduction of a drug outside of the gastrointestinal tract; generally in injectable form

Parkinsonism Any of several neurological conditions that resemble Parkinson's disease and that result from a deficiency or blockage of dopamine caused by degenerative disease, drugs, or toxins

Partial response Relating to chemotherapy, a 50% or greater decrease in the tumor size, or other objective disease markers, and no evidence of any new disease for at least 1 month

Passive immunity The transfer of the effectors of immunity, which are called *immunoglobulins,* from an immune individual to another

Pathogenic (pah-thoh-JEH-nik) Disease-causing

Pathogens (PAH-tho-jenz) Bacteria or viruses that invade the body

Pediculicides (puh-DIK-yoo-lih-sydz) Pharmacologic agents that kill lice

Pellagra (peh-LEH-gruh) A condition caused by deficiency of vitamin B_3 and marked by dementia, dermatitis, diarrhea, and death

Percent A term meaning *hundredths* that can be expressed as a fraction, decimal, or ratio

Peripheral blood circulation Circulation in the body's extremities

Peripheral nervous system Part of the nervous system that is outside the brain and spinal cord

Peripheral resistance Friction in the arteries as blood flows through the vessels

Peristalsis (payr-ih-STALL-sis) The rhythmic movement of the intestine

Pharmacodynamics (far-muh-koh-dy-NAH-mix) The biochemical and physiologic effects of drugs and mechanisms of drug action

Pharmacognosy (far-muh-KOG-nuh-see) The study of drugs derived from herbal and other natural sources

Pharmacokinetics (far-muh-koh-kih-NEH-tix) The study of the absorption, distribution, biotransformation, metabolism, and excretion of drugs

Pharmacology The study of drugs, including their actions and effects in living body systems

Pharmacotherapeutics (far-muh-koh-thayr-ruh-PYOO-tix) The study of how drugs may best be used in the treatment of illnesses and which drug is most or least appropriate to use for a specific disease

Photoreceptors Visual receptor cells of the eye

Phylloquinone (fil-loh-KWIH-nohn) Dietary form of vitamin K_1, which aids in blood clotting and bone development; treatment for warfarin (Coumadin) overdose

Plant alkaloids Physiologically active organic bases containing nitrogen (and usually oxygen) that are found in seed plants; prevent cell division (or meiosis); also called *mitotic inhibitors*

Platelet plug (PLATE-let) Plug formed by platelets that become sticky and adhere to the inner lining of the injured vessel and to each other

Platelets (PLATE-lets) Megakaryocyte fragments important in the clotting of blood

Pneumonitis (new-moh-NY-tis) Inflammation of the lungs

Polypharmacy The practice of simultaneously prescribing multiple medicines to a single patient

Porphyria (por-FEE-ree-uh) A genetic disorder caused by deficiency of enzymes of the heme biosynthetic pathway

Preanesthetics (pree-an-ess-THEH-tiks) Agents used to partially sedate patients prior to surgery

Priapism (PRY-uh-pizm) Painful and prolonged erection

Primary hypertension Hypertension that has no known cause; accounts for 90% of cases

Productive cough A cough that brings up fluid or mucus from the lungs

Progesterones One of the major groups of female sex hormones; promote changes in the uterus during the reproductive cycle

Prophylaxis (pro-fih-LAK-sis) Prevention, as in drug treatment or other therapy that is given to prevent a disease

Proprietary name A drug's name assigned by the manufacturer and protected by copyright; brand or trade name

Prostaglandins (prah-stuh-GLAN-dinz) Hormone-like substances that control blood pressure, contract smooth muscle, and modulate inflammation

Protozoan (pro-toh-ZOH-un) A single-celled highly mobile microorganism

Pruritus (proo-RYE-tus) Itching

Psoriasis (soh-RY-uh-sis) A chronic, relapsing inflammatory skin disorder

Ptosis (TOE-sis) Drooping eyelid

Puberty The phase in development when an individual becomes reproductively functional

Pupil Circular opening in the iris of the eye

Purkinje fibers (pur-KIN-jee) Specialized conductive fibers located within the walls of the ventricles that conduct an electrical stimulus or impulse that enables the heart to contract in a coordinated fashion

Radical cure A treatment that eliminates a microorganism from both blood and tissue

Ratio A mathematical expression that compares the relationship of one number to another number, or expresses a part of a whole number

Receptor A specific protein in cell membranes that specific drugs bind to, producing a pharmacologic effect

Refractory (ree-FRAK-toh-ree) The period during repolarization when cells cannot respond normally to a second stimulus

Regional anesthesia Affects a large but limited part of the body and is often used in obstetrics (labor and delivery)

Reimportation Importation of a drug into the United States that was originally manufactured in the United States

Renal corpuscle (REE-nul KOR-pus-sul) A filtering unit of the nephron composed of a cluster of blood capillaries called a *glomerulus*

Renal tubule (REE-nul TOO-byool) The part of the nephron that leads away from the glomerular capsule and becomes highly coiled

Renin (REE-nin) A hormone secreted by the kidneys that converts angiotensinogen to angiotensin I

Retina The inner layer of eye that contains the visual receptor cells

Retinal detachment Separation of the retina from the corneal layer of the eye

Retinopathy (ret-tih-NOP-ah-thee) Degeneration of the blood vessels of the retina

Rickets A deficiency of calcitriol that is characterized by malformation of skeletal tissue in growing children

Roman numeral A number represented by a letter (for example, I = 1, V = 5, X = 10)

Salpingitis (sal-pin-JY-tis) Inflammation or infection of a fallopian tube

Sarcomas (sar-KO-muhs) Malignant growths of muscle or connective tissue

Scabicides (SKAY-bih-sydz) Pharmacologic drugs that kill mites

Scabies (SKAY-beez) A group of dermatologic conditions caused by mites that burrow into the skin, causing intense itching

Sclera The outer layer of eye

Scored Notched

Seizures Abnormal electrical activity in the brain

Serotonin (sayr-uh-TO-nin) A neurotransmitter that causes the blood vessel to go into spasms

Serum sickness A reaction to a foreign serum

Side effects Results of drug (or other) therapy in addition to, or in extension of, the desired therapeutic effects, which are usually (but not always) undesirable

Sinoatrial node (syn-oh-AY-tree-ull) The pacemaker; specialized cardiac muscle tissue that initiates one impulse after another; located just beneath the epicardium, in the right atrium, near the opening of the superior vena cava

Somnolence (SAHM-no-lents) A state of near-sleep, a strong desire for sleep, or sleeping for unusually long periods

Spasticity (spas-TIH-sih-tee) Inability of opposing muscle groups to move in a coordinated manner

Sperm male sex cells

Spina bifida (SPY-nuh BIFF-ih-duh) A condition wherein the spinal column is imperfectly closed, resulting in protrusion of the meninges or spinal cord

Spinal anesthesia Injection of anesthetic agent into the subarachnoid space through a spinal needle

Stable disease In terms of cancer, a tumor that neither grows nor shrinks in size

STAT Immediately

Steatorrhea (stee-at-oh-REE-ah) Elimination of large amounts of fat in the stool

Stroke Cerebrovascular accident

Stroke volume Amount of blood pumped by a ventricle in 1 minute

Subarachnoid (sub-uh-RAK-noyd) Area of spinal cord beneath the arachnoid membrane or between the arachnoid and pia mater, and filled with cerebrospinal fluid

Substantia nigra (sub-STAN-shee-uh NY-gra) A large cell mass involved in metabolic disturbances associated with Parkinson's disease

Subtherapeutic doses Drug doses that are below the level used to treat diseases

Subtrahend (SUB-truh-hend) In subtraction, the number that is to be deducted from another

Suspensions Dosage forms that contain undissolved drug particles and must be shaken to evenly distribute them

Sustained release Tablets and capsules that are specially coated and contain several doses so that they dissolve at specific times; also called *delayed release* or *timed release*

Sympathetic (sim-puh-THEH-tik) Relating to the sympathetic part of the autonomic nervous system, or the fight-or-flight response

Sympathetic nervous system The part of the nervous system that accelerates heart rate, constricts blood vessels, and raises blood pressure

Sympathomimetics (sim-path-oh-mi-MET-iks) Adrenergic agonists

Synapses (SIN-aps-eez) The point of contact between nerve cells and each other or other types of cells

Syndrome (SIN-drohm) A collection of signs and symptoms that together signify a specific disease

Systole Ventricles relax and heart stops ejecting blood

Tachycardia (tak-ee-KAR-dee-uh) An abnormally fast heartbeat

Tardive dyskinesia (TAR-div dis-kih-NEE-zhah) Slowed ability to make voluntary movements

Teratogenic (teh-rah-toh-JEN-ik) Able to cause birth defects in fetuses

Testosterone The most abundant androgen

Therapeutic Meant to treat a disease or disorder

Thiazides The most commonly prescribed class of diuretics

Thromboembolism (throm-bo-EM-bo-lizm) The blocking of a blood vessel by a particle that has broken away from a blood clot at its site of formation

Thrombi (THROM-by) Blood clots that form within a blood vessel and attach to the site of formation

Thrush A yeast infection in the mouth caused by *Candida albicans,* a normal resident of the GI tract and vagina

Thyrotoxicosis (thy-ro-toks-ih-KOH-sis) Graves' disease; a disorder in which the thyroid gland is overactive; characterized by numerous eye problems

Toddler A child from approximately 1 to 3 years of age

Tolerance The body's slow adaptation to a drug; higher and higher doses are required to achieve the same effect; reduced responsiveness to a drug

Tonic-clonic Contraction-relaxation

Total body water Amount of water in body

Toxic agent Poisonous or harmful substance

Toxicity (tok-SIH-sih-tee) The state of being noxious; refers to a drug's ability to poison the body

Toxicologists (tok-sih-KAW-loh-jistz) Those who study poisons and toxics agents and their treatments

Toxicology (tok-sih-KAW-luh-jee) The study of poisons and poisonings, including adverse drug reactions

Toxin (TOKS-in) A chemical produced by a microorganism that can be harmful

Toxoids (TOKS-oyds) Protein toxins that have been modified to reduce their hazardous properties without significantly altering their antigenic properties

Trade name A drug's proprietary or brand name

Tubular reabsorption The method by which the kidneys selectively reclaim just the right amounts of substances that the body requires, such as water, electrolytes, and glucose

Tubular secretion The method by which the cells of the tubules remove certain substances from the blood and deposit them into the fluid in the tubules

Tumor suppressor genes A category of genes involved in carcinogenesis; they regulate and inhibit inappropriate cellular growth and proliferation

Ulcers A break in skin or mucous membrane with loss of surface tissue, disintegration and necrosis of epithelial tissue, and often pus

Unit A standard of measure, weight, or any other similar quality

Universal antidote (AN-tih-doht) One agent that will counteract all poisons

Urea (yoo-REE-uh) The most abundant organic waste that results in breakdown of amino acids

Uric acid (YOO-rik) A type of waste molecule formed by the recycling of nitrogenous base from RNA molecules

Urticaria (er-tih-KAY-ree-uh) Vascular reaction of the skin characterized by a rash and severe itching

Vaccination (vak-sih-NAY-shun) Active immunization

Vaccine (vak-SEEN) A preparation of killed microorganisms, living attenuated organisms, or living virulent organisms that are administered to produce or artificially increase immunity to a particular disease

Vasodilation (vass-oh-dy-LAY-shun) Dilation of blood vessels; this action relaxes the smooth muscle of the peripheral arterioles

Vasopressin (vaz-oh-PRESS-in) A peptide hormone of the posterior pituitary gland; also called *antidiuretic hormone (ADH)*

Vasospasms (VAY-soh-spah-zims) Spasms of the blood vessels

Ventricles (VEN-trih-kuls) The lower heart chambers that pump blood out of the heart

Vertigo (VER-tih-go) A sensation of revolving, either of the patient themselves, or of their environment

Viruses Tiny genetic parasites that require the host cell to replicate and spread

Vitreous humor (VIT-ree-us) Transparent, jelly-like fluid in the posterior cavity of the eye; supports the internal parts of the eye and helps maintain the eye's shape

Volatile liquids Inhalation anesthetic agents that are easily vaporized liquids

Water deficit Low levels of body water; dehydration

Water of metabolism The volume of body water that is a byproduct of the oxidative metabolism of nutrients (about 10%)

Wheal A slightly reddened, raised lesion

Whole bowel irrigation Rapid administration of large volumes of an osmotically balanced polyethylene glycol solution given orally or via a nasogastric tube, to flush out the entire GI tract

Xanthine derivatives (ZAN-theen) A group of drugs chemically related to caffeine that dilate bronchioles in the lungs

Appendices

Appendix A

The 100 Most Commonly Used Drugs in the United States

(These drugs are listed in descending order beginning with the most commonly prescribed drug, hydrocodone w/APAP).

Trade Name	Generic Name
Hydrocodone w/APAP	hydrocodone with APAP
Lipitor	atorvastatin
Tenormin	atenolol
Synthroid	levothyroxine
Premarin	conjugated estrogens
Zithromax	azithromycin
Lasix	furosemide
Amoxil	amoxicillin
Norvasc	amlodipine
Hydro-Diuril	hydrochlorothiazide
Xanax	alprazolam
Proventil, Ventolin	albuterol
Zoloft	sertraline hydrochloride
Paxil	paroxetine hydrochloride
Zocor	simvastatin
Prevacid	lansoprazole
Motrin, Advil, Nuprin	ibuprofen
Dyrenium	triamterene
Toprol-XL	metoprolol succinate
Keflex	cephalexin monohydrate
Celebrex	celecoxib
Zyrtec	cetirizine hydrochloride
Levoxyl	levothyroxine sodium
Allegra	fexofenadine hydrochloride
Ortho Evra	norgestimate/ethinyl estradiol
Celexa	citalopram hydrobromide
Deltasone	prednisone
Prilosec	omeprazole
Claritin	loratadine

(continued)

Trade Name	Generic Name
Prozac	fluoxetine hydrochloride
Tylenol	acetaminophen
Ambien	zolpidem tartrate
Lopressor	metoprolol tartrate
Ativan	lorazepam
Fosamax	alendronate sodium
Darvon-N	propoxyphene N/APAP
Glucophage, Fortamet	metformin hydrochloride
Zantac	ranitidine hydrochloride
Elavil	amitriptyline hydrochloride
Viagra	sildenafil citrate
Prempro	conjugated estrogens/medroxyprogesterone
Trimox	amoxicillin
Neurontin	gabapentin
Wellbutrin	bupropion hydrochloride
Pravachol	pravastatin sodium
Augmentin	amoxicillin/clavulanate
Nexium	esomeprazole
Accupril	quinapril hydrochloride
Prinivil	lisinopril
Effexor XR	venlafaxine
Singulair	montelukast sodium
Zestril	lisinopril
potassium chloride, K-Lease, Klorvess	potassium chloride
Klonopin	clonazepam
Naprosyn	naproxen
Coumadin Sodium	warfarin sodium
Desyrel	trazodone hydrochloride
Cipro	ciprofloxacin hydrochloride
Flonase	fluticasone propionate
Flexeril	cyclobenzaprine hydrochloride
Calan, Isoptin	verapamil
Vasotec	enalapril maleate
Ismo, Imdur	isosorbide mononitrate
Levaquin	levofloxacin
Valium	diazepam
Glucotrol XL	glipizide
Panwarfin	warfarin sodium
Plavix	clopidogrel bisulfate

Trade Name	Generic Name
Diflucan	fluconazole
Serevent Diskus	salmeterol/xinafoate
Protonix	pantoprazole sodium
Diovan	valsartan
Micronase	glyburide
Altace	ramipril
Allopurinol Zyloprim	allopurinol
Estrogel	estradiol
Avandia	rosiglitazone maleate
Actos	pioglitazone hydrochloride
Lotensin	benazepril hydrochloride
Clarinex	desloratadine
Depo-Provera C-150, Provera	medroxyprogesterone acetate
Roxicodone	oxycodone hydrochloride
Vibramycin	doxycycline hyclate
Lanoxin	digoxin
Cozaar	losartan potassium
Nasonex	mometasone furoate
Cardizem	diltiazem hydrochloride
Catapres	clonidine hydrochloride
Digitek	digoxin
Medrol	methylprednisolone
Evista	raloxifene hydrochloride
Folvite	folic acid
Glucophage XR	metformin hydrochloride
Penicillin VK	penicillin V potassium
Risperdal	risperidone
Septra	trimethoprim sulfamethoxazole
Boniva	ibandronate sodium
Aciphex	rabeprazole sodium
Zyprexa	olanzapine
Crestor	rosuvastatin

Appendix B

The Most Common Poisonous Substances and Their Antidotes

Drug	Antidote
Acetaminophen	Acetylcysteine
Anticholinesterases (cholinergics)	Atropine, pralidoxime
Antidepressants (monoamine oxidase inhibitors and tyramine-containing foods)	Phentolamine
Benzodiazepines	Flumazenil
Cyanide	Amyl nitrite, sodium nitrite, sodium thiosulfate
Digoxin (digitoxin)	Digoxin immune Fab (Digibind)
Fluorouracil (5-FU)	Leucovorin calcium
Heparin	Protamine sulfate
Ifosfamide	Mesna
Iron	Deferoxamine
Lead	Edentate calcium disodium, dimercaprol, succimer
Methotrexate	Leucovorin calcium
Opioid analgesics, heroin	Nalmefene, naloxone
Thrombolytic agents	Aminocaproic acid (Amicar)
Tricyclic antidepressants	Physostigmine
Warfarin (Coumadin)	Phytonadione (vitamin K)

Appendix C

Common Sound-Alike Drug Names

The following is a list of common sound-alike drug names. Trade names are capitalized. In parentheses next to each drug name is the pharmacologic classification or use of the drug.

Accupril (ACE inhibitor)	Accutane (anti-acne drug)
Aciphex (proton pump inhibitor)	Accupril (ACE inhibitor)
Actos (oral hypoglycemic)	Actonel (bone growth regulator)
albuterol (sympathomimetic)	atenolol (beta-blocker)
Aldomet (antihypertensive)	Aldoril (antihypertensive)
allopurinol (antigout drug)	Apresoline (antihypertensive)
alprazolam (antianxiety agent)	lorazepam (antianxiety agent)
Ambien (sedative-hypnotic)	Amen (progestin)
amiodarone (antiarrhythmic)	amrinone (inotropic agent)
amitriptyline (antidepressant)	nortriptyline (antidepressant)
Apresazide (antihypertensive)	Apresoline (antihypertensive)
Aripiprazole (antipsychotic)	Lansoprazole (proton pump inhibitor)
Artane (cholinergic-blocking agent)	Altace (ACE inhibitor)
Atarax (antianxiety agent)	Ativan (antianxiety agent)
atenolol (beta-blocker)	timolol (beta-blocker)
Atrovent (cholinergic blocker)	Alupent (sympathomimetic)
Bacitracin (antibacterial)	Bactroban (anti-infective, topical)
Brevital (barbiturate)	Brevibloc (beta-blocker)
calciferol (vitamin D)	calcitriol (vitamin D)
carboplatin (antineoplastic agent)	cisplatin (antineoplastic agent)
Cardene (calcium channel blocker)	Cardizem (calcium channel blocker)
Cardura (antihypertensive)	Ridaura (gold-containing anti-inflammatory agent)
Cataflam (NSAID)	Catapres (antihypertensive)
cefuroxime (cephalosporin)	deferoxamine (iron chelator)
Celebrex (NSAID)	Cerebyx (anticonvulsant)
chlorpromazine (antipsychotic)	chlorpropamide (oral antidiabetic)
Clinoril (NSAID)	Clozaril (antipsychotic)
clomipramine (antidepressant)	clomiphene (ovarian stimulant)
clonidine (antihypertensive)	Klonopin (anticonvulsant)
Combivir (combination drug to treat AIDS)	Combivent (combination drug for COPD)
Cozaar (antihypertensive)	Zocor (antihyperlipidemic)

(continued)

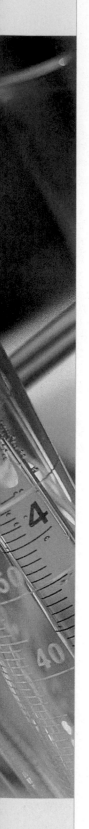

cyclosporine (immunosuppressant)   cycloserine (antineoplastic)

Cytovene (antiviral drug)   Cytosar (antineoplastic)

Cytoxan (antineoplastic)   Cytotec (prostaglandin derivative)

Dantrium (skeletal muscle relaxant)   danazol (gonadotropin inhibitor)

Darvocet-N (analgesic)   Darvon-N (analgesic)

daunorubicin (antineoplastic)   doxorubicin (antineoplastic)

desipramine (antidepressant)   diphenhydramine (antihistamine)

DiaBeta (oral hypoglycemic)   Zebeta (beta-blocker)

digitoxin (cardiac glycoside)   digoxin (cardiac glycoside)

diphenhydramine (antihistamine)   dimenhydrinate (antihistamine)

dopamine (sympathomimetic)   dobutamine (sympathomimetic)

Edecrin (diuretic)   Eulexin (antineoplastic)

enalapril (ACE inhibitor)   Eldepryl (anti-Parkinson agent)

Eryc (erythromycin base)   Ery-Tab (erythromycin base)

etidronate (bone-growth regulator)   etretinate (antipsoriatic)

etomidate (general anesthetic)   etidronate (bone-growth regulator)

E-Vista (antihistamine)   Evista (estrogen-receptor modulator)

Fioricet (analgesic)   Fiorinal (analgesic)

Flomax (alpha-adrenergic blocker)   Volmax (sympathomimetic)

flurbiprofen (NSAID)   fenoprofen (NSAID)

folinic acid (leucovorin calcium)   folic acid (vitamin B complex)

Gantrisin (sulfonamide)   Gantanol (sulfonamide)

glipizide (oral hypoglycemic)   glyburide (oral hypoglycemic)

glyburide (oral hypoglycemic)   Glucotrol (oral hypoglycemic)

Hycodan (cough preparation)   Hycomine (cough preparation)

hydralazine (antihypertensive)   hydroxyzine (antianxiety agent)

hydrocodone (narcotic analgesic)   hydrocortisone (corticosteroid)

Hydrogesic (analgesic combination)   hydroxyzine (antihistamine)

hydromorphone (narcotic analgesic)   morphine (narcotic analgesic)

Hydropres (antihypertensive)   Diupres (antihypertensive)

Hytone (topical corticosteroid)   Vytone (topical corticosteroid)

imipramine (antidepressant)   Norpramin (antidepressant)

Inderal (beta-blocker)   Inderide (antihypertensive)

Indocin (NSAID)   Minocin (antibiotic)

K-Phos Neutral (phosphorus-potassium   Neutra-Phos-K (phosphorus-potassium
   replenisher)   replenisher)

Lamictal (anticonvulsant)   Lamisil (antifungal)

Lamisil (antiviral)   Ludiomil (adrenergic blocker)

Lanoxin (cardiac glycoside)   Lasix (diuretic)

Lantus (insulin glargine)   Lente insulin (insulin zinc suspension)

Lioresal (muscle relaxant)   ·   lisinopril (ACE inhibitor)

Lithostat (lithium carbonate)   Lithobid (lithium carbonate)

Lithotabs (lithium carbonate)   Lithobid (lithium carbonate)

Lodine (NSAID)   codeine (narcotic analgesic)

Lopid (antihyperlipidemic)   Lorabid (beta-lactam antibiotic)

lovastatin (antihyperlipidemic)   Lotensin (ACE inhibitor)

Ludiomil (adrenergic blocker)   Lomotil (antidiarrheal)

Medrol (corticosteroid)   Haldol (antipsychotic)

metolazone (thiazide diuretic)   methotrexate (antineoplastic)

metoprolol (adrenergic blocker)   misoprostol (prostaglandin derivative)

Monopril (ACE inhibitor)   minoxidil (antihypertensive)

nicardipine (calcium channel blocker)   nifedipine (calcium channel blocker)

Norlutate (progestin)   Norlutin (progestin)

Noroxin (fluoroquinolone antibiotic)   Neurontin (anticonvulsant)

Norvir (antiviral)   Retrovir (antiviral)

Ocufen (NSAID)   Ocuflox (fluoroquinolone antibiotic)

Orinase (oral hypoglycemic)   Ornade (upper respiratory product)

Percocet (narcotic analgesic)   Percodan (narcotic analgesic)

paroxetine (antidepressant)   paclitaxel (antineoplastic)

Paxil (antidepressant)   paclitaxel (antineoplastic)

penicillamine (heavy metal antagonist)   penicillin (antibiotic)

pindolol (beta-blocker)   Parlodel (inhibitor of prolactin secretion)

Platinol (antineoplastic)   Paraplatin (antineoplastic)

Pravachol (antihyperlipidemic)   Prevacid (gastrointestinal drug)

prednisolone (corticosteroid)   prednisone (corticosteroid)

Prilosec (gastric acid inhibitor)   Prozac (antidepressant)

Prinivil (ACE inhibitor)   Proventil (sympathomimetic)

Procanbid (antidysrhythmic)   Procan SR (antidysrhythmic)

quinine (antimalarial)   quinidine (antiarrhythmic)

Regroton (antihypertensive)   Hygroton (diuretic)

Topamax (anticonvulsant)   Toprol-XL (antihypertensive)

tizanidine (skeletal muscle relaxant)   tiagabine (anticonvulsant)

tramadol (analgesic)   trazodone (prostaglandin)

Zantac (H_2-receptor antagonist)   Xanax (sedative-hypnotic)

Zantac (H_2-receptor antagonist)   Zyrtec (antihistamine)

Zocor (HMG-CoA reductase inhibitor)   Zyrtec (antihistamine)

Appendix D

Immunization Schedule

Table 1 ■ Childhood Immunization Schedule

DEPARTMENT OF HEALTH AND HUMAN SERVICES • CENTERS FOR DISEASE CONTROL AND PREVENTION

Recommended Childhood and Adolescent Immunization Schedule UNITED STATES • 2006

Vaccine ▼ / Age ▶	Birth	1 month	2 months	4 months	6 months	12 months	15 months	18 months	24 months	4–6 years	11–12 years	13–14 years	15 years	16–18 years
Hepatitis B[1]	HepB	HepB		HepB[1]		HepB					HepB Series			
Diphtheria, Tetanus, Pertussis[2]			DTaP	DTaP	DTaP		DTaP			DTaP	Tdap	Tdap		
Hemophilus influenzae type b[3]			Hib	Hib	Hib[3]	Hib								
Inactivated Poliovirus			IPV	IPV		IPV				IPV				
Measles, Mumps, Rubella[4]						MMR				MMR		MMR		
Varicella[5]						Varicella					Varicella			
Meningococcal[6]						Vaccines within broken line are for selected populations			MPSV4		MCV4		MCV4 / MCV4	
Pneumococcal[7]			PCV	PCV	PCV	PCV				PCV	PPV			
Influenza[8]					Influenza (Yearly)					Influenza (Yearly)				
Hepatitis A[9]										HepA Series				

This schedule indicates the recommended ages for routine administration of currently licensed childhood vaccines, as of December 1, 2005, for children through age 18 years. Any dose not administered at the recommended age should be administered at any subsequent visit when indicated and feasible. ▮ Indicates age groups that warrant special effort to administer those vaccines not previously administered. Additional vaccines may be licensed and recommended during the year. Licensed combination vaccines may be used whenever any components of the combination are indicated and other components of the vaccine are not contraindicated and if approved by the Food and Drug Administration for that dose of the series. Providers should consult the respective ACIP statement for detailed recommendations. Clinically significant adverse events that follow immunization should be reported to the Vaccine Adverse Event Reporting System (VAERS). Guidance about how to obtain and complete a VAERS form is available at www.vaers.hhs.gov or by telephone, 800-822-7967.

▮ Range of recommended ages ▮ Catch-up immunization ▮ 11–12 year old assessment

Courtesy of Centers for Disease Control and Prevention, National Immunization Program http://www.cdc.gov/Nip/. These recommendations must be read along with the footnotes.

1. **Hepatitis B vaccine (HepB).** *AT BIRTH:* **All newborns** should receive monovalent HepB soon after birth and before hospital discharge. **Infants born to mothers who are HBsAg-positive** should receive HepB and 0.5 mL of hepatitis B immune globulin (HBIG) within 12 hours of birth. **Infants born to mothers whose HBsAg status is unknown** should receive HepB within 12 hours of birth. The mother should have blood drawn as soon as possible to determine her HBsAg status; if HBsAg-positive, the infant should receive HBIG as soon as possible (no later than age 1 week). **For infants born to HBsAg-negative mothers,** the birth dose can be delayed in rare circumstances but only if a physician's order to withhold the vaccine and a copy of the mother's original HBsAg-negative laboratory report are documented in the infant's medical record. *FOLLOWING THE BIRTHDOSE:* The HepB series should be completed with either monovalent HepB or a combination vaccine containing HepB. The second dose should be administered at age 1–2 months. The final dose should be administered at age ≥24 weeks. It is permissible to administer 4 doses of HepB (e.g., when combination vaccines are given after the birth dose); however, if monovalent HepB is used, a dose at age 4 months is not needed. **Infants born to HbsAg-positive mothers** should be tested for HBsAg and antibody to HBsAg after completion of the HepB series, at age 9–18 months (generally at the next well-child visit after completion of the vaccine series).

2. **Diphtheria and tetanus toxoids and acellular pertussis vaccine (DTaP).** The fourth dose of DTaP may be administered as early as age 12 months, provided 6 months have elapsed since the third dose and the child is unlikely to return at age 15–18 months. The final dose in the series should be given at age ≥4 years.

   Tetanus and diphtheria toxoids and acellular pertussis vaccine (Tdap—adolescent preparation) is recommended at age 11–12 years for those who have completed the recommended childhood DTP/DTaP vaccination series and have not received a Td booster dose. Adolescents 13–18 years who missed the 11–12-year Td/Tdap booster dose should also receive a single dose of Tdap if they have completed the recommended childhood DTP/DTaP vaccination series. Subsequent **tetanus and diphtheria toxoids (Td)** are recommended every 10 years.

3. *Hemophilus influenzae* **type b conjugate vaccine (Hib).** Three Hib conjugate vaccines are licensed for infant use. If PRP-OMP (PedvaxHIB® or ComVax® [Merck]) is administered at ages 2 and 4 months, a dose at age 6 months is not required. DTaP/Hib combination products should not be used for primary immunization in infants at ages 2, 4 or 6 months but can be used as boosters after any Hib vaccine. The final dose in the series should be administered at age ≥12 months.

4. **Measles, mumps, and rubella vaccine (MMR).** The second dose of MMR is recommended routinely at age 4–6 years but may be administered during any visit, provided at least 4 weeks have elapsed since the first dose and both doses are administered beginning at or after age 12 months. Those who have not previously received the second dose should complete the schedule by age 11–12 years.

5. **Varicella vaccine.** Varicella vaccine is recommended at any visit at or after age 12 months for susceptible children (i.e., those who lack a reliable history of chickenpox). Susceptible persons aged ≥13 years should receive 2 doses administered at least 4 weeks apart.

6. **Meningococcal vaccine (MCV4).** Meningococcal conjugate vaccine (MCV4) should be given to all children at the 11–12 year old visit as well as to unvaccinated adolescents at high school entry (15 years of age). Other adolescents who wish to decrease their risk for meningococcal disease may also be vaccinated. All college freshmen living in dormitories should also be vaccinated, preferably with MCV4, although **meningococcal polysaccharide vaccine (MPSV4)** is an acceptable alternative. Vaccination against invasive meningococcal disease is recommended for children and adolescents aged ≥2 years with terminal complement deficiencies or anatomic or functional asplenia and certain other high risk groups (see *MMWR* 2005;54 [RR-7]:1-21); use MPSV4 for children aged 2–10 years and MCV4 for older children, although MPSV4 is an acceptable alternative.

7. **Pneumococcal vaccine.** The heptavalent **pneumococcal conjugate vaccine (PCV)** is recommended for all children aged 2–23 months and for certain children aged 24–59 months. The final dose in the series should be given at age ≥12 months. **Pneumococcal polysaccharide vaccine (PPV)** is recommended in addition to PCV for certain high-risk groups. See *MMWR* 2000; 49(RR-9):1-35.

8. **Influenza vaccine.** Influenza vaccine is recommended annually for children aged ≥6 months with certain risk factors (including, but not limited to, asthma, cardiac disease, sickle cell disease, human immunodeficiency virus [HIV], diabetes, and conditions that can compromise respiratory function or handling of respiratory secretions or that can increase the risk for aspiration), healthcare workers, and other persons (including household members) in close contact with persons in groups at high risk (see *MMWR* 2005;54[RR-8]:1-55). In addition, healthy children aged 6–23 months and close contacts of healthy children aged 0–5 months are recommended to receive influenza vaccine because children in this age group are at substantially increased risk for influenza-related hospitalizations. For healthy persons aged 5–49 years, the intranasally administered, live, attenuated influenza vaccine (LAIV) is an acceptable alternative to the intramuscular trivalent inactivated influenza vaccine (TIV). See *MMWR* 2005;54(RR-8):1-55. Children receiving TIV should be administered a dosage appropriate for their age (0.25 mL if aged 6–35 months or 0.5 mL if aged ≥3 years). Children aged ≤8 years who are receiving influenza vaccine for the first time should receive 2 doses (separated by at least 4 weeks for TIV and at least 6 weeks for LAIV).

9. **Hepatitis A vaccine (HepA).** HepA is recommended for all children at 1 year of age (i.e.,12–23 months). The 2 doses in the series should be administered at least 6 months apart. States, counties, and communities with existing HepA vaccination programs for children 2–18 years of age are encouraged to maintain these programs. In these areas, new efforts focused on routine vaccination of 1-year-old children should enhance, not replace, ongoing programs directed at a broader population of children. HepA is also recommended for certain high risk groups (see *MMWR* 1999; 48[RR-12]1-37).

The Childhood and Adolescent Immunization Schedule is approved by:
Advisory Committee on Immunization Practices www.cdc.gov/nip/acip • American Academy of Pediatrics www.aap.org • American Academy of Family Physicians www.aafp.org

Table 2 ■ Adult Immunization Schedule

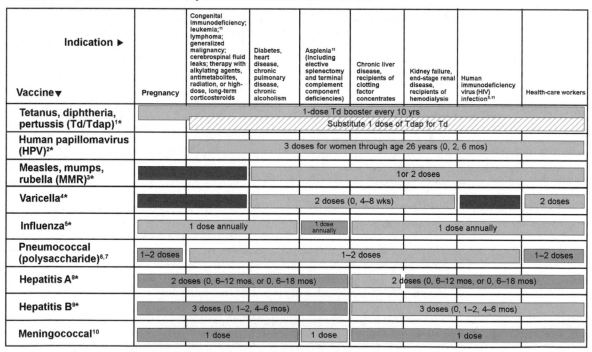

Recommended Adult Immunization Schedule
United States, October 2006–September 2007

Recommended adult immunization schedule, by vaccine and age group

Vaccine ▼ / Age group (yrs) ►	19–49 years	50–64 years	≥65 years
Tetanus, diphtheria, pertussis (Td/Tdap)[1]*	1-dose Td booster every 10 yrs / Substitute 1 dose of Tdap for Td		
Human papillomavirus (HPV)[2]*	3 doses (females)		
Measles, mumps, rubella (MMR)[3]*	1 or 2 doses	1 dose	
Varicella[4]*	2 doses (0, 4–8 wks)	2 doses (0, 4–8 wks)	
Influenza[5]*	1 dose annually	1 dose annually	
Pneumococcal (polysaccharide)[6,7]	1–2 doses		1 dose
Hepatitis A[8]*	2 doses (0, 6–12 mos, or 0, 6–18 mos)		
Hepatitis B[9]*	3 doses (0, 1–2, 4–6 mos)		
Meningococcal[10]	1 or more doses		

Recommended adult immunization schedule, by vaccine and medical and other indications

Vaccine ▼ / Indication ►	Pregnancy	Congenital immunodeficiency; leukemia;[11] lymphoma; generalized malignancy; cerebrospinal fluid leaks; therapy with alkylating agents, antimetabolites, radiation, or high-dose, long-term corticosteroids	Diabetes, heart disease, chronic pulmonary disease, chronic alcoholism	Asplenia[11] (including elective splenectomy and terminal complement component deficiencies)	Chronic liver disease, recipients of clotting factor concentrates	Kidney failure, end-stage renal disease, recipients of hemodialysis	Human immunodeficiency virus (HIV) infection[3,11]	Health-care workers
Tetanus, diphtheria, pertussis (Td/Tdap)[1]*	1-dose Td booster every 10 yrs / Substitute 1 dose of Tdap for Td							
Human papillomavirus (HPV)[2]*	3 doses for women through age 26 years (0, 2, 6 mos)							
Measles, mumps, rubella (MMR)[3]*	(Contraindicated)	1 or 2 doses						
Varicella[4]*	(Contraindicated)	2 doses (0, 4–8 wks)					(Contraindicated)	2 doses
Influenza[5]*	1 dose annually		1 dose annually	1 dose annually				
Pneumococcal (polysaccharide)[6,7]	1–2 doses	1–2 doses						1–2 doses
Hepatitis A[8]*	2 doses (0, 6–12 mos, or 0, 6–18 mos)			2 doses (0, 6–12 mos, or 0, 6–18 mos)				
Hepatitis B[9]*	3 doses (0, 1–2, 4–6 mos)			3 doses (0, 1–2, 4–6 mos)				
Meningococcal[10]	1 dose		1 dose	1 dose				

* Covered by the Vaccine Injury Compensation Program

These recommendations must be read along with the footnotes, which can be found in Appendix D.

☐ For all persons in this category who meet the age requirements and who lack evidence of immunity (e.g., lack documentation of vaccination or have no evidence of prior infection)

☐ Recommended if some other risk factor is present (e.g., on the basis of medical, occupational, lifestyle, or other indications)

■ Contraindicated

Courtesy of Centers for Disease Control and Prevention, National Immunization Program http://www.cdc.gov/Nip/

1. **Tetanus, diphtheria, and acellular pertussis (Td/Tdap) vaccination.** Adults with uncertain histories of a complete primary vaccination series with diphtheria and tetanus toxoid–containing vaccines should begin or complete a primary vaccination series. A primary series for adults is 3 doses; administer the first 2 doses at least 4 weeks apart and the third dose 6–12 months after the second. Administer a booster dose to adults who have completed a primary series and if the last vaccination was received ≥10 years previously. Tdap or tetanus and diphtheria (Td) vaccine may be used; Tdap should replace a single dose of Td for adults aged <65 years who have not previously received a dose of Tdap (either in the primary series, as a booster, or for wound management). Only one of two Tdap products (Adacel® [sanofi pasteur, Swiftwater, Pennsylvania]) is licensed for use in adults. If the person is pregnant and received the last Td vaccination ≥10 years previously, administer Td during the second or third trimester; if the person received the last Td vaccination in <10 years, administer Tdap during the immediate postpartum period. A onetime administration of 1-dose of Tdap with an interval as short as 2 years from a previous Td vaccination is recommended for postpartum women, close contacts of infants aged <12 months, and all health-care workers with direct patient contact. In certain situations, Td can be deferred during pregnancy and Tdap substituted in the immediate postpartum period, or Tdap can be given instead of Td to a pregnant woman after an informed discussion with the woman (see http://www.cdc.gov/nip/publications/acip-list.htm). Consult the ACIP statement for recommendations for administering Td as prophylaxis in wound management (http://www.cdc.gov/mmwr/preview/mmwrhtml/00041 645.htm).

2. **Human Papillomavirus (HPV) vaccination.** HPV vaccination is recommended for all women aged ≤26 years who have not completed the vaccine series. Ideally, vaccine should be administered before potential exposure to HPV through sexual activity; however, women who are sexually active should still be vaccinated. Sexually active women who have not been infected with any of the HPV vaccine types receive the full benefit of the vaccination. Vaccination is less beneficial for women who have already been infected with one or more of the four HPV vaccine types. A complete series consists of 3 doses. The second dose should be administered 2 months after the first dose; the third dose should be administered 6 months after the first dose. Vaccination is not recommended during pregnancy. If a woman is found to be pregnant after initiating the vaccination series, the remainder of the 3-dose regimen should be delayed until after completion of the pregnancy.

3. **Measles, Mumps, Rubella (MMR) vaccination.** *Measles component:* adults born before 1957 can be considered immune to measles. Adults born during or after 1957 should receive ≥1 dose of MMR unless they have a medical contraindication, documentation of > 1 dose, history of measles based on health-care provider diagnosis, or laboratory evidence of immunity. A second dose of MMR is recommended for adults who 1) have been recently exposed to measles or in an outbreak setting; 2) were previously vaccinated with killed measles vaccine; 3) have been vaccinated with an unknown type of measles vaccine during 1963–1967; 4) are students in postsecondary educational institutions; 5) work in a health-care facility, or 6) plan to travel internationally. Withhold MMR or other measles-containing vaccines from HIV-infected persons with severe immunosuppression. *Mumps component:* adults born before 1957 can generally be considered immune to mumps. Adults born during or after 1957 should receive 1 dose of MMR unless they have a medical contraindication, history of mumps based on health-care provider diagnosis, or laboratory evidence of immunity. A second dose of MMR is recommended for adults who 1) are in an age group that is affected during a mumps outbreak; 2) are students in postsecondary educational institutions; 3) work in a health care facility; or 4) plan to travel internationally. For unvaccinated health-care workers born before 1957 who do not have other evidence of mumps immunity, consider giving 1 dose on a routine basis and strongly consider giving a second dose during an outbreak. *Rubella component:* administer 1 dose of MMR vaccine to women whose rubella vaccination history is unreliable or who lack laboratory evidence of immunity. For women of childbearing age, regardless of birth year, routinely determine rubella immunity and counsel women regarding congenital rubella syndrome. Do not vaccinate women who are pregnant or who might become pregnant within 4 weeks of receiving vaccine. Women who do not have evidence of immunity should receive MMR vaccine upon completion or termination of pregnancy and before discharge from the health-care facility.

4. **Varicella vaccination.** All adults without evidence of immunity to varicella should receive 2 doses of varicella vaccine. Special consideration should be given to those who 1) have close contact with persons at high risk for severe disease (e.g., health-care workers and family contacts of immunocompromised persons) or 2) are at high risk for exposure or transmission (e.g., teachers of young children; child care employees; residents and staff members of institutional settings, including correctional institutions; college students; military personnel; adolescents and adults living in households with children; nonpregnant women of childbearing age; and international travelers). Evidence of immunity to varicella in adults includes any of the following: 1) documentation of 2 doses of varicella vaccine at least 4 weeks apart; 2) U.S.-born before 1980 (although for health-care workers and pregnant women, birth before 1980 should not be considered evidence of immunity); 3) history of varicella based on diagnosis or verification of varicella by a health-care provider (for a patient reporting a history of or presenting with an atypical case, a mild case, or both, health-care providers should seek either an epidemiologic link with a typical varicella case or evidence of laboratory confirmation, if it was performed at the time of acute disease); 4) history of herpes zoster based on health-care provider diagnosis; or 5) laboratory evidence of immunity or laboratory confirmation of disease. Do not vaccinate women who are pregnant or might become pregnant within 4 weeks of receiving the vaccine. Assess pregnant women for evidence of varicella immunity. Women who do not have evidence of immunity should receive dose 1 of varicella vaccine upon completion or termination of pregnancy and before discharge from the health-care facility. Dose 2 should be administered 4-8 weeks after dose 1.

5. **Influenza vaccination:** *Medical indications:* chronic disorders of the cardiovascular or pulmonary systems, including asthma; chronic metabolic diseases, including diabetes mellitus, renal dysfunction, hemoglobinopathies, or immunosuppression (including immunosuppression caused by medications or HIV); any condition that compromises respiratory function

or the handling of respiratory secretions or that can increase the risk of aspiration (e.g., cognitive dysfunction, spinal cord injury, or seizure disorder or other neuromuscular disorder); and pregnancy during the influenza season. No data exist on the risk for severe or complicated influenza disease among persons with asplenia; however, influenza is a risk factor for secondary bacterial infections that can cause severe disease among persons with asplenia. *Occupational indications:* health-care workers and employees of long-term–care and assisted living facilities. *Other indications:* residents of nursing homes and other long-term–care and assisted living facilities; persons likely to transmit influenza to persons at high risk (i.e., in-home household contacts and caregivers of children aged 0–59 months, or persons of all ages with high-risk conditions); and anyone who would like to be vaccinated. Healthy, nonpregnant persons aged 5–49 years without high-risk medical conditions who are not contacts of severely immunocompromised persons in special care units can receive either intranasally administered influenza vaccine (FluMist®) or inactivated vaccine. Other persons should receive the inactivated vaccine.

6. **Pneumococcal polysaccharide vaccination.** *Medical indications:* chronic disorders of the pulmonary system (excluding asthma); cardiovascular diseases; diabetes mellitus; chronic liver diseases, including liver disease as a result of alcohol abuse (e.g., cirrhosis); chronic renal failure or nephrotic syndrome; functional or anatomic asplenia (e.g., sickle cell disease or splenectomy [if elective splenectomy is planned, vaccinate at least 2 weeks before surgery]); immunosuppressive conditions (e.g., congenital immunodeficiency, HIV infection [vaccinate as close to diagnosis as possible when CD4 cell counts are highest], leukemia, lymphoma, multiple myeloma, Hodgkin disease, generalized malignancy, organ or bone marrow transplantation); chemotherapy with alkylating agents, antimetabolites, or high-dose, long-term corticosteroids; and cochlear implants. *Other indications:* Alaska Natives and certain American Indian populations and residents of nursing homes or other long-term–care facilities.

7. **Revaccination with pneumococcal polysaccharide vaccine.** One-time revaccination after 5 years for persons with chronic renal failure or nephrotic syndrome; functional or anatomic asplenia (e.g., sickle cell disease or splenectomy); immunosuppressive conditions (e.g., congenital immuno-deficiency, HIV infection, leukemia, lymphoma, multiple myeloma, Hodgkin disease, generalized malignancy, or organ or bone marrow transplantation); or chemotherapy with alkylating agents, antimetabolites, or high-dose, long-term corticosteroids. For persons aged ≥65 years, one-time revaccination if they were vaccinated 5 years previously and were aged <65 years at the time of primary vaccination.

8. **Hepatitis A vaccination.** *Medical indications:* persons with chronic liver disease and persons who receive clotting factor concentrates. *Behavioral indications:* men who have sex with men and persons who use illegal drugs. *Occupational indications:* persons working with hepatitis A virus (HAV)–infected primates or with HAV in a research laboratory setting. *Other indications:* persons traveling to or working in countries that have high or intermediate endemicity of hepatitis A (a list of countries is available at http://www.dc.gov/travel/diseases.htm) and any person who would like to obtain immunity. Current vaccines should be administered in a 2-dose schedule at either 0 and 6–12 months, or 0 and 6–18

months. If the combined hepatitis A and hepatitis B vaccine is used, administer 3 doses at 0, 1, and 6 months.

9. **Hepatitis B vaccination.** *Medical indications:* Persons with end-stage renal disease, including patients receiving hemodialysis; persons seeking evaluation or treatment for a sexually transmitted disease (STD); persons with HIV infection; persons with chronic liver disease; and persons who receive clotting factor concentrates. *Occupational indications:* health-care workers and public-safety workers who are exposed to blood or other potentially infectious body fluids. *Behavioral indications:* sexually active persons who are not in a long-term, mutually monogamous relationship (i.e., persons with >1 sex partner during the previous 6 months); current or recent injection-drug users; and men who have sex with men. *Other indications:* household contacts and sex partners of persons with chronic hepatitis B virus (HBV) infection; clients and staff members of institutions for persons with developmental disabilities; all clients of STD clinics; international travelers to countries with high or intermediate prevalence of chronic HBV infection (a list of countries is available at http://www.cdc.gov/travel/diseases.htm); and any adult seeking protection from HBV infection. Settings where hepatitis B vaccination is recommended for all adults: STD treatment facilities; HIV testing and treatment facilities; facilities providing drug-abuse treatment and prevention services; health-care settings providing services for injection-drug users or men who have sex with men; correctional facilities; end-stage renal disease programs and facilities for chronic hemodialysis patients; and institutions and nonresidential daycare facilities for persons with developmental disabilities. *Special formulation indications:* for adult patients receiving hemodialysis and other immunocompromised adults, 1 dose of 40 μg/mL (Recombivax HB®) or 2 doses of 20 μg/mL (Engerix-B®).

10. **Meningococcal vaccination.** *Medical indications:* adults with anatomic or functional asplenia, or terminal complement component deficiencies. *Other indications:* first-year college students living in dormitories; microbiologists who are routinely exposed to isolates of *Neisseria meningitidis;* military recruits; and persons who travel to or live in countries in which meningococcal disease is hyperendemic or epidemic (e.g., the "meningitis belt" of Sub-Saharan Africa during the dry season [December–June]), particularly if contact with local populations will be prolonged. Vaccination is required by the government of Saudi Arabia for all travelers to Mecca during the annual Hajj. Meningococcal conjugate vaccine is preferred for adults with any of the proceeding indications who are aged ≤55 years, although meningococcal polysaccharide vaccine (MPSV4) is an acceptable alternative. Revaccination after 5 years might be indicated for adults previously vaccinated with MPSV4 who remain at high risk for infection (e.g., persons residing in areas in which disease is epidemic).

11. **Selected conditions for which *Haemophilus influenzae* type b (Hib) vaccination may be used.** Hib conjugate vaccines are licensed for children aged 6 week–71 months. No efficacy data are available on which to base a recommendation concerning use of Hib vaccine for older children and adults with the chronic conditions associated with an increased risk for Hib disease. However, studies suggest good immunogenicity in patients who have sickle cell disease, leukemia, or HIV infection or have had splenectomies; administering vaccine to these patients is not contraindicated.

This schedule indicates the recommended age groups and medical indications for routine administration of currently licensed vaccines for persons aged >19 years, as of October 1, 2006. Licensed combination vaccines may be used whenever any components of the combination are indicated and when the vaccine's other components are not contraindicated. For detailed recommendations on all vaccines, including those used primarily for travelers or that are issued during the year, consult the manufacturers' package inserts and the complete statements from the Advisory Committee on Immunization Practices (http://www.cdc.gov/nip/publications/acip-list.htm).

Report all clinically significant postvaccination reactions to the Vaccine Adverse Event Reporting System (VAERS). Reporting forms and instructions on filing a VAERS report are available at http://www.vaers.hhs.gov or by telephone, 800-822-7967.

Information on how to file a Vaccine Injury Compensation Program claim is available at http://www.hrsa.gov/vaccinecompensation or by telephone, 800-338-2382.To file a claim for vaccine injury, contact the U.S. Court of Federal Claims, 717 Madison Place, N.W., Washington, DC. 20005; telephone, 202-357-6400.

Additional information about the vaccines in this schedule and contraindications for vaccination is also available at http://www.cdc.gov/nip or from the CDC-INFO Contact Center at 800-CDC-INFO (800-232-4636) in English and Spanish, 24 hours a day, 7 days a week.

**Approved by the Advisory Committee on Immunization Practices,
the American College of Obstetricians and Gynecologists, the American Academy of Family Physicians,
and the American College of Physicians**

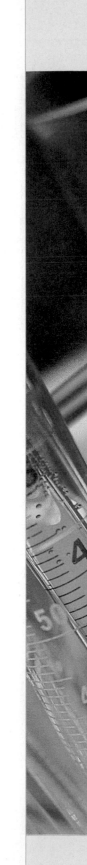

Appendix E

Answers to Apply Your Knowledge Exercises and Checkpoint Reviews

Chapter 1

APPLY YOUR KNOWLEDGE 1.1

Multiple Choice

1. c
2. a
3. b
4. b
5. c

Fill in the Blank

1. absorption, metabolism, reabsorption, excretion, and site of action
2. receptor
3. drug concentration
4. men; longer; body fat
5. detoxification; elimination

APPLY YOUR KNOWLEDGE 1.2

Multiple Choice

1. b
2. d
3. a
4. b
5. c

Fill in the Blank

1. absorption; distribution; metabolism; excretion
2. food; physiochemical; routes
3. excretion; kidneys
4. oxidation; reduction; hydrolysis; conjugation

APPLY YOUR KNOWLEDGE 1.3

Matching

1. a, d, f, g
2. h
3. b
4. e
5. c

Fill in the Blank

1. antibody-dependent
2. immediate hypersensitivity
3. complex-mediated
4. delayed hypersensitivity
5. life-threatening

Chapter 2

APPLY YOUR KNOWLEDGE 2.1

Fill in the Blank

1. Pure Food and Drug Act
2. interstate commerce; safe; effective
3. diethylene glycol; antifreeze
4. prescription
5. deformities; first

APPLY YOUR KNOWLEDGE 2.2

Multiple Choice

1. d
2. c
3. a
4. a
5. c

Fill in the Blank

1. Drug Abuse Control Amendment of 1965
2. designer drugs
3. analogue
4. Controlled Substance Act
5. I; V
6. II
7. III
8. V
9. monopoly
10. Prescription Drug Marketing Act of 1987

APPLY YOUR KNOWLEDGE 2.3

Fill in the Blank

1. Occupational Safety and Health Administration (OSHA)
2. Occupational Safety and Health Administration (OSHA)
3. Health Insurance Portability and Accountability Act (HIPAA)
4. protected
5. Drug Enforcement Administration (DEA); violence; coercion

Name That Acronym

1. Occupational Safety and Health Administration
2. Health Insurance Portability and Accountability Act
3. Food, Drug, and Cosmetic Act
4. Food and Drug Administration
5. Controlled Substances Act
6. Drug Enforcement Administration
7. over the counter
8. acquired immunodeficiency syndrome
9. Bureau of Narcotics and Dangerous Drugs
10. Omnibus Budget Reconciliation Act

APPLY YOUR KNOWLEDGE 2.4

Matching

1. f
2. e
3. a
4. b
5. c
6. d

Multiple Choice

1. b
2. a
3. c
4. d
5. a

Chapter 3

APPLY YOUR KNOWLEDGE 3.1

Fill in the Blank

1. central meaning
2. o
3. beginning; root
4. o
5. root

Matching

1. c
2. d
3. b
4. a
5. f
6. e

APPLY YOUR KNOWLEDGE 3.2

Multiple Choice

1. c
2. a
3. c
4. b
5. b

Fill in the Blank

1. NPO; Tx
2. write on the label, times, immediately, four times a day
3. PULV
4. twice a day
5. microgram

APPLY YOUR KNOWLEDGE 3.3

Fill in the Blank

1. plant, animal, mineral, synthetic, engineering
2. brand; trade
3. insulin; pepsin
4. generic
5. bitter

Multiple Choice

1. c
2. d
3. c
4. b
5. a

APPLY YOUR KNOWLEDGE 3.4

Matching

1. d
2. e
3. b
4. c
5. a

Multiple Choice

1. b
2. a
3. c
4. d
5. b

APPLY YOUR KNOWLEDGE 3.5

Fill in the Blank

1. prescription

2. properly written, dated, signed
3. drug chart
4. separate IV orders chart
5. physician

Matching

1. c
2. d
3. e
4. a
5. b

Chapter 4

APPLY YOUR KNOWLEDGE 4.1

Fill in the Blank

1. three; dose
2. stat
3. date; time
4. patient information
5. route of administration

Multiple Choice

1. d
2. b
3. a
4. d
5. c

APPLY YOUR KNOWLEDGE 4.2

Fill in the Blank

1. formulation; manufacturing
2. 44,000
3. dosage
4. signature
5. (a) prescribing; ordering (b) dispensed (c) administered; monitored

Matching

1. c
2. e
3. a
4. d
5. b

APPLY YOUR KNOWLEDGE 4.3

Multiple Choice

1. d
2. a
3. c
4. d
5. a

Matching

1. e
2. c
3. d
4. a
5. b

APPLY YOUR KNOWLEDGE 4.4

Multiple Choice

1. d
2. b
3. c
4. c
5. c
6. d

Matching

1. c
2. e
3. a
4. b
5. d

APPLY YOUR KNOWLEDGE 4.5

Fill in the Blank

1. transdermal
2. gelatin, cocoa butter
3. atomization; aerosolization
4. toxicity
5. decongestants
6. transdermal
7. inhalation
8. nebulizer

Matching

1. b
2. c
3. a
4. d
5. e

CHECKPOINT REVIEW 1

1. d
2. b
3. c
4. a
5. d
6. c
7. a
8. b

9. c
10. c
11. b
12. a
13. a
14. b
15. b
16. d
17. d
18. c
19. b
20. c
21. d
22. a
23. c
24. b
25. b
26. d
27. a
28. c
29. a
30. c
31. b
32. c
33. b
34. d
35. d
36. b
37. d
38. a
39. b
40. b
41. d
42. c
43. b
44. b
45. b
46. e
47. c
48. a
49. d
50. b
51. e
52. d
53. b
54. c
55. a

Case Studies

56. No, the father would not be allowed by law (the Privacy Act) to have access to the medical records because the child is a minor and the father doesn't have custody.

57. The pharmacy technician should look for the Comprehensive Drug Abuse Prevention and Control Act of 1970.

Chapter 5

APPLY YOUR KNOWLEDGE 5.1

Do the Math

1. 8
2. 25
3. 15
4. 6
5. 21
6. XIV
7. XV
8. XVI
9. XXVII
10. VII
11. XI
12. VI
13. X

Matching

1. b
2. b
3. a
4. a
5. b

APPLY YOUR KNOWLEDGE 5.2

Fill in the Blank

1. smaller
2. top number
3. combined
4. smaller; larger
5. invert; multiply
6. 35
7. 100
8. 88
9. 60
10. numerator

Multiple Choice

1. b
2. a
3. d

APPLY YOUR KNOWLEDGE 5.3

Calculation of Decimals

1. 32.95
2. 57.96
3. 13.506
4. 7.269
5. 28.212
6. $7.15
7. $15.59

8. 9.569
9. 21.6
10. 324.03
11. 0.15
12. 403.144
13. 75,100.75
14. 348.58
15. 0.016
16. 300
17. 5.45
18. 3.74
19. 4,120
20. 400

APPLY YOUR KNOWLEDGE 5.4

Fill in the Blank

1. colon; :
2. solution
3. 100 units:1 mL
4. unit

Do the Math

1. 1/3
2. 3/4
3. 1/50
4. 3/5
5. 4/7
6. 1/2

APPLY YOUR KNOWLEDGE 5.5

Do the Math

1. 16
2. 9
3. 65
4. 8
5. 4
6. 35
7. 20
8. 100

APPLY YOUR KNOWLEDGE 5.6

Fill in the Blank

1. whole number
2. hundredths
3. fraction
4. denominator
5. percent; decimal

Do the Math

1. 0.02
2. 0.18

3. 0.4
4. 1.06
5. 0.008
6. 0.245
7. 1.5075
8. 0.045
9. 8%
10. 3,200%
11. 44%
12. 50%
13. 1.9%
14. 570%
15. 1,300%
16. 99%

Chapter 6

APPLY YOUR KNOWLEDGE 6.1

Fill in the Blank

1. 25 g
2. 8 mL
3. 55/100 mg
4. 100 mcg
5. 7-2/10 mcg
6. 16 L
7. 2,000 mL
8. 4 m
9. 19 mm
10. 3-1/2 cm

Multiple Choice

1. c
2. b
3. b
4. c
5. b

APPLY YOUR KNOWLEDGE 6.2

Fill in the Blank

1. ʒ*
2. gr
3. dr or ʒ*
4. qt
5. pt
6. m or ♏*

*Although students should be aware of these abbreviations for apothecary measurements, they should not use these abbreviations in clinical practice. Their use has been linked to medication errors.

APPLY YOUR KNOWLEDGE 6.3

Fill in the Blank

1. 4
2. 15
3. 1
4. 6
5. 450 drops
6. 2
7. 4
8. 2
9. length
10. volume
11. weight
12. 24
13. 3

APPLY YOUR KNOWLEDGE 6.4

1. 160
2. 8
3. 0.625
4. 0.375
5. 120
6. 255
7. 15
8. 2
9. 5
10. 1/2
11. 80
12. 8
13. 0.16
14. 0.19
15. 0.09
16. 240
17. 90
18. 450
19. 2.5
20. 1/2
21. 0.25

APPLY YOUR KNOWLEDGE 6.5

1. 55.4°F
2. 69.8°F
3. 97.2°F
4. 113°F
5. 156.6°F
6. 206.6°F
7. 211.82°F
8. 222.8°F
9. −10.9°C
10. −3.1°C
11. 10.2°C
12. 22.4°C
13. 25.8°C
14. −23.1°C

Chapter 7

APPLY YOUR KNOWLEDGE 7.1

Matching

1. d
2. e
3. a
4. f
5. c
6. b

Drug Dosage Calculations

1. 1/2 tablet
2. 3 mL
3. 2 tablets
4. 4 mL

APPLY YOUR KNOWLEDGE 7.2

Labeling

1. 6.125
2. 3
3. 3
4. 2
5. 4

Drug Dosage Calculation

1. 2 capsules
2. 2 tablets
3. 10 mL
4. 12.5 mL or 2-1/2 tsp
5. 1 tablet

APPLY YOUR KNOWLEDGE 7.3

Labeling

1. 62.5
2. 1–4 tsp 3–4 times daily
3. 19,200
4. 12.5
5. 15
6. 118.5

Drug Dosage Calculations

1. 0.16 mL
2. 1.5 mL
3. 0.5 mL
4. 2 mL
5. 0.5 mL
6. 1.2 mL
7. 2 mL

APPLY YOUR KNOWLEDGE 7.4

Multiple Choice

1. c
2. b
3. a
4. d
5. a

Do the Math

1. 25 kg
2. 5 kg
3. 71.3 kg
4. 8 kg
5. 95 kg
6. 12.2 kg
7. 42.2 kg
8. 61.3 kg

CHECKPOINT REVIEW 2

1. 2-5/8, 4/4, 9/7
2. 1/100, 1/160
3. 1/3, 1/12
4. 1-1/16, 1-2/9, 7-7/9
5. 3/4
6. 1
7. 3-1/3
8. 2-3/4
9. 1-1/3
10. 13/2
11. 47/6
12. 6/5
13. 32/3
14. 411/4
15. 1/1,000
16. 1/10
17. 3/10
18. 5/9
19. 1-5/12
20. 1-1/24
21. 1-1/13
22. 53/132
23. 5-118/119
24. 1-7/15
25. 1/40
26. 3/100
27. 1/2
28. 35/48
29. 3/32
30. 254-1/16
31. 1/30
32. 3/14
33. 3-1/13
34. 1/3
35. volume
36. 1/1,000

37. 1,000
38. 1
39. 1,000
40. milligram
41. kilogram
42. weight
43. 4 kg
44. 0.6 g
45. 2.5 mm
46. 20 mg
47. gram(s)
48. millimeter(s)
49. centimeter(s)
50. kilogram(s)
51. microgram(s)
52. milliliter(s)
53. quart(s)
54. grain(s)
55. minim(s)
56. dram(s)
57. 1
58. 32
59. gr x
60. 2 pt
61. 1/2 oz
62. 16 pt
63. 4 oz
62. gr iii
65. 3 T
66. 10 t
67. 6 gtt
68. 25 mEq
69. 2
70. 1
71. 8
72. 3
73. 20 milliequivalents
74. 15 pounds
75. 50 drops
76. 8 tablespoons
77. 1/2
78. 2
79. 2
80. 1
81. 4
82. 2.5
83. 2
84. 5
85. 1
86. 2
87. 15
88. 1-1/2
89. 7.5
90. 3
91. 2
92. 7.5
93. 1/2

94. 1/2
95. 3
96. 1
97. 1
98. 1.5
99. 2.5
100. 0.7
101. 6
102. desired dose
103. dosage unit
104. dose on hand
105. amount to administer
106. tuberculin syringe
107. 3.0
108. 70/30
109. USP
110. continuous
111. nomogram
112. Young's; Fried's
113. weight
114. Young's
115. Fried's

Chapter 8

APPLY YOUR KNOWLEDGE 8.1

Matching

1. c
2. d
3. a
4. e
5. b

Fill in the Blank

1. solid; liquid
2. animal muscles; organs
3. weight loss; protein loss; fatigue
4. simple sugars; complex carbohydrates
5. soluble; insoluble

APPLY YOUR KNOWLEDGE 8.2

Fill in the Blank

1. vitamin C; vitamin B complex
2. beri-beri
3. vitamin B_3; niacin
4. megaloblastic
5. vitamin C
6. blindness; burning and itching
7. vitamin K
8. vitamin C

Matching

1. d
2. a
3. c
4. b

APPLY YOUR KNOWLEDGE 8.3

Multiple Choice

1. d
2. a
3. b
4. c
5. c
6. b

Matching

1. d
2. b
3. a
4. c

APPLY YOUR KNOWLEDGE 8.4

Multiple Choice

1. c
2. b
3. c
4. a
5. b

Fill in the Blank

1. recommended dietary allowance
2. modified consistency diets
3. GI tract
4. dextrose, amino acid
5. central venous

APPLY YOUR KNOWLEDGE 8.5

Matching

1. e
2. c
3. a
4. d
5. b

Fill in the Blank

1. 280
2. carbohydrate
3. sodium
4. 7.3
5. 1.8

Chapter 9

APPLY YOUR KNOWLEDGE 9.1

Matching

1. h
2. f
3. e
4. g
5. c
6. a
7. d
8. b

Multiple Choice

1. c
2. a
3. b
4. d

APPLY YOUR KNOWLEDGE 9.2

Fill in the Blank

1. folic acid
2. penicillins
3. estrogen
4. bactericidal
5. sulfonamides
6. gram-positive; gram-negative

Multiple Choice

1. d
2. c
3. b
4. a
5. d

APPLY YOUR KNOWLEDGE 9.3

Matching

1. j
2. i
3. e
4. h
5. b
6. a
7. f
8. g
9. d
10. c

Multiple Choice

1. c
2. d
3. b
4. b
5. c

APPLY YOUR KNOWLEDGE 9.4

Multiple Choice

1. b
2. e
3. a
4. e
5. c

Labeling

1. clarithromycin
2. Abbott Laboratories
3. Biaxin
4. tablets
5. 03-2126-2/R4
6. 250 mg
7. Cipro
8. ciprofloxacin hydrochloride
9. The tablets are now marked "CIP 250" and "BAYER."
10. Bayer HealthCare

APPLY YOUR KNOWLEDGE 9.5

Matching

1. e
2. d
3. a
4. c
5. b

Fill in the Blank

1. typhoid fever
2. lincomycin
3. *Neisseria gonorrhoeae*
4. lincomycin
5. gray-baby syndrome

APPLY YOUR KNOWLEDGE 9.6

Fill in the Blank

1. isoniazid
2. conjunction
3. lungs; lymph nodes
4. rifampin
5. pyrazinamide

Matching

1. e
2. c
3. b
4. d
5. a

APPLY YOUR KNOWLEDGE 9.7

Matching

1. c

2. e
3. d
4. a
5. b

Multiple Choice

1. c
2. d
3. b
4. a
5. c

Chapter 10

APPLY YOUR KNOWLEDGE 10.1

Multiple Choice

1. b
2. a
3. c
4. b
5. d

Matching

1. a, c
2. b
3. a
4. b
5. d
6. b
7. d
8. c

APPLY YOUR KNOWLEDGE 10.2

Fill in the Blank

1. malaria; vivax, malariae, ovale
2. DNA
3. falciparum
4. decrease; rabies
5. falciparum; deaths

Multiple Choice

1. b
2. d
3. a
4. e
5. c

APPLY YOUR KNOWLEDGE 10.3

Multiple Choice

1. c
2. a
3. d
4. b
5. d

Fill in the Blank

1. dysentery
2. trichomoniasis
3. giardiasis
4. metronidazole
5. iodine

Chapter 11

APPLY YOUR KNOWLEDGE 11.1

Fill in the Blank

1. immunity
2. T cells
3. antibodies
4. humoral immunity
5. lymphocytes

Matching

1. e
2. c
3. a
4. b
5. d
6. f

APPLY YOUR KNOWLEDGE 11.2

Fill in the Blank

1. microorganisms
2. antigen
3. immunoglobins; antibodies
4. smallpox
5. active
6. killed; attenuated; living
7. protein
8. vaccinations
9. increased
10. potency

APPLY YOUR KNOWLEDGE 11.3

Fill in the Blank

1. diphtheria, tetanus, pertussis
2. *Hemophilus influenzae* type b
3. measles, mumps, rubella
4. chickenpox
5. childhood

Matching

1. d
2. a
3. b
4. c
5. f
6. e

APPLY YOUR KNOWLEDGE 11.4

Multiple Choice

1. a
2. d
3. d
4. d
5. b

APPLY YOUR KNOWLEDGE 11.5

Matching

1. b
2. e
3. a
4. d
5. c

Fill in the Blank

1. anaphylactic reaction
2. rapid; short
3. injection; muscle
4. asplenia
5. plasma

Chapter 12

APPLY YOUR KNOWLEDGE 12.1

Fill in the Blank

1. prostaglandin
2. anemia, occult bleeding, or massive GI hemorrhage
3. analgesic; antipyretic
4. epilepsy; parkinsonism; hepatic; renal
5. aspirin; viral

Multiple Choice

1. c
2. d
3. a
4. b
5. c

APPLY YOUR KNOWLEDGE 12.2

Multiple Choice

1. a
2. c
3. c
4. a
5. d

Matching

1. d
2. e
3. a
4. b
5. c

APPLY YOUR KNOWLEDGE 12.3

Multiple Choice

1. b
2. c
3. d
4. d
5. b

Fill in the Blank

1. endogenous
2. morphine
3. opioid alkaloids
4. heroin
5. mu; kappa; delta

APPLY YOUR KNOWLEDGE 12.4

Matching

1. c
2. d
3. b
4. a

Fill in the Blank

1. not established
2. narcotic overdosage
3. naltrexone
4. somnolence; lethargy
5. opioid antagonists

APPLY YOUR KNOWLEDGE 12.5

Matching

1. b
2. d
3. f
4. c
5. a
6. e

Fill in the Blank

1. analgesia and sedation
2. head injuries, increased intracranial pressure, or a history of drug abuse
3. 30; 3
4. synthetic
5. sedation, drowsiness, vertigo, dizziness, headache, amnesia, euphoria, and insomnia

Chapter 13

APPLY YOUR KNOWLEDGE 13.1

Fill in the Blank

1. oma
2. U.S.; 500,000; annually
3. surgery; radiation
4. tumor suppressor genes
5. G_1 phase
6. splits into two new cells
7. mechanism of action
8. benign; malignant

Matching

1. e
2. a
3. b
4. c
5. d

APPLY YOUR KNOWLEDGE 13.2

Matching

1. e
2. d
3. b
4. c
5. a

Fill in the Blank

1. oral mucosa ulceration
2. acute and chronic myelocytic leukemia
3. severe cardiac disease
4. rapidly growing cells
5. bones and muscles

Multiple Choice

1. b
2. a
3. c
4. d
5. d

APPLY YOUR KNOWLEDGE 13.3

Fill in the Blank

1. connective tissue cells
2. kidney; melanoma
3. white blood cells
4. proteins
5. monoclonal antibodies
6. kidneys; lungs; liver
7. physician

CHECKPOINT REVIEW 3

1. d
2. c
3. b
4. c
5. d
6. c
7. b
8. a
9. b
10. c
11. a
12. d
13. b
14. a
15. c
16. d
17. c
18. b
19. a
20. d
21. a
22. c
23. d
24. b
25. a
26. c
27. a
28. c
29. c
30. d
31. c
32. b
33. c
34. d
35. b
36. a
37. a
38. c
39. b
40. c
41. c
42. d
43. d
44. d
45. b
46. a
47. b
48. b
49. e
50. d
51. a
52. c
53. b
54. e
55. c

56. d
57. a
58. b
59. metronidazole
60. antiprotozoal
61. antibiotics
62. bacteria
63. bactericidal
64. SMZ/TMP
65. penicillins
66. gram-positive
67. nephrotoxicity
68. large amounts
69. 50; 60
70. beri-beri
71. nausea
72. immunity
73. antigen
74. B-lymphocytes
75. antitoxin

Chapter 14

APPLY YOUR KNOWLEDGE 14.1

Fill in the Blank

1. norepinephrine, dopamine, acetylcholine, serotonin, and gamma-aminobutyric acid
2. withdrawal
3. sensory, integrative, and motor
4. Parkinson's disease
5. attention deficit–hyperactivity disorder (ADHD), narcolepsy, and obesity

Matching

1. e
2. b
3. c
4. a
5. d

Multiple Choice

1. b
2. d
3. c
4. a
5. c

APPLY YOUR KNOWLEDGE 14.2

Multiple Choice

1. d
2. a
3. c
4. b
5. d
6. c

Matching

1. d
2. e
3. b
4. a
5. c

APPLY YOUR KNOWLEDGE 14.3

Fill in the Blank

1. basal ganglia of the brain
2. levodopa
3. dopamine
4. 1%; 60
5. acetylcholine
6. dyskinesia
7. dopamine; acetylcholine
8. muscarinic

Matching

1. e
2. b
3. d
4. c
5. a

APPLY YOUR KNOWLEDGE 14.4

Matching

1. g
2. d
3. f
4. b
5. h
6. e
7. c
8. a

Fill in the Blank

1. schizophrenia
2. 1 to 2 weeks
3. phenothiazines
4. atypical; typical
5. 2 to 3 liters

APPLY YOUR KNOWLEDGE 14.5

Multiple Choice

1. c
2. c
3. a
4. d
5. a

Fill in the Blank

1. reactive
2. antimuscarinic
3. serotonin
4. SSRIs
5. orthostatic hypotension
6. MAOIs

Chapter 15

APPLY YOUR KNOWLEDGE 15.1

Fill in the Blank

1. central; peripheral
2. sympathetic
3. parasympathetic
4. neuron
5. synapse
6. norepinephrine
7. cholinergic
8. adrenergic; norepinephrine; noradrenaline

Multiple Choice

1. b
2. d
3. c
4. c

APPLY YOUR KNOWLEDGE 15.2

Fill in the Blank

1. tyrosine
2. epinephrine
3. sympathetic
4. vasoconstriction
5. antagonists
6. dilation

Matching

1. b
2. a, c
3. d, e
4. f

APPLY YOUR KNOWLEDGE 15.3

Matching

1. e
2. g
3. b
4. a
5. f
6. c
7. h
8. d

Fill in the Blank

1. hypotension, nasal congestion, and subjunctival hemorrhage
2. smooth muscle
3. hypertension
4. dizziness, lethargy, insomnia, and diarrhea
5. ophthalmology
6. anticholinergic drug

Chapter 16

APPLY YOUR KNOWLEDGE 16.1

Fill in the Blank

1. rapid; pleasant; withdrawal; skeletal muscle; therapeutic index
2. unconscious
3. dentistry; minor
4. anesthetic accident
5. 1; 2

Matching

1. d
2. e
3. c
4. a
5. b

APPLY YOUR KNOWLEDGE 16.2

Fill in the Blank

1. ester agents
2. sevoflurane
3. reliability; faster; less
4. central nervous system
5. diagnostic; therapeutic; surgical

Matching

1. i
2. h
3. j
4. f
5. b
6. e
7. d
8. c
9. g
10. a

APPLY YOUR KNOWLEDGE 16.3

Fill in the Blank

1. ester agents
2. biopsy; vasectomy; neonatal circumcision; dental procedures; drainage of abscesses

3. toxic effects
4. esters; amides
5. amide

Matching

1. f
2. b
3. e
4. d
5. c
6. a
7. g

APPLY YOUR KNOWLEDGE 16.4

Matching

1. d
2. c
3. a
4. e
5. b

Chapter 17

APPLY YOUR KNOWLEDGE 17.1

Multiple Choice

1. d
2. a
3. b
4. d
5. c

APPLY YOUR KNOWLEDGE 17.2

Fill in the Blank

1. psoriasis
2. ultraviolet light
3. acne
4. benzoyl peroxide
5. corns; calluses; plantar warts
6. unknown
7. vitamin A; vitamin D
8. epidermis

APPLY YOUR KNOWLEDGE 17.3

Multiple Choice

1. d
2. c
3. a
4. c
5. a

Chapter 18

APPLY YOUR KNOWLEDGE 18.1

Fill in the Blank

1. oxygen; nutrients
2. mediastinum; epicardium
3. endocardium
4. arteries; veins; capillaries
5. heart; arteries; veins; lymphatic system

Labeling

1. right atrium
2. left ventricle
3. bicuspid valve
4. epicardium
5. myocardium
6. aortic valve
7. aorta
8. inferior vena cava

APPLY YOUR KNOWLEDGE 18.2

Fill in the Blank

1. angina
2. classical (stable)
3. variant or vasospastic
4. dilate coronary blood vessels
5. nitroglycerin
6. glaucoma
7. myocardial ischemia; pain

Matching

1. f
2. a, c
3. a, b, e
4. a
5. e,
6. a, c, e
7. e
8. e, f

APPLY YOUR KNOWLEDGE 18.3

Fill in the Blank

1. oxygenated coronary blood
2. intravenous fluids
3. hemorrhage (specifically in the brain)
4. 50%
5. damage
6. morphine
7. respiration; myocardial contractility
8. workload; blood supply

APPLY YOUR KNOWLEDGE 18.4

Fill in the Blank

1. ventricular tachycardia
2. beta-blockers
3. Ib
4. quinidine
5. lidocaine
6. phenytoin
7. propranolol
8. amiodarone
9. verapamil
10. ibutilide

Labeling

1. metoprolol succinate
2. beta-blocker
3. extended-release tablets
4. Rx
5. hypertension: 25–100 mg/d; angina: 100 mg/d; heart failure class II; 25 mg/d for 2 weeks; more severe heart failure; 12.5 mg/d
6. hypertension, angina, heart failure
7. cardiovascular
8. AstraZeneca
9. Store at 25°C (77°F)
10. pregnancy category C

Chapter 19

APPLY YOUR KNOWLEDGE 19.1

Fill in the Blank

1. pressure, resistance
2. arterial, capillary, venous
3. aorta
4. hypertension
5. hypertensive crisis
6. unknown
7. corticosteroids, cocaine
8. 90 to 99, 140 to 159

Matching

1. e
2. f
3. g
4. a
5. c
6. d
7. b

APPLY YOUR KNOWLEDGE 19.2

Multiple Choice

1. a
2. b
3. b
4. c
5. a

Matching

1. d
2. e
3. c
4. a
5. b

APPLY YOUR KNOWLEDGE 19.3

Multiple Choice

1. c
2. a
3. b
4. d
5. c

Matching

1. e
2. d
3. a
4. c
5. b

APPLY YOUR KNOWLEDGE 19.4

Fill in the Blank

1. cholesterol
2. diet modification; exercise, LDL
3. statins
4. niacin, unpleasant side effects
5. triglycerides, VLDL

Matching

1. c
2. e
3. d
4. b
5. a

CHECKPOINT REVIEW 4

1. b
2. d
3. c

4. b
5. b
6. a
7. a
8. c
9. d
10. b
11. d
12. b
13. d
14. a
15. b
16. c
17. d
18. b
19. d
20. d
21. b
22. d
23. a
24. c
25. b
26. b
27. d
28. c
29. a
30. c
31. b
32. d
33. b
34. a
35. d
36. b
37. c
38. a
39. c
40. c
41. b
42. d
43. c
44. d
45. c
46. a
47. c
48. d
49. b
50. c
51. neurotransmitters
52. ocular
53. muscarinic
54. cholinergic
55. cooling
56. irreversible
57. nicotinic
58. catecholamines
59. parasympatholytics
60. balanced

Chapter 20

APPLY YOUR KNOWLEDGE 20.1

Fill in the Blank

1. hemorrhaging
2. fibrin
3. hemostasis
4. serotonin
5. platelets
6. injury

Matching

1. e
2. a
3. d
4. b
5. c
6. f

APPLY YOUR KNOWLEDGE 20.2

Fill in the Blank

1. prolong
2. dissolve; larger
3. oral
4. thrombolytics
5. standard (unfractionated) heparin
6. bioavailability; effects

Multiple Choice

1. c
2. b
3. a
4. b
5. d
6. a

APPLY YOUR KNOWLEDGE 20.3

Fill in the Blank

1. arterial thrombosis
2. platelet activation
3. GI ulceration, hypertension, asthma, allergies, and nasal polyps
4. bleeding time
5. platelets

Matching

1. c
2. d
3. e
4. b
5. a

APPLY YOUR KNOWLEDGE 20.4

Fill in the Blank

1. surgical sites
2. plasminogen; plasmin; fibrin; thrombi
3. bleeding
4. feverfew, galling, ginger, and ginkgo
5. fibrinolysis; fibrinogenolysis
6. pregnancy; lactation
7. dissolve (or lyse)

Matching

1. c
2. d
3. b
4. e
5. a

Chapter 21

APPLY YOUR KNOWLEDGE 21.1

Multiple Choice

1. b
2. d
3. a
4. d
5. c

Fill in the Blank

1. glomerular filtration; reabsorption; excretion
2. nephron
3. renal pyramids
4. collecting tubule
5. distal convoluted tubule; collecting tubule
6. balance
7. water of metabolism

APPLY YOUR KNOWLEDGE 21.2

Fill in the Blank

1. electrolytes
2. 2,500 mL
3. urine
4. sodium, potassium, calcium, magnesium, chloride, sulfate, bicarbonate, hydrogen
5. cations
6. aldosterone

Matching

1. d
2. a
3. e
4. b
5. c

APPLY YOUR KNOWLEDGE 21.3

Multiple Choice

1. c
2. b
3. a
4. d
5. a
6. a
7. d
8. c

Matching

1. g
2. b
3. e
4. a
5. c
6. d
7. f

Chapter 22

APPLY YOUR KNOWLEDGE 22.1

Matching

1. h
2. d
3. e
4. a
5. g
6. b
7. f
8. c

Multiple Choice

1. d
2. a
3. c
4. c
5. b

APPLY YOUR KNOWLEDGE 22.2

Multiple Choice

1. c
2. c
3. b
4. a
5. d
6. d

Matching

1. f
2. d
3. a
4. e
5. c
6. b

APPLY YOUR KNOWLEDGE 22.3

Fill in the Blank

1. glucagon
2. diabetes mellitus
3. lispro
4. hypoglycemic reaction
5. both type 1 and type 2 diabetes
6. 70% NPH and 30% regular insulin
7. sulfonylureas
8. first-generation; second-generation

Labeling

1. regular human insulin
2. 100 mL/mL
3. Eli Lilly and Company
4. rDNA origin
5. Keep in a cold place. Avoid freezing.

APPLY YOUR KNOWLEDGE 22.4

Multiple Choice

1. c
2. d
3. a
4. d
5. c
6. b

Fill in the Blank

1. mineralocorticoids
2. androgens
3. glucocorticoids
4. Addison's disease
5. sodium, potassium

Chapter 23

APPLY YOUR KNOWLEDGE 23.1

Matching

1. c
2. a
3. f
4. b
5. e
6. d

Multiple Choice

1. e
2. b
3. a
4. b
5. e

APPLY YOUR KNOWLEDGE 23.2

Multiple Choice

1. c
2. b
3. d
4. a
5. d

Fill in the Blank

1. feminization
2. corpus luteum
3. vagina, uterus, uterine tubes, ovaries, external reproductive structures
4. anterior pituitary; gonadotropins FSH and LH
5. endometrial hyperplasia; endometrial carcinoma

Matching

1. e
2. c
3. d
4. a
5. b

APPLY YOUR KNOWLEDGE 23.3

Matching

1. e
2. d
3. a
4. c
5. b

Multiple Choice

1. d
2. a
3. d
4. b
5. d

Chapter 24

APPLY YOUR KNOWLEDGE 24.1

Fill in the Blank

1. salivary glands, liver, gallbladder, pancreas
2. digestion, absorption, metabolism
3. ulcers
4. 8 meters, 186
5. peptic ulcer

6. 2 to 3 quarts (about 2 to 3 liters)
7. metabolism of food and drugs
8. small intestine

Multiple Choice

1. d
2. a
3. b
4. a
5. c

APPLY YOUR KNOWLEDGE 24.2

Sound-Alike Drug Names

1. difenoxin hydrochloride with atropine sulfate
2. Kao-Span
3. paregoric
4. loperamide
5. bismuth subsalicylate

Multiple Choice

1. d
2. c
3. a
4. c
5. b

APPLY YOUR KNOWLEDGE 24.3

Multiple Choice

1. a
2. c
3. d
4. c
5. d

Fill in the Blank

1. paralytic ileus
2. antimuscarinic
3. short-term treatment
4. emollients, surfactants
5. nausea, vomiting, diarrhea, abdominal cramps

APPLY YOUR KNOWLEDGE 24.4

Fill in the Blank

1. unabsorbed ingested poisons
2. medulla oblongata of the brain
3. comatose, semicomatose, deeply sedated, shock, seizures
4. 6 months old
5. in decline

Matching

1. h
2. e
3. g
4. f
5. d
6. a
7. c
8. b

Chapter 25

APPLY YOUR KNOWLEDGE 25.1

Multiple Choice

1. d
2. c
3. c
4. b
5. b

Fill in the Blank

1. 16 million Americans
2. bronchodilators
3. oxygen and removing carbon dioxide
4. nose, nasal cavity, paranasal sinuses, and pharynx
5. larynx, trachea, bronchial tree, and lungs

APPLY YOUR KNOWLEDGE 25.2

Fill in the Blank

1. relaxing smooth muscles of the bronchial tree
2. bronchospasm; bronchitis
3. emphysema
4. chronic; acute
5. connective tissue

Matching

1. d
2. c
3. e
4. a
5. b

APPLY YOUR KNOWLEDGE 25.3

Fill in the Blank

1. reduce coughing
2. opioid; nonopioid
3. congestion
4. tracheostomy; atelectasis
5. swollen mucous membranes

Matching

1. f
2. c
3. b
4. a
5. e
6. d

CHECKPOINT REVIEW 5

1. d
2. b
3. a
4. c
5. b
6. b
7. c
8. a
9. a
10. d
11. b
12. a
13. c
14. c
15. d
16. b
17. c
18. c
19. a
20. c
21. d
22. a
23. d
24. b
25. b
26. d
27. a
28. b
29. d
30. a
31. d
32. c
33. b
34. b
35. a
36. d
37. b
38. a
39. b
40. d
41. d
42. a
43. a
44. d
45. d
46. a

47. b
48. b
49. d
50. b
51. e
52. d
53. c
54. a
55. b
56. d
57. c
58. e
59. a
60. b
61. gastric upsets
62. testosterone
63. estrogen
64. estrogens
65. mouth
66. duodenal ulcer
67. motility
68. beta$_2$; xanthenes
69. antagonists
70. digestive system

Chapter 26

APPLY YOUR KNOWLEDGE 26.1

Fill in the Blank

1. support, storage of minerals and lipids, blood cell production, protection, leverage
2. skeletal, cardiac, smooth
3. osteopenia
4. parathyroid hormone, calcitonin
5. estrogen-receptor modulator

Matching

1. e
2. d
3. b
4. c
5. a

APPLY YOUR KNOWLEDGE 26.2

Multiple Choice

1. d
2. b
3. c
4. d
5. c

Matching

1. g
2. c
3. e
4. f
5. b
6. d
7. a

APPLY YOUR KNOWLEDGE 26.3

Fill in the Blank

1. urate deposition
2. overproduction, underexcretion
3. gout
4. xanthine oxidase
5. acute gouty attacks
6. gout
7. hyperuricemia
8. anti-inflammatory drug therapy, acute attack
9. probenecid, sulfinpyrazone
10. acute, gouty arthritis

Matching

1. d
2. a
3. c
4. b

APPLY YOUR KNOWLEDGE 26.4

Matching

1. f
2. d
3. c
4. e
5. b
6. a

Multiple Choice

1. a
2. c
3. d
4. b
5. d

Chapter 27

APPLY YOUR KNOWLEDGE 27.1

Fill in the Blank

1. smooth muscle fibers

2. posterior cavity
3. cataract
4. cornea
5. pigment
6. retina
7. autonomic
8. lens in position
9. corticosteroids
10. more common

APPLY YOUR KNOWLEDGE 27.2

Matching

1. h
2. j
3. e
4. i
5. a
6. d
7. g
8. f
9. c
10. b

Multiple Choice

1. d
2. a
3. c
4. b
5. a

Chapter 28

APPLY YOUR KNOWLEDGE 28.1

Fill in the Blank

1. child-resistant
2. poison control center
3. cyanide
4. toxic (poisonous) agent
5. carbon monoxide
6. aversive agents
7. insecticides

APPLY YOUR KNOWLEDGE 28.2

Matching

1. e
2. c
3. a
4. b
5. d

Fill in the Blank

1. presentation; exposure
2. emesis; gastric lavage; hemoperfusion
3. emetine
4. medulla; chemoreceptor
5. discarded
6. sorbitol
7. osmotic pressure; retaining
8. salts; poorly
9. renal

APPLY YOUR KNOWLEDGE 28.3

Multiple Choice

1. d
2. a
3. c
4. b
5. d
6. a

Fill in the Blank

1. common
2. 8
3. acetaminophen
4. 8 to 12
5. acetone
6. ethylene glycol

APPLY YOUR KNOWLEDGE 28.4

Fill in the Blank

1. bleeding
2. methamphetamine; crystal meth; cocaine; crack
3. phenobarbital; diazepam
4. coma; respiratory depression
5. activated charcoal

Matching

1. c
2. d
3. a
4. d
5. b

APPLY YOUR KNOWLEDGE 28.5

Multiple Choice

1. b
2. b
3. a
4. c

5. d
6. c

Matching

1. a
2. d
3. e
4. b
5. c

APPLY YOUR KNOWLEDGE 28.6

Matching

1. c
2. a
3. e
4. d
5. f
6. b
7. g

Fill in the Blank

1. renal; pneumonia
2. lithium; hemodialysis
3. chelating agents
4. less
5. whole bowel irrigation
6. hyperkalemia
7. depressant
8. magnesium
9. potassium
10. lead

APPLY YOUR KNOWLEDGE 28.7

Fill in the Blank

1. central; sympathetic
2. contaminated clothing
3. cellular lipids
4. alcohol intoxication
5. aspirin
6. vertigo; hearing impairment
7. seizures; hypotension; dysrhythmias; cardiac arrest
8. endotracheal intubation; gastric lavage

APPLY YOUR KNOWLEDGE 28.8

Multiple Choice

1. a
2. b
3. c
4. c
5. d

Chapter 29

APPLY YOUR KNOWLEDGE 29.1

Multiple Choice

1. c
2. d
3. b
4. a
5. d

Fill in the Blank

1. 10
2. renal
3. body fat, laboratory, serum protein
4. OTC medications
5. 35

APPLY YOUR KNOWLEDGE 29.2

Matching

1. c
2. d
3. b
4. a

Fill in the Blank

1. P450
2. famotidine; nizatidine
3. hypokalemia
4. respiratory
5. bleeding

Chapter 30

APPLY YOUR KNOWLEDGE 30.1

Fill in the Blank

1. few weeks after birth
2. water
3. kernicterus
4. older children and adults
5. clearance rates

Multiple Choice

1. c
2. c
3. b
4. d
5. b

APPLY YOUR KNOWLEDGE 30.2

Fill in the Blank

1. stain the incoming teeth of an infant
2. pyridoxine deficiency
3. thyroid cancer
4. receptors; inadequate drug-receptor binding
5. body weight

Matching

1. d
2. e
3. a
4. b
5. c

CHECKPOINT REVIEW 6

1. d
2. b
3. d
4. a
5. b
6. c
7. a
8. d
9. b
10. c
11. b
12. c
13. a
14. b
15. d
16. c
17. b
18. a
19. c
20. d
21. c
22. b
23. d
24. b
25. a
26. d
27. a
28. c
29. c
30. a
31. d
32. b
33. d
34. b
35. b
36. c
37. b

38. d
39. b
40. b
41. c
42. b
43. c
44. d
45. c
46. b
47. b
48. c
49. c
50. a
51. e
52. c
53. b
54. a

55. d
56. e
57. d
58. c
59. b
60. a
61. thyroid
62. human body
63. retina
64. beta-blockers
65. lower
66. filtration rate
67. elderly
68. coral
69. ethanol
70. activated charcoal

Index

A

aa abbreviation, 40
Abbokinase, 437, 444, 445t
abbreviations
 in apothecary system, 111
 defined, 40
 general medical, 42t
 in household system, 112
 incorrect, and medication
  errors, 65
 metric system, 109t
 review questions on, 42–43
 used for measurements, 41t
 used in prescriptions, 40–41
abciximab, 442, 443t
Abilify, 315t
absorption, drug
 factors affecting, 11–12
 in geriatric patients, 628–629
 in infants and children, 641–642
abuse potential, 25
ac abbreviation, 40
acarbose, 489t, 491
accessory sex organs
 female, 506
 male, 501
Accolate, 550t, 554
accommodation, 590
Accupril, 398, 408t
acebutolol, 338t, 392t, 407t
ACE inhibitors. *See* angiotensin-
  converting enzyme (ACE)
  inhibitors
Aceon, 408t
acetaminophen, 253
acetaminophen overdose, 609
acetaminophen poisoning, 611
acetazolamide, 461t, 594t
acetohexamide, 489t
acetylcholine (ACh), 295, 309, 327
acetylcysteine, 558, 559t, 611
acetylsalicylic acid, 11
Achromycin, 191t, 371t, 636
acid-forming salts, 459
acid glycoproteins, 12
acidity of the stomach, 11
ACIP, 236
AcipHex, 525t
acitretin, 369, 370t
Aclovate, 367t
acne, 370–371
acromegaly, 473
Acticin, 376
Actinex, 372t
actinic keratoses, 371
Activase, 444, 445t
activated charcoal, 608, 609
active immunity, 232
active immunizing agents, 233
Activelle, 510t

active metabolites, 12
Actonel, 571t
Actos, 489t, 492
acute angle-closure glaucoma, 592
acute diarrhea, 530
acute gouty arthritis, 580
acute myocardial infarction
  (AMI), 390
acute pain, 246
acyclovir, 202t, 203–204
ad abbreviation, 40
Adalat, 408t
adalimumab, 575t, 577
adapalene, 371t
addiction, to sedatives, 298
Addison's disease, 477, 493, 495
addition
 of decimal fractions, 100
 of fractions, 96–97
 of fractions with dissimilar
  denominators, 97–98
additives, food, 169
adenocarcinoma, 271
adenohypophysis, 472
adenomas, 271
adenosine antagonists, 277
ADHD (attention-hyperactivity
  disorder), 298
adipose tissues, 366
adjuvant treatment, 270
ad lib abbreviation, 40
administration, drug. *See* drug
  administration
AdoMet, 334t
adrenal glands, 470, 493–495
Adrenalin (drug), 334t, 355, 360
adrenaline, 8, 44
adrenal medulla, 327–328
adrenergic agonists, 333–337
adrenergic antagonists, 337–342
 alpha-receptor antagonists, 339
 beta-receptor antagonists,
  339–340
 classification of, 338t
adrenergic blockers, 333
adrenergic neurons, 328
adrenergic receptors, 331–332
adrenocortical hormones (glucocorticoids), 493–494
adrenocortical steroids, 493–497
 glucocorticoids, 493–494
 major, 494t
 mineralocorticoids, 495
 review questions on, 496–497
adrenocorticotropic hormone
  (ACTH), 472, 472t,
  473, 493
adrenoreceptors, 334
Adriamycin, 275t, 281
Adrucil, 275t, 278

adsorbents, 531–532, 608
adults, immunizations for, 237–239
adverse drug reactions (ADR), 6,
  15–16
 of analgesics/anti-inflammatory
  drugs, 248, 249, 250, 252,
  253, 256, 258, 260, 261,
  262, 263–264, 265
 of anesthetics, 351, 353, 356
 of antibacterial/antiviral agents,
  178, 180, 182, 185, 186,
  189, 190, 194, 195, 196,
  198, 199, 200, 201, 203,
  204, 205, 206
 of anticoagulants, 437, 439, 440,
  442, 444
 of antidiabetic therapies, 485,
  486, 487, 488, 490, 491,
  494, 495
 of antifungal agents, 214, 215, 216
 of antihyperlipidemics, 423,
  424, 425
 of antihypertensive agents, 410,
  411, 412, 414
 of antimalarial agents, 218,
  219, 220
 of antiprotozoal agents, 223, 224
 of autonomic drugs, 335, 336,
  337, 339, 341, 342
 of cancer therapies, 277, 278, 279,
  280, 281, 284
 of cardiac drugs, 387, 394, 395,
  396, 398, 418
 of central nervous system drugs,
  297, 299, 300–301, 304,
  305, 306, 307, 310, 311,
  314, 315–316, 318,
  319, 320
 of diuretics, 459, 460, 461, 463, 464
 of eye disorder drugs, 595, 598,
  599, 601
 of gastrointestinal disorder drugs,
  526, 527, 528, 530, 535,
  536, 537, 539
 of immunoglobulins/immunizing
  agents, 234, 241
 of musculoskeletal disorder
  drugs, 572, 573, 575, 576,
  577, 580, 581, 582, 584
 of reproductive system drugs,
  503, 508, 509, 511,
  515, 516
 of respiratory disorder drugs, 552,
  553, 554, 555, 557,
  559, 560
 of skin medications, 367, 369,
  371, 372, 376
 of thyroid/antithyroid drugs, 477,
  478, 479
Advil, 249, 636

Credits

Chapter 1

Page 5, Michal Heron/Pearson Education/PH College.

Chapter 2

Page 22, Laima Druskis/Pearson Education/PH College; Page 23, Pearson Education/PH College; Page 25, Pearson Education/PH College; Page 30, Michal Heron/Pearson Education/PH College; Page 31, Mike Gallitelli/Pearson Education/PH College; Page 33, Michal Heron/Pearson Education/PH College.

Chapter 3

Page 38, Darryl Bush/Pearson Education/PH College; Page 46, Al Dodge; Page 47, Fig. 2: Al Dodge; Page 47, Fig. 3: Al Dodge; Page 49, Al Dodge.

Chapter 4

Page 61, Pearson Education/PH College; Page 72, Michal Heron/Pearson Education/PH College; Page 73, Fig 6: Michal Heron/Pearson Education/PH College; Page 73, Fig 7a: Michal Heron/Pearson Education/PH College; Page 73, Fig 7c: Michal Heron/Person Education/PH College; Page 80, Michal Heron/Pearson Education/PH College.

Chapter 5

Page 93, Multi-Med-Media.

Chapter 6

Page 108, George Dodson/Pearson Education/PH College.

Chapter 9

Page 174, Brian Warling/Pearson Education/PH College.

Chapter 10

Page 211, Michal Heron/Pearson Education/PH College; Page 222, Centers for Disease Control and Prevention (CDC).

Chapter 11

Page 229, Pearson Education/PH College.

Chapter 12

Page 246, Pearson Education/PH College; Page 247, Pearson Education/Benjamin Cummings Publishing Company.

Chapter 13

Page 270, Mark Harmel/Getty Images Inc.–Stone Allstock.

Chapter 14

Page 295, Michal Heron/Pearson Education/PH College.

Chapter 15

Page 325, Laima Druskis/Pearson Education/PH College.

Chapter 16

Page 347, Michal Heron/Pearson Education/PH College.

Chapter 17

Page 365, Network Graphics/Pearson Education/PH College.

Chapter 18

Page 381, Michal Heron/Pearson Education/PH College.

Chapter 19

Page 403, Michal Heron/Pearson Education/PH College; Page 416, Fig 3: © Dorling Kindersley; Page 416, Fig 4: Pearson Education/PH College.

Chapter 20

Page 433, Michal Heron/Pearson Education/PH College; Page 434, Pearson Education/Benjamin Cummings Publishing Company.

Chapter 21

Page 449, Prentice Hall School Division.

Chapter 22

Page 470, UPI/Corbis/Bettmann.

Chapter 25

Page 545, Michal Heron/Pearson Education/PH College.

Chapter 27

Page 590, Robert Harbison.

Chapter 29

Page 627, Bill Aron/PhotoEdit Inc.

Pearson Education, Inc.

YOU SHOULD CAREFULLY READ THE TERMS AND CONDITIONS BEFORE USING THE CD-ROM PACKAGE. USING THIS CD-ROM PACKAGE INDICATES YOUR ACCEPTANCE OF THESE TERMS AND CONDITIONS.

Pearson Education, Inc. provides this program and licenses its use. You assume responsibility for the selection of the program to achieve your intended results, and for the installation, use, and results obtained from the program. This license extends only to use of the program in the United States or countries in which the program is marketed by authorized distributors.

LICENSE GRANT

You hereby accept a nonexclusive, nontransferable, permanent license to install and use the program ON A SINGLE COMPUTER at any given time. You may copy the program solely for backup or archival purposes in support of your use of the program on the single computer. You may not modify, translate, disassemble, decompile, or reverse engineer the program, in whole or in part.

TERM

The License is effective until terminated. Pearson Education, Inc. reserves the right to terminate this License automatically if any provision of the License is violated. You may terminate the License at any time. To terminate this License, you must return the program, including documentation, along with a written warranty stating that all copies in your possession have been returned or destroyed.

LIMITED WARRANTY

THE PROGRAM IS PROVIDED "AS IS" WITHOUT WARRANTY OF ANY KIND, EITHER EXPRESSED OR IMPLIED, INCLUDING, BUT NOT LIMITED TO, THE IMPLIED WARRANTIES OR MERCHANTABILITY AND FITNESS FOR A PARTICULAR PURPOSE. THE ENTIRE RISK AS TO THE QUALITY AND PERFORMANCE OF THE PROGRAM IS WITH YOU. SHOULD THE PROGRAM PROVE DEFECTIVE, YOU (AND NOT PRENTICE-HALL, INC. OR ANY AUTHORIZED DEALER) ASSUME THE ENTIRE COST OF ALL NECESSARY SERVICING, REPAIR, OR CORRECTION. NO ORAL OR WRITTEN INFORMATION OR ADVICE GIVEN BY PRENTICE-HALL, INC., ITS DEALERS, DISTRIBUTORS, OR AGENTS SHALL CREATE A WARRANTY OR INCREASE THE SCOPE OF THIS WARRANTY.

SOME STATES DO NOT ALLOW THE EXCLUSION OF IMPLIED WARRANTIES, SO THE ABOVE EXCLUSION MAY NOT APPLY TO YOU. THIS WARRANTY GIVES YOU SPECIFIC LEGAL RIGHTS AND YOU MAY ALSO HAVE OTHER LEGAL RIGHTS THAT VARY FROM STATE TO STATE.

Pearson Education, Inc. does not warrant that the functions contained in the program will meet your requirements or that the operation of the program will be uninterrupted or error-free.

However, Pearson Education, Inc. warrants the diskette(s) or CD-ROM(s) on which the program is furnished to be free from defects in material and workmanship under normal use for a period of ninety (90) days from the date of delivery to you as evidenced by a copy of your receipt.

The program should not be relied on as the sole basis to solve a problem whose incorrect solution could result in injury to person or property. If the program is employed in such a manner, it is at the user's own risk and Pearson Education, Inc. explicitly disclaims all liability for such misuse.

LIMITATION OF REMEDIES

Pearson Education, Inc.'s entire liability and your exclusive remedy shall be:

1. the replacement of any diskette(s) or CD-ROM(s) not meeting Pearson Education, Inc.'s "LIMITED WARRANTY" and that is returned to Pearson Education, or

2. if Pearson Education is unable to deliver a replacement diskette(s) or CD-ROM(s) that is free of defects in materials or workmanship, you may terminate this agreement by returning the program.

IN NO EVENT WILL PRENTICE-HALL, INC. BE LIABLE TO YOU FOR ANY DAMAGES, INCLUDING ANY LOST PROFITS, LOST SAVINGS, OR OTHER INCIDENTAL OR CONSEQUENTIAL DAMAGES ARISING OUT OF THE USE OR INABILITY TO USE SUCH PROGRAM EVEN IF PRENTICE HALL, INC. OR AN AUTHORIZED DISTRIBUTOR HAS BEEN ADVISED OF THE POSSIBILITY OF SUCH DAMAGES, OR FOR ANY CLAIM BY ANY OTHER PARTY.

SOME STATES DO NOT ALLOW FOR THE LIMITATION OR EXCLUSION OF LIABILITY FOR INCIDENTAL OR CONSEQUENTIAL DAMAGES, SO THE ABOVE LIMITATION OR EXCLUSION MAY NOT APPLY TO YOU.

GENERAL

You may not sublicense, assign, or transfer the license of the program. Any attempt to sublicense, assign, or transfer any of the rights, duties, or obligations hereunder is void.

This Agreement will be governed by the laws of the State of New York.

Should you have any questions concerning this Agreement, you may contact Pearson Education, Inc. by writing to:

Director of New Media
Higher Education Division
Pearson Education, Inc.
One Lake Street
Upper Saddle River, NJ 07458

Should you have any questions concerning technical support, you may contact:

Product Support Department: Monday–Friday 8:00 A.M.-8:00 P.M. and Sunday 5:00 P.M.-12:00 A.M. (All times listed are Eastern). 1-800-677-6337

You can also get support by filling out the web form located at http://247.prenhall.com

YOU ACKNOWLEDGE THAT YOU HAVE READ THIS AGREEMENT, UNDERSTAND IT, AND AGREE TO BE BOUND BY ITS TERMS AND CONDITIONS. YOU FURTHER AGREE THAT IT IS THE COMPLETE AND EXCLUSIVE STATEMENT OF THE AGREEMENT BETWEEN US THAT SUPERSEDES ANY PROPOSAL OR PRIOR AGREEMENT, ORAL OR WRITTEN, AND ANY OTHER COMMUNICATIONS BETWEEN US RELATING TO THE SUBJECT MATTER OF THIS AGREEMENT.